A Visual Guide to Clinical Anatomy

A Visual Guide to Clinical Anatomy

Robert H. Whitaker, MA, MD, MCHIR, FRCS

University of Cambridge
Cambridge, UK

WILEY Blackwell

This edition first published 2021
© 2021 Robert H. Whitaker. Published 2021 by John Wiley & Sons Ltd.

Registered Office(s)
John Wiley & Sons, Inc., 111 River Street, Hoboken, NJ 07030, USA
John Wiley & Sons Ltd, The Atrium, Southern Gate, Chichester, West Sussex, PO19 8SQ, UK

Editorial Office
9600 Garsington Road, Oxford, OX4 2DQ, UK

For details of our global editorial offices, customer services, and more information about Wiley products visit us at www.wiley.com.

Wiley also publishes its books in a variety of electronic formats and by print-on-demand. Some content that appears in standard print versions of this book may not be available in other formats.

Library of Congress Cataloging-in-Publication Data

Names: Whitaker, R. H. (Robert H.), author, illustrator.
Title: A visual guide to clinical anatomy / Robert H. Whitaker.
Description: Hoboken, NJ : Wiley-Blackwell, 2021.
Identifiers: LCCN 2020027865 (print) | LCCN 2020027866 (ebook) |
  ISBN 9781119708100 (paperback) | ISBN 9781119708162 (adobe pdf) |
  ISBN 9781119708148 (epub)
Subjects: MESH: Body Regions–anatomy & histology | Clinical Medicine |
  Pictorial Work
Classification: LCC QM25 (print) | LCC QM25 (ebook) | NLM QS 17 | DDC
  611.0022/2–dc23
LC record available at https://lccn.loc.gov/2020027865
LC ebook record available at https://lccn.loc.gov/2020027866

Cover Design: Wiley
Cover Image: Courtesy of Robert H. Whitaker

Set in 10/12pt Sabon by SPi Global, Pondicherry, India
Printed and bound in Singapore by Markono Print Media Pte Ltd

10 9 8 7 6 5 4 3 2 1

Contents

Preface

Robert H. Whitaker

It is easier to say what this book is not, rather than what it is. It is definitely not a textbook or an atlas but simply a series of images that I have used for teaching over the last 30 years as an Anatomy Lecturer and Demonstrator in The University of Cambridge, UK. The images have also been used for numerous lectures, courses and meetings elsewhere.

Each image is designed to give a synopsis of anatomical and clinical information about an individual topic or clinical condition for both medical students and those in clinical practice. I have drawn each image myself using *Adobe Illustrator*, a graphics programme that I can recommend to all aspiring anatomical artists.

Anatomists have often been accused of teaching students too much detail that is not clinically relevant and I have been very much aware of this. I have strived only to teach anatomy that will be pertinent to their varied clinical careers and constantly endeavoured to find easy ways to learn and remember the vast amount of information that anatomy comprises.

I make no apology for a lack of neuroanatomy as it is outside my field. There is relatively little embryology amongst these images but six concise podcasts in embryology in the form of lectures with images can be found on www.instantanatomy.co.uk (a subscription website) which includes a panacea of descriptive anatomy. www.instantanatomy.net is a free, similar website with fewer lectures. I also make no apology that you will find duplication of both illustrations and text on two or more images throughout. This is intentional as often the same information is needed for any individual teaching slide.

I would be delighted if some of you wish to use the images in this book for your own lectures or teaching and you are very welcome to do so with an acknowledgement.

I am most grateful to Mr John Fergus FRCS who very kindly helped me to check every image for anatomical and clinical accuracy. I took advice from a team of experts for the sections on the heart (Professor John Wallwork, CBE, FRCS, FMedSci), the eye (Mr. Nick Sarkis, FRCS) and ear, nose and throat (Mr. Roger Gray, FRCS). To each of them I am eternally grateful.

Robert H. Whitaker
2020

Foreword

By Professor Harold Ellis

Human Anatomy is intrinsically interesting - surely everyone likes to know how he or she is constructed. However, it is, of course, of immense practical importance to people in the healing professions. Just as the London taxi driver needs to learn "the knowledge" of the streets of the metropolis, so health workers need to know what lies below their palpating fingers. Of course, surgeons need to be especially competent anatomists.

The early anatomy textbooks had no or few illustrations, and these were mostly crude and grossly inaccurate. In 1543 came a revolution; the publication by the young anatomist Andreas Vesalius, of Padua, of "*De Humani Corpora Fabrica*", (the structure of the human body). Its revolutionary contribution was not so much the text but the magnificent illustrations – good enough and often still used today. Interestingly, there is still debate about who some of these anonymous artists were.

Good teachers of Anatomy, without exception, can produce clear and accurate diagrams; those that are most appreciated are ones that the student can reproduce. Robert H. Whitaker, a retired urologist and now Anatomy teacher, is well known for his Anatomy texts and his lectures, which are illustrated by his own clearly reproducible illustrations. This new publication will prove useful to both undergraduate and graduate students in reinforcing their anatomy studies. I only wish a book like this had been available all those years ago, when I was an Anatomy student!

Professor Harold Ellis, CBE, DM, MCh, FRCS
Emeritus Professor of Surgery, University of London; Clinical Anatomist,
Guy's Campus London SE1 1US, UK

Foreword

By Professor Sir Roy Calne

I have known Robert H. Whitaker for nearly 50 years as a surgical colleague, friend and fellow artist working together at Addenbrooke's Hospital in Cambridge, UK. We have shared Surgical Grand Rounds, Committee Meetings and many other hospital and social activities. We have an underlying mutual respect. With the production of this unique anatomical book he has introduced us to a new approach to teaching in that it is neither an atlas nor is it a textbook. When you delve into this beautifully illustrated book you will be impressed with its fund of knowledge and bright, colourful images.

Robert has produced some 920 annotated anatomical images that provide a concise synopsis of what is important for students and others to know and retain in order to undertake safe and competent clinical practice in any branch of medicine. These clear and beautiful images are a feat indeed!

A knowledge of anatomy is as relevant today as it was a century ago and I remember a comment I made in the Christmas Edition of the British Medical Journal many years ago when endoscopic surgery was in its infancy, that there was a risk of endoscopic surgeons not being able to get out of trouble with an open operation if they did not have an accurate working knowledge of the anatomy of the region.

Each image tells a story of a particular aspect of anatomy and its relevance to clinical practice. This brings the subject to light and its beautiful presentation makes it interesting, enjoyable and memorable.

Professor Sir Roy Calne, MA, MS, FRS, FRCS, FRCP
Emeritus Professor of Surgery, University of Cambridge and Addenbrooke's
Hospital, Cambridge CB2 0QQ, UK

About the Author

Robert H. Whitaker, MA, MD, MChir, FRCS, FMAA graduated from Selwyn College, Cambridge before undertaking his clinical training at University College Hospital, London. He spent a year at Johns Hopkins Hospital, Baltimore in the Urological Research Laboratories before returning to the St Peters Hospital Group in London to train as a urologist. He was a Senior Lecturer at the London Hospital Medical School before being appointed as a Consultant Urological Surgeon at Addenbrooke's Teaching Hospital in Cambridge, UK in 1973.

He spent 20 years practising mostly paediatric urology during which time he co-founded the British Association of Paediatric Urologists. He was an examiner for the Primary FRCS and later the MRCS at all four Colleges of Surgeons in the UK and a Hunterian Professor at the Royal College of Surgeons of England in 1973. He retired in 1990 to teach anatomy in the Department of Anatomy in Cambridge for the next 30 years. He is an Honorary Fellow and Examiner for the Medical Artists' Association of Great Britain and was awarded the Farquharson Teaching Award by the Royal College of Surgeons of Edinburgh in 2013. He was awarded the St Peter's Medal of the British Association of Urological Surgeons in 1994 and was made an Honorary Member of the European Society of Paediatric Urology in 2019.

Robert H. Whitaker is author of the anatomy textbook *Instant Anatomy*, now in its fifth edition (co-authored by Neil Borley), and has anatomy teaching websites – *www.instantanatomy.net and www.instantanatomy.co.uk*

Cambridge, UK
2020

SECTION 1

Upper Limb

A Visual Guide to Clinical Anatomy, First Edition. Robert H. Whitaker.
© 2021 Robert H. Whitaker. Published 2021 by John Wiley & Sons Ltd.

1.1 General Anatomy

SURFACE ANATOMY

Function of any bone:

- To give form
- For muscle attachments
- Movement
- Protection of internal organs
- Metabolic
  - Calcium, phosphorus
  - Haemopoiesis

CLASSIFICATION OF JOINTS 1

FIBROUS	CARTILAGINOUS	
	Primary	Secondary
Skull sutures	Costochondral	Midline symphyses
Interosseous membranes	1st sternochondral	Intervertebral
Inferior tibiofibular	Spheno-occipital	
11th, 12th costotransverse		Hyaline cartilage

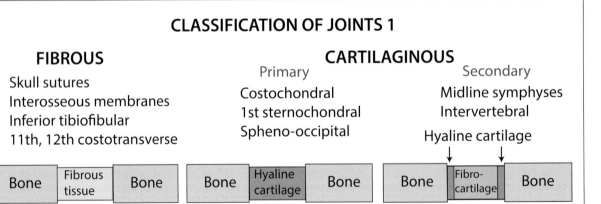

SYNOVIAL

ATYPICAL SYNOVIAL
Articular surface covered with fibrocartilage
Tempormandibular
Sternoclavicular
Acromioclavicular
2-7 Sternochondral

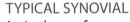

TYPICAL SYNOVIAL
Articular surface covered with hyaline cartilage
All other synovial joints

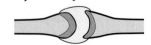

CLASSIFICATION OF JOINTS 2

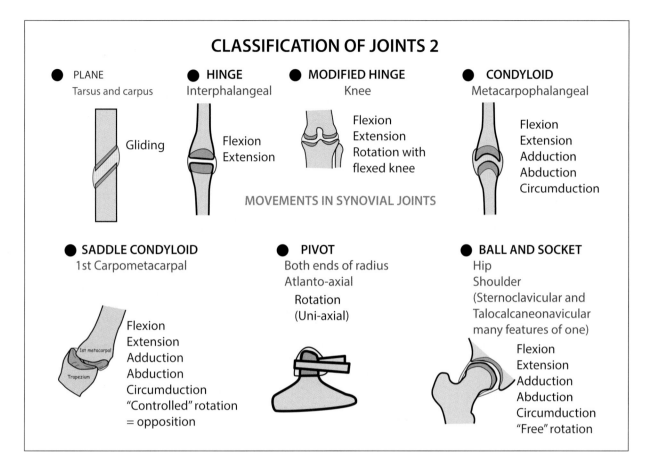

● PLANE
Tarsus and carpus

Gliding

● HINGE
Interphalangeal

Flexion
Extension

● MODIFIED HINGE
Knee

Flexion
Extension
Rotation with
flexed knee

MOVEMENTS IN SYNOVIAL JOINTS

● CONDYLOID
Metacarpophalangeal

Flexion
Extension
Adduction
Abduction
Circumduction

● SADDLE CONDYLOID
1st Carpometacarpal

Flexion
Extension
Adduction
Abduction
Circumduction
"Controlled" rotation
= opposition

1st metacarpal

Trapezium

● PIVOT
Both ends of radius
Atlanto-axial

Rotation
(Uni-axial)

● BALL AND SOCKET
Hip
Shoulder
(Sternoclavicular and
Talocalcaneonavicular
many features of one)

Flexion
Extension
Adduction
Abduction
Circumduction
"Free" rotation

LANDMARKS AROUND SHOULDER

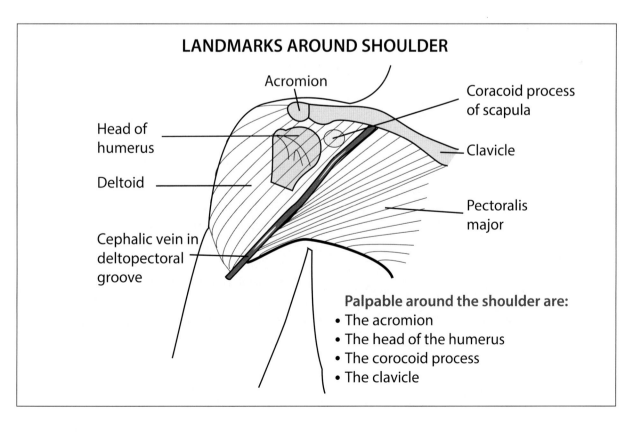

Acromion

Coracoid process
of scapula

Head of
humerus

Clavicle

Deltoid

Pectoralis
major

Cephalic vein in
deltopectoral
groove

Palpable around the shoulder are:
- The acromion
- The head of the humerus
- The corocoid process
- The clavicle

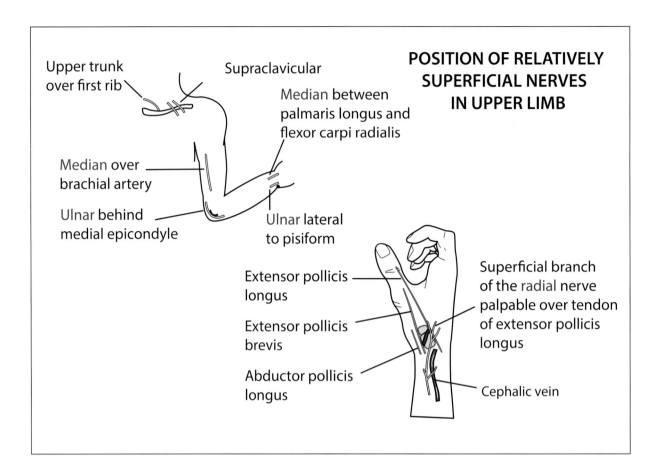

POSITION OF RELATIVELY SUPERFICIAL NERVES IN UPPER LIMB

Upper trunk over first rib

Supraclavicular

Median between palmaris longus and flexor carpi radialis

Median over brachial artery

Ulnar behind medial epicondyle

Ulnar lateral to pisiform

Extensor pollicis longus

Extensor pollicis brevis

Abductor pollicis longus

Superficial branch of the radial nerve palpable over tendon of extensor pollicis longus

Cephalic vein

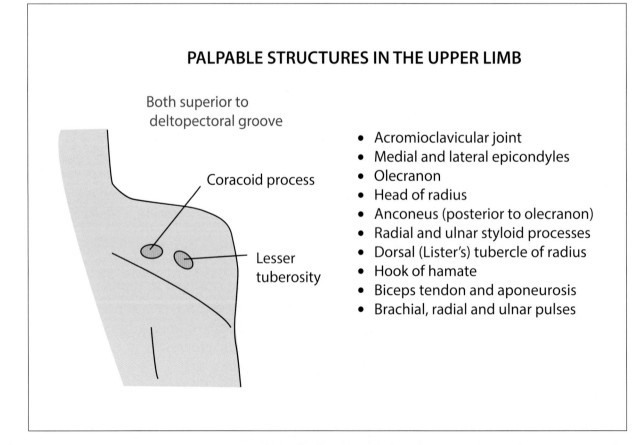

PALPABLE STRUCTURES IN THE UPPER LIMB

Both superior to deltopectoral groove

Coracoid process

Lesser tuberosity

- Acromioclavicular joint
- Medial and lateral epicondyles
- Olecranon
- Head of radius
- Anconeus (posterior to olecranon)
- Radial and ulnar styloid processes
- Dorsal (Lister's) tubercle of radius
- Hook of hamate
- Biceps tendon and aponeurosis
- Brachial, radial and ulnar pulses

VULNERABLE NERVES IN THE ARM

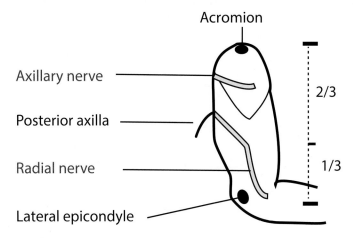

Acromion

Axillary nerve

Posterior axilla

Radial nerve

Lateral epicondyle

2/3

1/3

RADIAL NERVE
Passes from where the posterior axilla meets the arm to a point 2/3 down a line from acromion to the lateral epicondyle then it passes anterior to the lateral epicondyle

LEFT SCAPULA

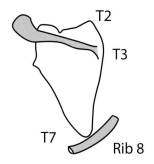

T2

T3

T7

Rib 8

- Covers half the ribs 2-7
- 8th rib is first below
- Upper border at T2
- Medial spine at T3
- Lower border at T7

DERMATOMES IN THE OUTSTRETCHED UPPER LIMB
(Anterior view)

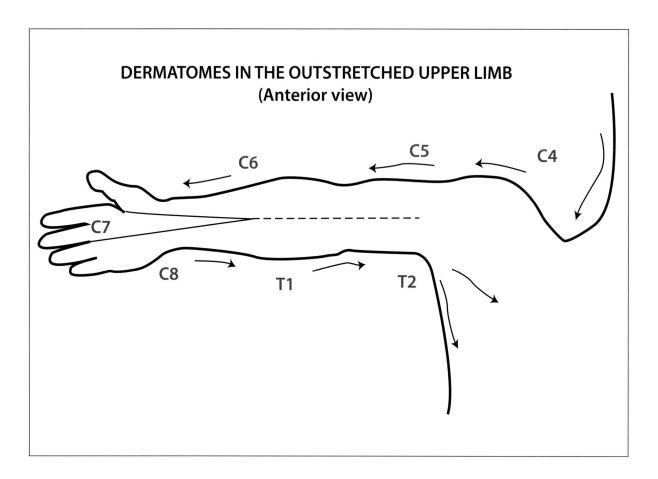

UPPER LIMB DERMATOMES

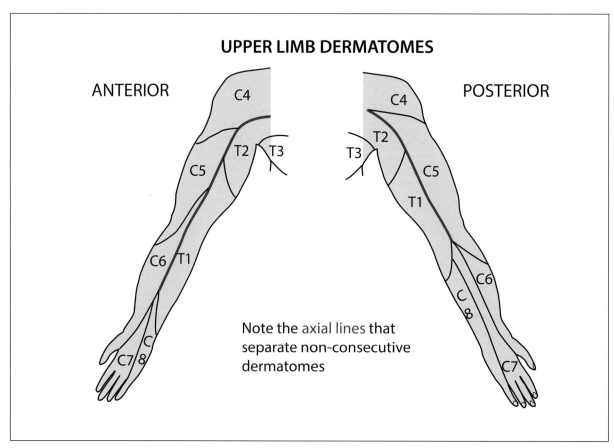

Note the axial lines that separate non-consecutive dermatomes

UPPER LIMB DERMATOMES

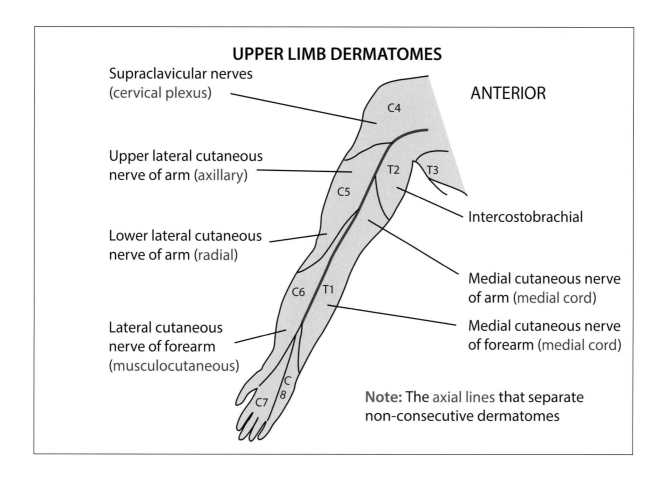

Supraclavicular nerves
(cervical plexus)

ANTERIOR

Upper lateral cutaneous
nerve of arm (axillary)

Lower lateral cutaneous
nerve of arm (radial)

Lateral cutaneous
nerve of forearm
(musculocutaneous)

Intercostobrachial

Medial cutaneous nerve
of arm (medial cord)

Medial cutaneous nerve
of forearm (medial cord)

Note: The axial lines that separate
non-consecutive dermatomes

CUTANEOUS NERVES OF THE UPPER LIMB

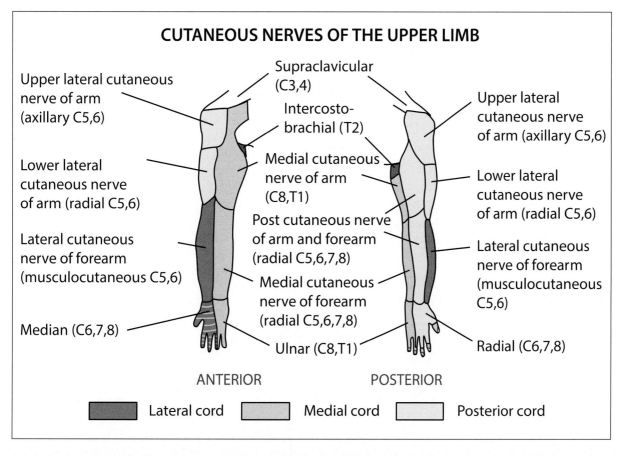

Upper lateral cutaneous
nerve of arm
(axillary C5,6)

Supraclavicular
(C3,4)

Upper lateral
cutaneous nerve
of arm (axillary C5,6)

Intercosto-
brachial (T2)

Lower lateral
cutaneous nerve
of arm (radial C5,6)

Medial cutaneous
nerve of arm
(C8,T1)

Lower lateral
cutaneous nerve
of arm (radial C5,6)

Lateral cutaneous
nerve of forearm
(musculocutaneous C5,6)

Post cutaneous nerve
of arm and forearm
(radial C5,6,7,8)

Lateral cutaneous
nerve of forearm
(musculocutaneous
C5,6)

Median (C6,7,8)

Medial cutaneous
nerve of forearm
(radial C5,6,7,8)

Radial (C6,7,8)

Ulnar (C8,T1)

ANTERIOR   POSTERIOR

Lateral cord   Medial cord   Posterior cord

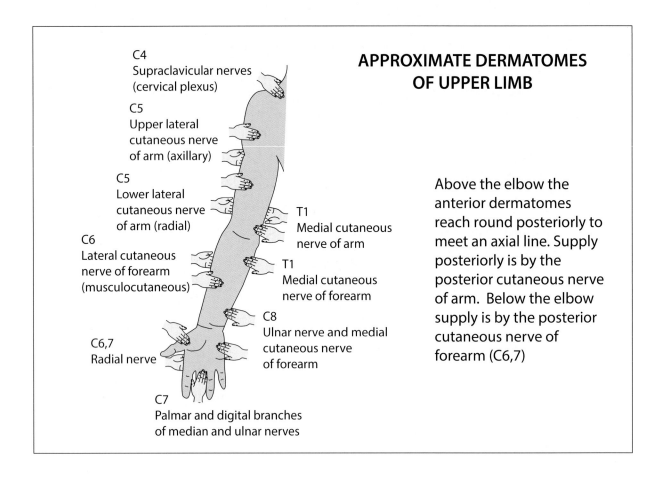

C4
Supraclavicular nerves
(cervical plexus)

C5
Upper lateral
cutaneous nerve
of arm (axillary)

C5
Lower lateral
cutaneous nerve
of arm (radial)

C6
Lateral cutaneous
nerve of forearm
(musculocutaneous)

C6,7
Radial nerve

C7
Palmar and digital branches
of median and ulnar nerves

T1
Medial cutaneous
nerve of arm

T1
Medial cutaneous
nerve of forearm

C8
Ulnar nerve and medial
cutaneous nerve
of forearm

APPROXIMATE DERMATOMES OF UPPER LIMB

Above the elbow the anterior dermatomes reach round posteriorly to meet an axial line. Supply posteriorly is by the posterior cutaneous nerve of arm. Below the elbow supply is by the posterior cutaneous nerve of forearm (C6,7)

SEGMENTAL NERVE SUPPLY IN UPPER LIMB

SHOULDER:
Flexion/abduction/lateral rotation	C5
Extension/adduction/medial rotation	C6,7,8

ELBOW:
Flexion (biceps reflex)	C5,6
Extension (triceps reflex)	C6,7,8

FOREARM:
Pronation	C7,8
Supination	C6

WRIST:
Flexion/extension	C7,8

FINGERS/THUMB (LONG TENDONS):
Flexion/extension	C7,8

HAND (SMALL MUSCLES):
All movements	T1

LIMB TENDON REFLEXES

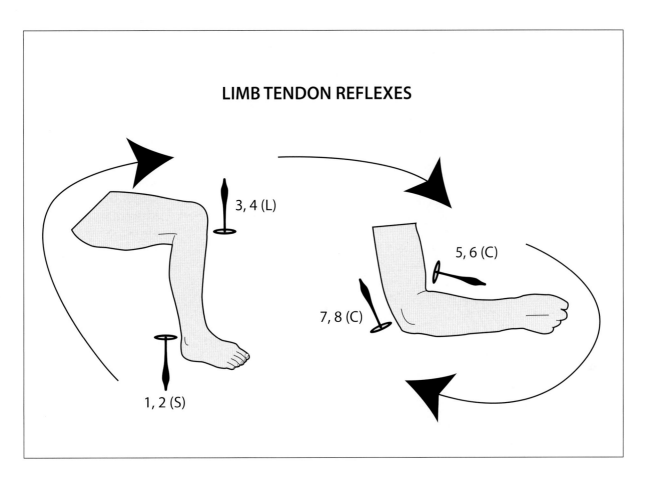

UPPER LIMB MYOTOMES

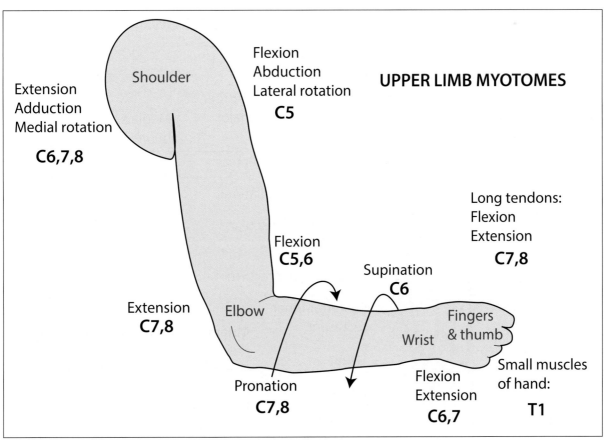

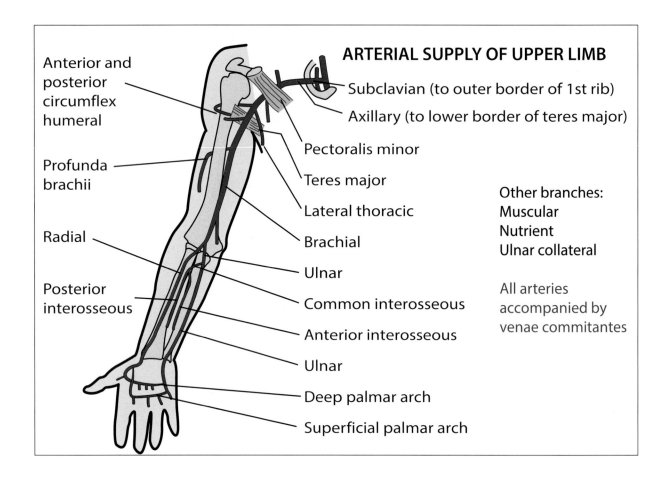

ARTERIAL SUPPLY OF UPPER LIMB

Anterior and posterior circumflex humeral

Profunda brachii

Radial

Posterior interosseous

Subclavian (to outer border of 1st rib)

Axillary (to lower border of teres major)

Pectoralis minor

Teres major

Lateral thoracic

Brachial

Ulnar

Common interosseous

Anterior interosseous

Ulnar

Deep palmar arch

Superficial palmar arch

Other branches:
Muscular
Nutrient
Ulnar collateral

All arteries accompanied by venae commitantes

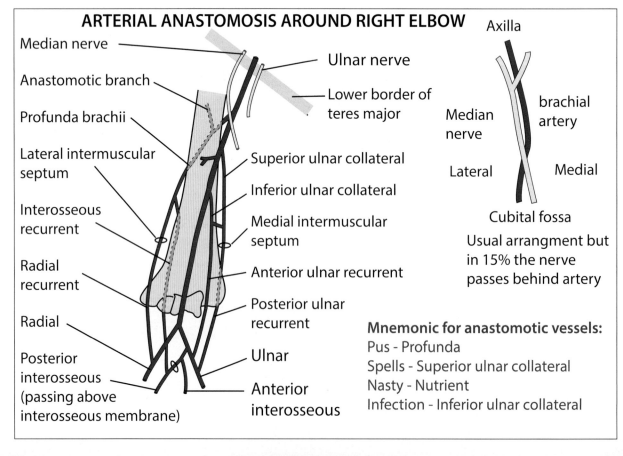

ARTERIAL ANASTOMOSIS AROUND RIGHT ELBOW

Median nerve

Anastomotic branch

Profunda brachii

Lateral intermuscular septum

Interosseous recurrent

Radial recurrent

Radial

Posterior interosseous (passing above interosseous membrane)

Ulnar nerve

Lower border of teres major

Superior ulnar collateral

Inferior ulnar collateral

Medial intermuscular septum

Anterior ulnar recurrent

Posterior ulnar recurrent

Ulnar

Anterior interosseous

Axilla

Median nerve

brachial artery

Lateral

Medial

Cubital fossa

Usual arrangment but in 15% the nerve passes behind artery

Mnemonic for anastomotic vessels:
Pus - Profunda
Spells - Superior ulnar collateral
Nasty - Nutrient
Infection - Inferior ulnar collateral

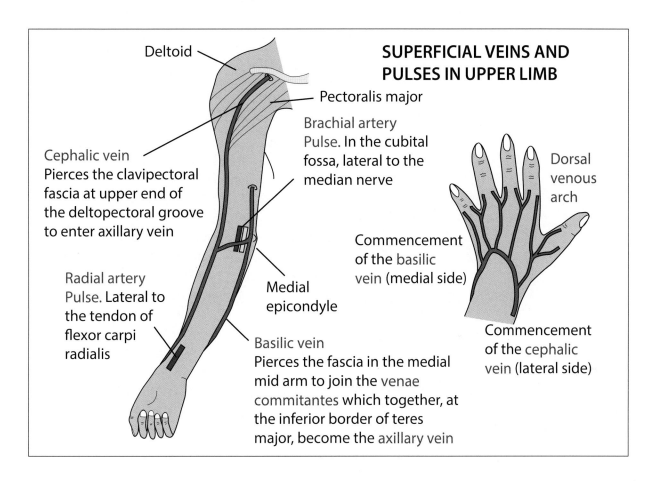

SUPERFICIAL VEINS AND PULSES IN UPPER LIMB

Deltoid

Pectoralis major

Brachial artery
Pulse. In the cubital fossa, lateral to the median nerve

Dorsal venous arch

Cephalic vein
Pierces the clavipectoral fascia at upper end of the deltopectoral groove to enter axillary vein

Commencement of the basilic vein (medial side)

Radial artery
Pulse. Lateral to the tendon of flexor carpi radialis

Medial epicondyle

Commencement of the cephalic vein (lateral side)

Basilic vein
Pierces the fascia in the medial mid arm to join the venae commitantes which together, at the inferior border of teres major, become the axillary vein

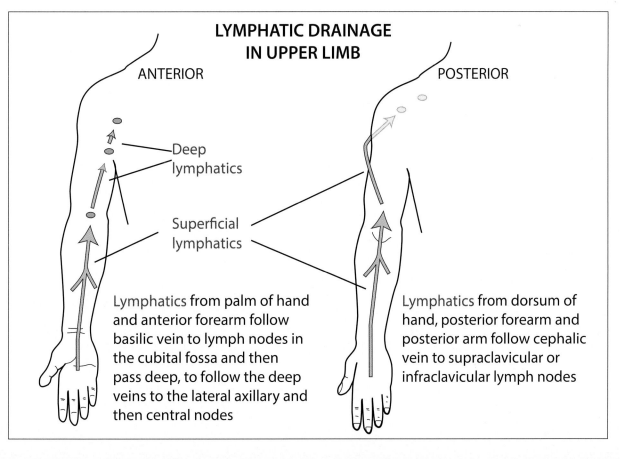

LYMPHATIC DRAINAGE IN UPPER LIMB

ANTERIOR

POSTERIOR

Deep lymphatics

Superficial lymphatics

Lymphatics from palm of hand and anterior forearm follow basilic vein to lymph nodes in the cubital fossa and then pass deep, to follow the deep veins to the lateral axillary and then central nodes

Lymphatics from dorsum of hand, posterior forearm and posterior arm follow cephalic vein to supraclavicular or infraclavicular lymph nodes

AXILLARY LYMPH NODES

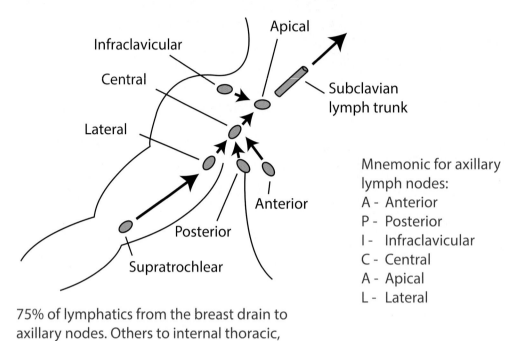

Infraclavicular

Central

Lateral

Apical

Subclavian
lymph trunk

Anterior

Posterior

Supratrochlear

Mnemonic for axillary
lymph nodes:
A - Anterior
P - Posterior
I - Infraclavicular
C - Central
A - Apical
L - Lateral

75% of lymphatics from the breast drain to
axillary nodes. Others to internal thoracic,
abdominal nodes or to other breast

1.2   Shoulder and Arm

SHOULDER JOINT (GLENOHUMERAL)

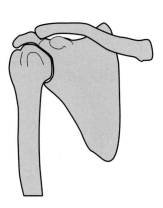

Blood: Circumflex humeral arteries
Nerves: Subscapular, suprascapular, axillary (Hilton's law)
Bursae: Subscapular, subacromial, infraspinatus, supraspinatus
Stability: Bones (poor), Capsule (relatively poor), Muscles +++, ligaments +++
Support: Rotator cuff (subscapularis, supraspinatus, infraspinatus, teres minor), long head biceps, triceps in abduction, muscles from chest to arm

SHOULDER JOINT (GLENOHUMERAL)

LIGAMENTS:

1,2,3: Glenohumeral
Anterior: superior, middle, inferior (weak thickenings of capsule)
4: Subscapularis
5: Teres major
6: Supraspinatus
7: Short head biceps
8: Pectoralis minor

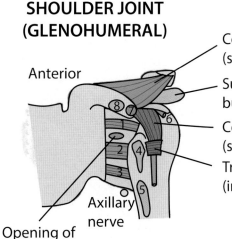

Anterior

Coraco-acromial (strong ++)
Subacromial bursa (large)
Coracohumeral (strong)
Transverse humeral (intertubercular)

Axillary nerve

Opening of subscapular bursa

Shallow glenoid fossa - deepened by glenoid labrum. Synovial, Ball and socket. Humeral head is 1/3 hemisphere
Capsule: Strong and taut superiorly (anti-sag), inferiorly lax and inserted lower to allow wide abduction, flexion and extension. Synovium: Envelops biceps tendon, communicates with bursae anteriorly and posteriorly

SHOULDER JOINT AND ROTATOR CUFF MUSCLES

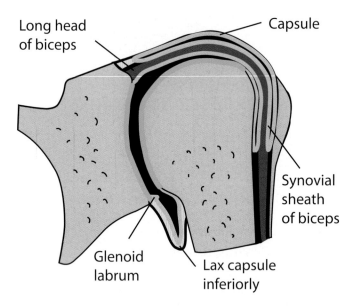

Long head of biceps

Capsule

Synovial sheath of biceps

Glenoid labrum

Lax capsule inferiorly

Rotator Cuff Muscles:
Subscapularis (anterior)
Infraspinatus (posterior)
Teres minor (posterior)
Supraspinatus (superior)

All blend with capsule of shoulder joint

Lax capsule inferiorly allows dislocation of head of humerus inferiorly and usually anteriorly

The tendon of the long head of biceps lies within the capsule but not within the synovial membrane. It attaches to the supraglenoid tubercle

SUBACROMIAL BURSA AND PAINFUL ARC SYNDROME

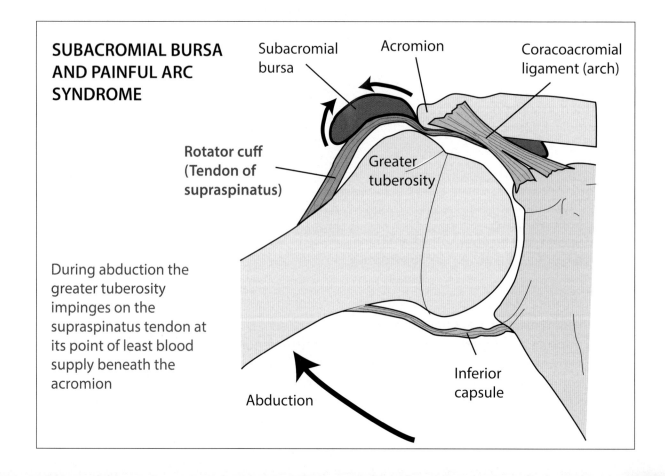

Subacromial bursa

Acromion

Coracoacromial ligament (arch)

Rotator cuff (Tendon of supraspinatus)

Greater tuberosity

During abduction the greater tuberosity impinges on the supraspinatus tendon at its point of least blood supply beneath the acromion

Abduction

Inferior capsule

ACROMIOCLAVICULAR JOINT

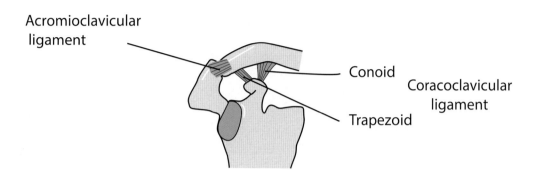

- Synovial
- Atypical
- Thick superior capsule (acromioclavicular ligament)
- Incomplete fibrocartilaginous disc in upper joint
- Strong coracoclavicular ligament
- **Nerve:** Lateral supraclavicular (C4)
- **Movements:** Gliding (passive) and 20° of rotation of scapula

ACROMIOCLAVICULAR JOINT AND CORACOCLAVICULAR LIGAMENTS

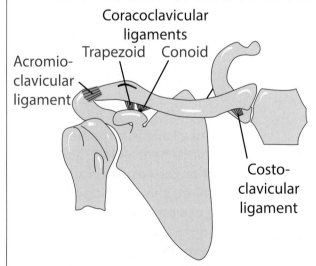

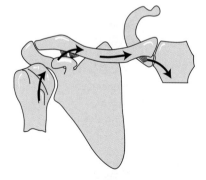

The acromioclavicular joint can dislocate but forces usually pass through coracoclavicular ligament to the clavicle then via the costoclavicular ligament to the manubrium and sternum. Excessive force will fracture the clavicle

ACROMIOCLAVICULAR JOINT
- Synovial, Atypical, Plane (passive gliding)
- Thick superior capsule (acromioclavicular ligament)
- Incomplete fibrocartilaginous disc in upper joint
- Strong coracoclavicular ligament
- Nerve: Lateral supraclavicular (C4)
- Movements: gliding (passive) and 20° of rotation of scapula

STERNOCLAVICULAR JOINT

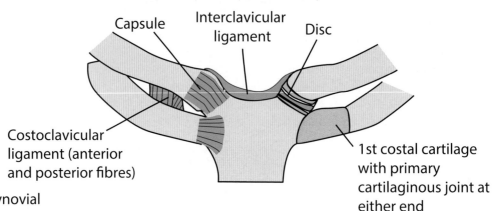

Capsule

Interclavicular ligament

Disc

Costoclavicular ligament (anterior and posterior fibres)

1st costal cartilage with primary cartilaginous joint at either end

- Synovial
- Atypical (fibrocartilage on joint surfaces)
- Fibrocartilaginous disc dividing it into 2 cavities
- Manubrial surface is concave
- All the features of a ball and socket joint
- Disc attached to capsule, acts as shock absorber
- Capsule thick above and posteriorly
- Fulcrum at costoclavicular ligament
- Clavicle rotates 40 degrees
- Nerves: supraclavicular (C3,4)

Ligaments:
- Thickening of capsule (above and posteriorly) = anterior and posterior sternoclavicular ligaments
- Interclavicular
- Costoclavicular (strong)

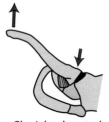

Clavicle elevated At distal end, medial end depresses

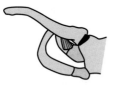

At rest

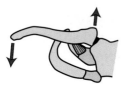

Clavicle depressed at distal end, medial end elevates

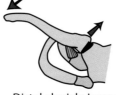

Distal clavicle is pushed forwards, medial end retracts

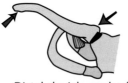

Distal clavicle pushed posteriorly, medial end protrudes

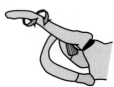

Distal and medial clavicle can rotate together

MOVEMENTS AT THE STERNOCLAVICULAR JOINT

In view of all the movements described here and the ability to pivot on the costoclavicular ligament, the sternoclavicular joint can be regarded has having many the features of a ball and socket joint

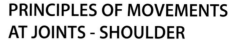

PRINCIPLES OF MOVEMENTS AT JOINTS - SHOULDER

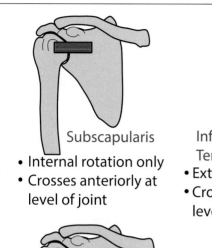

Subscapularis
- Internal rotation only
- Crosses anteriorly at level of joint

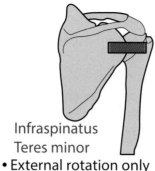

Infraspinatus
Teres minor
- External rotation only
- Crosses posteriorly at level of joint

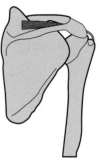

Supraspinatus
Deltoid
- Abduction only
- Crosses superorly at level of joint

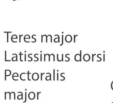

Teres major
Latissimus dorsi
Pectoralis major
- Internal rotation and adduction
- Crosses both anteriorly and inferior to level of joint

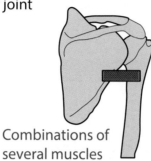

Combinations of several muscles
- External rotation and adduction
- Crosses both posteriorly and inferior to level of joint

SUPRASPINATUS

Origin: 3/4 supraspinous fossa and upper spine of scapula
Insertion: Superior facet of greater tuberosity of humerus and joint capsule
Action: Abducts and stabilises shoulder
Nerve supply: Suprascapular (C5,6 upper trunk)

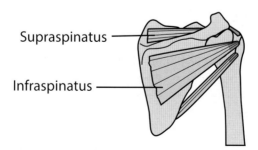

Supraspinatus

Infraspinatus

INFRASPINATUS

Origin: Medial 3/4 infraspinous fossa and intermuscular septum
Insertion: Medial facet of greater tuberosity of humerus and joint capsule
Action: Lateral rotation and stabilisation of shoulder
Nerve supply: Suprascapular (C5,6 upper trunk)

DELTOID

Origin: Lateral third clavicle, acromion, spine of scapula as far as deltoid tubercle of scapula
Insertion: Deltoid tubercle of humerus
Action: Abducts arm. Anterior fibres flex and medially rotate. Posterior fibres extend and laterally rotate
Nerve supply: Axillary (C5,6 posterior cord)

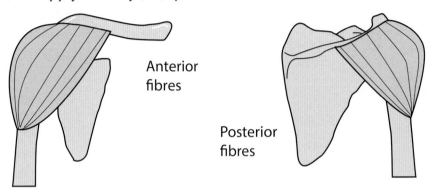

Anterior fibres

Posterior fibres

Special note: There is little doubt that the lateral fibres of deltoid help supraspinatus to initiate abduction of the shoulder but from the images above it is obvious that the anterior and posterior fibres cross the joint more effectively as soon as abduction begins and thus give more power to abduction

RHOMBOID MAJOR

Origin: Spines of T2-5 and supraspinous ligaments
Insertion: Lower half posterior medial scapula
Action: Retracts and rotates scapula to rest position
Nerve supply: Dorsal scapular (C5 from root)

RHOMBOID MINOR

Origin: Spines C7 and T1 and lower ligamentum nuchae
Insertion: Posteromedial scapula level with spine
Action: Retracts and rotates scapula to rest
Nerve supply: Dorsal scapular (C5 from root)

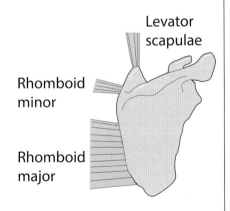

Levator scapulae

Rhomboid minor

Rhomboid major

LEVATOR SCAPULAE

Origin: Posterior tubercles of transverse processes C1-4
Insertion: Upper medial border of scapula
Action: Raises medial end of scapula
Nerve supply: Dorsal scapular (C5 root)

SUBSCAPULARIS

Origin: Medial 2/3 subscapular fossa
Insertion: Lesser tuberosity of humerus, half medial lip of bicipital groove, shoulder joint capsule
Action: Medial rotation stabilisation of shoulder
Nerve supply: Upper and lower subscapular (posterior cord C6,7)

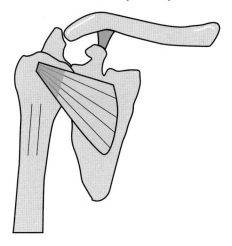

PECTORALIS MAJOR

Clavicular head
Origin: Medial half of clavicle
Insertion: Anterior lamina (of trilaminar insertion) and lateral lip of bicipital groove, deep fascia, anterior lip of deltoid tuberosity

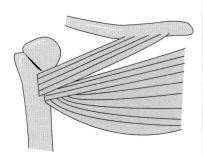

Sternocostal head
Origin: Anterior and lateral manubrium, body of sternum, aponeurosis of external oblique, upper 7 costal cartilages (not always 1st or 7th)
Insertion: Manubrial fibres to intermediate lamina. Sternocostal fibres to posterior lamina with highest fibres into capsule of shoulder
Action: Flexion, adduction, internal rotation
Nerve supply: lateral and medial pectoral nerves

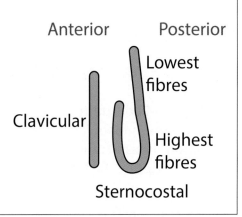

Anterior   Posterior

Lowest fibres

Clavicular

Highest fibres

Sternocostal

PECTORALIS MINOR

Origin: Ribs 3,4,5
Insertion: Coracoid process
Action: Protracts scapula with serratus anterior
Nerve supply: Medial and lateral pectoral nerves

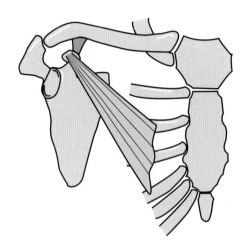

TERES MAJOR

Origin: Oval area on lower third lateral side of inferior angle of scapula
Insertion: Medial lip of bicipital groove
Action: Medial rotation, adduction, stabilisation of shoulder
Nerve supply: Lower subscapular (posterior cord C5,6)

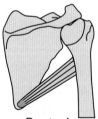

Posterior

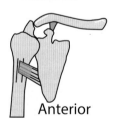

Anterior

TERES MINOR

Origin: Middle third lateral border of scapula
Insertion: Inferior facet of greater tuberosity and joint capsule
Action: Lateral rotation and stabilisation of shoulder
Nerve supply: Axillary nerve (C5,6 (posterior cord)

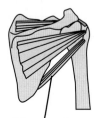

Teres minor

SERRATUS ANTERIOR

Origin: Upper 8 ribs and intercostal membranes
Insertion: Inner, medial border of scapula
Action: Protracts and laterally rotates scapula
Nerve supply: Long thoracic nerve of Bell
C5 to slips 1 and 2
C6 to slips 3 and 4
C7 to slips 5, 6, 7, and 8

1st slip visible in posterior triangle of neck

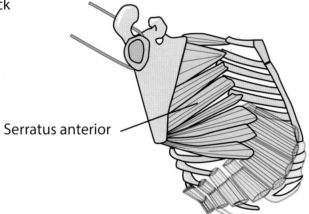

Serratus anterior

Note: If slips 5, 6, 7, 8, under the control of C7 act alone, the scapula is rotated with minimal protraction as in abduction of the upper limb.

TRAPEZIUS

Origin: Superior nuchal line and crest, occiput, nuchal ligament, spines and supraspinous ligaments T1-12.
Insertion: Lateral 1/3 clavicle, medial acromion, spine of scapula around to deltoid tubercle.
Action: Lateral rotation, elevation, depression and retraction of scapula (lowest fibres elevate body when arm is fixed. Upper fibres extend and laterally flex head and neck. Rotation is aided by serratus anterior).
Nerve supply: Spinal root of accessory nerve (XI).

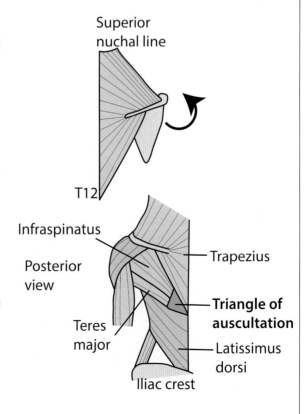

Superior nuchal line

T12

Infraspinatus

Posterior view

Trapezius

Triangle of auscultation

Teres major

Latissimus dorsi

Iliac crest

LATISSIMUS DORSI

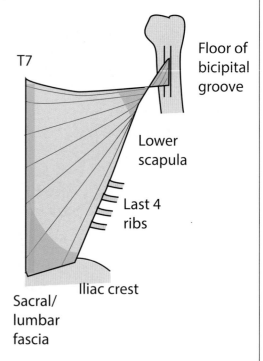

Origin: Spines and supraspinous ligament T7 down to sacrum, lumbar fascia, posterior third of iliac crest, last 4 ribs and inferior angle of scapula.
Insertion: Flat tendon into floor of bicipital groove.
Action: Adducts, extends and medially rotates shoulder. Aids both inspiration and expiration.
Nerve supply: Thoracodorsal nerve from posterior cord.

T7

Floor of bicipital groove

Lower scapula

Last 4 ribs

Iliac crest

Sacral/ lumbar fascia

MUSCLES ATTACHED TO RIBS

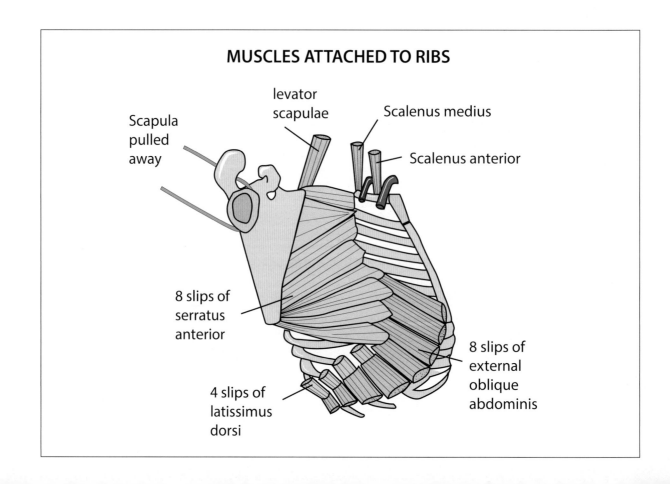

Scapula pulled away

levator scapulae

Scalenus medius

Scalenus anterior

8 slips of serratus anterior

8 slips of external oblique abdominis

4 slips of latissimus dorsi

LOOKING DOWN ON RIGHT SHOULDER

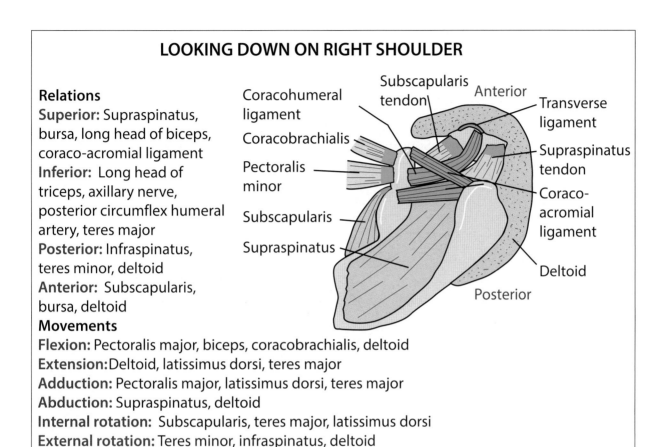

Relations
Superior: Supraspinatus, bursa, long head of biceps, coraco-acromial ligament
Inferior: Long head of triceps, axillary nerve, posterior circumflex humeral artery, teres major
Posterior: Infraspinatus, teres minor, deltoid
Anterior: Subscapularis, bursa, deltoid

Movements
Flexion: Pectoralis major, biceps, coracobrachialis, deltoid
Extension: Deltoid, latissimus dorsi, teres major
Adduction: Pectoralis major, latissimus dorsi, teres major
Abduction: Supraspinatus, deltoid
Internal rotation: Subscapularis, teres major, latissimus dorsi
External rotation: Teres minor, infraspinatus, deltoid

(Labels in figure: Coracohumeral ligament, Coracobrachialis, Pectoralis minor, Subscapularis, Supraspinatus, Subscapularis tendon, Anterior, Transverse ligament, Supraspinatus tendon, Coraco-acromial ligament, Deltoid, Posterior)

ANTERIOR ARM

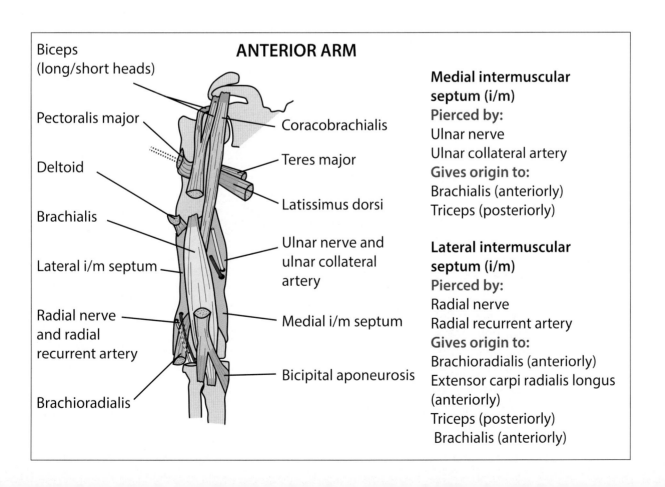

(Labels in figure: Biceps (long/short heads), Pectoralis major, Deltoid, Brachialis, Lateral i/m septum, Radial nerve and radial recurrent artery, Brachioradialis, Coracobrachialis, Teres major, Latissimus dorsi, Ulnar nerve and ulnar collateral artery, Medial i/m septum, Bicipital aponeurosis)

Medial intermuscular septum (i/m)
Pierced by:
Ulnar nerve
Ulnar collateral artery
Gives origin to:
Brachialis (anteriorly)
Triceps (posteriorly)

Lateral intermuscular septum (i/m)
Pierced by:
Radial nerve
Radial recurrent artery
Gives origin to:
Brachioradialis (anteriorly)
Extensor carpi radialis longus (anteriorly)
Triceps (posteriorly)
Brachialis (anteriorly)

SUBCLAVIUS

Origin: 1st rib, costochondral junction
Insertion: Subclavian groove inferior middle clavicle
Action: Stabilises clavicle
Nerve supply: Nerve to subclavius (C5,6 off roots)

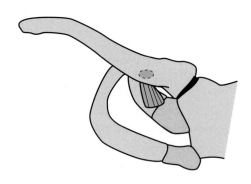

AXIAL (CROSS) SECTION OF MID RIGHT ARM

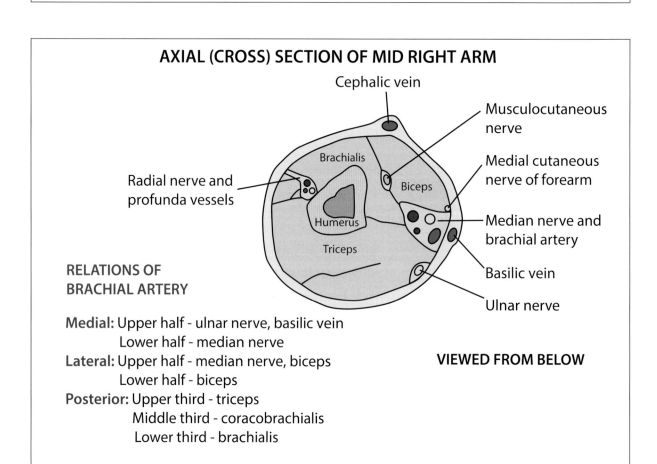

Cephalic vein

Musculocutaneous nerve

Brachialis

Biceps

Radial nerve and profunda vessels

Medial cutaneous nerve of forearm

Humerus

Median nerve and brachial artery

Triceps

Basilic vein

Ulnar nerve

VIEWED FROM BELOW

RELATIONS OF BRACHIAL ARTERY

Medial: Upper half - ulnar nerve, basilic vein
Lower half - median nerve
Lateral: Upper half - median nerve, biceps
Lower half - biceps
Posterior: Upper third - triceps
Middle third - coracobrachialis
Lower third - brachialis

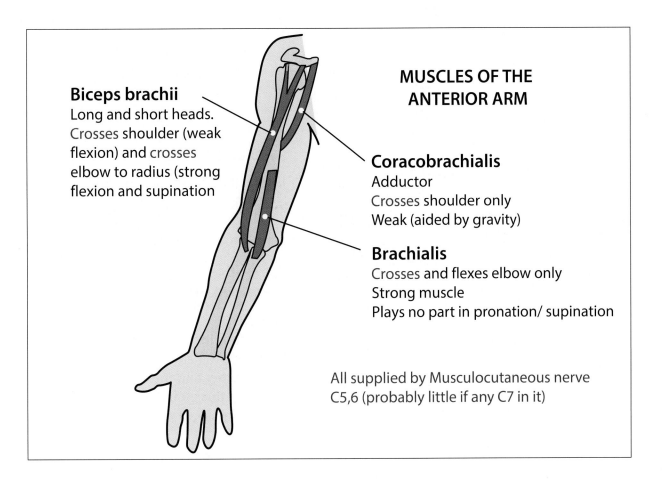

MUSCLES OF THE ANTERIOR ARM

Biceps brachii
Long and short heads.
Crosses shoulder (weak flexion) and crosses elbow to radius (strong flexion and supination

Coracobrachialis
Adductor
Crosses shoulder only
Weak (aided by gravity)

Brachialis
Crosses and flexes elbow only
Strong muscle
Plays no part in pronation/ supination

All supplied by Musculocutaneous nerve C5,6 (probably little if any C7 in it)

ANTERIOR ARM MUSCLES

Biceps
Origin:
Long head - Supraglenoid tubercle
Short head - coracoid
Insertion: Radial tuberosity and bicipital aponeurosis
Action: Flexes shoulder and elbow. Supinates
Nerve supply: Musculocutaneous

Brachialis
Origin: Anterior/lower 1/2 humerus and medial and lateral intermuscular septum
Insertion: Coronoid process and tubercle of ulna
Action: Flexes elbow
Nerve supply: Musculocutaneous and twig from radial

Coracobrachialis
Origin: Coracoid process
Insertion: Anteromedial humerus - mid shaft
Action: Adducts and flexes shoulder
Nerve supply: Musculocutaneous
Note: Coracobrachialis is the equivalent to the three adductors in the leg. It is thus vestigially tripartite and a third head may remain as a supratrochlear spur (ligament of Struthers)

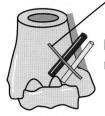

Brachial artery and median nerve

MUSCLES OF THE POSTERIOR ARM (EXTENSORS)

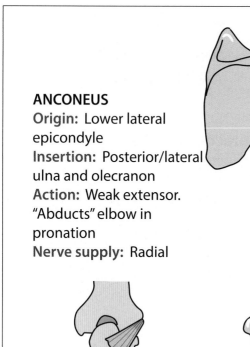

ANCONEUS
Origin: Lower lateral epicondyle
Insertion: Posterior/lateral ulna and olecranon
Action: Weak extensor. "Abducts" elbow in pronation
Nerve supply: Radial

3 HEADS OF TRICEPS

Lateral (lateral to spiral groove)

Medial (medial to spiral groove)

Long (infraglenoid tubercle)

Spiral groove begins between the medial and lateral heads

TRICEPS:
All 3 heads insert into the olecranon. It extends the elbow, weakly extends the shoulder and the long head stabilises the shoulder.
Nerve: Radial (C7,8)

QUADRANGULAR AND TRIANGULAR SPACES

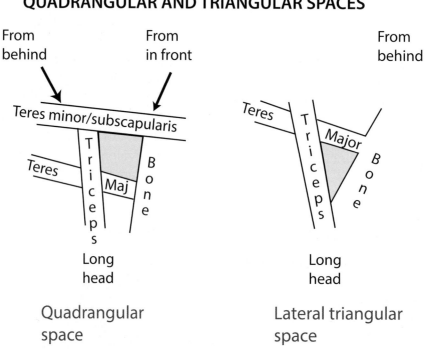

Quadrangular space

Lateral triangular space

POSTERIOR ARM MUSCLES AND SPACES

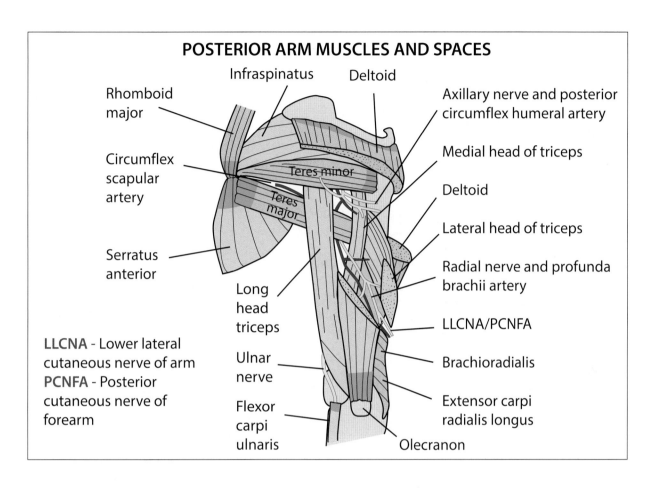

Rhomboid major

Infraspinatus

Deltoid

Axillary nerve and posterior circumflex humeral artery

Circumflex scapular artery

Teres minor

Teres major

Medial head of triceps

Deltoid

Lateral head of triceps

Serratus anterior

Radial nerve and profunda brachii artery

Long head triceps

LLCNA/PCNFA

LLCNA - Lower lateral cutaneous nerve of arm
PCNFA - Posterior cutaneous nerve of forearm

Ulnar nerve

Brachioradialis

Flexor carpi ulnaris

Extensor carpi radialis longus

Olecranon

QUADRANGULAR AND TRIANGULAR SPACES

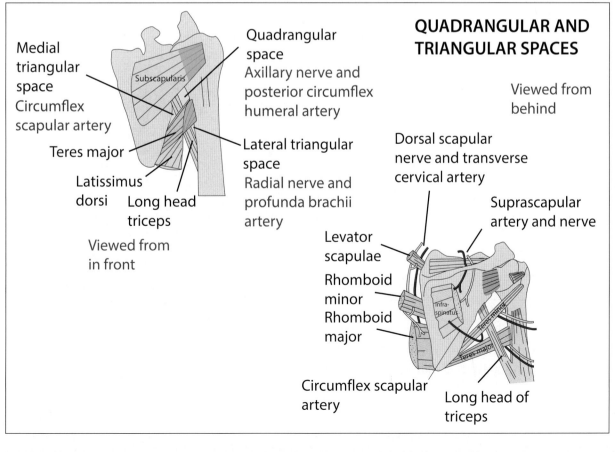

Medial triangular space
Circumflex scapular artery

Subscapularis

Quadrangular space
Axillary nerve and posterior circumflex humeral artery

Viewed from behind

Teres major

Lateral triangular space
Radial nerve and profunda brachii artery

Dorsal scapular nerve and transverse cervical artery

Suprascapular artery and nerve

Latissimus dorsi

Long head triceps

Viewed from in front

Levator scapulae

Rhomboid minor

Rhomboid major

Infra-spinatus

Teres minor

Teres major

Circumflex scapular artery

Long head of triceps

HUMERUS
(MUSCLE ATTACHMENTS)

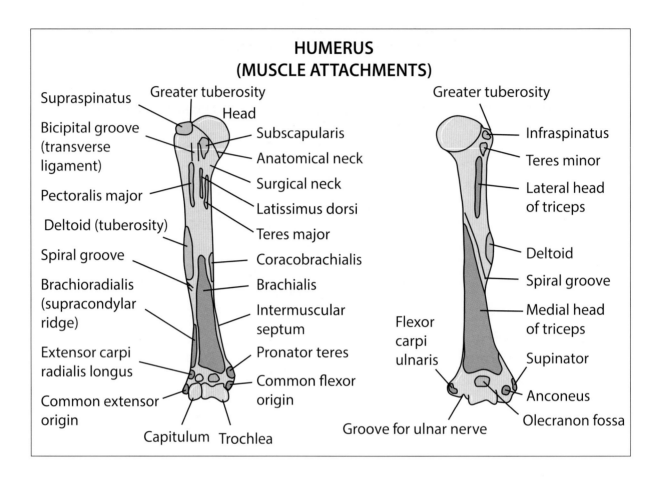

Supraspinatus

Bicipital groove (transverse ligament)

Pectoralis major

Deltoid (tuberosity)

Spiral groove

Brachioradialis (supracondylar ridge)

Extensor carpi radialis longus

Common extensor origin

Greater tuberosity

Head

Subscapularis

Anatomical neck

Surgical neck

Latissimus dorsi

Teres major

Coracobrachialis

Brachialis

Intermuscular septum

Pronator teres

Common flexor origin

Capitulum   Trochlea

Greater tuberosity

Infraspinatus

Teres minor

Lateral head of triceps

Deltoid

Spiral groove

Medial head of triceps

Supinator

Anconeus

Olecranon fossa

Flexor carpi ulnaris

Groove for ulnar nerve

ABDUCTION AT SHOULDER

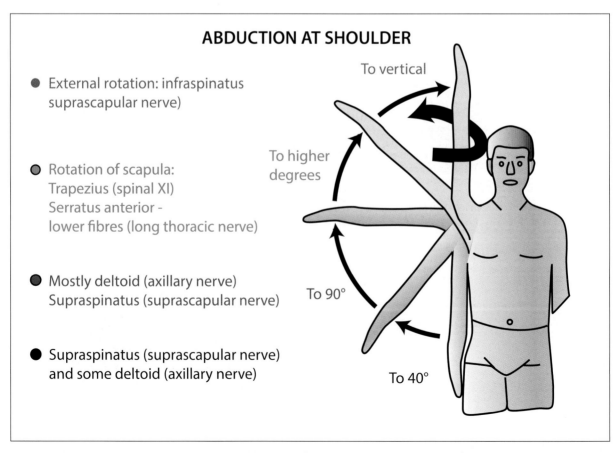

- External rotation: infraspinatus suprascapular nerve)

- Rotation of scapula: Trapezius (spinal XI) Serratus anterior - lower fibres (long thoracic nerve)

- Mostly deltoid (axillary nerve) Supraspinatus (suprascapular nerve)

- Supraspinatus (suprascapular nerve) and some deltoid (axillary nerve)

To vertical

To higher degrees

To 90°

To 40°

ARTERIAL ANASTOMOSIS AROUND SHOULDER

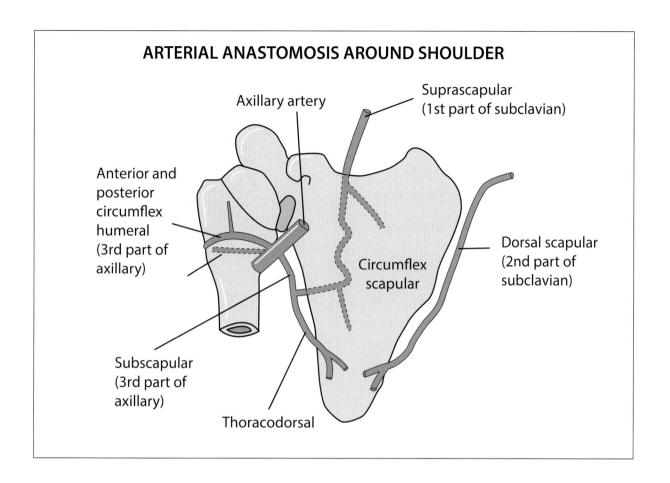

Axillary artery

Suprascapular
(1st part of subclavian)

Anterior and
posterior
circumflex
humeral
(3rd part of
axillary)

Dorsal scapular
(2nd part of
subclavian)

Circumflex
scapular

Subscapular
(3rd part of
axillary)

Thoracodorsal

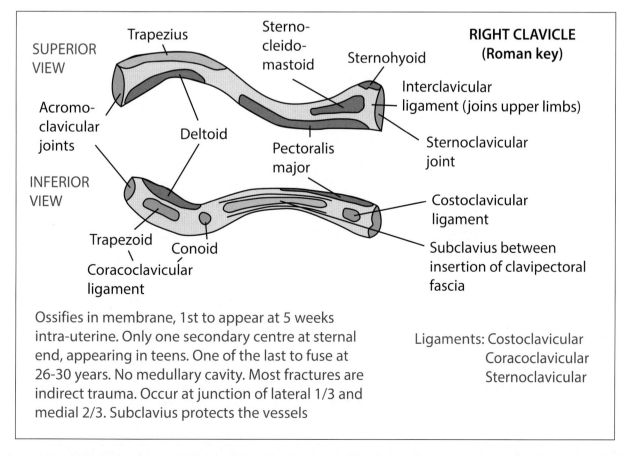

SUPERIOR
VIEW

Trapezius

Sterno-
cleido-
mastoid

Sternohyoid

**RIGHT CLAVICLE
(Roman key)**

Acromo-
clavicular
joints

Deltoid

Interclavicular
ligament (joins upper limbs)

Pectoralis
major

Sternoclavicular
joint

INFERIOR
VIEW

Costoclavicular
ligament

Trapezoid

Conoid

Coracoclavicular
ligament

Subclavius between
insertion of clavipectoral
fascia

Ossifies in membrane, 1st to appear at 5 weeks
intra-uterine. Only one secondary centre at sternal
end, appearing in teens. One of the last to fuse at
26-30 years. No medullary cavity. Most fractures are
indirect trauma. Occur at junction of lateral 1/3 and
medial 2/3. Subclavius protects the vessels

Ligaments: Costoclavicular
Coracoclavicular
Sternoclavicular

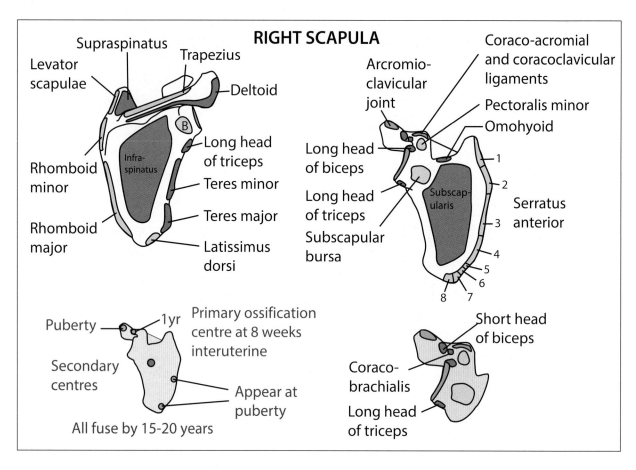

RIGHT SCAPULA

Levator scapulae
Supraspinatus
Trapezius
Deltoid
Long head of triceps
Infra-spinatus
Rhomboid minor
Teres minor
Teres major
Rhomboid major
Latissimus dorsi
B

Arcromio-clavicular joint
Coraco-acromial and coracoclavicular ligaments
Pectoralis minor
Omohyoid
Long head of biceps
Long head of triceps
Subscap-ularis
Subscapular bursa
Serratus anterior
1
2
3
4
5
6
7
8

Puberty
1yr
Secondary centres
Appear at puberty
Primary ossification centre at 8 weeks interuterine
All fuse by 15-20 years

Short head of biceps
Coraco-brachialis
Long head of triceps

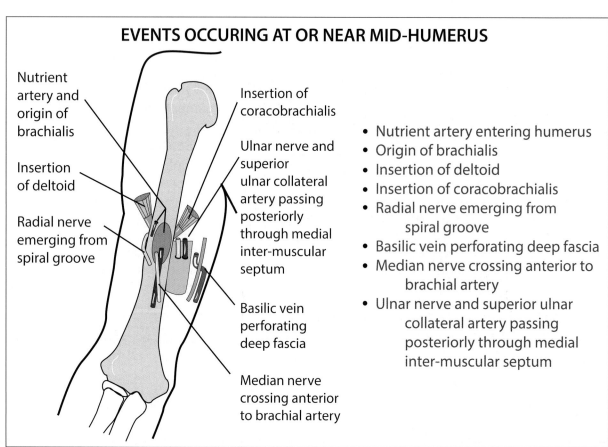

EVENTS OCCURING AT OR NEAR MID-HUMERUS

Nutrient artery and origin of brachialis

Insertion of deltoid

Radial nerve emerging from spiral groove

Insertion of coracobrachialis

Ulnar nerve and superior ulnar collateral artery passing posteriorly through medial inter-muscular septum

Basilic vein perforating deep fascia

Median nerve crossing anterior to brachial artery

- Nutrient artery entering humerus
- Origin of brachialis
- Insertion of deltoid
- Insertion of coracobrachialis
- Radial nerve emerging from spiral groove
- Basilic vein perforating deep fascia
- Median nerve crossing anterior to brachial artery
- Ulnar nerve and superior ulnar collateral artery passing posteriorly through medial inter-muscular septum

1.3 Axilla, Brachial Plexus and Nerve Lesions

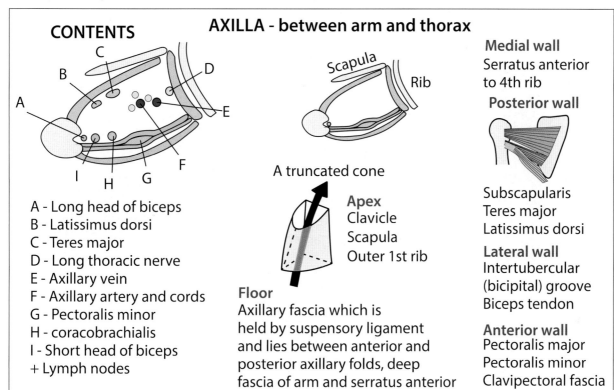

CONTENTS

AXILLA - between arm and thorax

A - Long head of biceps
B - Latissimus dorsi
C - Teres major
D - Long thoracic nerve
E - Axillary vein
F - Axillary artery and cords
G - Pectoralis minor
H - coracobrachialis
I - Short head of biceps
+ Lymph nodes

A truncated cone

Apex
Clavicle
Scapula
Outer 1st rib

Floor
Axillary fascia which is
held by suspensory ligament
and lies between anterior and
posterior axillary folds, deep
fascia of arm and serratus anterior

Medial wall
Serratus anterior
to 4th rib

Posterior wall
Subscapularis
Teres major
Latissimus dorsi

Lateral wall
Intertubercular
(bicipital) groove
Biceps tendon

Anterior wall
Pectoralis major
Pectoralis minor
Clavipectoral fascia

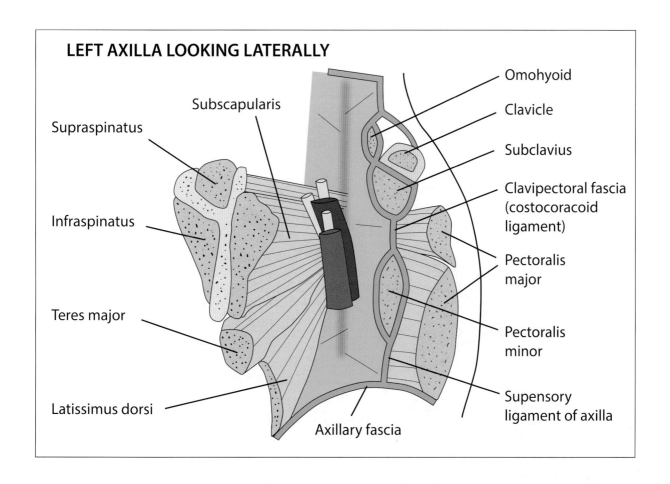

LEFT AXILLA LOOKING LATERALLY

Supraspinatus

Subscapularis

Infraspinatus

Teres major

Latissimus dorsi

Axillary fascia

Omohyoid

Clavicle

Subclavius

Clavipectoral fascia
(costocoracoid
ligament)

Pectoralis
major

Pectoralis
minor

Supensory
ligament of axilla

CLAVIPECTORAL FASCIA

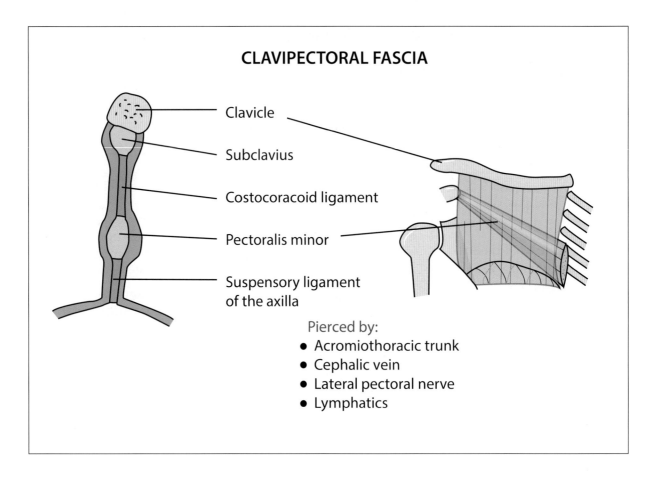

Clavicle

Subclavius

Costocoracoid ligament

Pectoralis minor

Suspensory ligament of the axilla

Pierced by:
- Acromiothoracic trunk
- Cephalic vein
- Lateral pectoral nerve
- Lymphatics

AXILLARY ARTERY 1
(branches from parts 1-2-3)

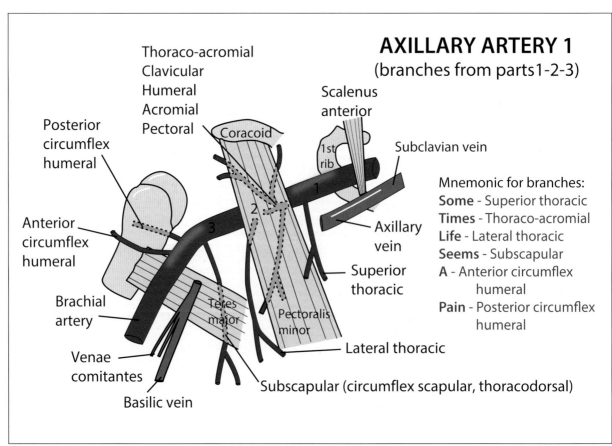

Thoraco-acromial
Clavicular
Humeral
Acromial
Pectoral

Scalenus anterior

Coracoid

1st rib

Subclavian vein

Posterior circumflex humeral

Anterior circumflex humeral

Brachial artery

Venae comitantes

Basilic vein

Teres major

Pectoralis minor

Axillary vein

Superior thoracic

Lateral thoracic

Subscapular (circumflex scapular, thoracodorsal)

Mnemonic for branches:
Some - Superior thoracic
Times - Thoraco-acromial
Life - Lateral thoracic
Seems - Subscapular
A - Anterior circumflex humeral
Pain - Posterior circumflex humeral

AXILLARY ARTERY 2
(branches from parts 1-2-3)

1st part: Outer border of 1st rib to medial edge of pectoralis minor
        1 branch: Superior thoracic
Relations: 3 cords of brachial plexus lie laterally
2nd part: Behind pectoralis minor
        2 branches: Thoraco-acromial, lateral thoracic
Relations: 3 cords around it according to their names
3rd part: lateral edge of pectoralis minor to lower border of teres major
        3 branches: Subscapular, anterior and posterior circumflex humeral
Relations: Median nerve forming from its two heads anterior to artery

Distal   Proximal

3rd part of artery with 2
heads of median nerve
forming anterior to it.

BRACHIAL PLEXUS

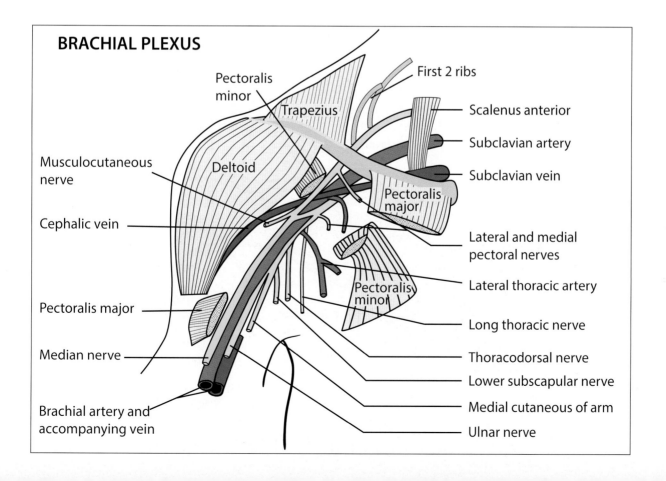

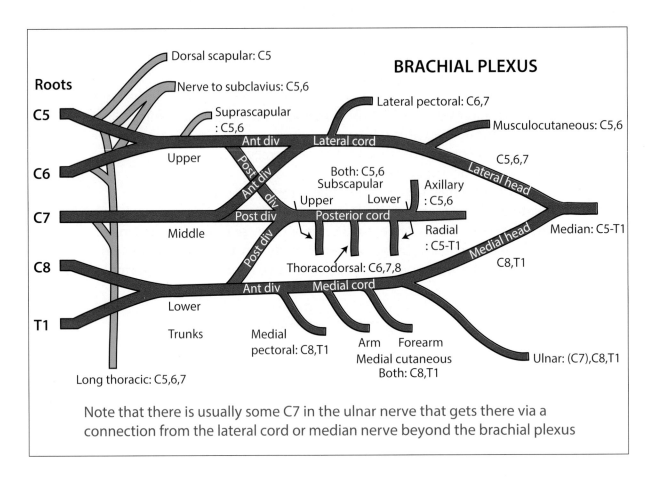

Note that there is usually some C7 in the ulnar nerve that gets there via a connection from the lateral cord or median nerve beyond the brachial plexus

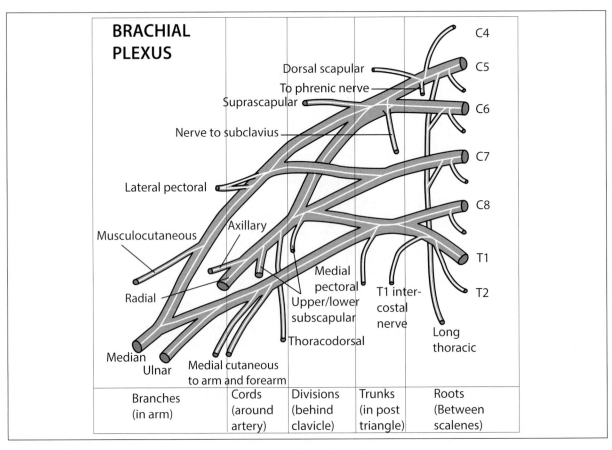

NERVE LESIONS IN THE UPPER LIMB

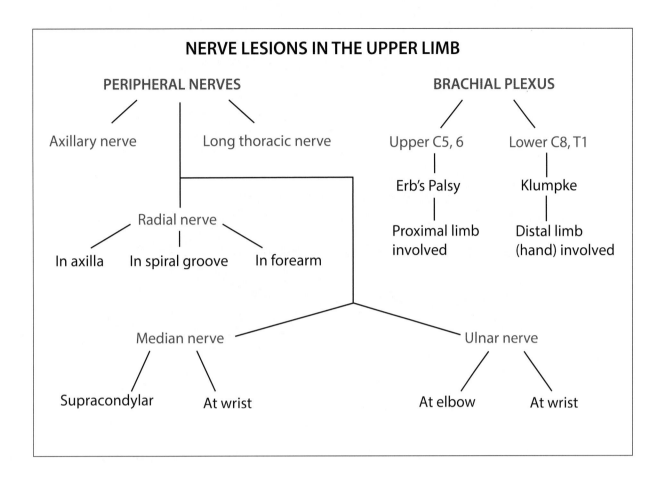

PERIPHERAL NERVES

Axillary nerve

Long thoracic nerve

Radial nerve

In axilla   In spiral groove   In forearm

Median nerve

Supracondylar   At wrist

BRACHIAL PLEXUS

Upper C5, 6

Lower C8, T1

Erb's Palsy

Klumpke

Proximal limb involved

Distal limb (hand) involved

Ulnar nerve

At elbow   At wrist

NERVE LESIONS IN THE UPPER LIMB

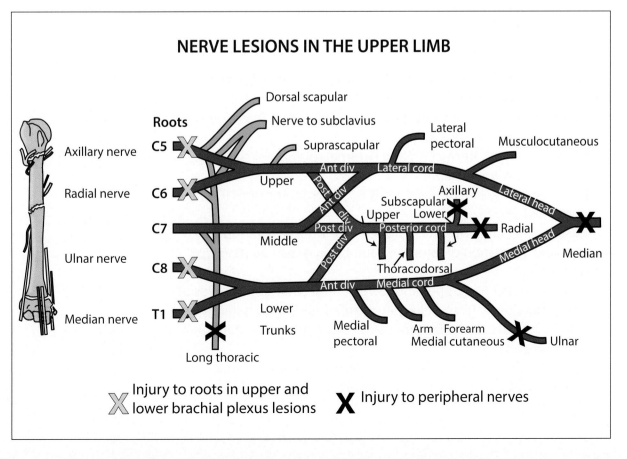

Roots

Axillary nerve

Radial nerve

Ulnar nerve

Median nerve

C5
C6
C7
C8
T1

Dorsal scapular
Nerve to subclavius
Suprascapular
Ant div   Lateral cord
Upper
Post div
Ant div
Post div
Post div   Posterior cord
Middle
Post div
Ant div   Medial cord
Lower
Trunks

Lateral pectoral
Musculocutaneous
Lateral cord
Axillary   Lateral head
Subscapular
Upper   Lower
Posterior cord   Radial
Thoracodorsal
Medial head   Median
Medial cord
Medial pectoral
Arm   Forearm
Medial cutaneous   Ulnar

Long thoracic

Injury to roots in upper and lower brachial plexus lesions

Injury to peripheral nerves

NERVE LESIONS: UPPER BRACHIAL PLEXUS - C5,6: 1

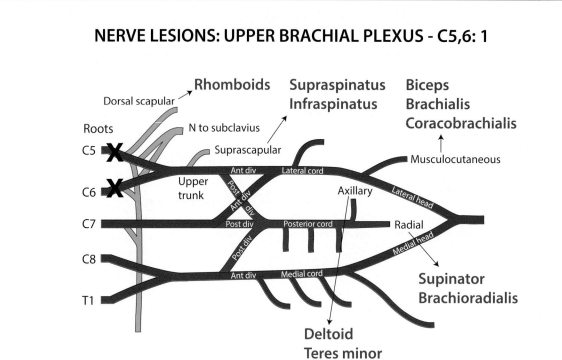

NERVE LESIONS: UPPER BRACHIAL PLEXUS - C5,6: 2

Aetiology: Birth traction (Erb Duchenne palsy) or adult trauma, (Erb's palsy) e.g. motorbike accident.

Muscle loss: Deltoid, short shoulder muscles, brachialis, biceps, supinator, brachioradialis.

Movement loss: Abduction and external rotation of shoulder, supination, elbow flexion.

Dominated by: Latissimus dorsi (C6,7,8), pronator teres (C6,7), pectorals (C6,7,8).

Result: Atrophy, limpness of upper arm, internal rotation of shoulder, pronation of forearm, palm backwards - 'waiter's tip deformity'.

Sensory loss: C5 in upper and lower lateral cutaneous nerves of arm (respectively from axillary and radial). Only if C6 is involved will the lateral cutaneous nerve of forearm (musculocutaneous) be affected.

Summary: C5 controls shoulder flexion, abduction, lateral rotation and elbow flexion. C6 controls supination including supinator.

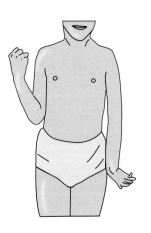

Left Erb's palsy

NERVE LESIONS: LOWER BRACHIAL PLEXUS - C8, T1: 1

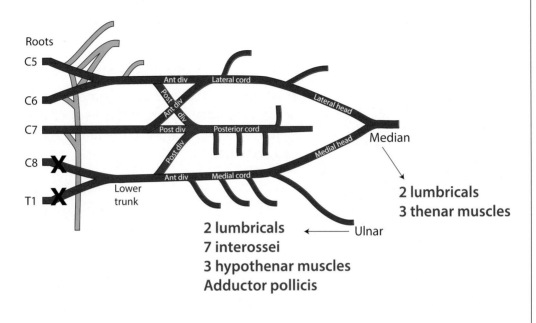

Roots
C5
C6
C7
C8
T1

Ant div
Lateral cord
Lateral head
Post div
Ant div
Post div
Posterior cord
Medial head
Median
Post div
Lower trunk
Ant div
Medial cord

2 lumbricals
3 thenar muscles

2 lumbricals
7 interossei
3 hypothenar muscles
Adductor pollicis

Ulnar

NERVE LESIONS: LOWER BRACHIAL PLEXUS - C8, T1: 2

Aetiology: Klumpke's palsy. Pull on arm at breech delivery (hyperabduction at shoulder), apical carcinoma of lung.
Muscle loss: Small muscles of hand - lumbricals and interossei, hypothenar, adductor pollicis.
Movement loss: Flexion at metacarpophalangeal joints and diminished extension at interphalangeal joints.
Dominated by: Long extensors acting on metacarpophalangeal joints and long flexors acting on interphalangeal joints.
Result: Clawed hand ('main en griffe'). Associated damage to sympathetic chain may give Horner's syndrome with ptosis, small pupil (miosis), flushed, dry face (anhydrosis).
Sensory loss: T1 distribution - lower (+ or - upper) inner arm and hand.
Test: Loss of bulk of 1st dorsal interosseous, inability to hold paper between outstretched fingers (see ulnar nerve lesions).
Note: C8 and T1 involvement by a cervical rib (see cervical rib image)

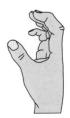

Look for evidence of a complete clawed-hand involving all fingers

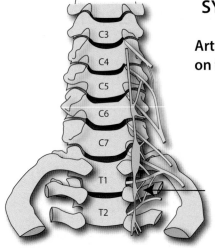

SYMPATHETIC CHAIN IN LOWER NECK

Arterial spasm may result from irritation of sympathetics on the subclavian artery from a cervical rib

SYMPATHECTOMY

Treatment of Raynaud's phenomenon by cutting the preganglionic sympathetic fibres at T2 and T3 to increase the blood flow to the fingers by preventing vasoconstriction

Small pupil
Mild ptosis
Flushed face
Dry face
Apparent enophthalmos

LEFT HORNER'S SYNDROME

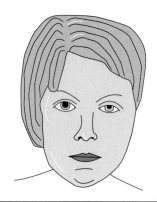

PERIPHERAL NERVE INJURY

Causes: Direct trauma, ischaemia, traction, compression
Classification of nerve injury:
1. Neurotmesis. Complete or partial division of a nerve
2. Axonotmesis. Interruption of the axons without interruption of the sheath
3. Neuropraxia. Bruising or concussion of a nerve without damage to the axon or sheath, leading to temporary loss of function

Classification of muscle power:
0. No contraction
1. Flicker or trace of contraction
2. Active movement with gravity eliminated
3. Active movement against gravity
4. Active movement against gravity and resistance
5. Normal power

Axon with myelin sheath and neurolemma which is composed of Schwann cells

Structure of a nerve

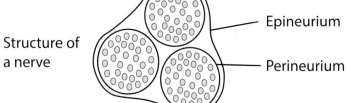

Epineurium

Perineurium

NERVE LESIONS: LONG THORACIC NERVE (OF BELL) -C5, 6, 7

Aetiology: Damage during surgery in the axilla for axillary node clearance or sentinel node biopsy for breast cancer, or placement of a chest drain. Occasionally congenital.

Result: Loss of serratus anterior leading to 'winging' of scapula. Decreased flexion and abduction of arm due to loss of scapular rotation. Varying degrees of disability according to the site of the lesion.

Sensory loss: Nil.

Test: Patient presses against wall and scapula on side of lesion will 'wing' (protrude posteriorly).

Anatomy: Passes down on serratus anterior in the mid-axillary line.

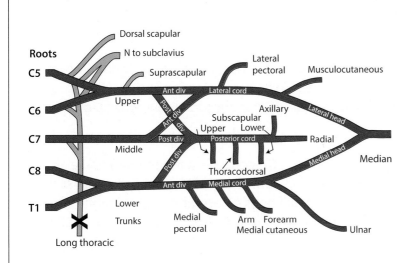

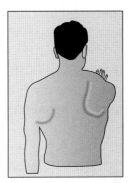

Right "winged" scapula whilst patient is pushing against wall

NERVE LESIONS: AXILLARY NERVE

Aetiology: Fractured neck of humerus or dislocation of shoulder (in 5% of dislocations)

Muscle: Loss of deltoid and teres minor

Movement loss: Diminished flexion, extension and abduction of shoulder.

Result: Wasting of deltoid

Sensory loss: Upper lateral cutaneous nerve of arm from its posterior branch. The autonomous area for this nerve is an area the size of a 'regimental patch' (A)

Test: For loss of sensation as indicated. In the acute clinical situation it is not practical to test for motor activity in deltoid

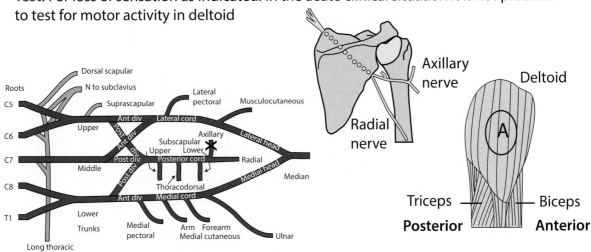

MEDIAN NERVE

FORMED: From two 'heads' in axilla, anterior to 3rd part of axillary artery. Crosses artery, usually anteriorly, from lateral to medial to lie medial to brachial artery in cubital fossa.

PASSES: Under biceps and onto or medial to brachialis, then between two heads of pronator teres, supplying it, and then under fibrous arch of flexor digitorum superficialis with ulnar artery. Under flexor digitorum superficialis, emerging from its lateral border to lie between tendons of flexor carpi radialis and palmaris longus. Passes deep to flexor retinaculum to reach palm of hand.

BRANCHES IN FOREARM: To flexor carpi radialis, palmaris longus and flexor digitorum superficialis. Via its anterior interosseous branch to flexor pollicis longus, half flexor digitorum profundus and pronator quadratus. Joint branches to elbow, wrist, superior and inferior radio-ulnar.

BRANCHES IN HAND: Sensory: Palmar cutaneous branch leaves the median nerve above the wrist and runs superficial to the flexor retinaculum to supply lateral palm skin. Main nerve in hand supplies palmar skin and dorsal nail beds of lateral 3 and half digits. Motor: lateral 2 lumbricals, abductor pollicis brevis, opponens pollicis and usually flexor pollicis brevis

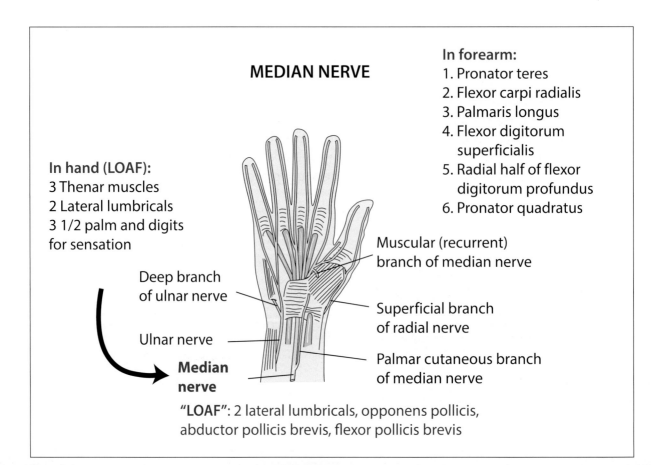

MEDIAN NERVE

In forearm:
1. Pronator teres
2. Flexor carpi radialis
3. Palmaris longus
4. Flexor digitorum superficialis
5. Radial half of flexor digitorum profundus
6. Pronator quadratus

In hand (LOAF):
3 Thenar muscles
2 Lateral lumbricals
3 1/2 palm and digits for sensation

Deep branch of ulnar nerve

Ulnar nerve

Median nerve

Muscular (recurrent) branch of median nerve

Superficial branch of radial nerve

Palmar cutaneous branch of median nerve

"LOAF": 2 lateral lumbricals, opponens pollicis, abductor pollicis brevis, flexor pollicis brevis

NERVE LESIONS: MEDIAN NERVE - SUPRACONDYLAR - C5 - T1

Aetiology: Supracondylar fracture/dislocation. (very rarely a tight bicipital aponeurosis, presence of a Struthers' Ligament or pronator syndrome where the median nerve is trapped between the two heads of pronator teres).

Muscle loss: Pronator teres, pronator quadratus, flexors of wrist/fingers (except flexor carpi ulnaris and ulnar half flexor digitorum profundus). Palmaris longus, two radial lumbricals and the 3 thenar muscles. Adductor pollicis is spared (ulnar nerve). Damage to the anterior interosseous nerve alone gives loss of flexor pollicis longus, flexor digitorum profundus to the index finger and middle fingers and pronator quadratus.

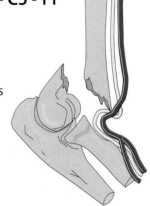

Supracondylar
Fracture at elbow

Movement loss: Loss of pronation, weak wrist flexion and abduction. Abduction of thumb is weak from loss of abductor pollicis brevis (abductor pollicis longus is intact). Loss of opposition of thumb (flexor pollicis longus). The thumb is virtually useless. Loss of flexor digitorum profundus to index and middle fingers and flexor digitorum superficialis to all four fingers.

Result: Ulnar deviation of wrist, thenar wasting, Papal benediction on attempting to make a "fist".

Sensory loss: Radial side of palm, radial 3 1/2 fingers and nail beds.

Test: Sensory - loss of pulp of index finger (autonomous area). Motor – loss of pronation of forearm, wrist flexion on the radial side, ability of thumb to abduct at right angles to palm (abductor pollicis brevis), opposition of thumb to index finger, flexion of interphalangeal joints of index and middle fingers and flexor pollicis longus by touching tip of thumb pulp to pulp of index. Flexion of the interphalangeal joints by flexor digitorum superficialis of index and middle fingers is assessed.

NERVE LESIONS: MEDIAN NERVE – AT WRIST– T1

Aetiology: Wrist laceration, carpal tunnel syndrome and injury during surgery for it.

Muscle loss: 2 radial lumbricals and thenar muscles except adductor pollicis (ulnar nerve).

Movement loss: Abduction, opposition and flexion of thumb is impaired or lost making the thumb virtually useless. Adduction of thumb is intact. Some abduction of thumb is possible as abductor pollicis longus (radial nerve) is intact.

Result: Thenar wasting and some clawing of index and middle fingers.

Sensory loss: Radial side of palm, fingers and nail beds of radial 3 1/2 fingers. The palmar cutaneous branch of median nerve is usually spared if the compression is in the carpal tunnel leading to intact sensation of thenar skin. A more proximal lesion may well damage this palmar cutaneous nerve with loss of sensation over the thenar eminence. Any numbness is often preceded by periods of paraesthesia, a tingling sensation as a result of nerve compression.

Test: Sensory - loss of pulp of index finger (autonomous area). Motor - inability of thumb to abduct at right angles to palm (abductor pollicis brevis) and oppose thumb to index finger.

VOLKMANN'S ISCHAEMIC CONTRACTURE

Aetiology: Damage to brachial artery in supracondylar fracture. Ischaemia leading to contracture of long flexors and extensors in the forearm.
Result: Deformed hand. Muscles are replaced with fibrous tissue.
Wrist flexed - bulkier flexors therefore more contracture.
Extension of metacarpophalangeal joints because of insertion of extensor tendons into these joints.
Flexed interphalangeal joints because of insertion of long flexor tendons into these joints.

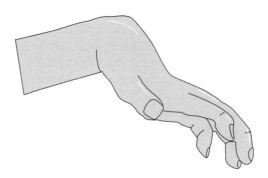

MEDIAN NERVE TESTING 1

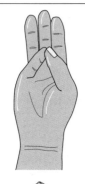

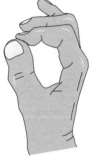

Inability to oppose index to thumb or little finger (loss of opponens pollicis).

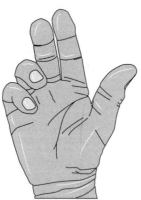

Note: Trying to make a fist

Papal benediction:
1. Thenar wasting
2. Ulnar deviation
3. Minimal flexion of digits 1-3

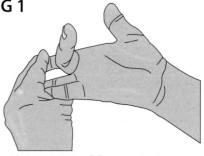

Testing the action of flexor digitorum superficialis (FDS) on the proximal interphalangeal joint (PIP). By stretching the tendons of flexor digitorum profundus (FDP) and the inter-tendinous connections to the other three fingers, the tendon of FDP to the middle finger is also effectively disabled. If FDS is intact the proximal interphalangeal joint can be flexed but there is inability to move the distal interphalangeal joint. This is the Quadriga phenomenon which shows that FDS is working normally.

MEDIAN NERVE TESTING 2

Testing abductor pollicis brevis by asking patient to touch pen with thumb

Assessment of the ability of abductor pollicis brevis to abduct the thumb at right angles to the palm. The muscle is always supplied by the median nerve

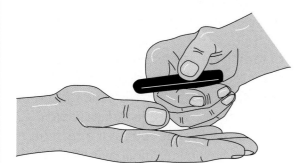

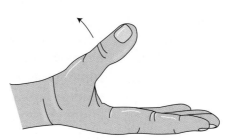

RADIAL NERVE 1

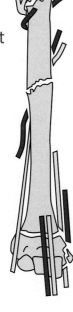

Midshaft fracture

Damage to radial nerve

Leaves: Axilla via lateral triangular space with profunda brachii artery

Spirals: Around posterior to upper fibres of the medial head of triceps, touching the humerus only in lower groove

Covered by: Upper fibres of brachialis

Passes through: Lateral intermuscular septum to reach the anterior compartment between brachialis and brachioradialis

To lie: Just lateral to the cubital fossa

Supplies: 3 cutaneous branches - posterior cutaneous nerves of arm and forearm; lower lateral cutaneous nerve of arm. Muscular branches to triceps, branchioradialis, extensor carpi radialis longus, anconeus and often a small twig to brachialis

Divides into: Posterior interosseus and superficial branch as it reaches supinator

RADIAL NERVE 2

Midshaft fracture

Damage to radial nerve

Main branches:

Posterior interosseous: Off radial under branchioradialis, passes between the two heads of supinator and into extensor compartment. Lies on abductor pollicis longus then interosseous membrane.

Supplies all muscles in the extensor compartment of forearm (except those supplied by the radial nerve - see above) also sensory to deep structures but no cutaneous branches.

Superficial branch of radial: Lies under brachioradialis, over supinator, pronator teres and flexor digitorum superficialis. Passes out lateral/posterior to brachioradialis tendon, lateral to radial artery, posterior to radial styloid and then tendon of extensor pollicis longus as it forms the dorsal side of the snuff box. Several terminal branches to skin of the back of the hand and 3 1/2 fingers short of the nail beds.

NERVE LESIONS: RADIAL NERVE IN AXILLA – C5 – T1

Aetiology: Surgical damage, trauma and classically, but now rarely, crutch pressure.

Muscle loss: Triceps, extensors of wrist, fingers and thumb.

Movement loss: Extensor weakness at elbow, wrist and metacarpophalangeal joints. Minimal loss of supination as biceps is intact.

Result: Wrist drop with loss of power grip as digit extensors are held elongated and flexors shortened.

Sensory loss: Over first dorsal web space (autonomous area), dorsal aspect of the radial 3 1/2, +/- lower lateral cutaneous nerve of arm. There may also be detectable sensory loss over posterior aspect of arm and forearm.

Test: Sensation as above. Power of brachioradialis, extension of wrist and elbow against resistance.

Anatomy: Branches of the radial nerve are mostly given off well before they reach the muscles that they supply.

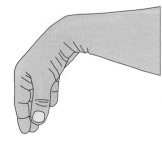

Wrist drop

NERVE LESIONS: RADIAL NERVE IN SPIRAL GROOVE – C5 – T1

Aetiology: Fracture mid-shaft humerus, Saturday night palsy and injections.

Muscle loss: Extensors of wrist, fingers and thumb, but triceps is spared. Extensor carpi radialis longus (ECRL) and brachioradialis may also be spared depending on the exact level of the injury. Loss of anconeus would probably be clinically insignificant but may give some instability in pronation and supination.

Movement loss: Extensor weakness of wrist and digits.

Result: Extension of elbow is normal, but the presence of wrist drop and loss of power grip will depend on whether ECRL is lost.

Sensory loss: Over 1st dorsal web space as for higher lesion. Lower lateral cutaneous nerve of arm is usually spared.

Test: Power of wrist extension.

Anatomy: ECRL is the most important muscle for wrist extension and is the first wrist extensor to be innervated by the radial nerve. Its fate determines the presence or absence of wrist drop.

Wrist drop is likely

NERVE LESIONS: RADIAL NERVE (POSTERIOR INTEROSSEOUS N) IN FOREARM – C7, 8

Aetiology: Lateral or posterior forearm trauma, surgical mishap or fracture/dislocation of radial head.

Muscle loss: Extensors of wrist and fingers, but extensor carpi radialis longus is spared.

Movement loss: Extensor weakness of metacarpophalangeal joints. Interphalangeal joints are normal because of intact interossei and lumbricals.

Result: No wrist drop. Grip is normal as extensor carpi radialis longus is intact. Extension of elbow is normal.

Sensory loss: No sensory loss if superficial radial nerve is intact.

Test: Power of extension of metacarpophalangeal joints.

No wrist drop

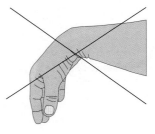

ULNAR NERVE

IN ARM AND FOREARM

Passes: Posterior to the axillary vessels and through the medial intermuscular septum with the superior ulnar collateral artery and branches of the radial nerve which supply the medial head of triceps.

Progresses: Posterior to medial epicondyle of humerus and between the two heads of flexor carpi ulnaris and against the medial ligament of the elbow.

Continues: Under flexor carpi ulnaris and on flexor digitorum profundus with the ulnar artery lateral to it. It emerges lateral to the tendon of flexor carpi ulnaris at the wrist and passes into the hand superficial to the flexor retinaculum (Canal of Guyon) as a deep and superficial branch.

Gives: Dorsal cutaneous branch whilst still under the flexor carpi ulnaris which supplies the medial skin of dorsum of hand and one and a half digits. Also give a palmar cutaneous branch to the medial palmar skin.

Supplies: Flexor carpi ulnaris, the elbow joint and the medial half of flexor digitorum profundus in the forearm.

IN HAND

Superficial branch: Supplies palmaris brevis and skin of palmar one and a half digits.

Deep branch: Passes over the hook of hamate and supplies: wrist joint, flexor digiti minimi, abductor digiti minimi, opponens digiti minimi, all 7 interossei, 2 medial lumbricals and ends in and supplies adductor pollicis. It sometimes supplies flexor pollicis brevis.

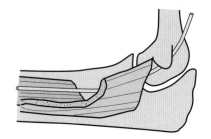

ULNAR NERVE

In forearm:
Flexor carpi ulnaris
Ulnar 1/2 flexor digitorum profundus

In hand:
3 Hypothenar muscles
2 Medial lumbricals
7 Interossei
1 Adductor pollicis
= **13 muscles**

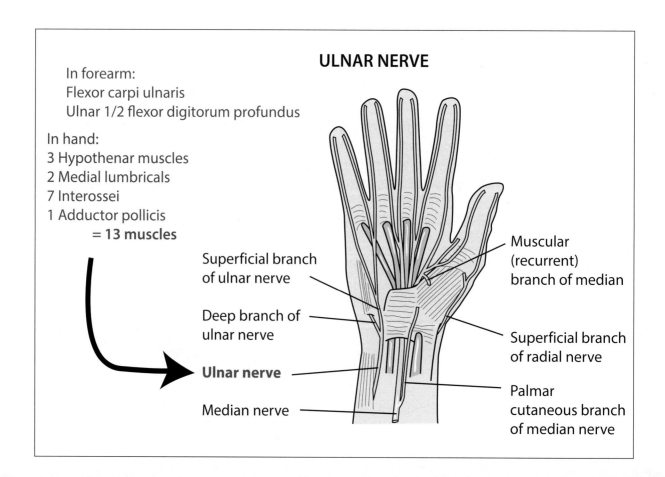

Superficial branch of ulnar nerve

Deep branch of ulnar nerve

Ulnar nerve

Median nerve

Muscular (recurrent) branch of median

Superficial branch of radial nerve

Palmar cutaneous branch of median nerve

NERVE LESIONS: ULNAR AT ELBOW – (C7), C8, T1

Aetiology: Present or previous fractures or dislocation of elbow, damage behind medial epicondyle. Pressure on operating table. Entrapment between the two heads of flexor carpi ulnaris.

Muscle loss: All intrinsic muscles of hand (except radial 2 lumbricals and three thenar muscles), flexor digitorum profundus to ring and little fingers, flexor carpi ulnaris.

Result: Clawing, loss of grip and loss of abduction and adduction of fingers BUT less clawing of index and middle fingers because of intact two radial lumbricals. Note also that there is less clawing of ring and little fingers than with a lesion at the wrist due to loss of flexor digitorum profundus to these fingers. There is also radial deviation.

Sensory loss: Ulnar side of palmar and dorsal aspects of the hand and ulnar one and a half fingers.

Test: Assess grip of paper between fingers and ability to splay fingers under resistance. Froment's test to judge power of adductor pollicis. Assess wasting of 1st dorsal interosseous muscle. Test distal interphalangeal joint of little finger for ulnar 1/2 of flexor digitorum profundus.
Test sensation of little finger pulp (autonomous area).

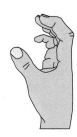

Claw
Hand

NERVE LESIONS: ULNAR AT WRIST -T1

Aetiology: Lacerations at wrist, damage within Canal of Guyon or direct trauma to palm of hand damaging deep motor branch.

Muscle loss: All intrinsic muscles of hand except radial 2 lumbricals and three thenar muscles. Flexor digitorum profundus and flexor carpi ulnaris are intact.

Result: Clawed hand (no interossei therefore no flexion of metacarpophalangeal joints but instead they are extended at the metacarpophalangeal joints by long extensors. There is flexion of interphalangeal joints by long flexors. Absent radial deviation.

Note: LESS clawing of index and middle fingers because of intact median nerve to radial lumbricals but MORE clawing of ring and little fingers because of intact ulnar 1/2 flexor digitorum profundus than for an ulnar lesion at elbow (**ulnar paradox**).

Sensory loss: Ulnar 1 1/2 fingers. Dorsal and palmar cutaneous branches may be spared depending on the exact level of the injury.

Test: Assess grip of paper between fingers and ability to splay fingers under resistance. Froment's test to judge power of adductor pollicis. Assess wasting of 1st dorsal interosseous muscle. Test sensation of pulp of little finger (autonomous area).

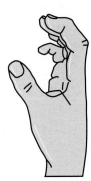

Clawed
Hand

EXPLANATION OF CLAWING

The key to understanding clawing is to appreciate that the first attachment of extensor digitorum to the dorsal hood is at the dorsal base of the proximal phalanx (see later image). The primary action of this muscle is to extend the metacarpophalangeal joint. Whereas extension of the proximal and distal interphalangeal joints is mediated predominantly by the dorsal and palmar interossei and lumbricals. If these small muscles of the hand are no longer active, as in an ulnar nerve lesion, then the extensor digitorum, unopposed, will forcefully overextend the metacarpophalangeal joint (see left lower image). Meanwhile the long flexor tendons flex the interphalangeal joints as they are powerful and overcome any attempted extension at these joints by extensor digitorum.

ACTION OF THE INTEROSSEI AND LUMBRICALS

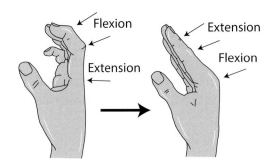

LUMBRICAL AND INTEROSSEI MUSCLES

Note: The lumbricals reach the fingers on their radial side and they cross the metacarpophalangeal joints on their palmar aspect at an angle that allows flexion of these joints. Their attachments to the extensor expansions (dorsal hoods) allows simultaneously extension of the interphalangeal joints.

However, as the interossei are more in line with the metacarpals (see image below) they can only achieve the same actions as the lumbricals by having two tendons – one to the dorsal hood and the other to the base of the proximal phalanx.

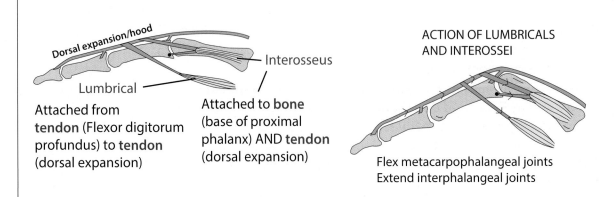

Attached from **tendon** (Flexor digitorum profundus) to **tendon** (dorsal expansion)

Attached to **bone** (base of proximal phalanx) AND **tendon** (dorsal expansion)

ACTION OF LUMBRICALS AND INTEROSSEI

Flex metacarpophalangeal joints
Extend interphalangeal joints

INTEROSSEI

LUMBRICALS

ACTION OF THE INTEROSSEI AND LUMBRICALS

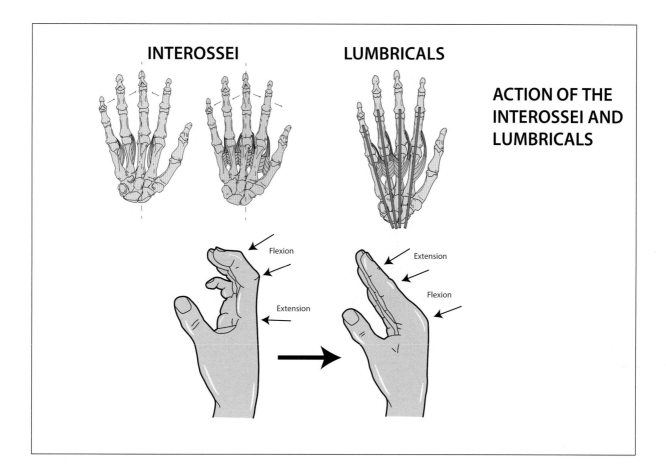

ULNAR NERVE TESTING 1

FROMENT'S TEST

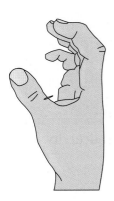

Clawing of hand is more marked in an ulnar lesion at the wrist as the long flexors are intact.
"Ulnar paradox"

Paper is pinched in the first web space between the proximal phalanx of the thumb and the metacarpophalangeal joint of the index finger, with the digits extended. Adductor pollicis is being tested. The patient may "cheat" by using flexor pollicis longus (median nerve)

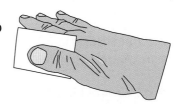

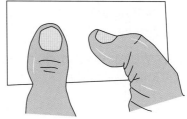

ULNAR NERVE TESTING 2

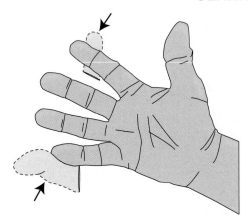

Attempt to splay (abduct) fingers against resistance using dorsal interossei

Testing the ability of the palmar interossei to adduct the fingers

EXAMINATION FOR CERVICAL RIB

1. Diminution of pulse

2. Paraesthesia in shaded area

3. Reproduction of symptoms on pulling arm downwards

4. Weakness of small muscles of the hand

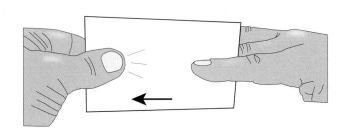

Cervical rib

SUMMARY OF MYOTOMES IN UPPER LIMB

SHOULDER:

Flexion/abduction/lateral rotation	C5
Extension/adduction/medial rotation	C6,7,8

ELBOW:

Flexion (biceps reflex)	C5,6
Extension (triceps reflex)	C6,7,8

FOREARM:

Pronation	C7,8
Supination	C6

WRIST:

Flexion/extension	C7,8

FINGERS/THUMB (LONG TENDONS):

Flexion/extension	C7,8

HAND (SMALL MUSCLES)

All movements	T1

MUSCULOCUTANEOUS NERVE

PASSES:

Between conjoined heads of coracobrachialis then between biceps and brachialis

SUPPLIES:

Motor - coracobrachialis, biceps and brachialis

Sensory - elbow joint and then lateral cutaneous nerve of forearm after emerging on lateral side of biceps

1.4 Elbow and Forearm

Capsule attachments

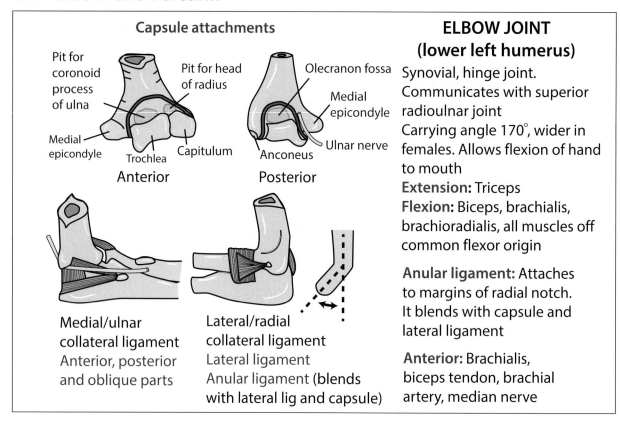

Pit for coronoid process of ulna
Pit for head of radius
Medial epicondyle
Trochlea
Capitulum

Anterior

Olecranon fossa
Medial epicondyle
Ulnar nerve
Anconeus

Posterior

Medial/ulnar collateral ligament
Anterior, posterior and oblique parts

Lateral/radial collateral ligament
Lateral ligament
Anular ligament (blends with lateral lig and capsule)

ELBOW JOINT (lower left humerus)

Synovial, hinge joint. Communicates with superior radioulnar joint

Carrying angle 170°, wider in females. Allows flexion of hand to mouth

Extension: Triceps

Flexion: Biceps, brachialis, brachioradialis, all muscles off common flexor origin

Anular ligament: Attaches to margins of radial notch. It blends with capsule and lateral ligament

Anterior: Brachialis, biceps tendon, brachial artery, median nerve

OSSIFICATION OF THE HUMERUS

Primary centre in mid shaft at 8 weeks intra-uterine. Secondary centre in head, greater and lesser tuberosities at 1 year. Note: Bone growth in upper limb is at upper humerus and at lower radius and ulna

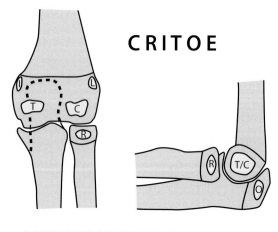

CRITOE

Lower end and elbow is more complex and is remembered best with the following mnemonic in the order in which they appear:

2 years	**C**apitulum
4 years	**R**adial head
6 years	**I**nternal (medial) epicondyle
8 years	**T**rochlea
10 years	**O**lecranon
12 years	**E**xternal (lateral) epicondyle

OSSIFICATION CENTRES AT ELBOW

RIGHT CUBITAL FOSSA

* Radial nerve entering between heads of supinator to become post interosseous nerve and superficial branch passing down under brachioradialis

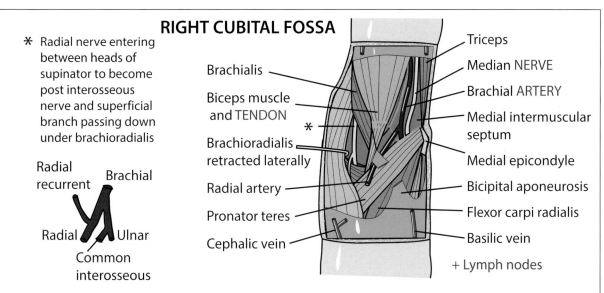

Radial recurrent

Brachial

Radial

Ulnar

Common interosseous

Brachialis

Biceps muscle and TENDON

*

Brachioradialis retracted laterally

Radial artery

Pronator teres

Cephalic vein

Triceps

Median NERVE

Brachial ARTERY

Medial intermuscular septum

Medial epicondyle

Bicipital aponeurosis

Flexor carpi radialis

Basilic vein

+ Lymph nodes

Site: Triangular space in anterior aspect of arm.

Borders: superior - intercondylar line: medial - lateral border of pronator teres: lateral - medial border of brachioradialis: floor - brachialis, supinator: roof - fascia.

Contains: From lateral to medial: biceps **T**endon, brachial **A**rtery and its accompanying veins, median **N**erve (i.e. **T.A.N.** - Tendon - Artery - Nerve), radial and post interosseous and superficial radial nerves under edge of brachioradialis. In fascia of roof are median basilic and cephalic veins, medial and lateral cutaneous nerves of forearm

PRONATION AND SUPINATION

AXIS: RADIAL HEAD - ULNAR STYLOID - LITTLE FINGER

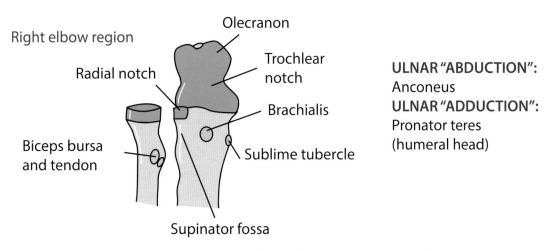

Right elbow region

Radial notch

Biceps bursa and tendon

Olecranon

Trochlear notch

Brachialis

Sublime tubercle

Supinator fossa

ULNAR "ABDUCTION":
Anconeus
ULNAR "ADDUCTION":
Pronator teres
(humeral head)

Note that the true axis of the forearm is through the mid-intercondylar point and the mid-interstyloid point - Thus, through the middle finger. Therefore in FREE pronation and supination the ulna is adducted and abducted whilst the radius rotates around it. This allows the hand to remain still in space

RADIO-ULNAR JOINTS

SUPERIOR
Continuous with elbow joint
Nerve supply: Anterior and posterior interosseous and median nerves
Anular ligament: Around neck, attached to edges of radial notch on ulna, not attached to radius. Blends with capsule above
Quadrate ligament: Neck of radius to supinator fossa of ulna. Criss-cross fibres
Relations: Anterior - Supinator and radial nerve
                  Posterior - Supinator

INFERIOR
- Separated from wrist joint by triangle of fibrocartilage attached at its base to the radius and its apex to the ulnar styloid
- Loose capsule pouches upwards to give a sacciform recess by pronator quadratus

PASSAGE OF NERVES AND ARTERIES IN THE RIGHT ELBOW REGION

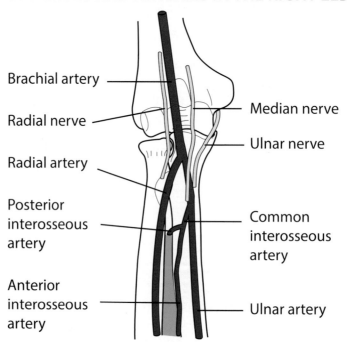

Brachial artery

Radial nerve

Radial artery

Posterior interosseous artery

Anterior interosseous artery

Median nerve

Ulnar nerve

Common interosseous artery

Ulnar artery

Arteries may pass <u>between</u> two bones (posterior interosseous artery passes between ulna and radius) Nerves always pass <u>around</u> bones.

LEFT SUPINATOR AND ITS
RELATION TO THE RADIAL NERVE

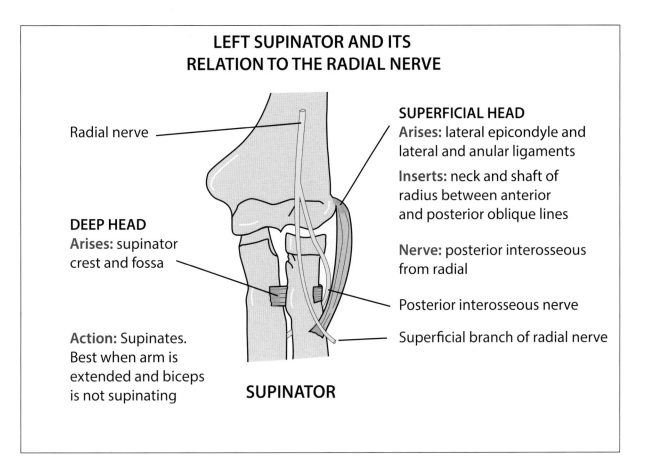

Radial nerve

SUPERFICIAL HEAD
Arises: lateral epicondyle and lateral and anular ligaments

Inserts: neck and shaft of radius between anterior and posterior oblique lines

Nerve: posterior interosseous from radial

DEEP HEAD
Arises: supinator crest and fossa

Posterior interosseous nerve

Superficial branch of radial nerve

Action: Supinates. Best when arm is extended and biceps is not supinating

SUPINATOR

RELATIONSHIPS OF NERVES AND ARTERIES
TO RIGHT PRONATOR TERES

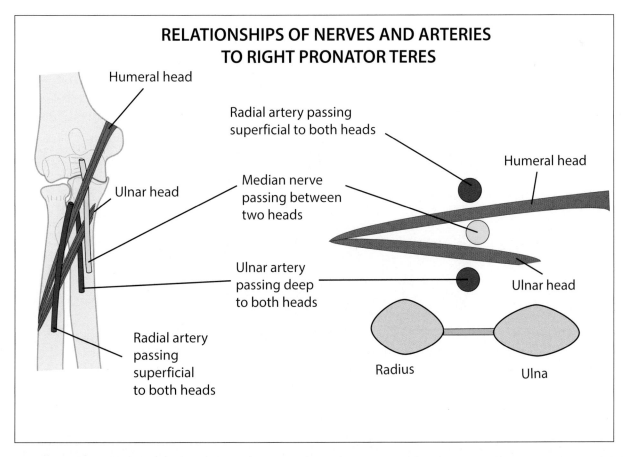

Humeral head

Radial artery passing superficial to both heads

Humeral head

Median nerve passing between two heads

Ulnar head

Ulnar artery passing deep to both heads

Ulnar head

Radial artery passing superficial to both heads

Radius

Ulna

NERVES PASSING BETWEEN TWO HEADS OF MUSCLES IN THE RIGHT ELBOW REGION

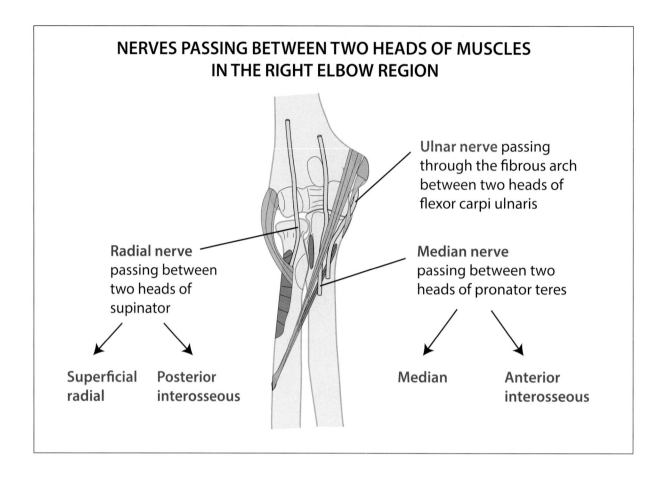

Ulnar nerve passing through the fibrous arch between two heads of flexor carpi ulnaris

Radial nerve passing between two heads of supinator

Median nerve passing between two heads of pronator teres

Superficial radial

Posterior interosseous

Median

Anterior interosseous

SURFACE ANATOMY OF POSTERIOR INTEROSSEOUS NERVE

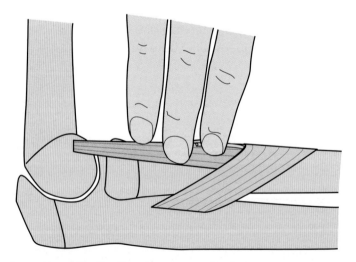

Henry's method for finding the posterior interosseous nerve:
3 fingers inferior to head of radius as the nerve passes into supinator

4 CATEGORIES OF ACTION OF THE ANTERIOR FOREARM MUSCLES

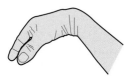

WRIST FLEXION

Flexor carpi ulnaris
Flexor carpi radialis

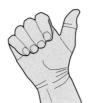

FINGER FLEXION

Flexor digitorum superficialis
Flexor digitorum profundus

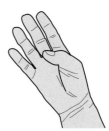

THUMB FLEXION

Flexor pollicis longus

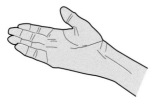

FROM
SUPINATION → TO
PRONATION

Pronator teres
Pronator quadratus

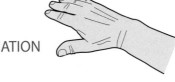

All supplied by MEDIAN nerve except FCU and 1/2 FDP - ULNAR nerve

Instead of learning a list of forearm muscles, it is best to consider the muscles that are needed to perform the movements shown above

RIGHT ANTERIOR FOREARM MUSCLES

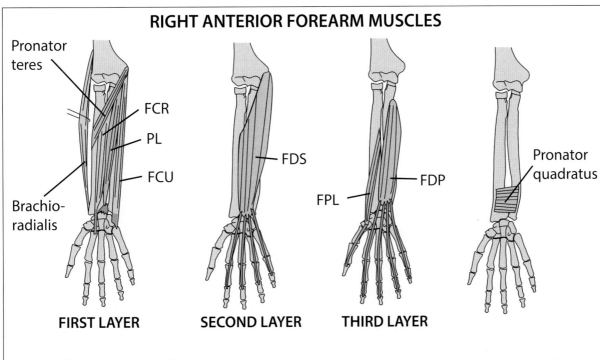

Pronator teres

FCR
PL
FCU

Brachio-radialis

FDS

FDP
FPL

Pronator quadratus

FIRST LAYER   **SECOND LAYER**   **THIRD LAYER**

FCR- Flexor carpi radialis
FCU- Flexor carpi ulnaris
FDP- Flexor digitorum profundus

FDS- Flexor digitorum superficialis
FPL- Flexor pollicis longus
PL- Palmaris longus

POSTERIOR ARM MUSCLES

TRICEPS

Origin: Long head -infraglenoid tubercle
Medial head - Medial spiral groove, posterior humerus, medial and lateral intermuscular septum
Lateral head - Superior/posterior humerus (linear)

Insertion: Long and lateral heads - flat tendon to posterior olecranon
Medial head - deep part of flat tendon and posterior capsule of elbow

Action: Extends elbow, weak extensor of shoulder. Long head stabilises the abducted shoulder

Nerve supply: Radial (C7,8)

ANCONEUS

Origin: Lower lateral epicondyle
Insertion: Posterior/lateral ulna and olecranon
Action: Weak extensor. "Abducts" elbow in pronation
Nerve supply: Radial

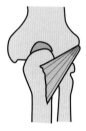

MUSCLES OF POSTERIOR FOREARM

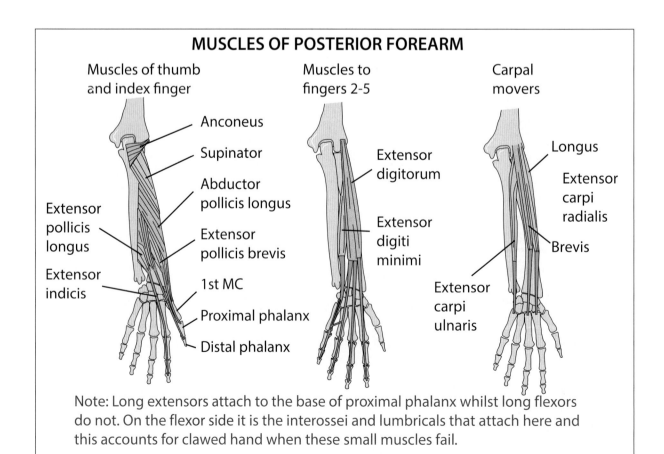

Muscles of thumb and index finger

- Anconeus
- Supinator
- Abductor pollicis longus
- Extensor pollicis brevis
- 1st MC
- Proximal phalanx
- Distal phalanx

Extensor pollicis longus
Extensor indicis

Muscles to fingers 2-5

- Extensor digitorum
- Extensor digiti minimi

Carpal movers

- Longus
- Extensor carpi radialis
- Brevis
- Extensor carpi ulnaris

Note: Long extensors attach to the base of proximal phalanx whilst long flexors do not. On the flexor side it is the interossei and lumbricals that attach here and this accounts for clawed hand when these small muscles fail.

EXTENSOR COMPARTMENT MUSCLES

SUPINATION:
Supinator
(Biceps)

EXTENSION OF FINGERS

EXTENSION AND ABDUCTION OF THUMB

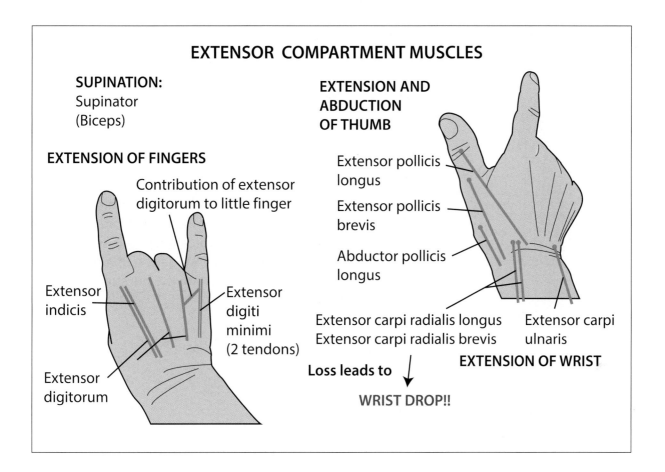

Contribution of extensor digitorum to little finger

Extensor indicis

Extensor digiti minimi (2 tendons)

Extensor digitorum

Extensor pollicis longus

Extensor pollicis brevis

Abductor pollicis longus

Extensor carpi radialis longus
Extensor carpi radialis brevis

Extensor carpi ulnaris

EXTENSION OF WRIST

Loss leads to

WRIST DROP!!

RULES FOR EXTENSOR TENDONS

In addition to tendons of extensor digitorum these two fingers have an extra tendon of their own

Four muscles arise deep in the posterior forearm and have tendons that pass to these two digits in the ratio of 3 to the thumb and 1 to the index finger

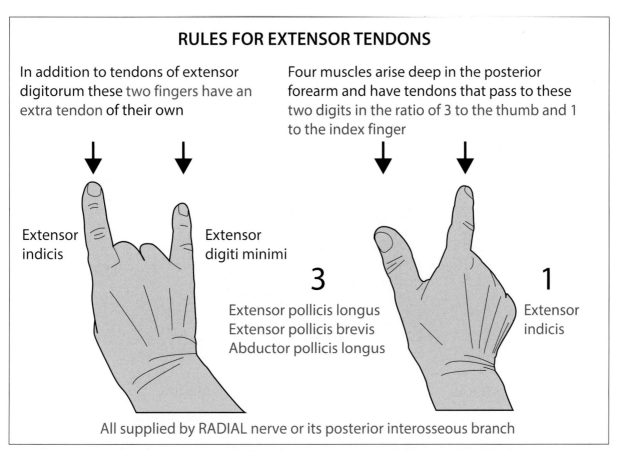

Extensor indicis

Extensor digiti minimi

3

Extensor pollicis longus
Extensor pollicis brevis
Abductor pollicis longus

1

Extensor indicis

All supplied by RADIAL nerve or its posterior interosseous branch

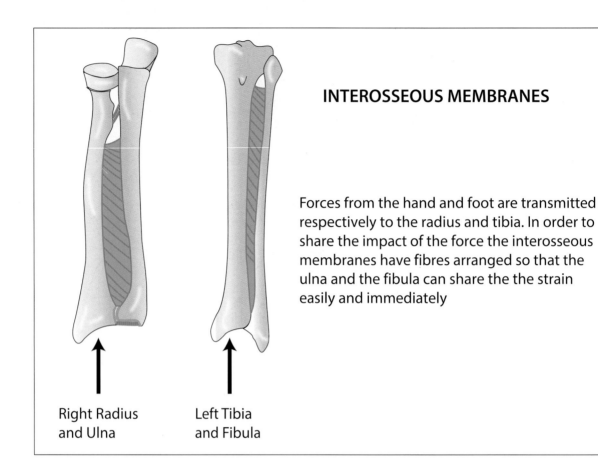

INTEROSSEOUS MEMBRANES

Forces from the hand and foot are transmitted respectively to the radius and tibia. In order to share the impact of the force the interosseous membranes have fibres arranged so that the ulna and the fibula can share the the strain easily and immediately

Right Radius
and Ulna

Left Tibia
and Fibula

CROSS SECTION OF RIGHT MID FOREARM LOOKING UP

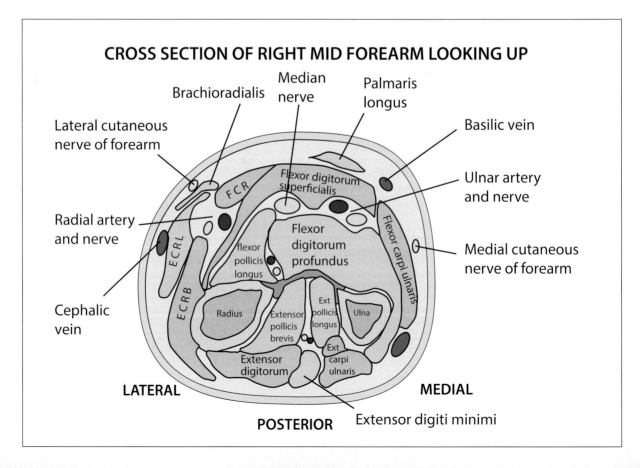

RADIAL ARTERY

Starts: Midline in cubital fossa
On to: Supinator and tendon of pronator teres, flexor pollicis longus, insertion of pronator quadratus and lower radius
Lateral to: Flexor digitorum superficialis
Under: Flexor carpi radialis, brachioradialis and snuff box tendons
On: Trapezium
Between: Heads of 1st dorsal interosseus and heads of adductor pollicis
Medial to: Radial nerve in forearm and superficial branch of radial nerve
Branches: Dorsal and palmar carpal; superficial palmar branch (anastomoses with superficial palmar arch); arteria princeps pollicis to thumb; arteria radialis indicis to index finger; and finishes as deep palmar arch with its palmar metacarpal branches

ULNAR ARTERY

Starts: Midline in cubital fossa
Passes deep to: Both heads of pronator teres and fibrous arch of flexor digitorum superficialis
On: Flexor digitorum profundus
Lateral to: Ulnar nerve
Superficial to: Flexor retinaculum
Ends as: Superficial palmar arch with its palmar digital branches and a branch to the deep arch
Branches: Common interosseous giving anterior and posterior branches

Anterior interosseous
Between: Flexor digitorum profundus and flexor pollicis longus
Supplies: Deep flexor muscles and bones
Passes: Posteriorly in lower forearm through interosseous membrane to supplement posterior interosseous artery
Ends as: Dorsal carpal anastomosis

Posterior interosseous
Passes: Into posterior compartment of forearm above the interosseous membrane
Supplies: Muscles of posterior forearm
Ends by: Anastomosing with anterior interosseous artery

1.5 Wrist and Hand

USE OF HAND

Grip
Percussion
Aggression/defence
Sensory
Expression

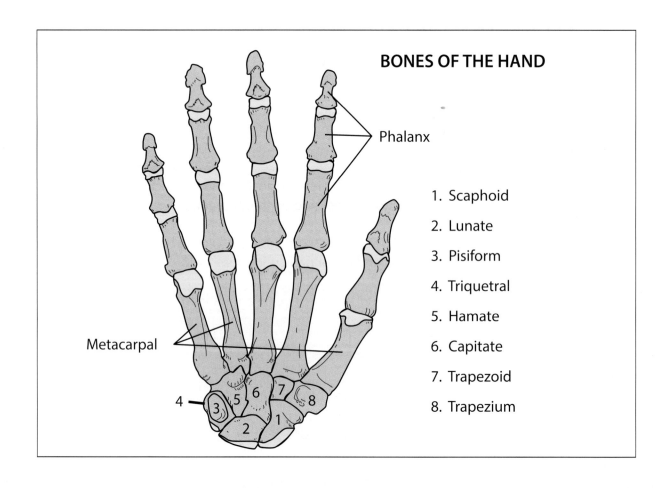

BONES OF THE HAND

Phalanx

Metacarpal

1. Scaphoid

2. Lunate

3. Pisiform

4. Triquetral

5. Hamate

6. Capitate

7. Trapezoid

8. Trapezium

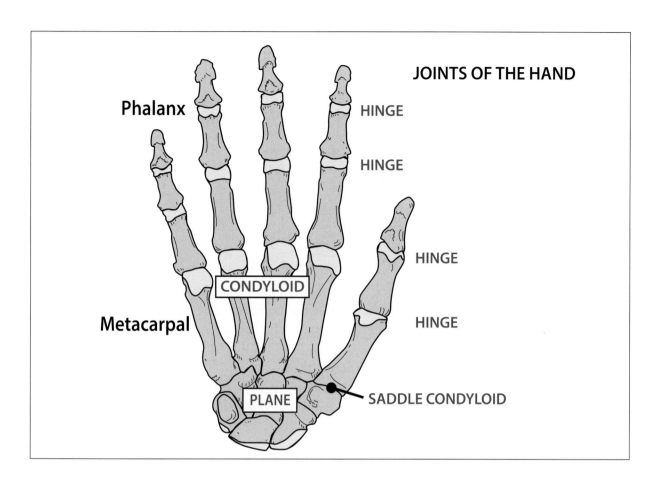

JOINTS OF THE HAND

Phalanx

HINGE

HINGE

HINGE

CONDYLOID

HINGE

Metacarpal

PLANE

SADDLE CONDYLOID

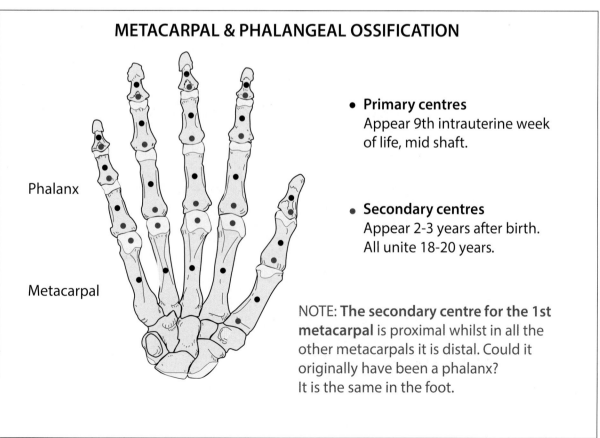

METACARPAL & PHALANGEAL OSSIFICATION

Phalanx

Metacarpal

- **Primary centres**
  Appear 9th intrauterine week
  of life, mid shaft.

- **Secondary centres**
  Appear 2-3 years after birth.
  All unite 18-20 years.

NOTE: **The secondary centre for the 1st metacarpal** is proximal whilst in all the other metacarpals it is distal. Could it originally have been a phalanx?
It is the same in the foot.

CARPAL BONES AND JOINTS

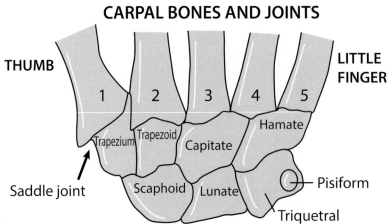

THUMB

LITTLE FINGER

1 2 3 4 5

Trapezium Trapezoid Capitate Hamate

Saddle joint

Scaphoid Lunate

Pisiform

Triquetral

JOINTS

1. Between 1st metacarpal and trapezium there is a saddle condyloid joint that allows flexion, extension, adduction, abduction and rotation. The rotation is not free and depends on the degree of opposition (i.e. it is "controlled").
2. All the other joints in the carpus are plane joints.
3. The carpometacarpal joints become progressively more mobile from thumb to little finger so that grip is more stable towards index finger and thumb.

OSSIFICATION OF BONES OF THE RIGHT HAND

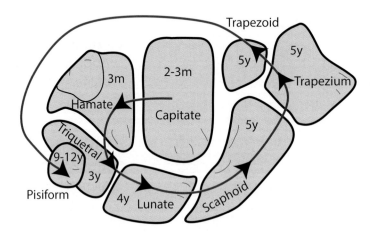

Trapezoid

5y

5y

Trapezium

3m

2-3m

Hamate

Capitate

5y

Triquetral

9-12y

3y

Pisiform

4y Lunate

Scaphoid

The red line with arrows indicates the order in which the **primary centres** appear from birth onwards. Anticlockwise in the right hand looking from the anterior surface

BLOOD SUPPLY OF THE SCAPHOID

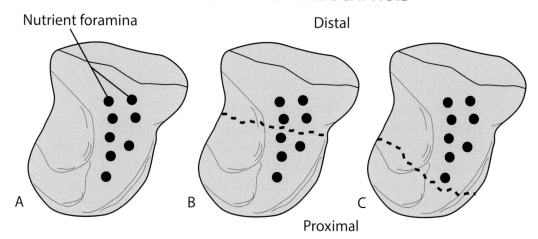

Nutrient foramina

Distal

Proximal

A   B   C

Blood vessels usually enter the bone distally with few or no nutrient foramina in the proximal segment. Avascular necrosis is less likely with a waist fracture (B) but very likely with a proximal fracture (C).

NOTE: The lunate may be dislocated ventrally either in association with a fracture of the scaphoid or separately. It may damage the median nerve by pushing it against the flexor retinaculum.

1st CARPOMETACARPAL JOINT
(Between trapezium and 1st metacarpal)

SADDLE CONDYLOID
Allows:
- Flexion
- Extension
- Adduction
- Abduction
- Circumduction
- "Controlled rotation"

All together = Opposition

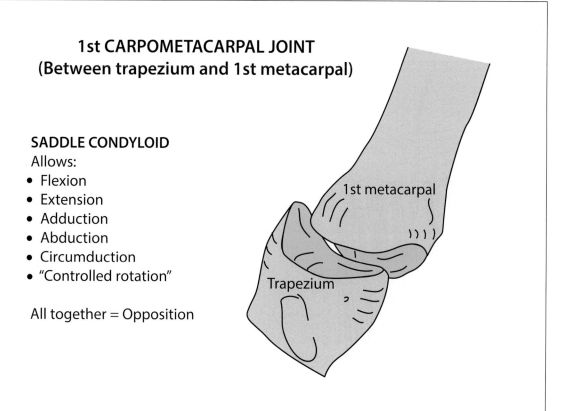

1st metacarpal

Trapezium

WRIST JOINT

Synovial. Strong+
Proximal: Radius and fibrocartilage
Distal: Scaphoid, lunate (triquetral in extreme adduction)
Triangular cartilage: Holds radius and ulna together and separates radiocarpal joint from inferior radio-ulnar joint
Capsular ligaments: Thick collateral at sides
Palmar radiocarpal ligaments: Radius to lunate and capitate
Movements: Flexion 80° (Mostly midcarpal)
Extension 60° (Mostly wrist)
Abduction 15°
Adduction 60°

VENTRAL ASPECT OF LEFT WRIST

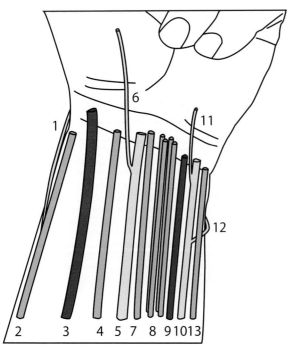

Structures from radial to ulnar side:
1 Superficial branch of the radial nerve (emerging posterior to brachioradialis)
2 Brachioradialis
3 Radial artery
4 Flexor carpi radialis
5 Median nerve with its palmar cutaneous branch (6)
7 Palmaris longus
8 Flexor digitorum superficialis (4 tendons)
9 Ulnar artery
10 Ulnar nerve with its palmar cutaneous branch (11) and dorsal cutaneous branch (12)
13 Flexor carpi ulnaris

RIGHT EXTENSOR RETINACULUM

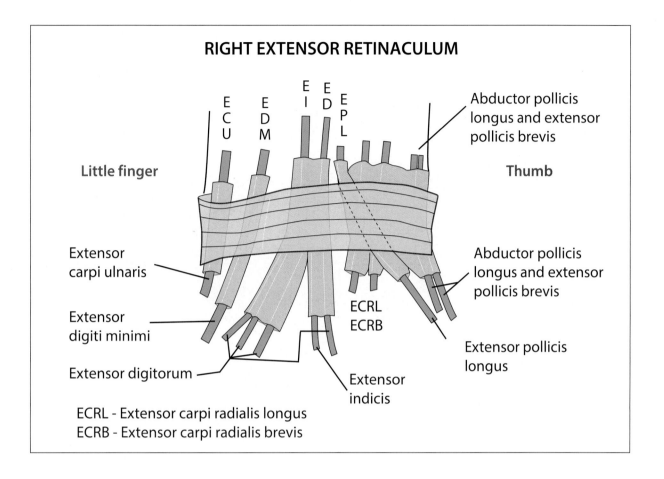

E E
C D E E E
U M I D P
L

Little finger

Thumb

Abductor pollicis longus and extensor pollicis brevis

Extensor carpi ulnaris

Extensor digiti minimi

Extensor digitorum

ECRL
ECRB

Extensor indicis

Abductor pollicis longus and extensor pollicis brevis

Extensor pollicis longus

ECRL - Extensor carpi radialis longus
ECRB - Extensor carpi radialis brevis

FLEXOR RETINACULUM

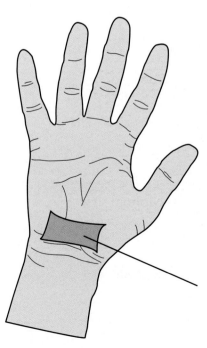

Arises: Tubercle of scaphoid and ridge of trapezium
Inserts: Pisiform and hook of hamate
Inserting into it: Palmaris longus and brevis
Arising from it: Thenar and hypothenar muscles
Superficial to it: Ulnar nerve and artery, palmar cutaneous branches of median and ulnar nerves
Deep to it: Contents of carpal tunnel and flexor carpi radialis in a separate compartment

Position of flexor retinaculum in hand. Proximal edge is level with distal wrist crease.

FLEXOR RETINACULUM

THUMB

LITTLE FINGER

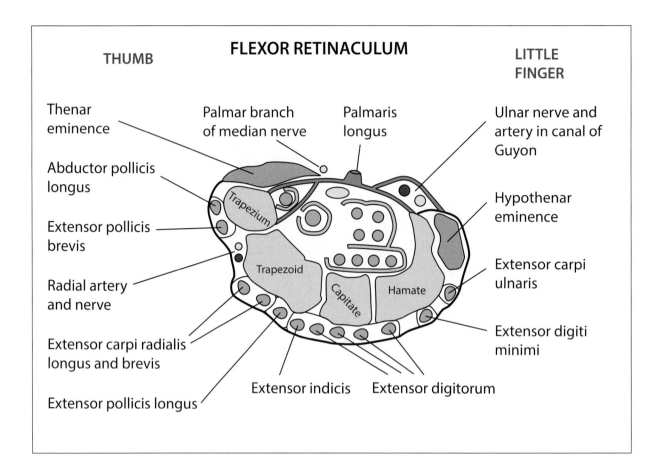

Thenar eminence

Palmar branch of median nerve

Palmaris longus

Ulnar nerve and artery in canal of Guyon

Abductor pollicis longus

Hypothenar eminence

Extensor pollicis brevis

Extensor carpi ulnaris

Radial artery and nerve

Extensor digiti minimi

Extensor carpi radialis longus and brevis

Extensor pollicis longus

Extensor indicis

Extensor digitorum

Trapezium

Trapezoid

Capitate

Hamate

MUSCLE ATTACHMENTS TO FLEXOR RETINACULUM

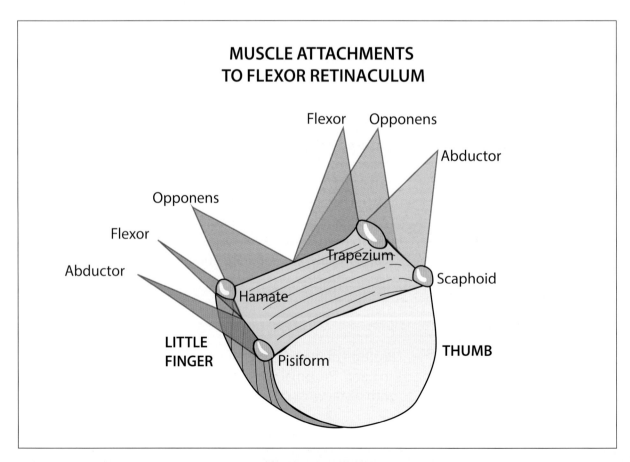

Flexor

Opponens

Abductor

Opponens

Flexor

Abductor

Trapezium

Scaphoid

Hamate

LITTLE FINGER

Pisiform

THUMB

FLEXOR RETINACULUM AND CARPAL TUNNEL

Medial aspect (ulnar)

Into palm of hand

Lateral aspect (radial)

Trapezium

Hamate

Scaphoid

Ulnar artery

Ulnar nerve in canal of Guyon

Pisiform

Flexor carpi radialis in separate compartment

R M I FPL
L I I
L M
L R

Beneath (deep to) the flexor retinaculum

1. Median nerve
2. 4 tendons of flexor digitorum profundus
3. 4 tendons of flexor digitorum superficialis
4. Tendon of flexor pollicis longus
5. Flexor carpi radialis (in its own compartment)

Superficial to the flexor retinaculum

1. Ulnar nerve and ulnar artery (in their own tunnel (Canal of Guyon)
2. Palmar cutaneous branch of median nerve

CARPAL TUNNEL SYNDROME

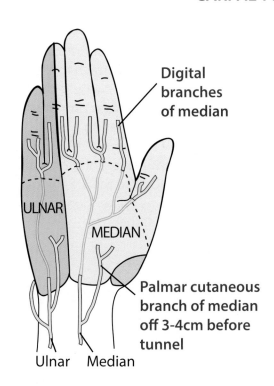

Digital branches of median

ULNAR

MEDIAN

Palmar cutaneous branch of median off 3-4cm before tunnel

Ulnar   Median

1. **Pain and paraesthesia** in lateral fingers and thumb, worse at night and waking patient.

2. **Sensory loss** similar distribution EXCEPT skin over thenar eminence spared (palmar cutaneous branch arising before carpal tunnel).

3. **Weakness** of abductor pollicis brevis.

4. **Associated with** hypothyroidism, pregnancy, arthritis, tenosynovitis, inflammation, old fractures but often idiopathic.

5. **Tinel's Test:** Tapping over flexor retinaculum gives tingling.

RIGHT EXTENSOR RETINACULUM
Attachments

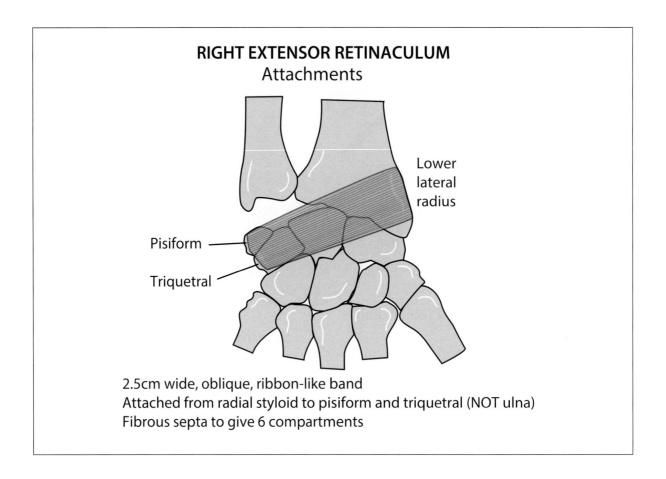

Lower lateral radius

Pisiform

Triquetral

2.5cm wide, oblique, ribbon-like band
Attached from radial styloid to pisiform and triquetral (NOT ulna)
Fibrous septa to give 6 compartments

EXTENSOR RETINACULUM OF WRIST

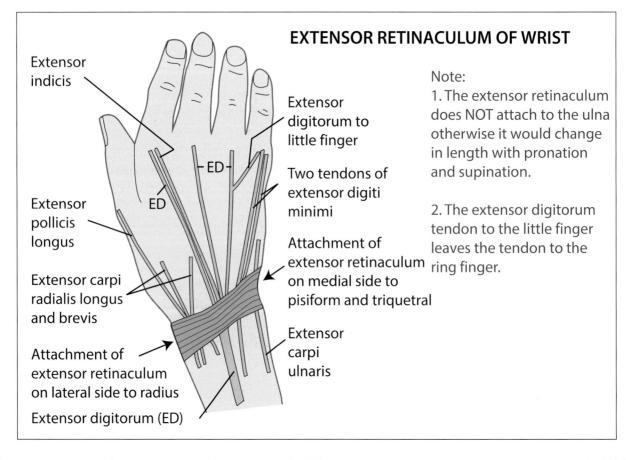

Extensor indicis

Extensor digitorum to little finger

ED

ED

Two tendons of extensor digiti minimi

Extensor pollicis longus

Attachment of extensor retinaculum on medial side to pisiform and triquetral

Extensor carpi radialis longus and brevis

Extensor carpi ulnaris

Attachment of extensor retinaculum on lateral side to radius

Extensor digitorum (ED)

Note:
1. The extensor retinaculum does NOT attach to the ulna otherwise it would change in length with pronation and supination.

2. The extensor digitorum tendon to the little finger leaves the tendon to the ring finger.

EXTENSOR TENDON COMPARTMENTS
JUST BEYOND THE LEFT EXTENSOR RETICULUM

LITTLE FINGER   THUMB

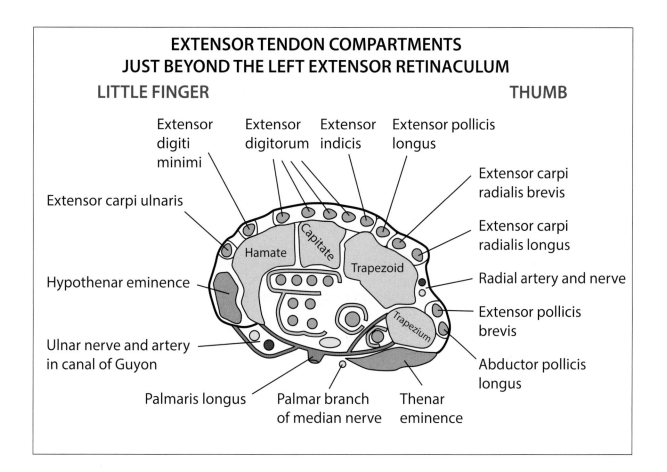

Extensor digiti minimi
Extensor digitorum
Extensor indicis
Extensor pollicis longus
Extensor carpi ulnaris
Extensor carpi radialis brevis
Extensor carpi radialis longus
Hypothenar eminence
Radial artery and nerve
Extensor pollicis brevis
Ulnar nerve and artery in canal of Guyon
Abductor pollicis longus
Palmaris longus
Palmar branch of median nerve
Thenar eminence

Capitate · Hamate · Trapezoid · Trapezium

ANATOMICAL SNUFF BOX

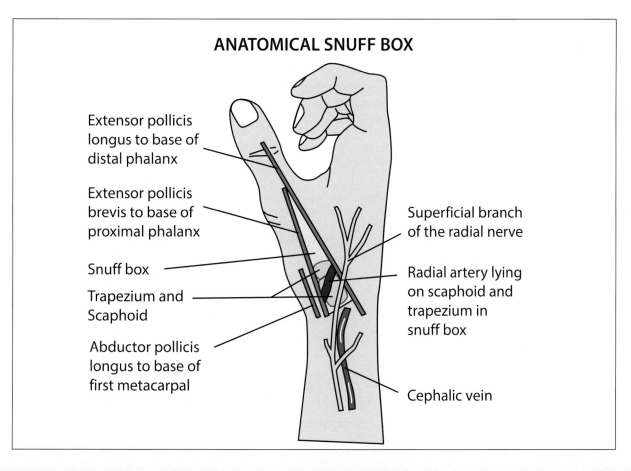

Extensor pollicis longus to base of distal phalanx
Extensor pollicis brevis to base of proximal phalanx
Snuff box
Trapezium and Scaphoid
Abductor pollicis longus to base of first metacarpal
Superficial branch of the radial nerve
Radial artery lying on scaphoid and trapezium in snuff box
Cephalic vein

CUTANEOUS NERVE SUPPLY OF HAND

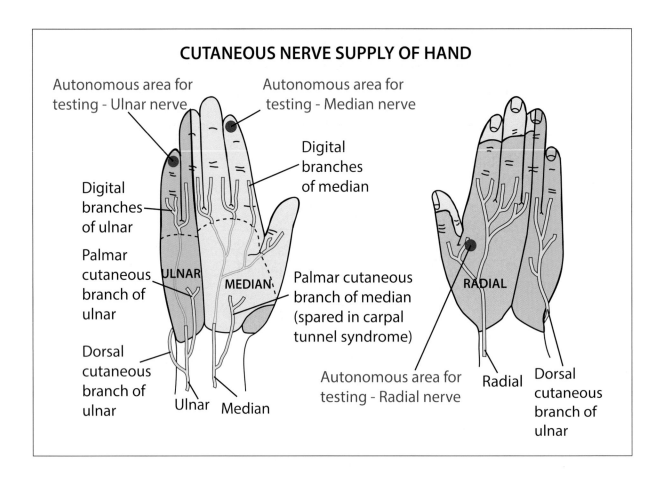

Autonomous area for testing - Ulnar nerve

Autonomous area for testing - Median nerve

Digital branches of median

Digital branches of ulnar

Palmar cutaneous branch of ulnar

ULNAR

MEDIAN

Palmar cutaneous branch of median (spared in carpal tunnel syndrome)

Dorsal cutaneous branch of ulnar

Ulnar   Median

RADIAL

Autonomous area for testing - Radial nerve

Radial

Dorsal cutaneous branch of ulnar

AUTONOMOUS SENSORY AREAS IN RIGHT HAND

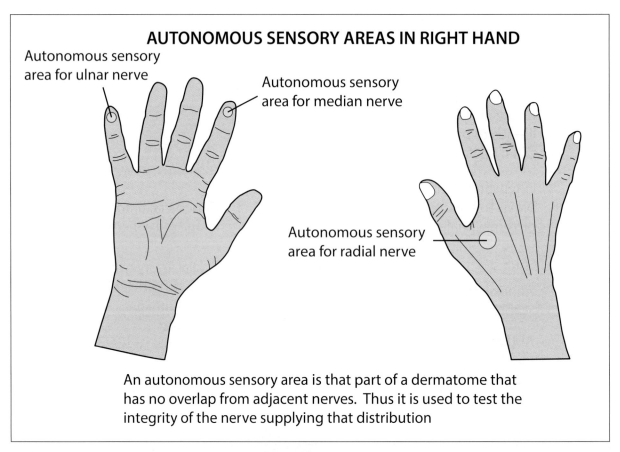

Autonomous sensory area for ulnar nerve

Autonomous sensory area for median nerve

Autonomous sensory area for radial nerve

An autonomous sensory area is that part of a dermatome that has no overlap from adjacent nerves. Thus it is used to test the integrity of the nerve supplying that distribution

PALMAR ARTERIAL ARCHES

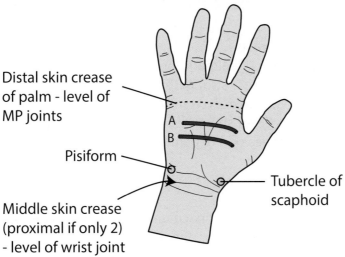

Distal skin crease of palm - level of MP joints

A

B

Pisiform

Tubercle of scaphoid

Middle skin crease (proximal if only 2) - level of wrist joint

A **Superficial palmar arch**
Level with base of outstretched thumb.
From ulnar artery.
1/2 way between distal palmar crease and distal wrist crease

B **Deep palmar arch**
From radial artery.
1cm proximal to superficial arch

PALMAR ARTERIAL ARCHES (left hand)

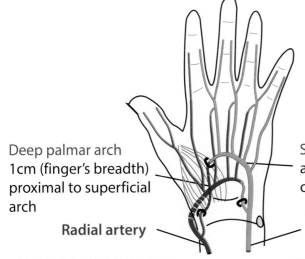

Allen's Test: Provides information as to which arch is dominant

Deep palmar arch 1cm (finger's breadth) proximal to superficial arch

Superficial palmar arch at level of base of outstretched thumb

Radial artery

Ulnar artery

DEEP PALMAR ARCH
From radial artery. Communicates with superficial arch
Branches:
    Princeps pollicis
    Radialis indicis
    3 palmar metacarpal
    3 perforating branches

SUPERFICIAL PALMAR ARCH
From ulnar artery.
Communicates with deep arch
Branches:
    Palmar digital arteries and communicating branches with metacarpal arteries of deep arch

PALMAR APONEUROSIS AND PALMAR BREVIS

Palmar aponeurosis
- Extension of palmaris longus via flexor retinaculum
- Central area is strong, thick and triangular
- **Inserts:** into deep transverse ligament of palm and fibrous flexor sheaths
- **Action:** ties skin of palm and fingers down

Palmaris brevis
- **Origin:** Flexor retinaculum and medial border of proximal palmar aponeurosis
- **Insertion:** Dermis of ulnar side of hand
- **Action:** Wrinkles skin
- **Nerve supply:** Superficial branch of ulnar nerve

DUPUYTREN'S CONTRACTURE

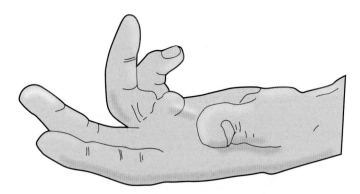

Typical appearances with maximal deformity of ring and little fingers due to fibrosis and shortening of palmar aponeurosis

During surgery for this condition, great care must be taken to avoid damage to the recurrent (muscular) branch of the median nerve which supplies the muscles of the thenar eminence

SYNOVIAL SHEATHS IN PALM OF HAND

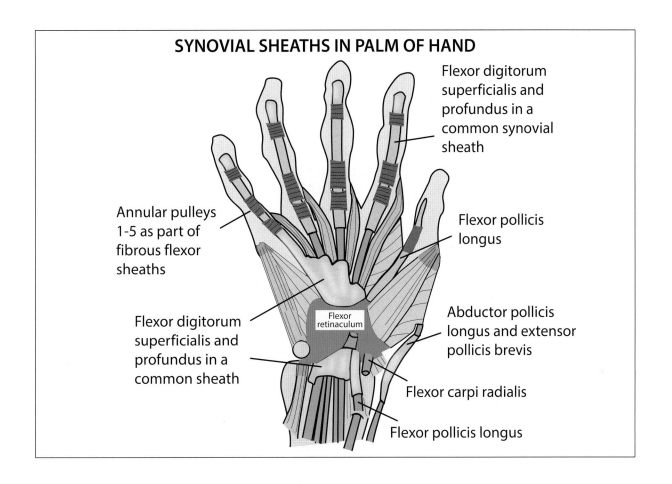

Flexor digitorum superficialis and profundus in a common synovial sheath

Annular pulleys 1-5 as part of fibrous flexor sheaths

Flexor pollicis longus

Flexor digitorum superficialis and profundus in a common sheath

Flexor retinaculum

Abductor pollicis longus and extensor pollicis brevis

Flexor carpi radialis

Flexor pollicis longus

DISSECTION OF PALM TO SHOW NERVES AND THENAR AND HYPOTHENAR MUSCLES

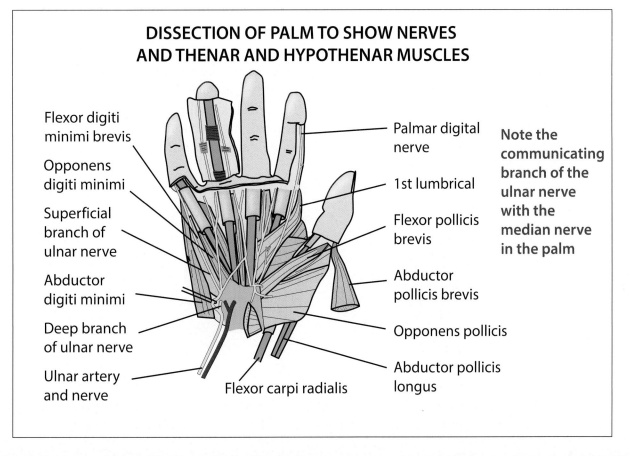

Flexor digiti minimi brevis

Opponens digiti minimi

Superficial branch of ulnar nerve

Abductor digiti minimi

Deep branch of ulnar nerve

Ulnar artery and nerve

Flexor carpi radialis

Palmar digital nerve

1st lumbrical

Flexor pollicis brevis

Abductor pollicis brevis

Opponens pollicis

Abductor pollicis longus

Note the communicating branch of the ulnar nerve with the median nerve in the palm

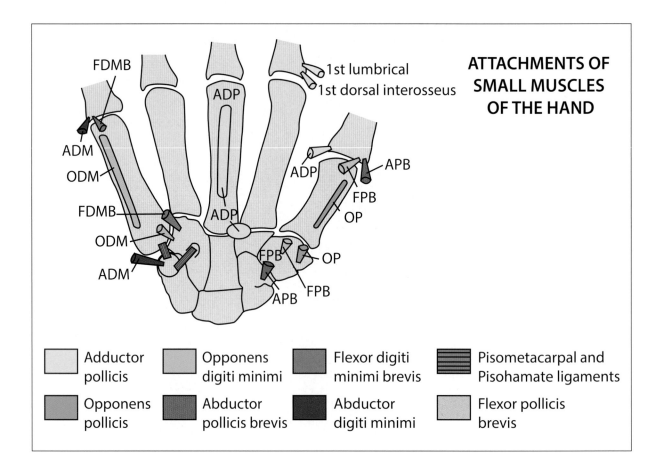

ATTACHMENTS OF SMALL MUSCLES OF THE HAND

Labels: FDMB, ADP, 1st lumbrical, 1st dorsal interosseus, ADM, ODM, ADP, APB, FDMB, FPB, OP, ODM, ADP, ADM, FPB, OP, APB, FPB

Legend:
- Adductor pollicis
- Opponens digiti minimi
- Flexor digiti minimi brevis
- Pisometacarpal and Pisohamate ligaments
- Opponens pollicis
- Abductor pollicis brevis
- Abductor digiti minimi
- Flexor pollicis brevis

INTEROSSEOUS MUSCLES

Origin: Anterior shafts of metacarpals 2,4,5
Insertion: Dorsal expansion and proximal phalanx
Action: Flex metacarpophalangeal and extend both interphalangeal joints. Adduct as per arrows

Origin: Inner shafts all metacarpals
Insertion: Dorsal expansion and proximal phalanx
Action: Flex metacarpophalangeal and extend both interphalangeal joints. Abduct as per arrows

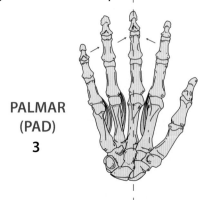

PALMAR (PAD)
3

UNIPENNATE

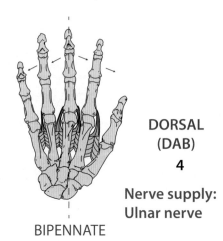

DORSAL (DAB)
4

Nerve supply: Ulnar nerve

BIPENNATE

They act by taking up the slack in the extensor expansion so that the pull of the long extensor is not wasted wholly on the metacarpophalangeal joints

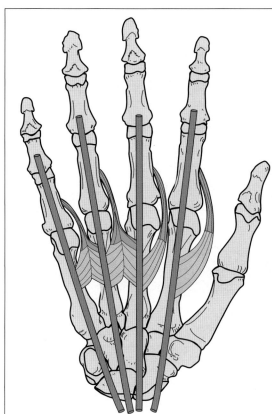

RIGHT LUMBRICALS

Origin: 4 tendons from flexor digitorum profundus, radial 2 are unipennate, ulnar 2 bipennate

Insertion: Extensor expansion over dorsum of proximal phalanx, distal to insertion of interossei, on radial side of fingers 2-5. NO bony attachments

Action: Flexion of metacarpophalangeal joints and extension of both interphalangeal joints of all fingers

Nerve supply: Ulnar nerve to ulnar 2, median nerve to radial 2 (can be 2:2, 3:1 or 1:3)

ACTION OF THE INTEROSSEI AND LUMBRICALS

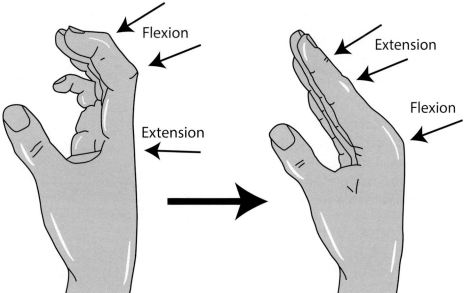

Both the interossei and the lumbicals act to flex the metacarpophalangeal joints and extend the two interphalangeal joints. Thus, if this action is disabled the hand is clawed (left hand image) due to the action of extensor digitorum on the metacarpophalangeal and the action of flexor digitorum profundus on the two interphalangeal joints. In addition, the interossei adduct and abduct the fingers but this is secondary to their main action above

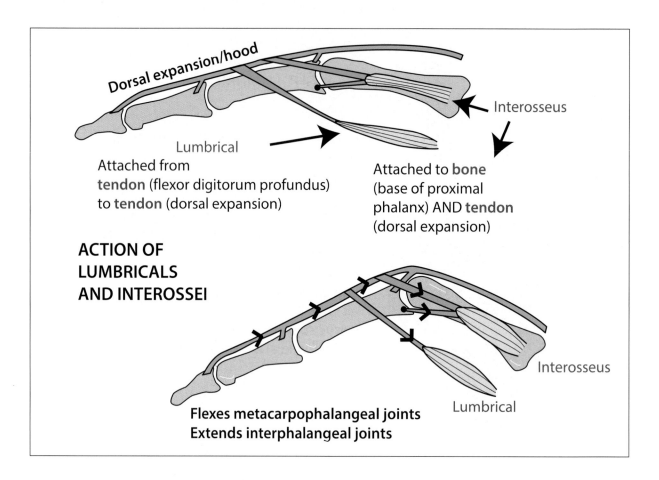

Dorsal expansion/hood

Interosseus

Lumbrical

Attached from tendon (flexor digitorum profundus) **to tendon** (dorsal expansion)

Attached to bone (base of proximal phalanx) AND **tendon** (dorsal expansion)

ACTION OF LUMBRICALS AND INTEROSSEI

Interosseus

Lumbrical

Flexes metacarpophalangeal joints
Extends interphalangeal joints

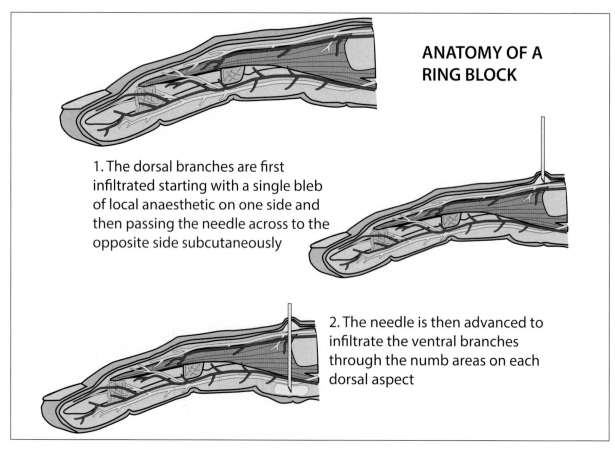

ANATOMY OF A RING BLOCK

1. The dorsal branches are first infiltrated starting with a single bleb of local anaesthetic on one side and then passing the needle across to the opposite side subcutaneously

2. The needle is then advanced to infiltrate the ventral branches through the numb areas on each dorsal aspect

FINGER TO SHOW TENDONS AND DIGITAL NERVES AND ARTERIES

CROSS SECTION
OF FINGER

Dorsal

Digital vessels
and dorsal and palmar
digital nerves

Dorsal (extensor)
expansion

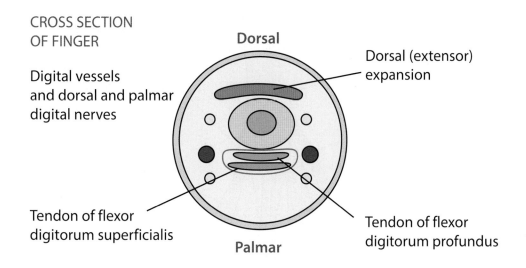

Tendon of flexor
digitorum superficialis

Palmar

Tendon of flexor
digitorum profundus

DETAILS OF LONG FLEXOR TENDONS IN FINGERS 1

Extensor digitorum

Extensor (dorsal) expansion

Metacarpal

Vincula brevia

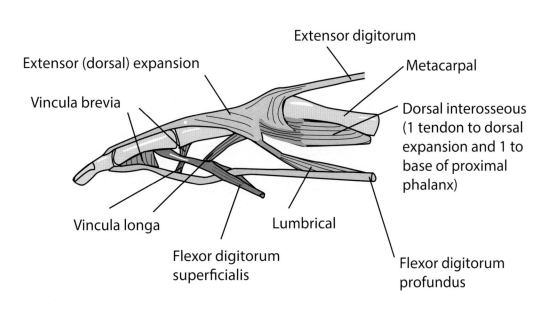

Dorsal interosseous
(1 tendon to dorsal
expansion and 1 to
base of proximal
phalanx)

Vincula longa

Lumbrical

Flexor digitorum
superficialis

Flexor digitorum
profundus

DETAILS OF LONG FLEXOR TENDONS IN FINGERS 2

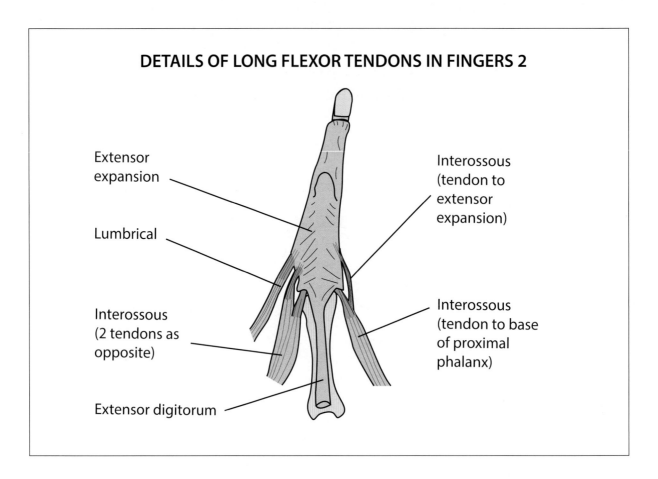

Extensor expansion

Lumbrical

Interossous (2 tendons as opposite)

Extensor digitorum

Interossous (tendon to extensor expansion)

Interossous (tendon to base of proximal phalanx)

NERVE DAMAGE IN WRIST AND HAND

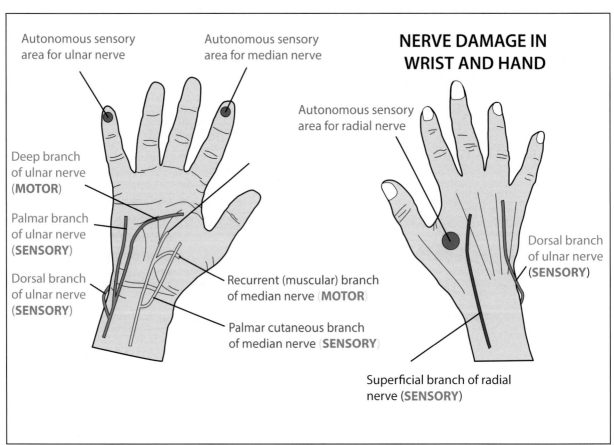

Autonomous sensory area for ulnar nerve

Autonomous sensory area for median nerve

Deep branch of ulnar nerve (**MOTOR**)

Palmar branch of ulnar nerve (**SENSORY**)

Dorsal branch of ulnar nerve (**SENSORY**)

Recurrent (muscular) branch of median nerve (**MOTOR**)

Palmar cutaneous branch of median nerve (**SENSORY**)

Autonomous sensory area for radial nerve

Dorsal branch of ulnar nerve (**SENSORY**)

Superficial branch of radial nerve (**SENSORY**)

SECTION 2

Lower Limb

2.1 Nerves, Vessels and Lymphatics

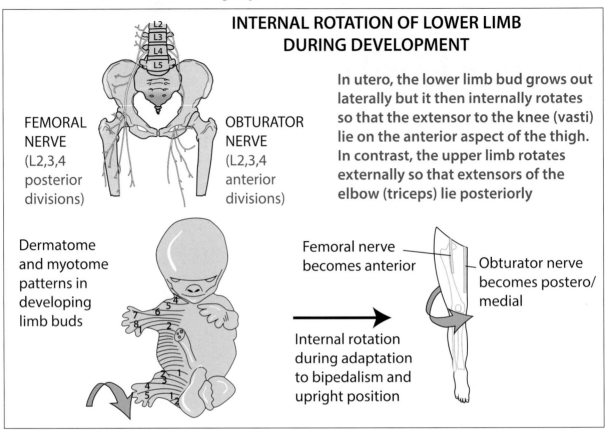

INTERNAL ROTATION OF LOWER LIMB DURING DEVELOPMENT

FEMORAL NERVE (L2,3,4 posterior divisions)

OBTURATOR NERVE (L2,3,4 anterior divisions)

In utero, the lower limb bud grows out laterally but it then internally rotates so that the extensor to the knee (vasti) lie on the anterior aspect of the thigh. In contrast, the upper limb rotates externally so that extensors of the elbow (triceps) lie posteriorly

Dermatome and myotome patterns in developing limb buds

Femoral nerve becomes anterior

Obturator nerve becomes postero/medial

Internal rotation during adaptation to bipedalism and upright position

SIMPLIFIED DERMATOMES OF LOWER LIMB

These are approximate dermatomes that are perfectly adequate for most clinical practice and for testing, for instance, in lumbar disc lesions. (See "dermatome dance" for an easy way of remembering and demonstrating them)

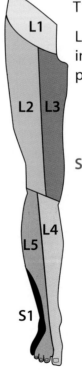

T12   Suprapubic area

L1   Hand's breadth below inguinal ligament, side of penis and scrotum

Stand on S1 - Sit on S3

Across foot on both dorsal and plantar surfaces from medial to lateral is **L4 - L5 - S1**

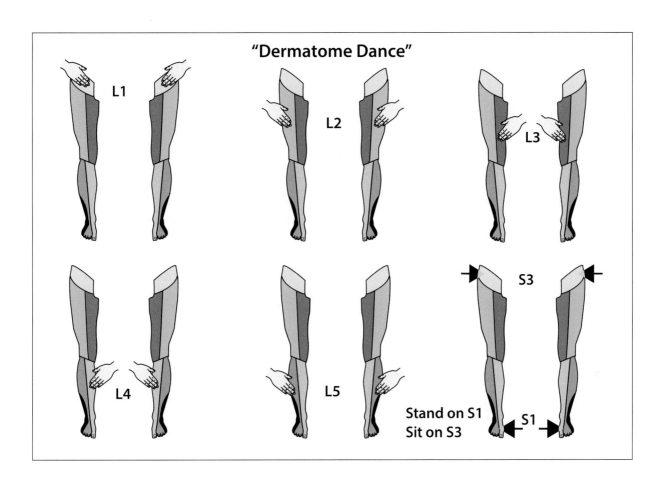

"Dermatome Dance"

L1

L2

L3

L4

L5

S3

S1

Stand on S1
Sit on S3

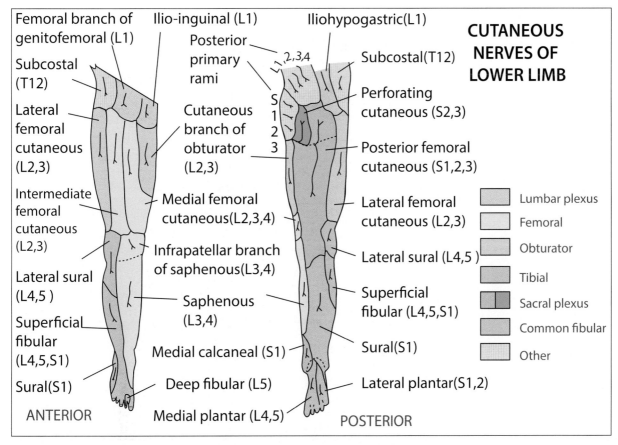

CUTANEOUS NERVES OF LOWER LIMB

Femoral branch of genitofemoral (L1)

Ilio-inguinal (L1)

Iliohypogastric(L1)

Posterior primary rami

Subcostal (T12)

Subcostal(T12)

Lateral femoral cutaneous (L2,3)

Cutaneous branch of obturator (L2,3)

Perforating cutaneous (S2,3)

Intermediate femoral cutaneous (L2,3)

Medial femoral cutaneous(L2,3,4)

Posterior femoral cutaneous (S1,2,3)

Infrapatellar branch of saphenous(L3,4)

Lateral femoral cutaneous (L2,3)

Lateral sural (L4,5)

Lateral sural (L4,5)

Saphenous (L3,4)

Superficial fibular (L4,5,S1)

Superficial fibular (L4,5,S1)

Medial calcaneal (S1)

Sural(S1)

Sural(S1)

Deep fibular (L5)

Lateral plantar(S1,2)

Medial plantar (L4,5)

ANTERIOR

POSTERIOR

	Lumbar plexus
	Femoral
	Obturator
	Tibial
	Sacral plexus
	Common fibular
	Other

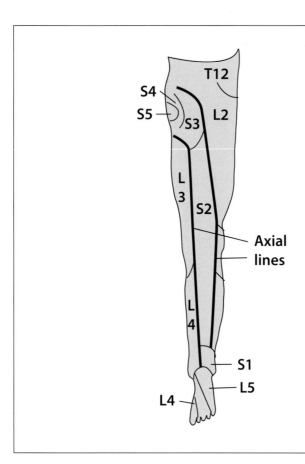

LOWER LIMB POSTERIOR DERMATOMES

Notes:
The final position of the dermatomes in the leg are affected by the internal rotation of the limb as we become upright.

The axial lines denote the separation of non-contiguous dermatomes where there is no overlap of sensation.

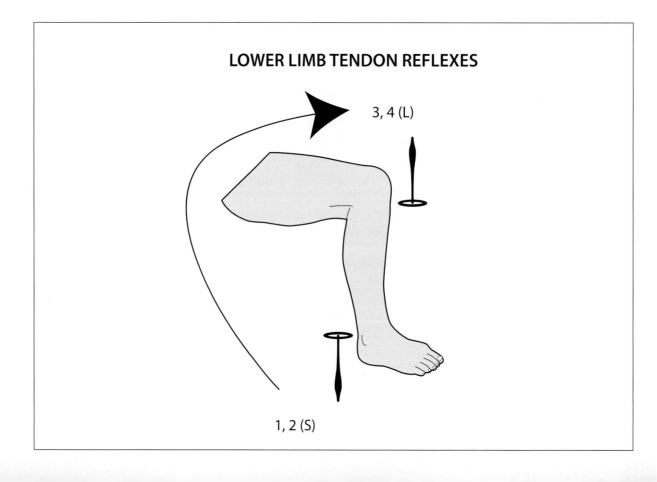

LOWER LIMB TENDON REFLEXES

3, 4 (L)

1, 2 (S)

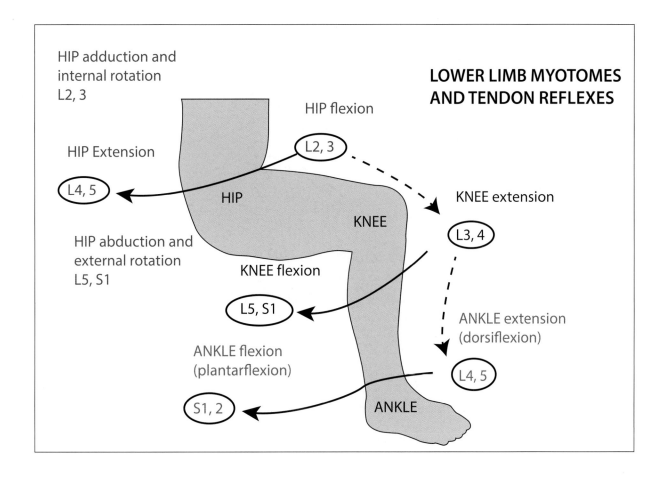

HIP adduction and internal rotation
L2, 3

LOWER LIMB MYOTOMES AND TENDON REFLEXES

HIP flexion

HIP Extension

L2, 3

L4, 5

HIP

KNEE extension

KNEE

L3, 4

HIP abduction and external rotation
L5, S1

KNEE flexion

L5, S1

ANKLE extension
(dorsiflexion)

ANKLE flexion
(plantarflexion)

L4, 5

S1, 2

ANKLE

SEGMENTAL NERVE SUPPLY FOR MOVEMENTS AND REFLEXES IN LOWER LIMB

HIP:	Flexion	L2,3
	Extension	L4,5
	Adduction/internal rotation	L1,2,3
	Abduction/external rotation	L5,S1
KNEE:	Flexion	L5,S1
	Extension	L3,4
ANKLE:	Dorsiflexion (extension)	L4,5
	Plantarflexion (flexion)	S1,2

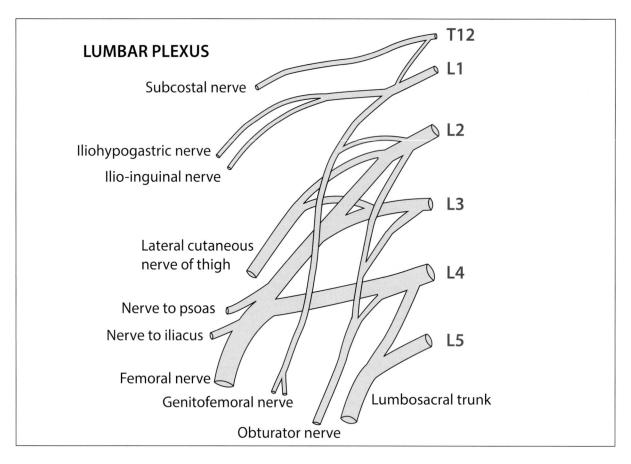

LUMBAR PLEXUS

T12
L1
Subcostal nerve
Iliohypogastric nerve
Ilio-inguinal nerve
L2
L3
Lateral cutaneous nerve of thigh
L4
Nerve to psoas
Nerve to iliacus
L5
Femoral nerve
Genitofemoral nerve
Lumbosacral trunk
Obturator nerve

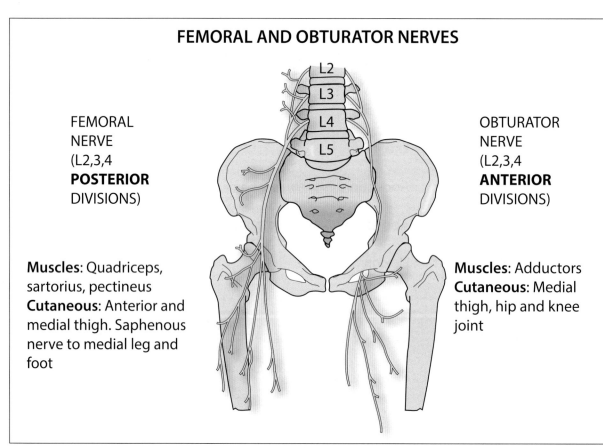

FEMORAL AND OBTURATOR NERVES

L2
L3
L4
L5

FEMORAL NERVE (L2,3,4 **POSTERIOR** DIVISIONS)

Muscles: Quadriceps, sartorius, pectineus
Cutaneous: Anterior and medial thigh. Saphenous nerve to medial leg and foot

OBTURATOR NERVE (L2,3,4 **ANTERIOR** DIVISIONS)

Muscles: Adductors
Cutaneous: Medial thigh, hip and knee joint

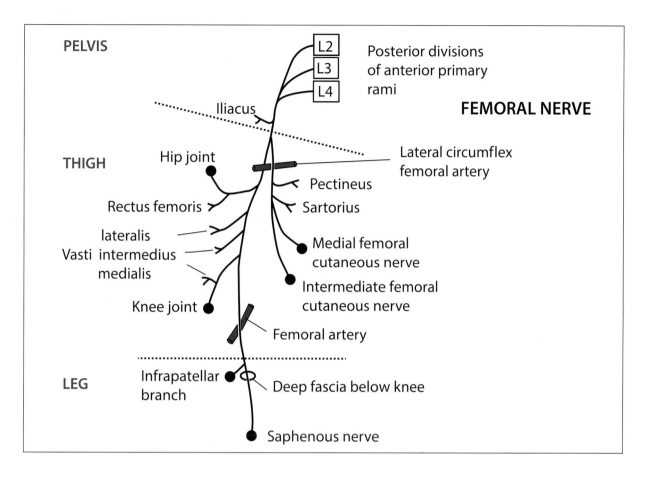

PELVIS

L2
L3
L4

Posterior divisions
of anterior primary
rami

FEMORAL NERVE

Iliacus

THIGH

Hip joint

Lateral circumflex
femoral artery

Pectineus

Rectus femoris

Sartorius

lateralis

Vasti intermedius

medialis

Medial femoral
cutaneous nerve

Intermediate femoral
cutaneous nerve

Knee joint

Femoral artery

LEG

Infrapatellar
branch

Deep fascia below knee

Saphenous nerve

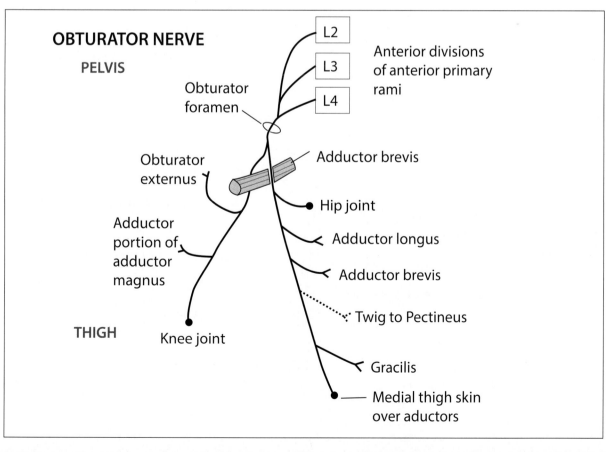

OBTURATOR NERVE

PELVIS

L2
L3
L4

Anterior divisions
of anterior primary
rami

Obturator
foramen

Obturator
externus

Adductor brevis

Hip joint

Adductor
portion of
adductor
magnus

Adductor longus

Adductor brevis

Twig to Pectineus

THIGH

Knee joint

Gracilis

Medial thigh skin
over aductors

SCIATIC NERVE

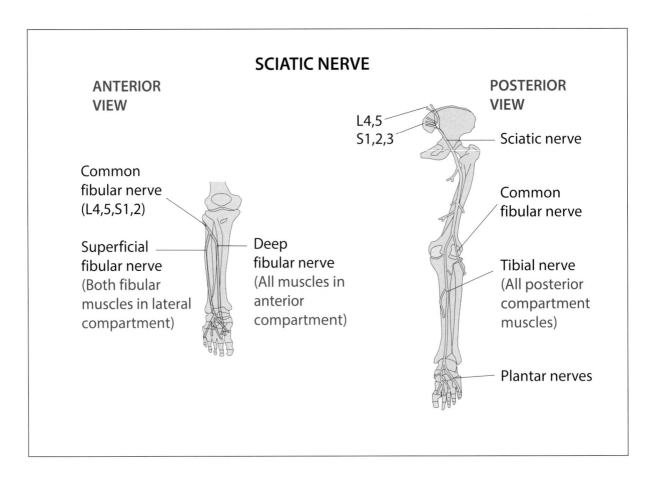

ANTERIOR VIEW

Common fibular nerve (L4,5,S1,2)

Superficial fibular nerve (Both fibular muscles in lateral compartment)

Deep fibular nerve (All muscles in anterior compartment)

POSTERIOR VIEW

L4,5 S1,2,3

Sciatic nerve

Common fibular nerve

Tibial nerve (All posterior compartment muscles)

Plantar nerves

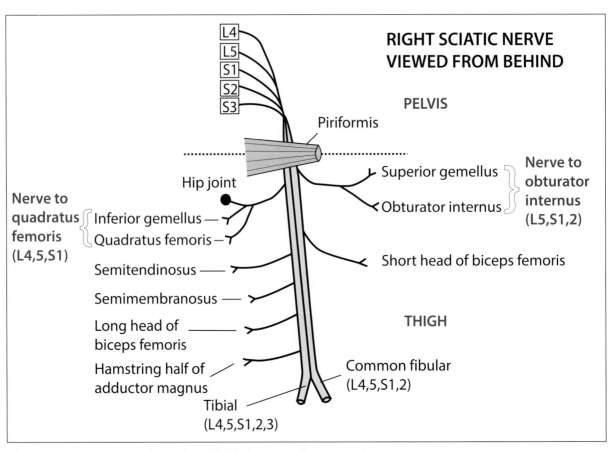

RIGHT SCIATIC NERVE VIEWED FROM BEHIND

L4
L5
S1
S2
S3

PELVIS

Piriformis

Hip joint

Superior gemellus

Obturator internus

Nerve to obturator internus (L5,S1,2)

Nerve to quadratus femoris (L4,5,S1)

Inferior gemellus

Quadratus femoris

Short head of biceps femoris

Semitendinosus

Semimembranosus

Long head of biceps femoris

THIGH

Hamstring half of adductor magnus

Common fibular (L4,5,S1,2)

Tibial (L4,5,S1,2,3)

TIBIAL NERVE
(L4,5,S1,2,3)

Leaves the sciatic nerve in lower thigh to lie centrally in popliteal fossa, between, and deep to, semitendinosus and biceps femoris. It passes into the lower leg under the fibrous arch of soleus, lies on tibialis posterior heading medially to pass posterior to the medial malleolus, beneath the flexor retinaculum.

BRANCHES IN THIGH TO:
Motor - gastrocnemius, popliteus, plantaris
Sensory - knee and superior tibiofibular joints, sural to posterolateral calf skin and lateral foot (sural communicating nerve from common fibular joins it)

BRANCHES IN LEG TO:
Motor - soleus, tibialis posterior, flexor digitorum longus, flexor hallucis longus
Sensory - ankle joint, medial calcaneal nerve to heel and medial sole skin

BRANCHES IN FOOT TO:
Motor and sensory - medial and lateral plantar nerves
(see other image for details)

COMMON FIBULAR NERVE - L4,5,S1,2

Leaves the sciatic nerve in lower thigh to lie laterally in popliteal fossa, deep to biceps femoris, then on plantaris and lateral head of gastrocnemius before winding around the neck of the fibula. It enters fibularis longus where it divides into its superficial and deep branches.

BRANCHES LEAVING IN THIGH TO:
Sensory - Sural communicating which joins sural (see tibial nerve), knee and superior tibiofibular joints, lateral sural to upper lateral calf skin.
Motor - Note that short head of biceps femoris is supplied by the common fibular portion of the sciatic nerve

BRANCHES LEAVING IN LEG AND FOOT TO:
Superficial fibular:
Motor - Fibularis longus and brevis
Sensory - Dorsal skin of foot excluding nail beds and first dorsal webspace
Deep fibular:
Motor - Tibialis anterior, extensor digitorum longus, extensor hallucis longus, fibularis tertius, extensor digitorum brevis
Sensory - Skin of first dorsal webspace

COMMON FIBULAR NERVE

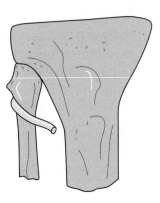

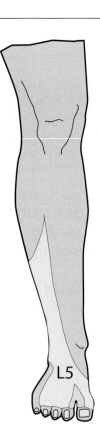

The common fibular nerve winds around the neck of the fibula before dividing into its deep ▨ and superficial ▨ branches. Pressure here from too tight a plaster or trauma can lead to **foot drop and sensory changes** in the skin of the lateral lower leg and foot as seen in a L4/5 disc lesion involving the L5 root.

L5

MEDIAL AND LATERAL PLANTAR NERVES

As the tibial nerve passes deep to the flexor retinaculum it gives off the medial and lateral plantar nerves

MEDIAL PLANTAR NERVE (L4,5,S1,2,3)
Motor - flexor digitorum brevis, flexor hallucis brevis, abductor hallucis, 1st lumbrical (all muscles supplied by S1,2 except 1st lumbrical which is S2,3)
Sensory - skin of most of sole and medial 3 and a half toes and nail beds (L4,5)

LATERAL PLANTAR NERVE (S1,2,3)
Motor - abductor digiti minimi, flexor digiti minimi brevis, flexor digitorum accessorius, all 7 interossei, 2nd, 3rd, 4th lumbricals, adductor hallucis (all muscles supplied by S2,3)
Sensory - skin of lateral sole and lateral one and a half toes and nail beds (S1)

NOTE: It is worth comparing the medial plantar nerve with the median in the hand and the lateral plantar nerve with the ulnar nerve in the hand. The similarities are obvious and the only significant differences are that the line of action of the interossei is along the second toe, a single lumbrical is supplied by the medial plantar nerve and that there is an extra muscle in the foot - flexor digitorum accessorius

SEGMENTAL NERVE SUPPLY TO MUSCLES 1

L1,2	Psoas minor	Segmental
L1,2,3	Psoas major	Segmental
L2,3	Adductor brevis	Obturator
L2,3	Gracilis	Obturator
L2,3	Sartorius	Femoral
L2,3	Iliacus	Femoral
L2,3	Pectineus	Femoral (+/- obturator)
L2,3,4	Rectus femoris	Femoral
L2,3,4	Adductor magnus	Obturator & sciatic (tibial portion)
L2,3,4	All 3 Vasti	Femoral
L2,3,4	Adductor longus	Obturator
L3,4	Obturator externus	Obturator
L4,5	Tibialis anterior	Deep fibular
L4,5	Tibialis posterior	Tibial

SEGMENTAL NERVE SUPPLY TO MUSCLES 2

L4,5,S1	Gluteus medius	Superior gluteal
L4,5,S1	Gluteus minimis	Superior gluteal
L4,5,S1	Inferior gemellus	N to quadratus femoris
L4,5,S1	Popliteus	Tibial
L4,5,S1	Quadratus femoris	N to quadratus femoris
L4,5,S1	Tensor fasciae latae	Superior gluteal
L5,S1	Extensor digitorum longus	Deep fibular
L5,S1	Extensor hallucis longus	Deep fibular
L5,S1	Fibularis tertius	Deep fibular
L5,S1	Extensor hallucis brevis	Deep fibular
L5,S1,2	Fibularis brevis	Superficial fibular
L5,S1,2	Fibularis longus	Superficial fibular
L5,S1,2	Semimembranosus	Sciatic (tibial portion)
L5,S1,2	Semitendinosus	Sciatic (tibial portion)
L5,S1,2	Gluteus maximus	Inferior gluteal
L5,S1,2	Obturator internus	N to obturator internus
L5,S1,2	Superior gemellus	N to obturator internus
L5,S1,2	Biceps femoris (both heads)	Sciatic (tibial & common fibular)

SEGMENTAL NERVE SUPPLY TO MUSCLES 3

S1,2	Extensor digitorum brevis	Deep fibular
S1,2	Soleus	Tibial
S1,2	Plantaris	Tibial
S1,2	Gastrocnemius	Tibial
S1,2	Piriformis	N to piriformis
S2,3	Abductor hallucis	Medial plantar
S2,3	Flexor digitorum brevis	Medial plantar
S2,3	Flexor hallucis brevis	Medial plantar
S2,3	Lumbricals	Medial & lateral plantar
S2,3	Abductor digiti minimi	Lateral plantar
S2,3	Adductor hallucis	Lateral plantar
S2,3	Flexor digiti minimi brevis	Lateral plantar
S2,3	Flexor digitorum longus	Tibial
S2,3	Flexor hallucis longus	Tibial
S2,3	Interossei	Lateral plantar
S2,3	Quadratus plantae (Flex. dig. accessorius)	Lateral plantar

NERVE LESIONS IN THE LOWER LIMB 1

NERVES TO PSOAS AND ILIACUS
No pelvic swing on walking
↓ in hip flexion

FEMORAL
↓ in hip flexion and loss of knee extension
Loss of sensation anterior thigh and medial leg

OBTURATOR
Loss of adduction of thigh
Loss of sensation inner thigh

SUPERIOR GLUTEAL
Loss of abduction at hip
Pelvic dip on walking

INFERIOR GLUTEAL
↓ in extension at hip
Buttock wasting

NERVE LESIONS IN THE LOWER LIMB 2

SCIATIC

Loss of all motor except adduction and flexion of thigh and extension of knee. Loss of sensation lower leg and foot

TIBIAL (HIGH)

Loss of flexion of toes and inversion of foot. Loss of sensation of sole of foot, inferior aspect of toes and nail beds

COMMON FIBULAR (HIGH)

Loss of extension of toes and foot (footdrop). Loss of sensation of lateral lower leg and upper foot

ROOT COMPRESSION

Prolapsed discs compresses nerve that emerges at the next intervertebral foramen and not usually the one at the same level as the disc. For example, disc lesion of the L4/5 space compresses L5 nerve

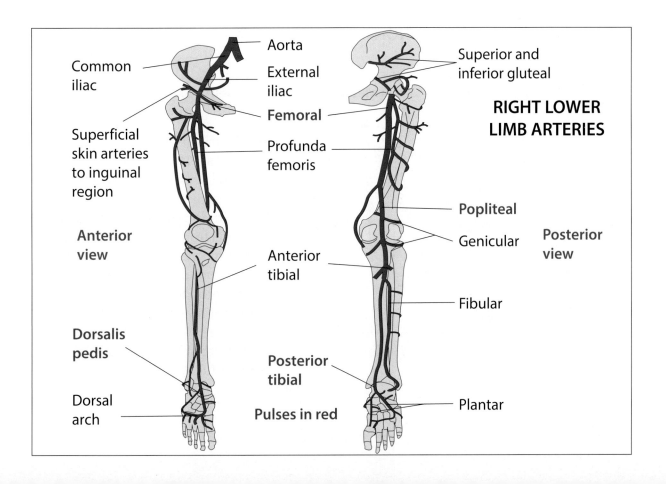

Common iliac

Aorta

External iliac

Femoral

Superior and inferior gluteal

RIGHT LOWER LIMB ARTERIES

Superficial skin arteries to inguinal region

Profunda femoris

Anterior view

Popliteal

Genicular

Posterior view

Anterior tibial

Fibular

Dorsalis pedis

Posterior tibial

Dorsal arch

Plantar

Pulses in red

RIGHT FEMORAL ARTERY

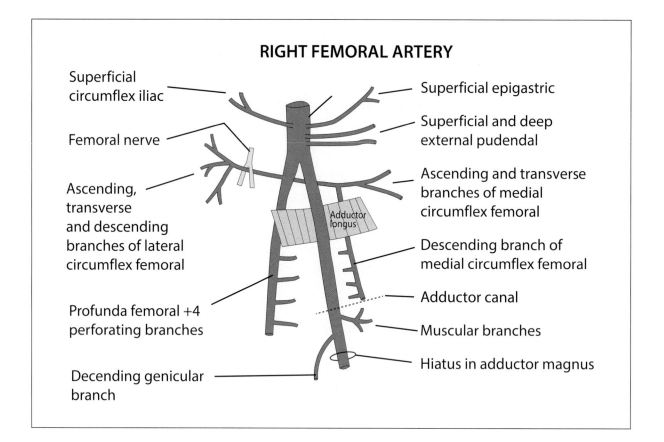

Superficial circumflex iliac

Femoral nerve

Ascending, transverse and descending branches of lateral circumflex femoral

Profunda femoral +4 perforating branches

Decending genicular branch

Superficial epigastric

Superficial and deep external pudendal

Ascending and transverse branches of medial circumflex femoral

Descending branch of medial circumflex femoral

Adductor canal

Muscular branches

Hiatus in adductor magnus

Adductor longus

PROFUNDA FEMORIS ARTERY

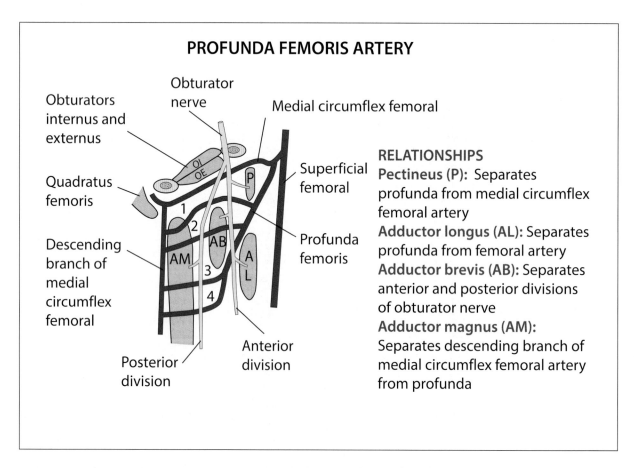

Obturators internus and externus

Quadratus femoris

Descending branch of medial circumflex femoral

Posterior division

Obturator nerve

Medial circumflex femoral

Superficial femoral

Profunda femoris

Anterior division

OI
OE
P
1
2
AB
AM
A
L
3
4

RELATIONSHIPS
Pectineus (P): Separates profunda from medial circumflex femoral artery
Adductor longus (AL): Separates profunda from femoral artery
Adductor brevis (AB): Separates anterior and posterior divisions of obturator nerve
Adductor magnus (AM): Separates descending branch of medial circumflex femoral artery from profunda

RIGHT ANTERIOR TIBIAL ARTERY VIEWED FROM IN FRONT

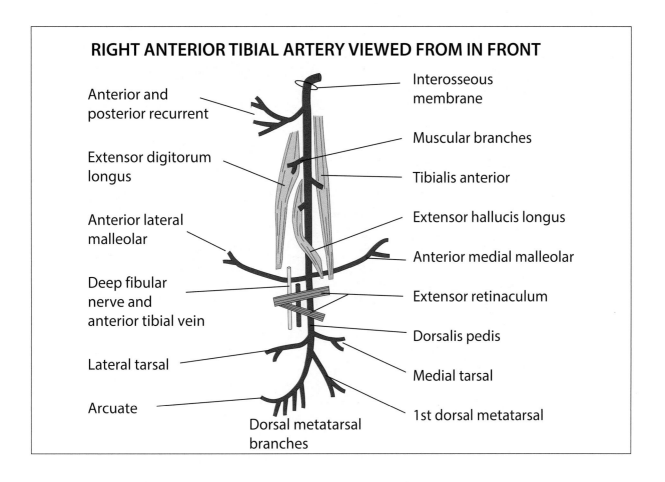

Anterior and posterior recurrent

Extensor digitorum longus

Anterior lateral malleolar

Deep fibular nerve and anterior tibial vein

Lateral tarsal

Arcuate

Dorsal metatarsal branches

Interosseous membrane

Muscular branches

Tibialis anterior

Extensor hallucis longus

Anterior medial malleolar

Extensor retinaculum

Dorsalis pedis

Medial tarsal

1st dorsal metatarsal

RIGHT POSTERIOR TIBIAL ARTERY VIEWED FROM BEHIND

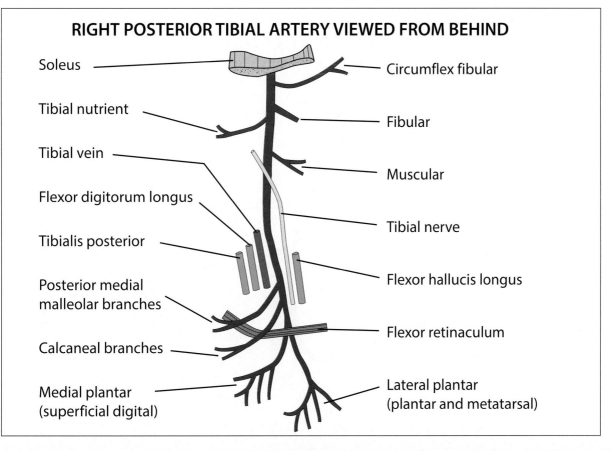

Soleus

Tibial nutrient

Tibial vein

Flexor digitorum longus

Tibialis posterior

Posterior medial malleolar branches

Calcaneal branches

Medial plantar (superficial digital)

Circumflex fibular

Fibular

Muscular

Tibial nerve

Flexor hallucis longus

Flexor retinaculum

Lateral plantar (plantar and metatarsal)

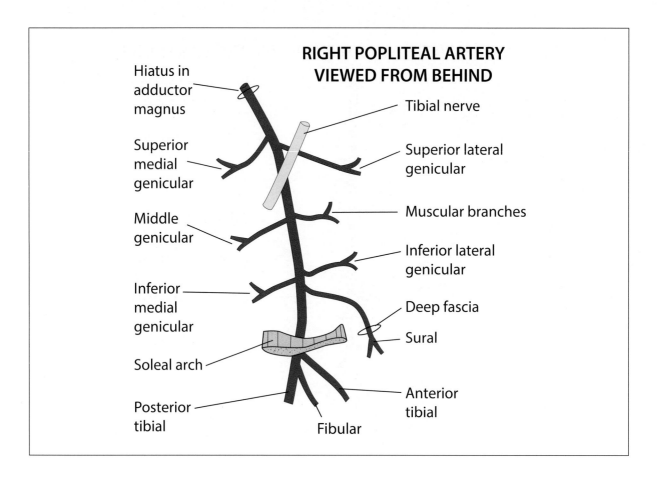

RIGHT POPLITEAL ARTERY VIEWED FROM BEHIND

Hiatus in adductor magnus

Tibial nerve

Superior medial genicular

Superior lateral genicular

Middle genicular

Muscular branches

Inferior lateral genicular

Inferior medial genicular

Deep fascia

Sural

Soleal arch

Posterior tibial

Anterior tibial

Fibular

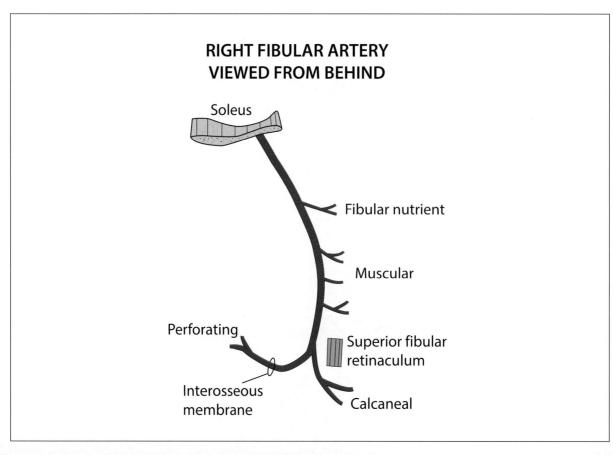

RIGHT FIBULAR ARTERY VIEWED FROM BEHIND

Soleus

Fibular nutrient

Muscular

Perforating

Superior fibular retinaculum

Interosseous membrane

Calcaneal

VEINS AND PULSES IN THE LOWER LIMB

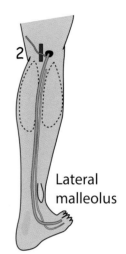

Anterior
GREAT (LONG) SAPHENOUS VEIN

Posterolateral
SMALL (SHORT) SAPHENOUS VEIN

Perforating veins at 3,6,9cm above ankle

Pulses
1. Femoral in groin
2. Popliteal in popliteal fossa
3. Posterior tibial behind medial malleolus
4. Dorsalis pedis on dorsum of foot

Lateral malleolus

Great saphenous vein
Starts: Medial side of dorsal venous arch
Passes: Anterior to medial malleolus with saphenous nerve then a hand's breadth posteromedial to patella

Small saphenous vein
Starts: Lateral side of dorsal venous arch
Passes: Behind lateral malleolus then upwards on post aspect of calf with sural nerve.
Perforates: Popliteal fascia and joins popliteal vein at a variable site

VENOUS RETURN FROM THE LEG

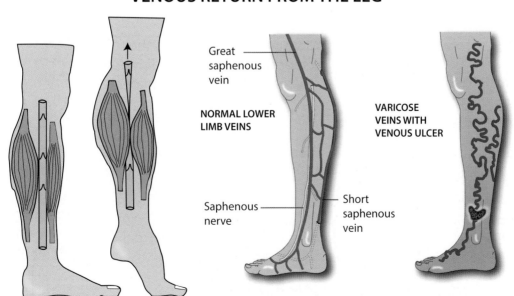

Great saphenous vein

NORMAL LOWER LIMB VEINS

Saphenous nerve

Short saphenous vein

VARICOSE VEINS WITH VENOUS ULCER

Venous blood in the superficial veins enters the deep veins via the perforator veins and is then pumped centrally by the muscle pumps (soleus and gastrocnemius) with the aid of valves. Failure of this mechanism leads to varicose veins and possible ulceration.

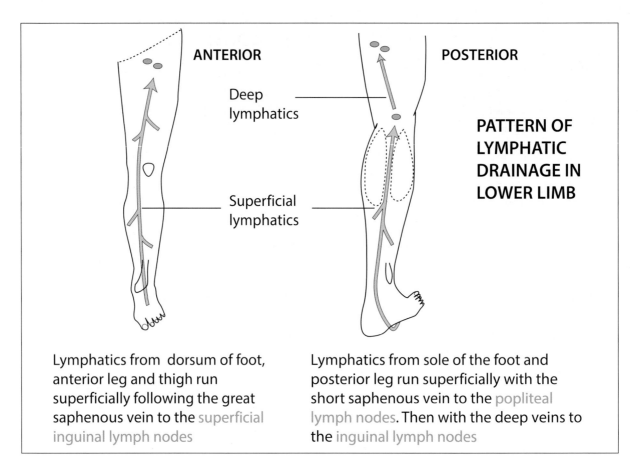

ANTERIOR

POSTERIOR

Deep lymphatics

Superficial lymphatics

PATTERN OF LYMPHATIC DRAINAGE IN LOWER LIMB

Lymphatics from dorsum of foot, anterior leg and thigh run superficially following the great saphenous vein to the superficial inguinal lymph nodes

Lymphatics from sole of the foot and posterior leg run superficially with the short saphenous vein to the popliteal lymph nodes. Then with the deep veins to the inguinal lymph nodes

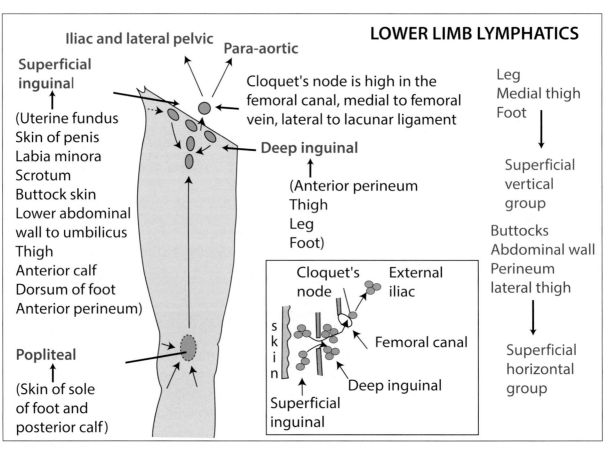

LOWER LIMB LYMPHATICS

Iliac and lateral pelvic

Para-aortic

Superficial inguinal

(Uterine fundus
Skin of penis
Labia minora
Scrotum
Buttock skin
Lower abdominal
wall to umbilicus
Thigh
Anterior calf
Dorsum of foot
Anterior perineum)

Cloquet's node is high in the femoral canal, medial to femoral vein, lateral to lacunar ligament

Deep inguinal

(Anterior perineum
Thigh
Leg
Foot)

Leg
Medial thigh
Foot

↓

Superficial vertical group

Buttocks
Abdominal wall
Perineum
lateral thigh

↓

Superficial horizontal group

Popliteal

(Skin of sole
of foot and
posterior calf)

Cloquet's node

External iliac

skin

Femoral canal

Deep inguinal

Superficial inguinal

2.2 Gluteal Region, Hip and Thigh

ATTACHMENTS TO HIP BONE (PUBIS - ISCHIUM - ILIUM)

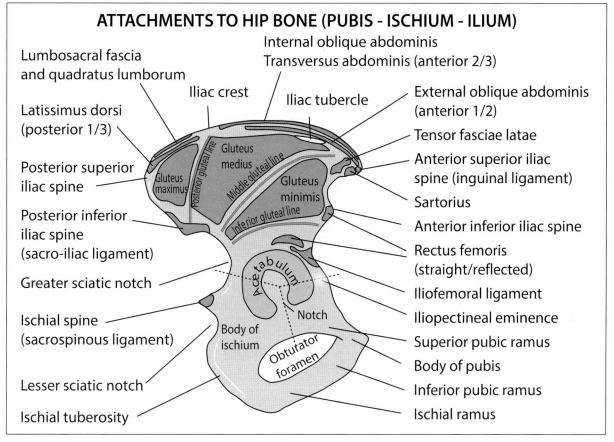

Lumbosacral fascia and quadratus lumborum

Internal oblique abdominis
Transversus abdominis (anterior 2/3)

Latissimus dorsi (posterior 1/3)

Iliac crest

Iliac tubercle

External oblique abdominis (anterior 1/2)

Tensor fasciae latae

Posterior superior iliac spine

Gluteus medius

Posterior gluteal line

Middle gluteal line

Gluteus maximus

Gluteus minimis

Anterior superior iliac spine (inguinal ligament)

Sartorius

Posterior inferior iliac spine (sacro-iliac ligament)

Inferior gluteal line

Anterior inferior iliac spine

Rectus femoris (straight/reflected)

Acetabulum

Greater sciatic notch

Iliofemoral ligament

Iliopectineal eminence

Notch

Ischial spine (sacrospinous ligament)

Body of ischium

Obturator foramen

Superior pubic ramus

Body of pubis

Lesser sciatic notch

Inferior pubic ramus

Ischial tuberosity

Ischial ramus

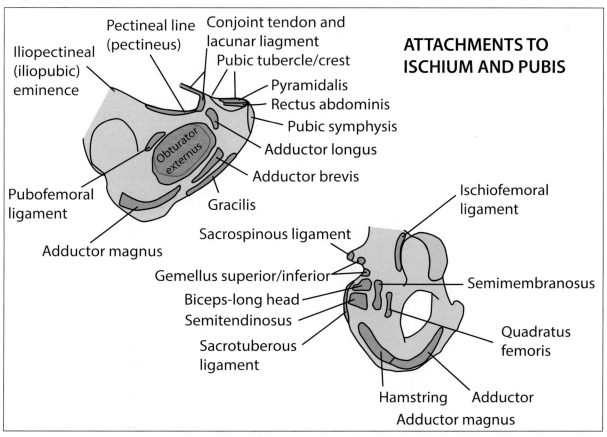

ATTACHMENTS TO ISCHIUM AND PUBIS

Iliopectineal (iliopubic) eminence

Pectineal line (pectineus)

Conjoint tendon and lacunar liagment

Pubic tubercle/crest

Pyramidalis

Rectus abdominis

Pubic symphysis

Obturator externus

Adductor longus

Adductor brevis

Pubofemoral ligament

Gracilis

Ischiofemoral ligament

Adductor magnus

Sacrospinous ligament

Gemellus superior/inferior

Semimembranosus

Biceps-long head

Semitendinosus

Quadratus femoris

Sacrotuberous ligament

Hamstring   Adductor
Adductor magnus

GLUTEAL REGION - PIRIFORMIS AND OBTURATOR INTERNUS

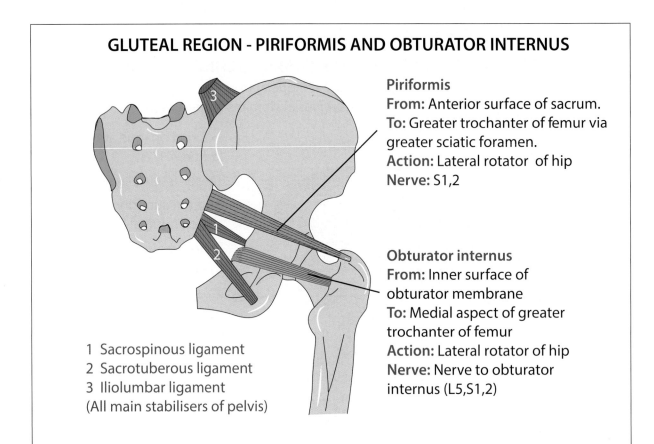

Piriformis
From: Anterior surface of sacrum.
To: Greater trochanter of femur via greater sciatic foramen.
Action: Lateral rotator of hip
Nerve: S1,2

Obturator internus
From: Inner surface of obturator membrane
To: Medial aspect of greater trochanter of femur
Action: Lateral rotator of hip
Nerve: Nerve to obturator internus (L5,S1,2)

1 Sacrospinous ligament
2 Sacrotuberous ligament
3 Iliolumbar ligament
(All main stabilisers of pelvis)

RIGHT GLUTEAL REGION

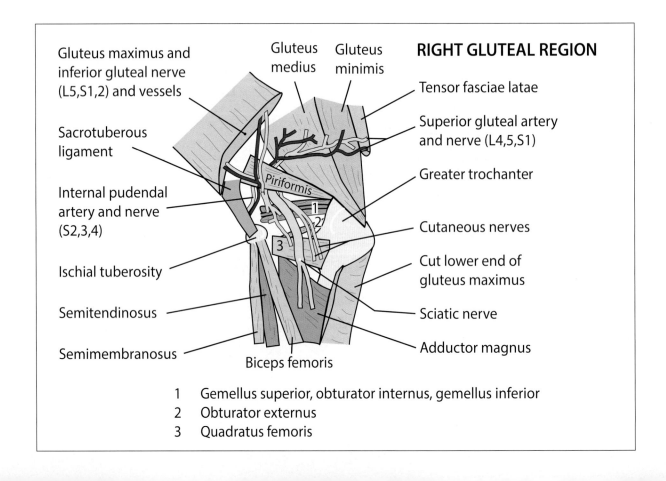

Gluteus maximus and inferior gluteal nerve (L5,S1,2) and vessels

Sacrotuberous ligament

Internal pudendal artery and nerve (S2,3,4)

Ischial tuberosity

Semitendinosus

Semimembranosus

Gluteus medius

Gluteus minimis

Piriformis

Biceps femoris

Tensor fasciae latae

Superior gluteal artery and nerve (L4,5,S1)

Greater trochanter

Cutaneous nerves

Cut lower end of gluteus maximus

Sciatic nerve

Adductor magnus

1 Gemellus superior, obturator internus, gemellus inferior
2 Obturator externus
3 Quadratus femoris

STRUCTURES PASSING THROUGH THE GREATER AND LESSER SCIATIC FORMINA

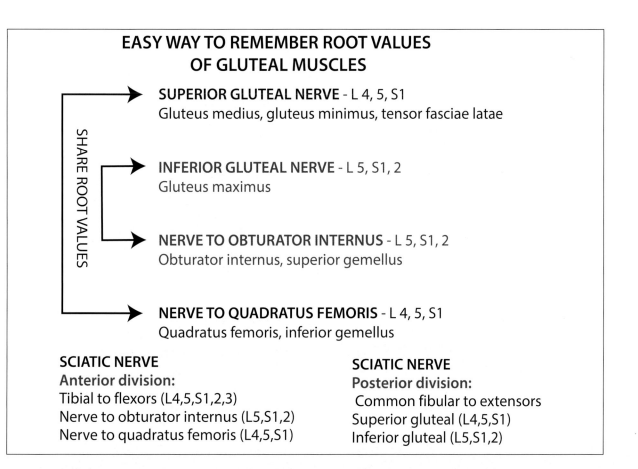

VIA GREATER SCIATIC FORAMEN
- Superior gluteal vessels
- Superior gluteal nerve (L4,5,S1)

PIRIFORMIS (S1,2)

- Inferior gluteal vessels
- Inferior gluteal nerve (L5,S1,2)
- Sciatic nerve (L4,5,S1,2,3)
- Perforating cutaneous nerve (S2,3)
- Posterior femoral cutaneous nerve (S1,2,3)
- Nerve to quadratus femoris (L4,5,S1)
- Nerve to obturator internus (L5,S1,2)
- Pudendal nerve (S2,3,4)
- Internal pudendal vessels

VIA LESSER SCIATIC FORAMEN

- Tendon of obturator internus
- Nerve to obturator internus
- Internal pudendal vessels
- Pudendal nerve

EASY WAY TO REMEMBER ROOT VALUES OF GLUTEAL MUSCLES

SHARE ROOT VALUES

SUPERIOR GLUTEAL NERVE - L 4, 5, S1
Gluteus medius, gluteus minimus, tensor fasciae latae

INFERIOR GLUTEAL NERVE - L 5, S1, 2
Gluteus maximus

NERVE TO OBTURATOR INTERNUS - L 5, S1, 2
Obturator internus, superior gemellus

NERVE TO QUADRATUS FEMORIS - L 4, 5, S1
Quadratus femoris, inferior gemellus

SCIATIC NERVE
Anterior division:
Tibial to flexors (L4,5,S1,2,3)
Nerve to obturator internus (L5,S1,2)
Nerve to quadratus femoris (L4,5,S1)

SCIATIC NERVE
Posterior division:
 Common fibular to extensors
Superior gluteal (L4,5,S1)
Inferior gluteal (L5,S1,2)

There are six nerves that arise from the roots of the sacral plexus that have the letter "P"

Piriformis, nerve to :	S1,2	Remains in pelvis to supply this muscle
Posterior femoral cutaneous nerve:	S1,2,3	Leaves pelvis via greater sciatic foramen
Perforating cutaneous nerve:	S2,3	Leaves pelvis via greater sciatic foramen
Pudendal nerve:	S2,3,4	Leaves pelvis via greater sciatic foramen
Pelvic splanchnic (parasympathetic) nerves:	S2,3,4	Remains in pelvis to supply pelvic organs
Perineal branch of S4:	S4	Remains in pelvis to supply levator ani

3 nerves remain in the pelvis and 3 exit via the greater sciatic foramen

VARIATIONS IN SCIATIC NERVE

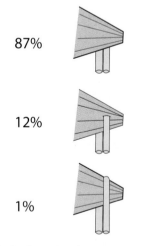

87%

12%

1%

Variations in the emergence of common fibular nerve in relation to piriformis

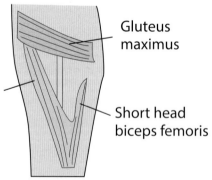

Covered by

Gluteus maximus

Long head biceps femoris

Short head biceps femoris

Nerve lies on:
- Superior gemellus
- Tendon of obturator internus
- Inferior gemellus
- Quadratus femoris
- Adductor magnus

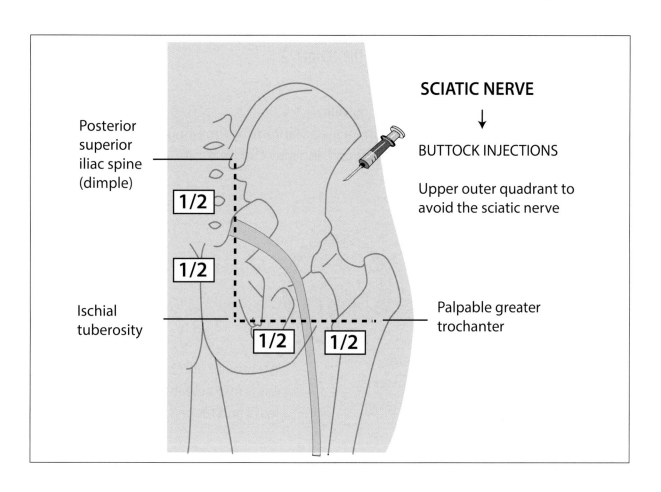

Posterior superior iliac spine (dimple)

SCIATIC NERVE

↓

BUTTOCK INJECTIONS

Upper outer quadrant to avoid the sciatic nerve

Ischial tuberosity

Palpable greater trochanter

HIP JOINT 1

Ball and socket

Synovial

Ligamentum teres in fovea

ANGLE OF NECK ON SHAFT

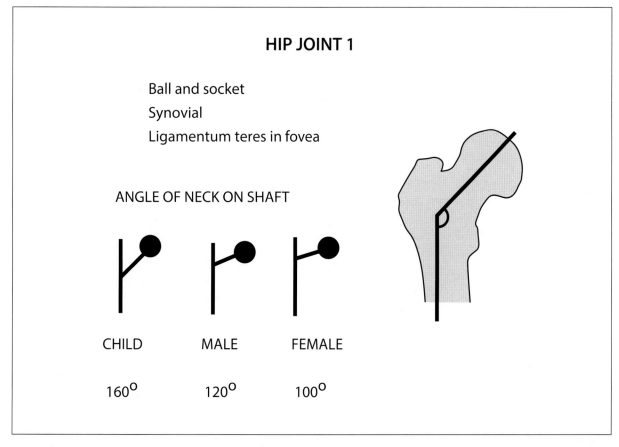

CHILD   MALE   FEMALE

160°   120°   100°

HIP JOINT 2

SYNOVIUM

From: Femoral articular margin

Covers: Intracapular femoral neck, labrum, ligamentum
   teres, Havesian fat pad and may communicate with
   psoas bursa

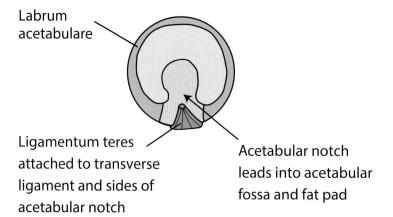

Labrum
acetabulare

Ligamentum teres
attached to transverse
ligament and sides of
acetabular notch

Acetabular notch
leads into acetabular
fossa and fat pad

ATTACHMENTS TO RIGHT FEMUR
GREATER TROCHANTER

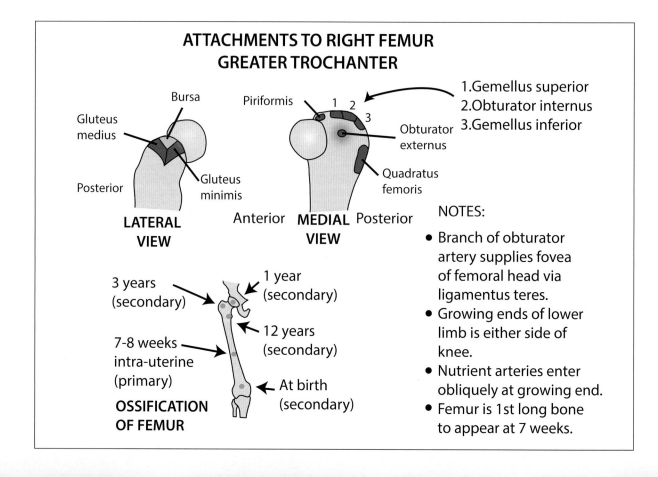

Bursa

Gluteus
medius

Posterior

Gluteus
minimis

**LATERAL
VIEW**

Piriformis   1   2

3

Obturator
externus

Quadratus
femoris

Anterior   **MEDIAL** Posterior
         VIEW

1.Gemellus superior
2.Obturator internus
3.Gemellus inferior

NOTES:

- Branch of obturator
  artery supplies fovea
  of femoral head via
  ligamentus teres.
- Growing ends of lower
  limb is either side of
  knee.
- Nutrient arteries enter
  obliquely at growing end.
- Femur is 1st long bone
  to appear at 7 weeks.

3 years
(secondary)

7-8 weeks
intra-uterine
(primary)

**OSSIFICATION
OF FEMUR**

1 year
(secondary)

12 years
(secondary)

At birth
(secondary)

HIP JOINT LIGAMENTS

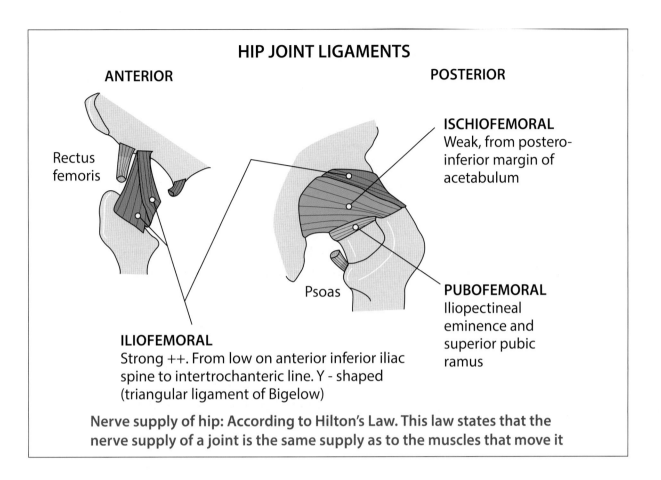

ANTERIOR

POSTERIOR

Rectus femoris

ISCHIOFEMORAL
Weak, from postero-inferior margin of acetabulum

Psoas

PUBOFEMORAL
Iliopectineal eminence and superior pubic ramus

ILIOFEMORAL
Strong ++. From low on anterior inferior iliac spine to intertrochanteric line. Y - shaped (triangular ligament of Bigelow)

Nerve supply of hip: According to Hilton's Law. This law states that the nerve supply of a joint is the same supply as to the muscles that move it

---

HIP JOINT 4

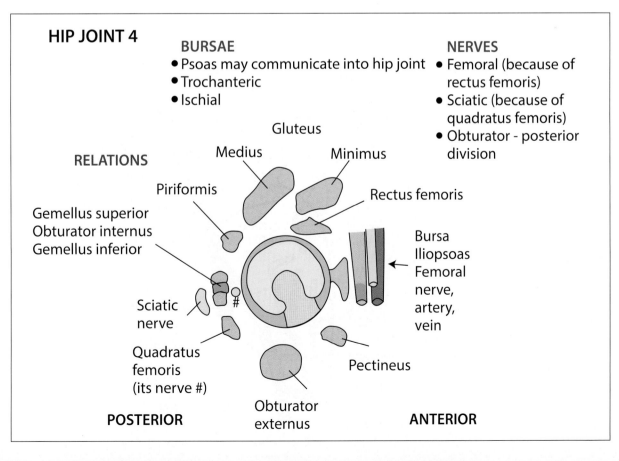

BURSAE
- Psoas may communicate into hip joint
- Trochanteric
- Ischial

NERVES
- Femoral (because of rectus femoris)
- Sciatic (because of quadratus femoris)
- Obturator - posterior division

RELATIONS

Gluteus

Medius   Minimus

Piriformis   Rectus femoris

Gemellus superior
Obturator internus
Gemellus inferior

Bursa
Iliopsoas
Femoral nerve, artery, vein

Sciatic nerve

#

Quadratus femoris (its nerve #)

Pectineus

Obturator externus

POSTERIOR

ANTERIOR

LOWER LIMB: SURFACE AND APPLIED ANATOMY

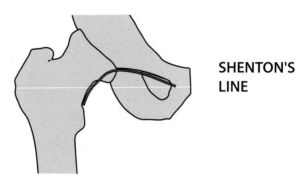

SHENTON'S LINE

Shenton's Line is a useful observation when looking at a radiograph of a pelvis/hip. In the normal appearances this line is smooth and unbroken

Note: When measuring to see if there is shortening of the lower limb it can be measured from the umbilicus to the medial malleolus. This may give an APPARENT shortening when the two sides are compared. However, only if the legs are measured from the anterior superior iliac spine to the medial malleolus will TRUE shortening be detected.

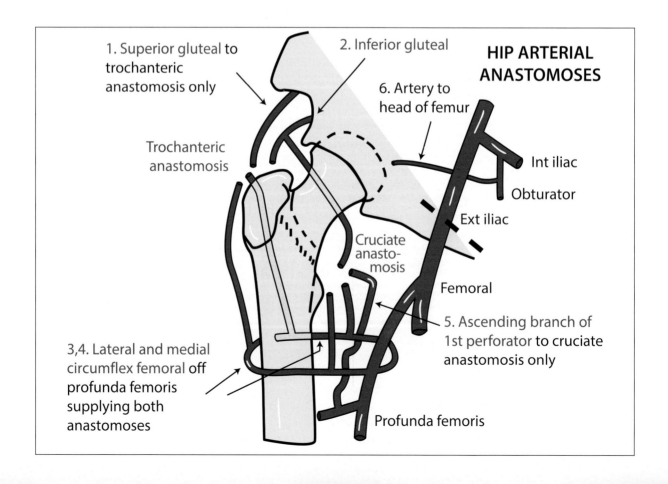

1. Superior gluteal to trochanteric anastomosis only

2. Inferior gluteal

HIP ARTERIAL ANASTOMOSES

6. Artery to head of femur

Trochanteric anastomosis

Int iliac

Obturator

Ext iliac

Cruciate anasto-mosis

Femoral

5. Ascending branch of 1st perforator to cruciate anastomosis only

3,4. Lateral and medial circumflex femoral off profunda femoris supplying both anastomoses

Profunda femoris

ARTERIAL SUPPLY TO HIP JOINT

Fracture lines.
A: Subcapital destroying virtually all supply to head of femur. Note that the vessels run beneath the retinacular fibres.
B: Intertrochanteric fracture which spares the majority of arterial supply to the head of the femur

Retinacular fibres

Small artery from obturator artery within the ligamentum teres. Probably minor contribution at any stage

A

Arteries from trochanteric and cruciate anastomoses reaching the head of the femur beneath the retinacular fibres

B

Arteries within marrow cavity

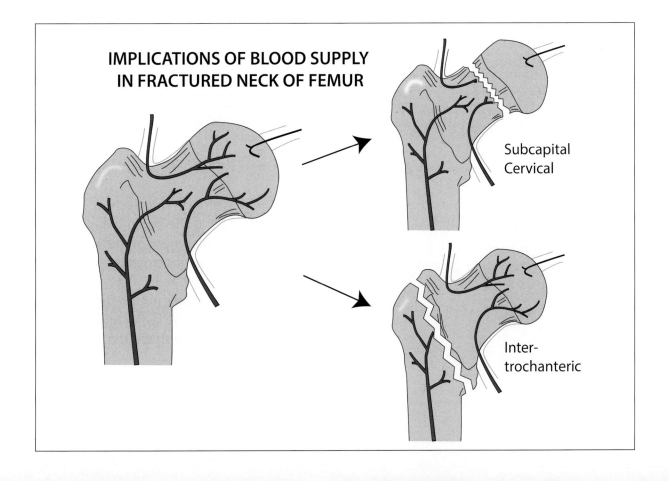

IMPLICATIONS OF BLOOD SUPPLY IN FRACTURED NECK OF FEMUR

Subcapital Cervical

Inter-trochanteric

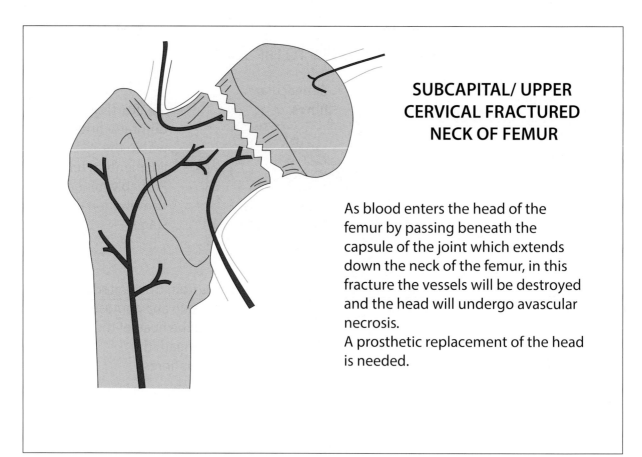

SUBCAPITAL/ UPPER CERVICAL FRACTURED NECK OF FEMUR

As blood enters the head of the femur by passing beneath the capsule of the joint which extends down the neck of the femur, in this fracture the vessels will be destroyed and the head will undergo avascular necrosis.
A prosthetic replacement of the head is needed.

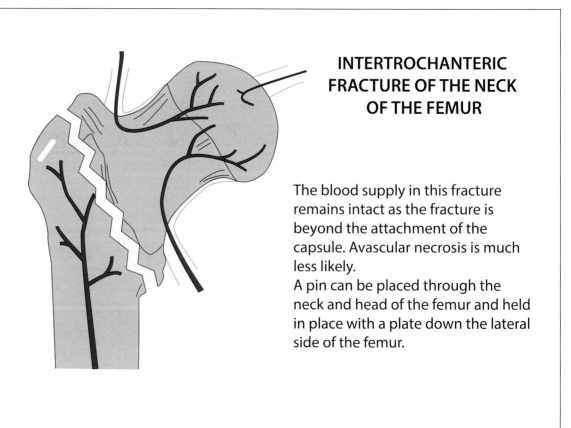

INTERTROCHANTERIC FRACTURE OF THE NECK OF THE FEMUR

The blood supply in this fracture remains intact as the fracture is beyond the attachment of the capsule. Avascular necrosis is much less likely.
A pin can be placed through the neck and head of the femur and held in place with a plate down the lateral side of the femur.

FRACTURE OF NECK OF LEFT FEMUR PHYSICAL SIGNS

Leg is externally rotated and shortened

External rotation due to:
- Multitude of external rotator muscles
- Weight of leg
- Change in axis of psoas pull (see next image)

Shortening due to pull of:
All muscles from pelvis to leg
- Psoas/iliacus
- Rectus femoris
- Adductors
- Hamstrings
- Sartorius

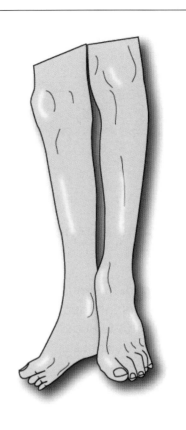

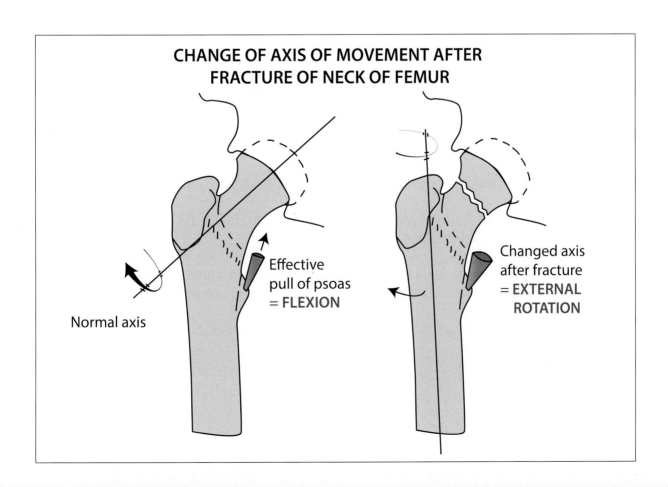

CHANGE OF AXIS OF MOVEMENT AFTER FRACTURE OF NECK OF FEMUR

Effective pull of psoas = FLEXION

Normal axis

Changed axis after fracture = EXTERNAL ROTATION

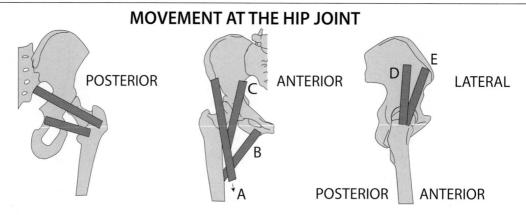

MOVEMENT AT THE HIP JOINT

EXTERNAL ROTATION
- Piriformis
- Gemelli
- Obturator externus
- Obturator internus
- Quadratus femoris
- Gluteus maximus
  (+ extension)
- Sartorius (A)
  (+ flexion)

ADDUCTION ONLY (B)
- Adductors: longus, brevis, magnus
- Gracilis
- (Pectineus)

FLEXION (C)
- Psoas and iliacus
- Rectus femoris

EXTENSION
- Hamstrings

ABDUCTION ONLY (D)
- Gluteus medius and minimus
  (posterior fibres)

INTERNAL ROTATION (E)
- Gluteus medius and minimus
  (anterior fibres)

HIP JOINT MOVEMENTS

Abduction
Gluteus medius, gluteus minimus, tensor fasciae latae
Adduction
Adductors brevis, longus, magnus (pectineus, gracilis, iliopsoas)
Flexion
Psoas, iliacius, rectus femoris, sartorius, (pectineus, tensor fasciae latae).
Note soft tissue limitation
Extension
Gluteus maximus, semitendinosus, semimembranosus, adductor
magnus, long head biceps femoris. Note, limited by capsule and ligaments
External rotation
Gluteus maximus, piriformis, obturators internus and externus, gemelli,
quadratus femoris
Internal rotation
Anterior fibres of gluteus medius and minimus

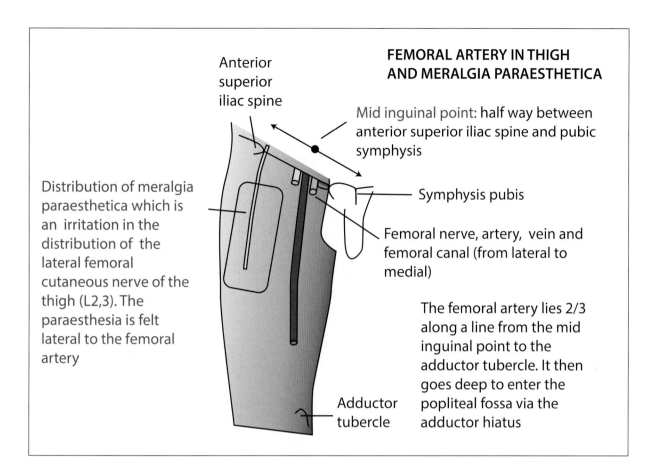

Anterior superior iliac spine

FEMORAL ARTERY IN THIGH AND MERALGIA PARAESTHETICA

Mid inguinal point: half way between anterior superior iliac spine and pubic symphysis

Distribution of meralgia paraesthetica which is an irritation in the distribution of the lateral femoral cutaneous nerve of the thigh (L2,3). The paraesthesia is felt lateral to the femoral artery

Symphysis pubis

Femoral nerve, artery, vein and femoral canal (from lateral to medial)

The femoral artery lies 2/3 along a line from the mid inguinal point to the adductor tubercle. It then goes deep to enter the popliteal fossa via the adductor hiatus

Adductor tubercle

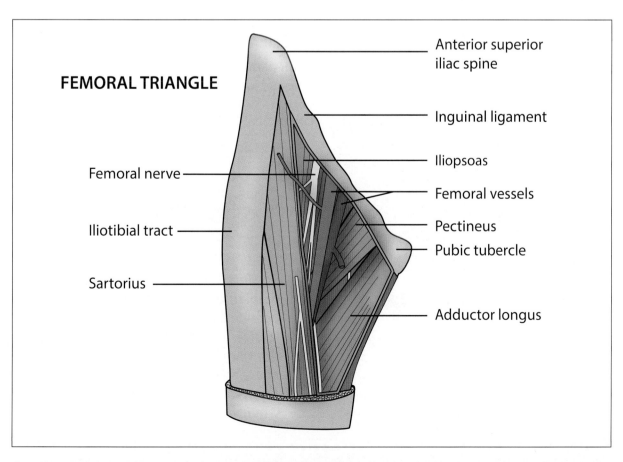

FEMORAL TRIANGLE

Anterior superior iliac spine

Inguinal ligament

Iliopsoas

Femoral nerve

Femoral vessels

Iliotibial tract

Pectineus

Pubic tubercle

Sartorius

Adductor longus

FEMORAL TRIANGLE

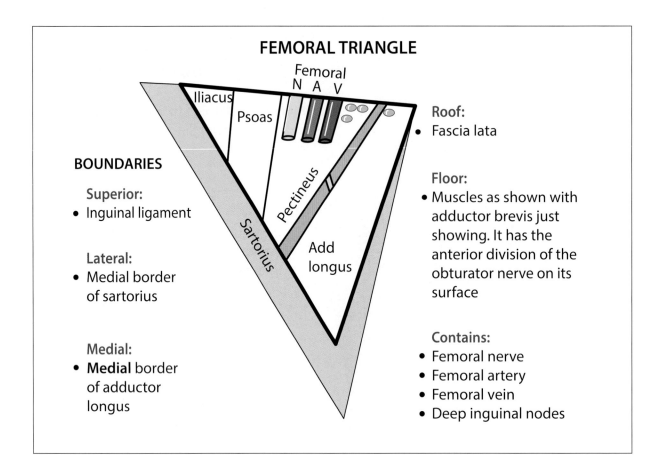

Femoral
N A V

Iliacus

Psoas

Pectineus

Sartorius

Add longus

Roof:
• Fascia lata

Floor:
• Muscles as shown with adductor brevis just showing. It has the anterior division of the obturator nerve on its surface

Contains:
• Femoral nerve
• Femoral artery
• Femoral vein
• Deep inguinal nodes

BOUNDARIES

Superior:
• Inguinal ligament

Lateral:
• Medial border of sartorius

Medial:
• **Medial** border of adductor longus

RIGHT FEMORAL CANAL, SHEATH AND RING

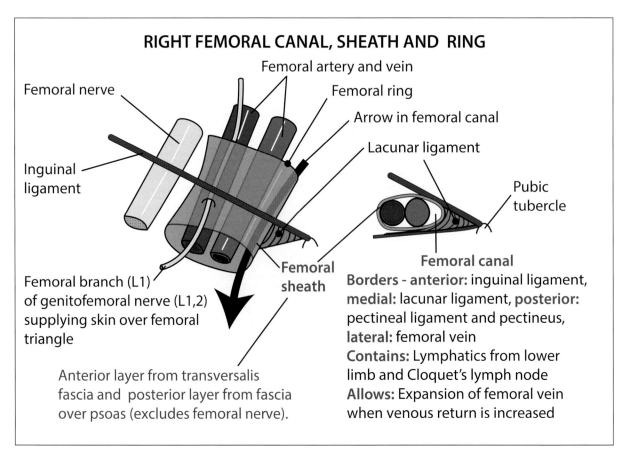

Femoral nerve

Inguinal ligament

Femoral artery and vein

Femoral ring

Arrow in femoral canal

Lacunar ligament

Pubic tubercle

Femoral sheath

Femoral branch (L1) of genitofemoral nerve (L1,2) supplying skin over femoral triangle

Anterior layer from transversalis fascia and posterior layer from fascia over psoas (excludes femoral nerve).

Femoral canal
Borders - anterior: inguinal ligament, **medial:** lacunar ligament, **posterior:** pectineal ligament and pectineus, **lateral:** femoral vein
Contains: Lymphatics from lower limb and Cloquet's lymph node
Allows: Expansion of femoral vein when venous return is increased

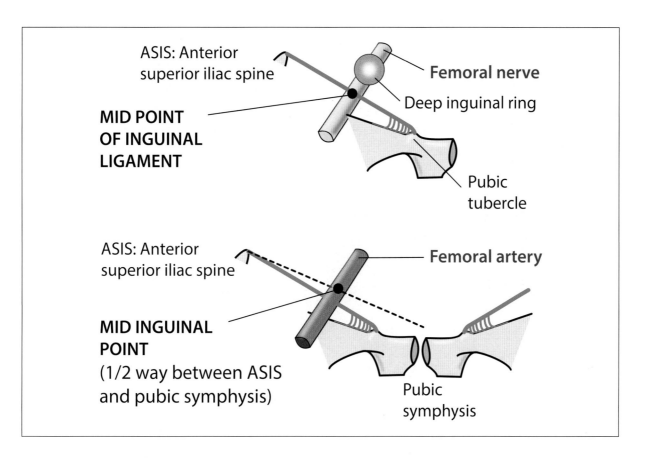

ASIS: Anterior superior iliac spine

Femoral nerve

MID POINT OF INGUINAL LIGAMENT

Deep inguinal ring

Pubic tubercle

ASIS: Anterior superior iliac spine

Femoral artery

MID INGUINAL POINT
(1/2 way between ASIS and pubic symphysis)

Pubic symphysis

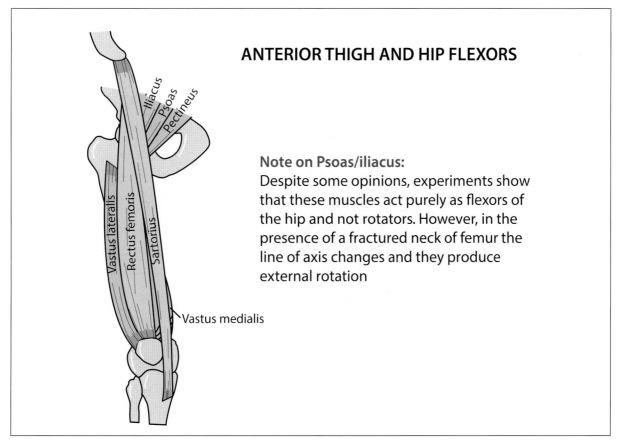

ANTERIOR THIGH AND HIP FLEXORS

Iliacus
Psoas
Pectineus

Vastus lateralis
Rectus femoris
Sartorius

Vastus medialis

Note on Psoas/iliacus:
Despite some opinions, experiments show that these muscles act purely as flexors of the hip and not rotators. However, in the presence of a fractured neck of femur the line of axis changes and they produce external rotation

THE "3 WATERSHED MUSCLES" WAY OF REMEMBERING THIGH MUSCLES

The 3 muscles with dual nerve supply are interposed between the three groups of muscles in the thigh. If you can recall these 3 then the groups are easily remembered

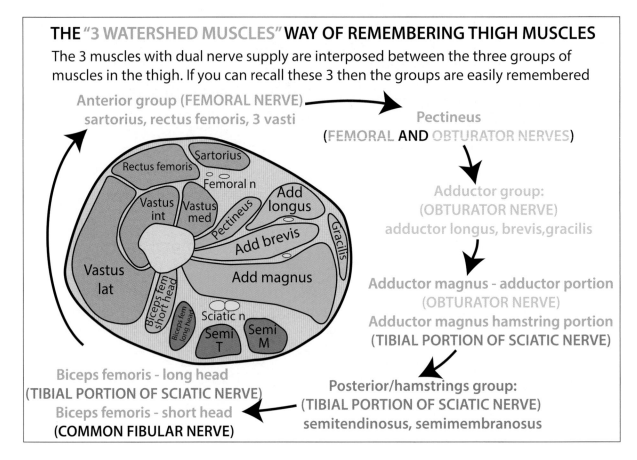

Anterior group (FEMORAL NERVE)
sartorius, rectus femoris, 3 vasti

Pectineus
(FEMORAL **AND** OBTURATOR NERVES)

Adductor group:
(OBTURATOR NERVE)
adductor longus, brevis, gracilis

Adductor magnus - adductor portion
(OBTURATOR NERVE)
Adductor magnus hamstring portion
(TIBIAL PORTION OF SCIATIC NERVE)

Posterior/hamstrings group:
(TIBIAL PORTION OF SCIATIC NERVE)
semitendinosus, semimembranosus

Biceps femoris - long head
(TIBIAL PORTION OF SCIATIC NERVE)
Biceps femoris - short head
(COMMON FIBULAR NERVE)

RIGHT ADDUCTOR (SUBSARTORIAL/HUNTER'S) CANAL
(viewed from below)

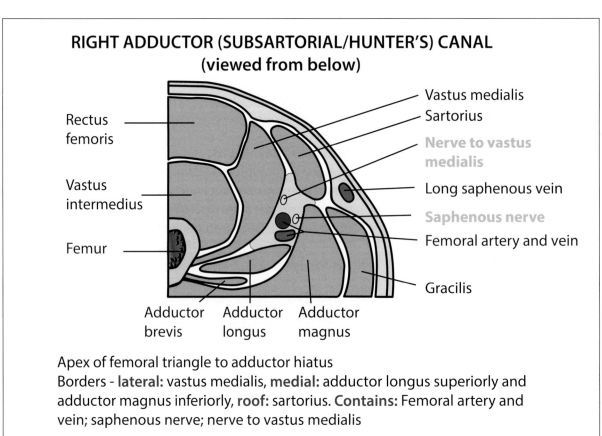

Rectus femoris

Vastus intermedius

Femur

Adductor brevis

Adductor longus

Adductor magnus

Vastus medialis

Sartorius

Nerve to vastus medialis

Long saphenous vein

Saphenous nerve

Femoral artery and vein

Gracilis

Apex of femoral triangle to adductor hiatus

Borders - **lateral:** vastus medialis, **medial:** adductor longus superiorly and adductor magnus inferiorly, **roof:** sartorius. **Contains:** Femoral artery and vein; saphenous nerve; nerve to vastus medialis

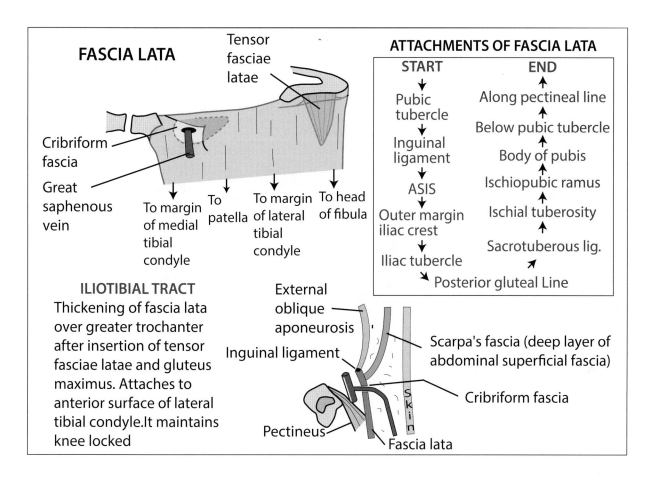

FASCIA LATA

Tensor fasciae latae

Cribriform fascia

Great saphenous vein

To margin of medial tibial condyle

To patella

To margin of lateral tibial condyle

To head of fibula

ATTACHMENTS OF FASCIA LATA

START	END
↓	↑
Pubic tubercle	Along pectineal line
↓	↑
Inguinal ligament	Below pubic tubercle
↓	↑
ASIS	Body of pubis
↓	↑
Outer margin iliac crest	Ischiopubic ramus
↓	↑
Iliac tubercle	Ischial tuberosity
↓	↑
Posterior gluteal Line	Sacrotuberous lig.

ILIOTIBIAL TRACT
Thickening of fascia lata over greater trochanter after insertion of tensor fasciae latae and gluteus maximus. Attaches to anterior surface of lateral tibial condyle.It maintains knee locked

External oblique aponeurosis

Inguinal ligament

Pectineus

Scarpa's fascia (deep layer of abdominal superficial fascia)

Cribriform fascia

Skin

Fascia lata

CUTANEOUS NERVE SUPPLY OF BUTTOCKS

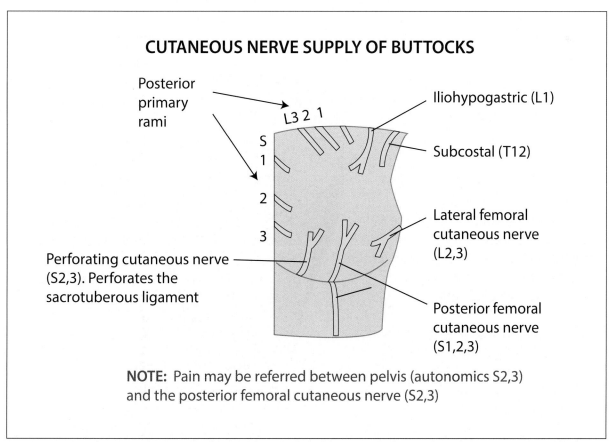

Posterior primary rami

L3 2 1

S 1

2

3

Iliohypogastric (L1)

Subcostal (T12)

Lateral femoral cutaneous nerve (L2,3)

Perforating cutaneous nerve (S2,3). Perforates the sacrotuberous ligament

Posterior femoral cutaneous nerve (S1,2,3)

NOTE: Pain may be referred between pelvis (autonomics S2,3) and the posterior femoral cutaneous nerve (S2,3)

2.3 Knee and Popliteal Fossa

ANTERIOR VIEW OF RIGHT KNEE

Anterior cruciate ligament - tight in extension, stops femur slipping backwards

Cordlike lateral collateral ligament - not attached to lateral meniscus

Posterior cruciate ligament - stops femur slipping forwards on tibia

Broad medial collateral ligament - attached to medial meniscus

ANTERIOR CRUCIATE LIGAMENT
From: Anterolateral tibia
To: Posterior on medial side of lateral femoral condyle
Limits: Extension and anterior draw and is taut on locking
Test: Pull tibia forwards on femur

PM - **Posterior goes medial**
AL - **Anterior goes lateral**

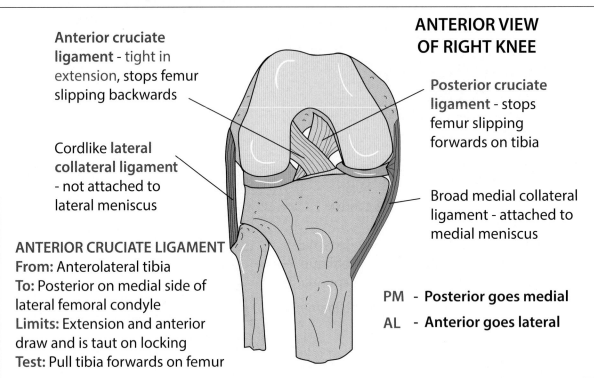

Broad medial collateral ligament - attached to medial meniscus

Posterior meniscofemoral ligament
Attached to medial femoral condyle

POSTERIOR VIEW OF RIGHT KNEE

Posterior cruciate ligament - stops femur slipping forwards on tibia

Anterior cruciate ligament - tight in extension, stops femur slipping backwards

POSTERIOR CRUCIATE LIGAMENT
From: Posteromedial tibia
To: Anterior on lateral side of medial femoral condyle
Limits: Posterior slide of tibia on femur.
Used: Down stairs and on hills
Test: Push tibia back on femur

Cordlike lateral collateral ligament - not attached to lateral meniscus

✳ Oblique popliteal ligament, a superficial structure, is one of the attachments of the semimembranosus tendon

PM - **Posterior goes medial**
AL - **Anterior goes lateral**

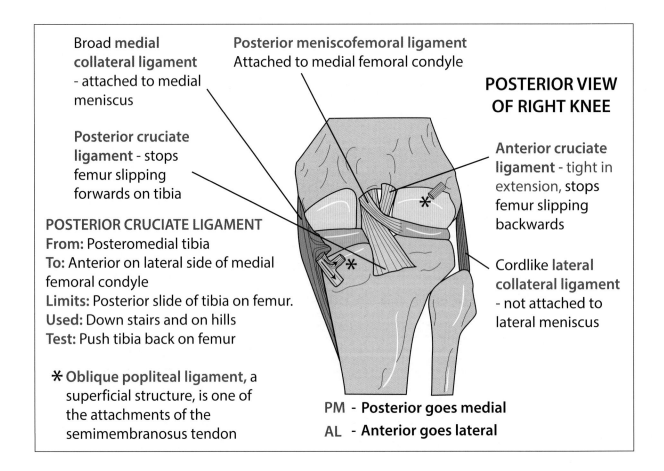

STRUCTURES ON RIGHT TIBIAL PLATEAU

T = Transverse ligament
IE = Intercondylar eminence
with medial and lateral
intercondylar tubercles

MENISCI
Liable to tears when flexed
knee is twisted.
Function: transfers forces,
keep bones together, helps
locking

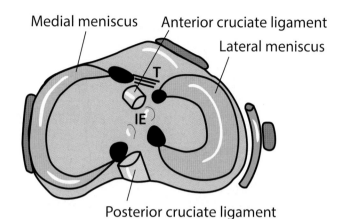

MEDIAL MENISCUS
- Wider "C"
- Medial lip slopes up
- Attaches as shown but also
  to medial collateral ligament
- More liable to damage than
  lateral meniscus

LATERAL MENISCUS
- Smaller, tighter "C"
- Lateral lip slopes down
- Not attached to lateral
  collateral ligament
- Attached as shown
- Lightly attached to popliteus
  and is retracted by it on flexion

ORDER OF STRUCTURES ON RIGHT TIBIAL PLATEAU
(Anterior to posterior)

M
A
L
L
M
P

Medial meniscus
(ant. attachment)

Ant. cruciate
ligament

Lateral meniscus
(ant. attachment)

Lateral meniscus
(post. attachment)

Post. cruciate
ligament

Medial meniscus
(post. attachment)

Note: The coronary ligaments of the knee are parts of the joint capsule that
connect the lower edges of the menisci to the edges of the tibial plateau

SUMMARY OF LIGAMENTS OF RIGHT KNEE

Medial 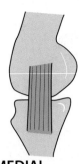 Lateral 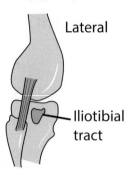 Posterior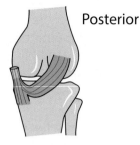

Iliotibial tract

MEDIAL COLLATERAL

- Broad, long, thick, strong
- Attached to capsule and medial meniscus
- Limits full extension and thus aids locking

LATERAL COLLATERAL

- Thick, cordlike.
- Not attached to joint structures.
- Limits full extension and thus aids locking

OBLIQUE POPLITEAL

- Upward extension of semimembranosus tendon.
- Limits extension and thus aids knee locking

NOTE

- Knee is largest joint in body
- It is a modified hinge joint
- The line of the body weight is anterior to the knee

BLOOD, NERVE SUPPLY AND MOVEMENTS OF KNEE JOINT

BLOOD SUPPLY

Genicular arteries from popliteal:
- Superior (medial and lateral)
- Middle
- Inferior (medial and lateral)

Femoral gives: Descending branch from profunda

NERVES

Posterior division of obturator

Femoral

Sciatic (both parts)

MOVEMENTS

Flexion: Semimembranosus, semitendinosus, biceps, gracilis, sartorius (gastrocnemius, plantaris, popliteus)

Extension: Quadriceps femoris, iliotibial tract (gluteus maximus, tensor fasciae latae)

Internal rotation(with knee flexed): Semimembranosus, semitendinosus, gracilis, sartorius

External rotation(with knee flexed): Biceps

Unlocking: Popliteus

Limb: 2.3 Knee and Popliteal Fossa | **119**

DRAWER TEST

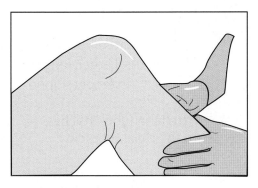 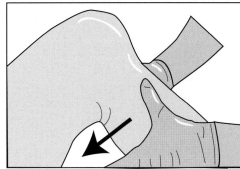

DRAWER TEST
Positive posterior drawer test showing a ruptured posterior cruciate ligament.
BUT beware - POSTERIOR SAG SIGN: if the dip below the patella is not noticed this might appear as a false positive anterior drawer test when the tibia is pulled anteriorly

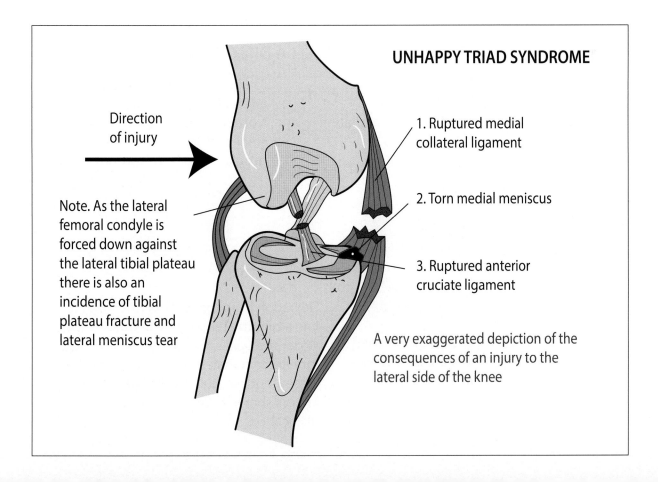

UNHAPPY TRIAD SYNDROME

Direction of injury

Note. As the lateral femoral condyle is forced down against the lateral tibial plateau there is also an incidence of tibial plateau fracture and lateral meniscus tear

1. Ruptured medial collateral ligament

2. Torn medial meniscus

3. Ruptured anterior cruciate ligament

A very exaggerated depiction of the consequences of an injury to the lateral side of the knee

RIGHT PATELLA

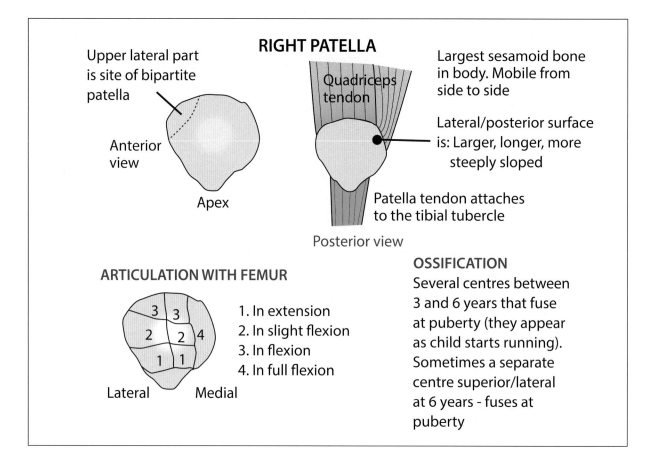

Upper lateral part is site of bipartite patella

Anterior view

Apex

Quadriceps tendon

Largest sesamoid bone in body. Mobile from side to side

Lateral/posterior surface is: Larger, longer, more steeply sloped

Patella tendon attaches to the tibial tubercle

Posterior view

ARTICULATION WITH FEMUR

1. In extension
2. In slight flexion
3. In flexion
4. In full flexion

Lateral   Medial

OSSIFICATION
Several centres between 3 and 6 years that fuse at puberty (they appear as child starts running). Sometimes a separate centre superior/lateral at 6 years - fuses at puberty

THE Q ANGLE AND PATELLA DISLOCATION

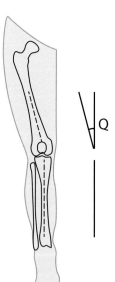

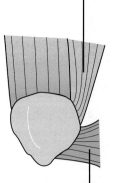

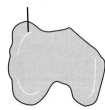

1. Insertion of lower fibres of vastus medialis into medial side of patella

2. Stronger medial retinacular fibres of knee capsule

3. More anteriorly protuberant lateral condyle of lower femur. Note that lateral condyle is smaller than medial one but it protrudes further anteriorly

Deviation from the vertical (the tibia) to a line along the femur (pull of quadriceps). Wider the pelvis, the greater the **Q angle** (greater in females).
Offset tends to pull patella laterally. 3 factors shown here help to avoid dislocation

PHYSIOLOGICAL LOCKING OF KNEE

LOCKING

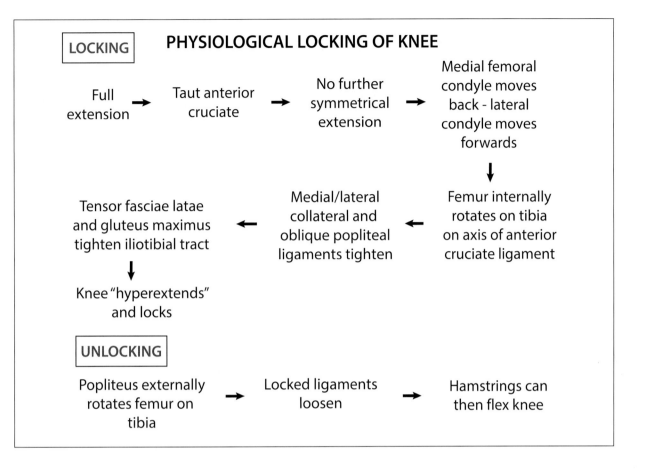

Full extension → Taut anterior cruciate → No further symmetrical extension → Medial femoral condyle moves back - lateral condyle moves forwards

↓

Tensor fasciae latae and gluteus maximus tighten iliotibial tract ← Medial/lateral collateral and oblique popliteal ligaments tighten ← Femur internally rotates on tibia on axis of anterior cruciate ligament

↓

Knee "hyperextends" and locks

UNLOCKING

Popliteus externally rotates femur on tibia → Locked ligaments loosen → Hamstrings can then flex knee

BURSAE AND SYNOVIUM OF KNEE

Tibial plateau showing attachment of synovium to its edges. The cruciate ligaments lie outside it but the menisci within it

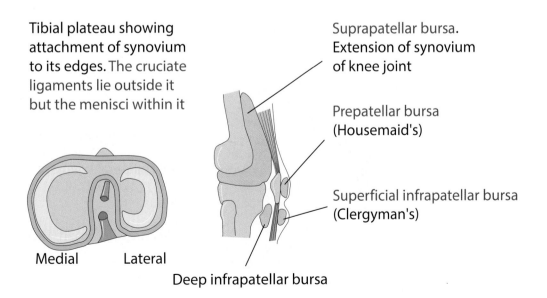

Suprapatellar bursa. Extension of synovium of knee joint

Prepatellar bursa (Housemaid's)

Superficial infrapatellar bursa (Clergyman's)

Medial   Lateral

Deep infrapatellar bursa

Synovium lines the inside of the capsule and is attached to the bony edges. It extends into the suprapatellar bursa

BURSAE AND SYNOVIUM OF KNEE

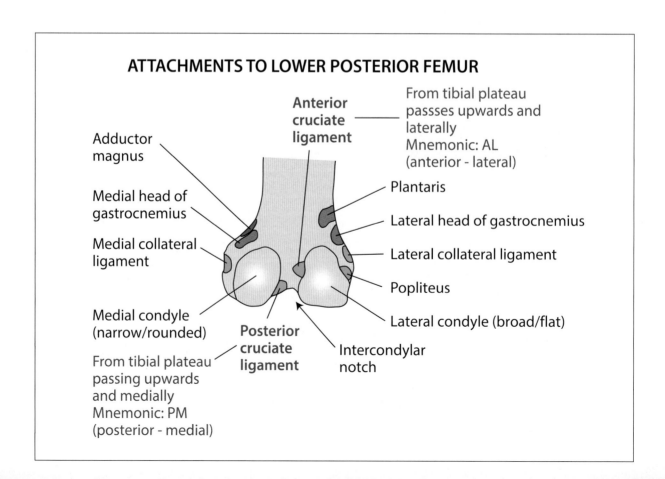

1. Under sartorius, gracilis, semitendinosus
2. Under medial head of gastrocnemius (often into joint)
3. Under lateral head of gastrocnemius (sometimes into joint)
4. Under lateral collateral ligament
5. Under popliteus (into joint)
6. Under semimembranosus

ATTACHMENTS TO LOWER POSTERIOR FEMUR

Anterior cruciate ligament — From tibial plateau passses upwards and laterally
Mnemonic: AL (anterior - lateral)

Adductor magnus

Plantaris

Medial head of gastrocnemius

Lateral head of gastrocnemius

Medial collateral ligament

Lateral collateral ligament

Popliteus

Medial condyle (narrow/rounded)

Posterior cruciate ligament

Lateral condyle (broad/flat)

Intercondylar notch

From tibial plateau passing upwards and medially
Mnemonic: PM (posterior - medial)

RIGHT KNEE JOINT CAPSULE

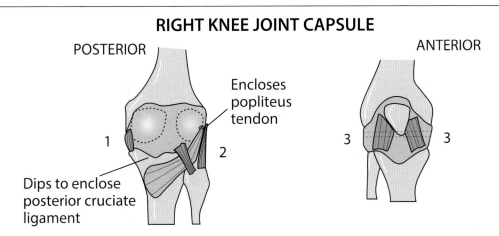

POSTERIOR

ANTERIOR

Encloses popliteus tendon

Dips to enclose posterior cruciate ligament

1   2

3   3

Capsule is attached to the bony margins of the tibia and femur. It has several thickenings shown below called internal ligaments.

1. Thickened medially to make the **Short Internal (medial) Ligament** which attaches to medial collateral ligament outside and to the medial meniscus inside as the **coronary ligaments.**

2. **Arcuate Popliteal Ligament.** This is Y shaped and the lateral part of it is often known as the **Short External (lateral) ligament.** Popliteus tendon passes medially to it.

3. **Medial and lateral Patellar Retinacular Fibres.** These reinforce the capsule anteriorly. The medial ones are important as they help to prevent the patella dislocating laterally.

MUSCLE ATTACHMENTS TO UPPER TIBIA AND FIBULA

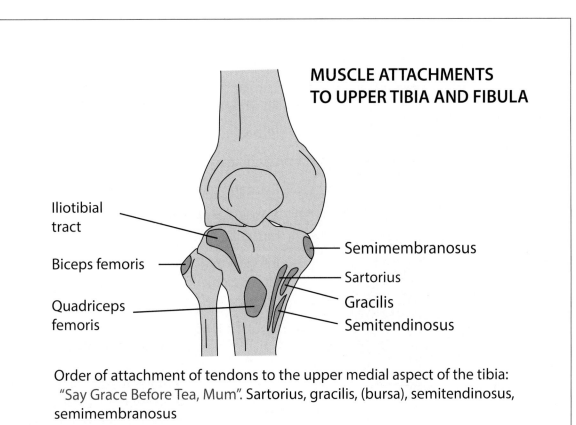

Iliotibial tract

Biceps femoris

Quadriceps femoris

Semimembranosus

Sartorius

Gracilis

Semitendinosus

Order of attachment of tendons to the upper medial aspect of the tibia:
"Say Grace Before Tea, Mum". Sartorius, gracilis, (bursa), semitendinosus, semimembranosus

RIGHT POPLITEAL REGION

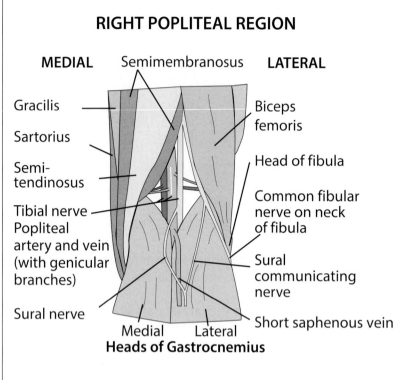

MEDIAL

Semimembranosus

LATERAL

Gracilis

Sartorius

Semi-tendinosus

Tibial nerve
Popliteal artery and vein (with genicular branches)

Sural nerve

Biceps femoris

Head of fibula

Common fibular nerve on neck of fibula

Sural communicating nerve

Short saphenous vein

Medial   Lateral
Heads of Gastrocnemius

The diamond shaped popliteal fossa is bounded inferiorly by two heads of **gastrocnemius** and superiorly by **hamstrings: biceps femoris** (laterally) and **semitendinosus** and **semimembranosus** (medially).

The popliteal artery is the deepest (most anterior) structure and may be difficult to palpate. Anterior to it are the posterior surface of the femur, capsule of knee joint and popliteus.

RIGHT POPLITEAL FOSSA (DEEP DISSECTION)

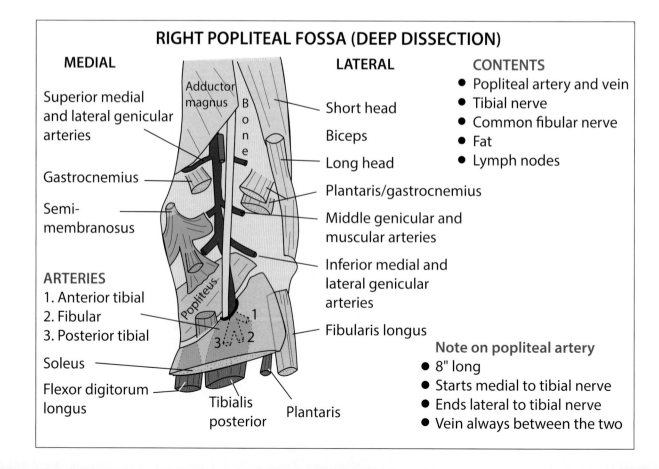

MEDIAL

Superior medial and lateral genicular arteries

Gastrocnemius

Semi-membranosus

ARTERIES
1. Anterior tibial
2. Fibular
3. Posterior tibial

Soleus

Flexor digitorum longus

Adductor magnus

Bone

Popliteus

Tibialis posterior

Plantaris

LATERAL

Short head

Biceps

Long head

Plantaris/gastrocnemius

Middle genicular and muscular arteries

Inferior medial and lateral genicular arteries

Fibularis longus

CONTENTS
- Popliteal artery and vein
- Tibial nerve
- Common fibular nerve
- Fat
- Lymph nodes

Note on popliteal artery
- 8" long
- Starts medial to tibial nerve
- Ends lateral to tibial nerve
- Vein always between the two

2.4 Lower Leg

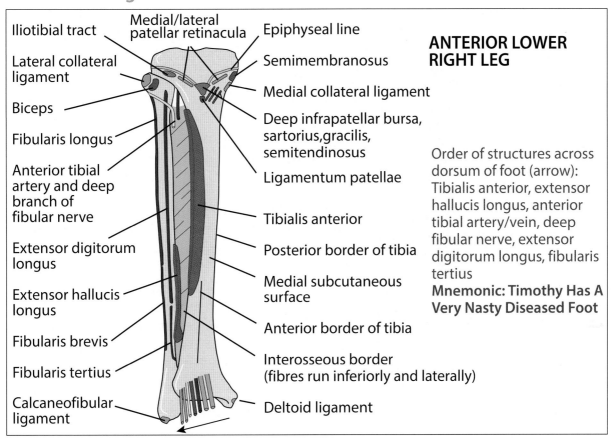

Iliotibial tract

Medial/lateral patellar retinacula

Epiphyseal line

Lateral collateral ligament

Semimembranosus

Biceps

Medial collateral ligament

Fibularis longus

Deep infrapatellar bursa, sartorius, gracilis, semitendinosus

Anterior tibial artery and deep branch of fibular nerve

Ligamentum patellae

Extensor digitorum longus

Tibialis anterior

Extensor hallucis longus

Posterior border of tibia

Medial subcutaneous surface

Fibularis brevis

Fibularis tertius

Anterior border of tibia

Calcaneofibular ligament

Interosseous border (fibres run inferiorly and laterally)

Deltoid ligament

ANTERIOR LOWER RIGHT LEG

Order of structures across dorsum of foot (arrow): Tibialis anterior, extensor hallucis longus, anterior tibial artery/vein, deep fibular nerve, extensor digitorum longus, fibularis tertius
Mnemonic: Timothy Has A Very Nasty Diseased Foot

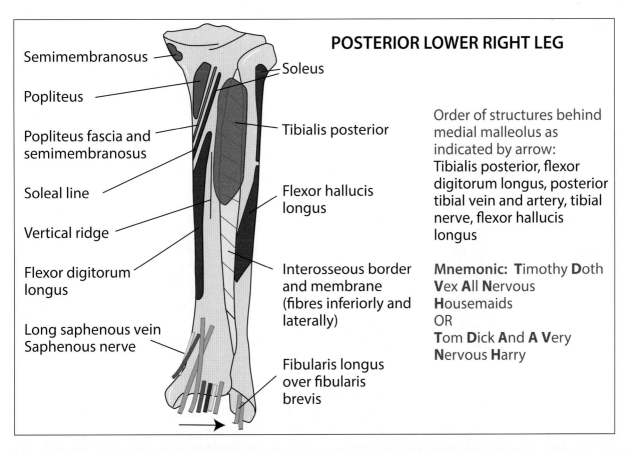

POSTERIOR LOWER RIGHT LEG

Semimembranosus

Soleus

Popliteus

Tibialis posterior

Popliteus fascia and semimembranosus

Soleal line

Flexor hallucis longus

Vertical ridge

Flexor digitorum longus

Interosseous border and membrane (fibres inferiorly and laterally)

Long saphenous vein
Saphenous nerve

Fibularis longus over fibularis brevis

Order of structures behind medial malleolus as indicated by arrow: Tibialis posterior, flexor digitorum longus, posterior tibial vein and artery, tibial nerve, flexor hallucis longus

Mnemonic: Timothy Doth Vex All Nervous Housemaids
OR
Tom Dick And A Very Nervous Harry

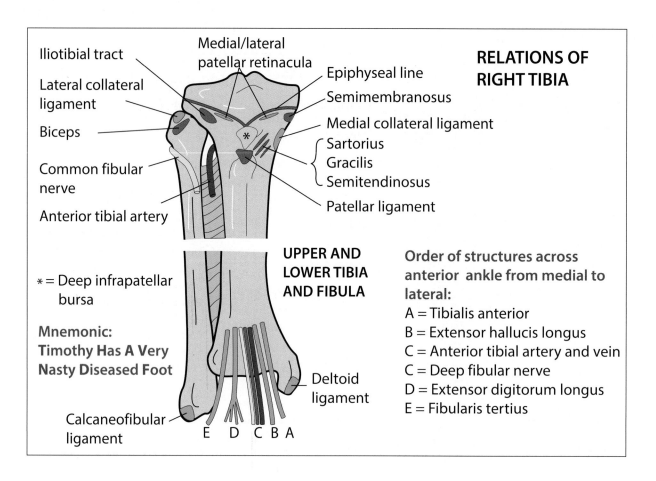

RELATIONS OF RIGHT TIBIA

Iliotibial tract

Lateral collateral ligament

Biceps

Common fibular nerve

Anterior tibial artery

Medial/lateral patellar retinacula

Epiphyseal line

Semimembranosus

Medial collateral ligament

Sartorius
Gracilis
Semitendinosus

Patellar ligament

UPPER AND LOWER TIBIA AND FIBULA

∗ = Deep infrapatellar bursa

Mnemonic:
Timothy Has A Very Nasty Diseased Foot

Deltoid ligament

Calcaneofibular ligament

E   D   C   B   A

Order of structures across anterior ankle from medial to lateral:
A = Tibialis anterior
B = Extensor hallucis longus
C = Anterior tibial artery and vein
C = Deep fibular nerve
D = Extensor digitorum longus
E = Fibularis tertius

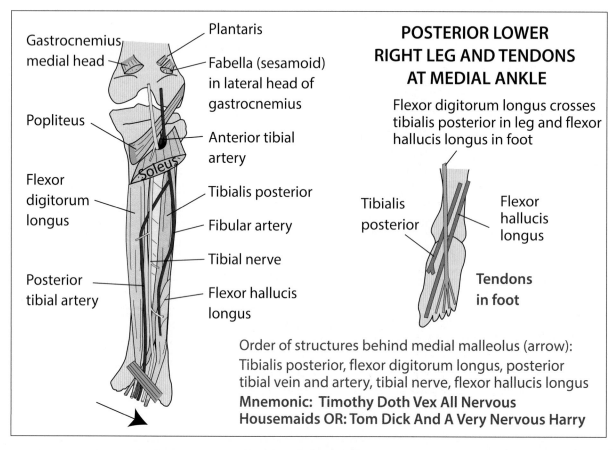

POSTERIOR LOWER RIGHT LEG AND TENDONS AT MEDIAL ANKLE

Gastrocnemius, medial head

Popliteus

Flexor digitorum longus

Posterior tibial artery

Plantaris

Fabella (sesamoid) in lateral head of gastrocnemius

Anterior tibial artery

Tibialis posterior

Fibular artery

Tibial nerve

Flexor hallucis longus

Soleus

Flexor digitorum longus crosses tibialis posterior in leg and flexor hallucis longus in foot

Tibialis posterior

Flexor hallucis longus

Tendons in foot

Order of structures behind medial malleolus (arrow):
Tibialis posterior, flexor digitorum longus, posterior tibial vein and artery, tibial nerve, flexor hallucis longus
Mnemonic: Timothy Doth Vex All Nervous Housemaids OR: Tom Dick And A Very Nervous Harry

POSTERIOR RIGHT LOWER LEG

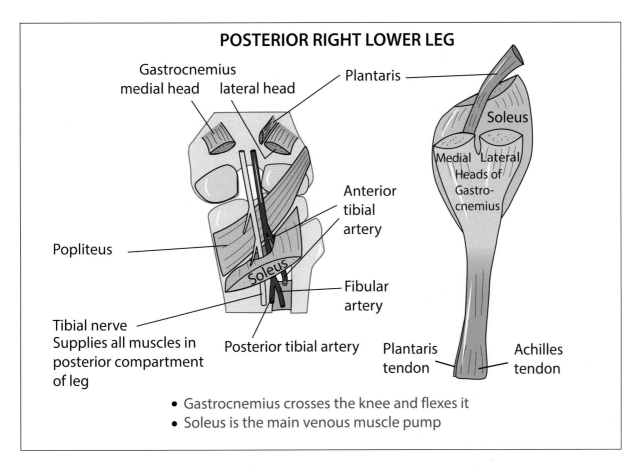

Gastrocnemius medial head lateral head

Plantaris

Soleus

Medial Lateral
Heads of
Gastro-
cnemius

Anterior tibial artery

Popliteus

Fibular artery

Soleus

Tibial nerve
Supplies all muscles in posterior compartment of leg

Posterior tibial artery

Plantaris tendon

Achilles tendon

- Gastrocnemius crosses the knee and flexes it
- Soleus is the main venous muscle pump

RIGHT LATERAL FIBULAR COMPARTMENT

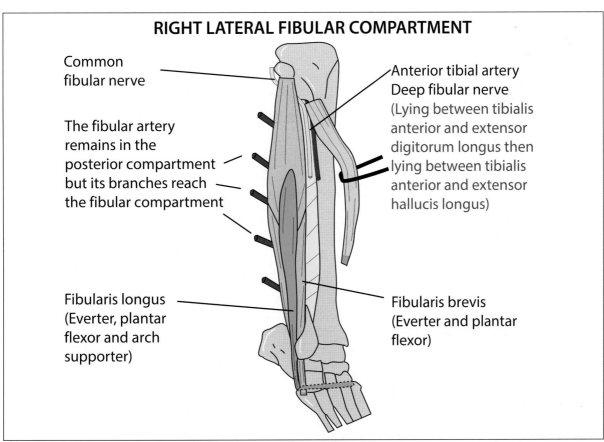

Common fibular nerve

Anterior tibial artery
Deep fibular nerve
(Lying between tibialis anterior and extensor digitorum longus then lying between tibialis anterior and extensor hallucis longus)

The fibular artery remains in the posterior compartment but its branches reach the fibular compartment

Fibularis longus
(Everter, plantar flexor and arch supporter)

Fibularis brevis
(Everter and plantar flexor)

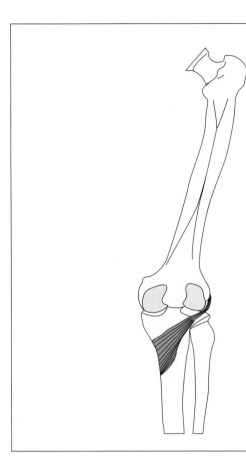

POPLITEUS

Arises: Upper posterior surface of tibia
Inserts: Lateral epicondyle of femur
Nerve: Tibial
Tendon: passes laterally, initially within the capsule of the knee then medial to the lateral collateral ligament and may lightly attach to lateral meniscus

Action: Laterally rotates femur on tibia to unlock the knee. It may be able to pull the lateral meniscus out of the way during the initial flexion of the knee after locking

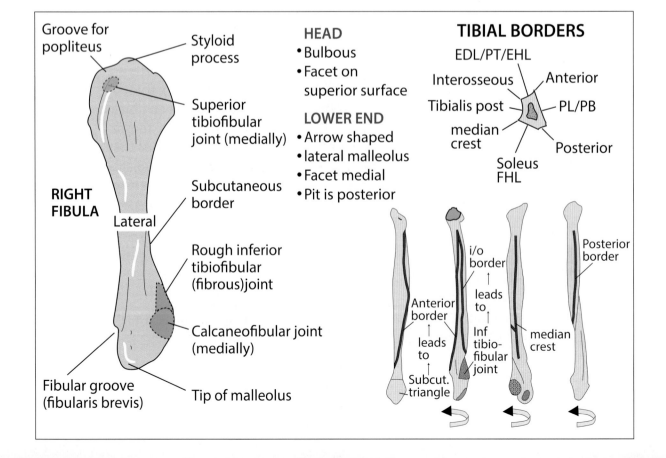

Groove for popliteus
Styloid process
Superior tibiofibular joint (medially)
Subcutaneous border
Rough inferior tibiofibular (fibrous) joint
Calcaneofibular joint (medially)
Tip of malleolus
Fibular groove (fibularis brevis)
RIGHT FIBULA
Lateral

HEAD
• Bulbous
• Facet on superior surface

LOWER END
• Arrow shaped
• lateral malleolus
• Facet medial
• Pit is posterior

TIBIAL BORDERS
EDL/PT/EHL
Interosseous
Tibialis post
median crest
Soleus FHL
Anterior
PL/PB
Posterior

Anterior border
leads to
Subcut. triangle

i/o border
leads to
Inf tibio-fibular joint

median crest

Posterior border

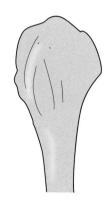

"SIDING" A FIBULA

HEAD
- Bulbous
- Facet on superior surface

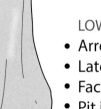

LOWER END
- Arrow shaped
- Lateral malleolus
- Facet medial
- Pit is posterior

TO "SIDE" A FIBULA
Hold the lower end of the fibula with the pulp of your thumb sitting comfortably in the pit. If it fits easily then the fibula is the same side as your hand. In this case it is a right fibula.
If it is not a comfortable fit then it belongs to the opposite side.

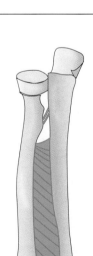

INTEROSSEOUS MEMBRANES

Forces from the hand and foot are transmitted respectively to the radius and tibia. In order to share the impact of the force the interosseous membranes have fibres arranged so that the ulna and the fibula can share the the strain easily and immediately

Right radius
and ulna

Left tibia
and fibula

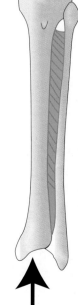

COMPARTMENT SYNDROMES OF LOWER LEG

SITE: Between tough deep fascia, intermuscular septa, bones and interosseous membrane

CAUSE: Trauma/infection leads to swelling, increased pressure, decreased perfusion, then ischaemia and tissue death

SYMPTOMS AND SIGNS: Pain, particularly on passive movement, decreased muscle and nerve function and loss of sensation. Pulse may be lost but often late in the course of events. A differential pressure between diastolic blood pressure and inter-compartmental pressure of 30mmHg or less is enough to cause damage and indicate the need for an operation

ANTERIOR: Pain, decreased dorsiflexion, extension of toes, loss of sensation in first dorsal skin cleft

LATERAL: Pain, decreased plantar flexion, inversion, loss of sensation of dorsal foot and toes

POSTERIOR: Divided by deep transverse intermuscular septum into superficial and deep syndromes. Superficial gives decreased plantar flexion and loss of sural nerve sensation. Deep gives decreased plantar and toe flexion, loss of tibial nerve sensation

COMPARTMENT SYNDROMES

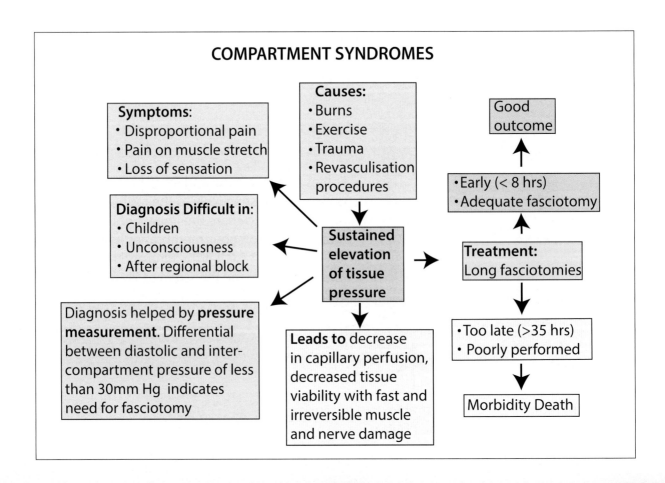

Symptoms:
- Disproportional pain
- Pain on muscle stretch
- Loss of sensation

Diagnosis Difficult in:
- Children
- Unconsciousness
- After regional block

Diagnosis helped by **pressure measurement**. Differential between diastolic and inter-compartment pressure of less than 30mm Hg indicates need for fasciotomy

Causes:
- Burns
- Exercise
- Trauma
- Revasculisation procedures

Sustained elevation of tissue pressure

Leads to decrease in capillary perfusion, decreased tissue viability with fast and irreversible muscle and nerve damage

Good outcome

- Early (< 8 hrs)
- Adequate fasciotomy

Treatment: Long fasciotomies

- Too late (>35 hrs)
- Poorly performed

Morbidity Death

COMPARTMENT SYNDROMES AND FASCIOTOMIES

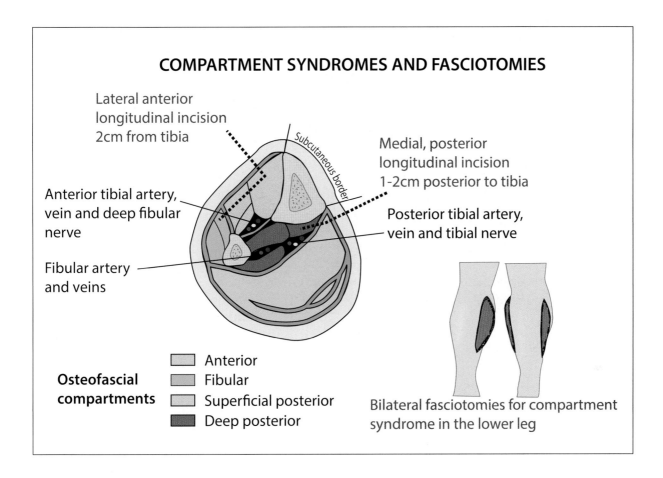

Lateral anterior longitudinal incision 2cm from tibia

Subcutaneous border

Medial, posterior longitudinal incision 1-2cm posterior to tibia

Anterior tibial artery, vein and deep fibular nerve

Posterior tibial artery, vein and tibial nerve

Fibular artery and veins

Osteofascial compartments

- Anterior
- Fibular
- Superficial posterior
- Deep posterior

Bilateral fasciotomies for compartment syndrome in the lower leg

2.5   Ankle and Foot

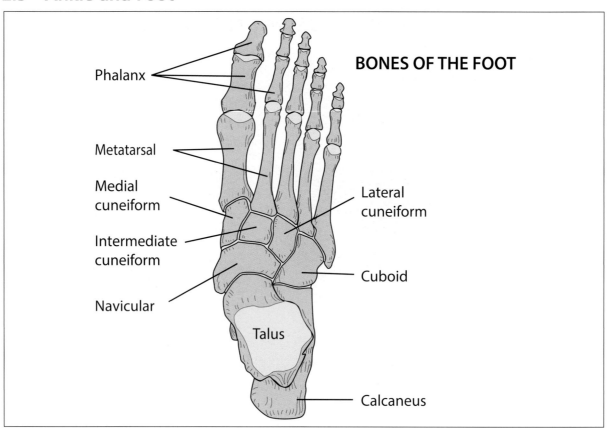

BONES OF THE FOOT

Phalanx

Metatarsal

Medial cuneiform

Intermediate cuneiform

Navicular

Lateral cuneiform

Cuboid

Talus

Calcaneus

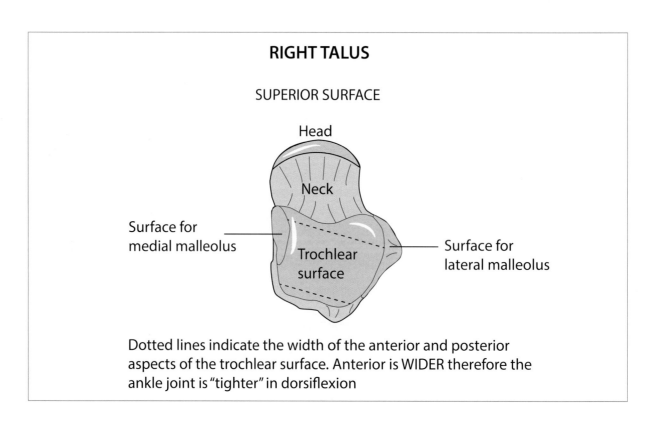

RIGHT TALUS

SUPERIOR SURFACE

Head

Neck

Surface for medial malleolus

Trochlear surface

Surface for lateral malleolus

Dotted lines indicate the width of the anterior and posterior aspects of the trochlear surface. Anterior is WIDER therefore the ankle joint is "tighter" in dorsiflexion

FRACTURE OF NECK OF TALUS

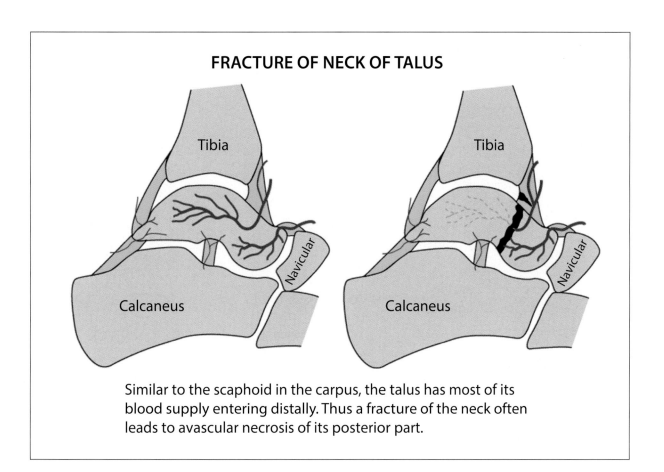

Similar to the scaphoid in the carpus, the talus has most of its blood supply entering distally. Thus a fracture of the neck often leads to avascular necrosis of its posterior part.

RIGHT CALCANEUS

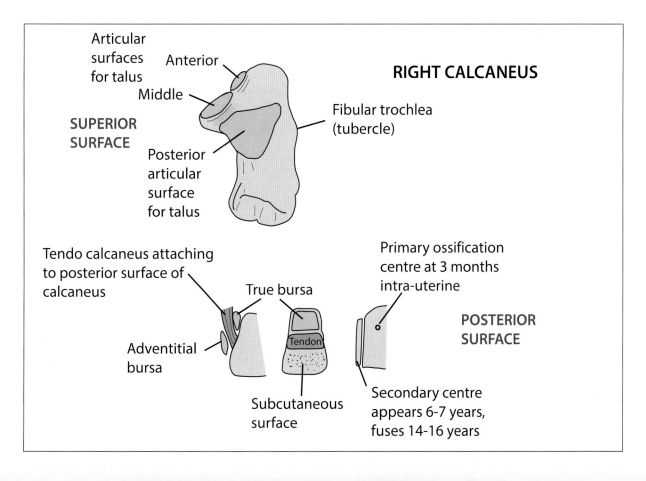

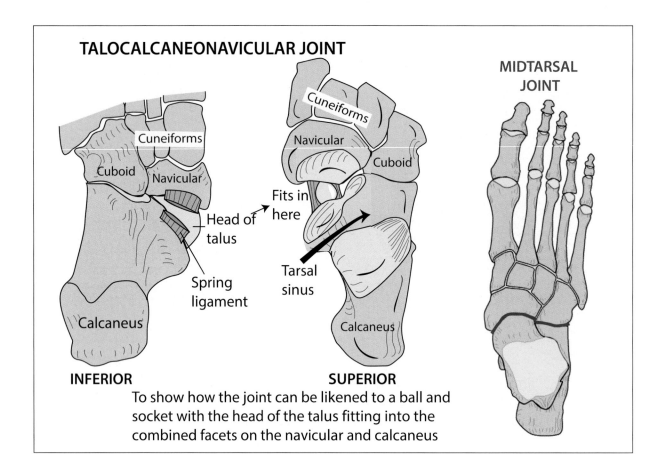

TALOCALCANEONAVICULAR JOINT

Cuneiforms

Navicular

Cuboid

Head of talus

Fits in here

Spring ligament

Tarsal sinus

Calcaneus

INFERIOR

Cuboid

Cuneiforms

Navicular

Calcaneus

SUPERIOR

To show how the joint can be likened to a ball and socket with the head of the talus fitting into the combined facets on the navicular and calcaneus

MIDTARSAL JOINT

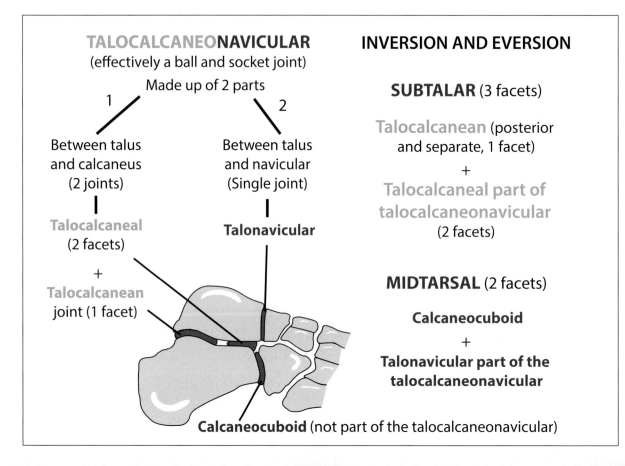

TALOCALCANEONAVICULAR
(effectively a ball and socket joint)

Made up of 2 parts

1

Between talus and calcaneus (2 joints)

Talocalcaneal (2 facets)

+

Talocalcanean joint (1 facet)

2

Between talus and navicular (Single joint)

Talonavicular

INVERSION AND EVERSION

SUBTALAR (3 facets)

Talocalcanean (posterior and separate, 1 facet)

+

Talocalcaneal part of talocalcaneonavicular (2 facets)

MIDTARSAL (2 facets)

Calcaneocuboid

+

Talonavicular part of the talocalcaneonavicular

Calcaneocuboid (not part of the talocalcaneonavicular)

ARCHES OF THE FOOT

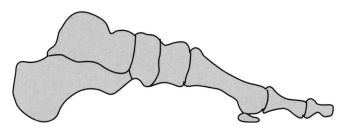

FOR:
Propulsion
Shock absorption
Resilience

FACTORS:
Shape of bones
Ligaments (+ plantar fascia)
Tendons
Tone of small muscles

There is varying dominance of each of these
factors in the medial, lateral and transverse arches

ARCHES OF THE FOOT

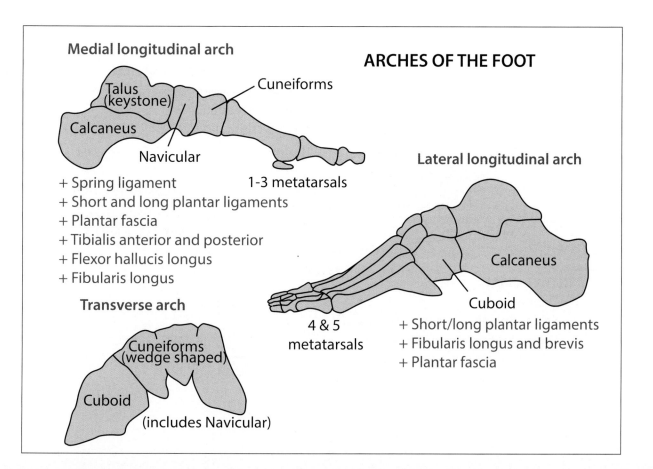

Medial longitudinal arch

Talus (keystone)

Cuneiforms

Calcaneus

Navicular

1-3 metatarsals

+ Spring ligament
+ Short and long plantar ligaments
+ Plantar fascia
+ Tibialis anterior and posterior
+ Flexor hallucis longus
+ Fibularis longus

Transverse arch

Cuneiforms (wedge shaped)

Cuboid

(includes Navicular)

Lateral longitudinal arch

Calcaneus

Cuboid

4 & 5 metatarsals

+ Short/long plantar ligaments
+ Fibularis longus and brevis
+ Plantar fascia

ACCESSORY OSSIFICATION OF FOOT BONES

Posterior process of talus may have its own ossification centre that fails to fuse = **OS TRIGONUM**

Both could be
mis-diagnosed as
a fracture

Similarly with the base of the
5th metatarsal = **OS VESALIANUM**

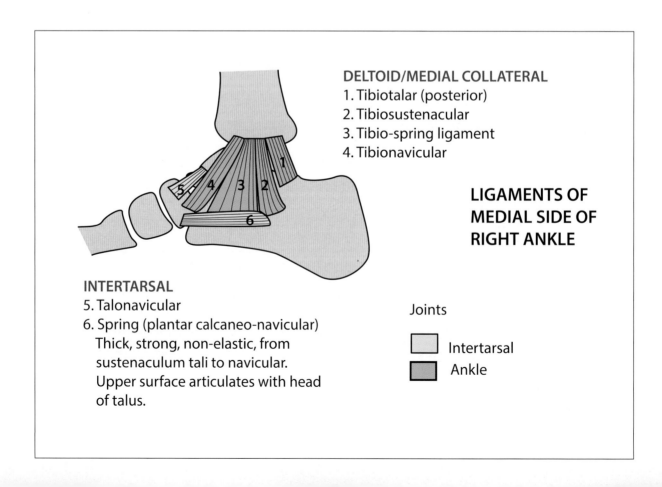

DELTOID/MEDIAL COLLATERAL
1. Tibiotalar (posterior)
2. Tibiosustenacular
3. Tibio-spring ligament
4. Tibionavicular

LIGAMENTS OF MEDIAL SIDE OF RIGHT ANKLE

INTERTARSAL
5. Talonavicular
6. Spring (plantar calcaneo-navicular)
   Thick, strong, non-elastic, from
   sustenaculum tali to navicular.
   Upper surface articulates with head
   of talus.

Joints

Intertarsal

Ankle

INFERIOR TIBIOFIBULAR LIGAMENT
1. Anterior tibiofibular
2. Posterior tibiofibular

LATERAL COLLATERAL LIGAMENT
3. Calcaneofibular
4. Anterior talofibular
5. Posterior talofibular

TARSAL/METATARSAL LIGAMENTS
6. Short/long plantar
7. Lateral talocalcaneal
8. Cervical
9. Bifurcate

LIGAMENTS ON LATERAL SIDE OF RIGHT ANKLE

Joints

- Inferior tibiofibular
- Ankle
- Intertarsal

POSTERIOR VIEW OF RIGHT ANKLE

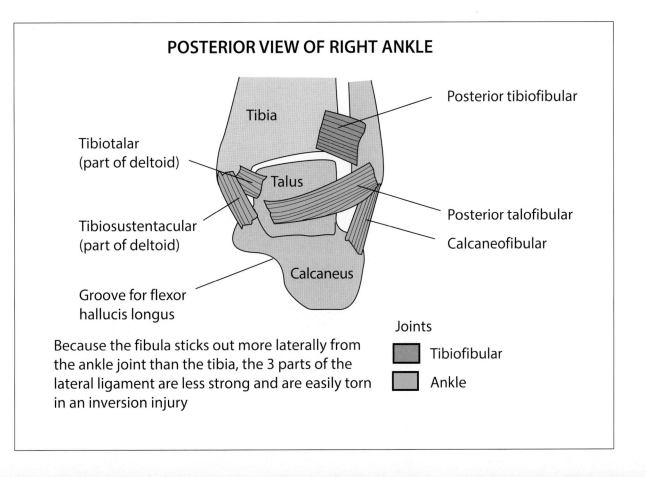

Posterior tibiofibular

Tibia

Tibiotalar
(part of deltoid)

Talus

Tibiosustentacular
(part of deltoid)

Posterior talofibular

Calcaneofibular

Calcaneus

Groove for flexor
hallucis longus

Joints

- Tibiofibular
- Ankle

Because the fibula sticks out more laterally from
the ankle joint than the tibia, the 3 parts of the
lateral ligament are less strong and are easily torn
in an inversion injury

INVERSION INJURIES OF ANKLE

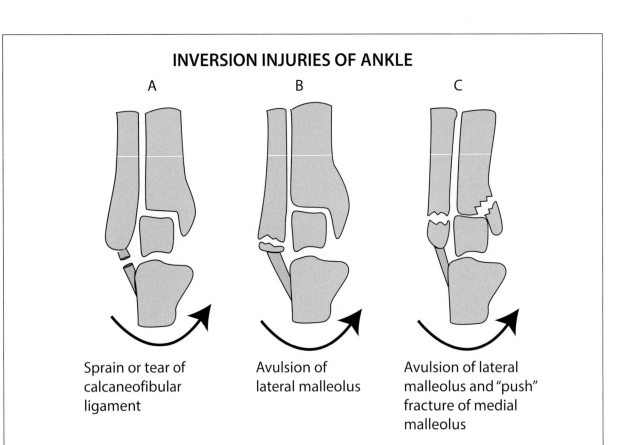

A

B

C

Sprain or tear of calcaneofibular ligament

Avulsion of lateral malleolus

Avulsion of lateral malleolus and "push" fracture of medial malleolus

TENDON AND NEUROVASCULAR RELATIONSHIPS ON MEDIAL ASPECTS OF ANKLE

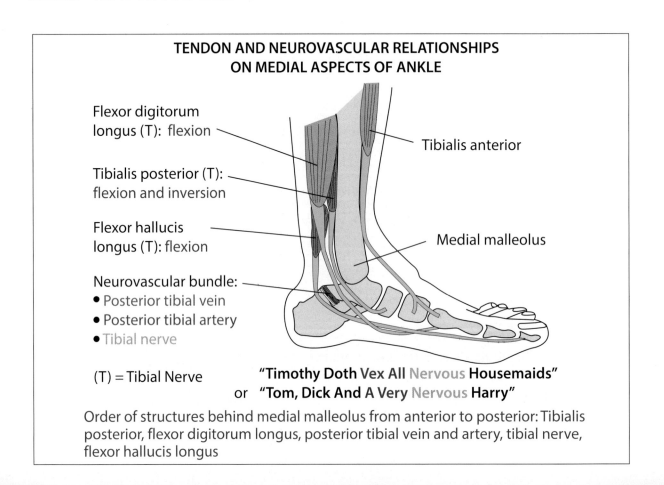

Flexor digitorum longus (T): flexion

Tibialis posterior (T): flexion and inversion

Flexor hallucis longus (T): flexion

Neurovascular bundle:
- Posterior tibial vein
- Posterior tibial artery
- Tibial nerve

Tibialis anterior

Medial malleolus

(T) = Tibial Nerve

"Timothy Doth Vex All Nervous Housemaids"
or **"Tom, Dick And A Very Nervous Harry"**

Order of structures behind medial malleolus from anterior to posterior: Tibialis posterior, flexor digitorum longus, posterior tibial vein and artery, tibial nerve, flexor hallucis longus

TENDON AND NEUROVASCULAR RELATIONSHIPS ON LATERAL ASPECTS OF RIGHT ANKLE

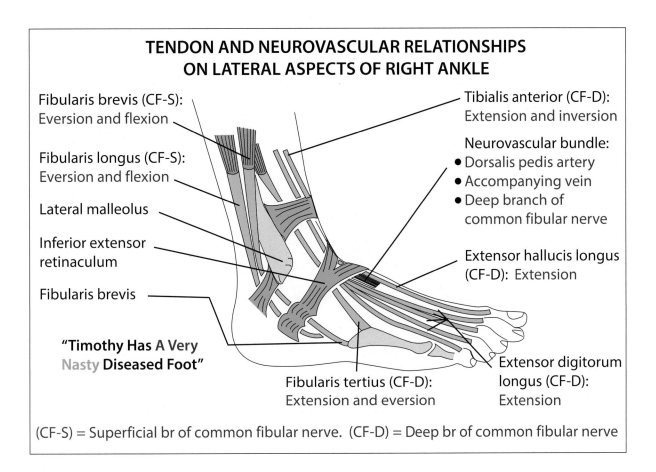

Fibularis brevis (CF-S): Eversion and flexion

Fibularis longus (CF-S): Eversion and flexion

Lateral malleolus

Inferior extensor retinaculum

Fibularis brevis

"Timothy Has A Very Nasty Diseased Foot"

Tibialis anterior (CF-D): Extension and inversion

Neurovascular bundle:
- Dorsalis pedis artery
- Accompanying vein
- Deep branch of common fibular nerve

Extensor hallucis longus (CF-D): Extension

Extensor digitorum longus (CF-D): Extension

Fibularis tertius (CF-D): Extension and eversion

(CF-S) = Superficial br of common fibular nerve. (CF-D) = Deep br of common fibular nerve

---

INVERSION AND EVERSION

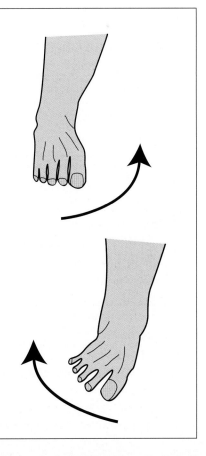

INVERSION
Always with some adduction of toes.
Muscles: Tibialis anterior/posterior (+/– extensor hallucis longus and flexor digitorum longus).

EVERSION
Always with some abduction of toes.
Muscles: Fibularis longus/brevis; fibularis tertius and extensor digitorum longus when foot is extended.

NOTE: As all these tendons insert distal to the midtarsal joint; this joint moves first and a little. But soon reaches its maximum and the torque is then transmitted to the subtalar joint which gives most of each movement.

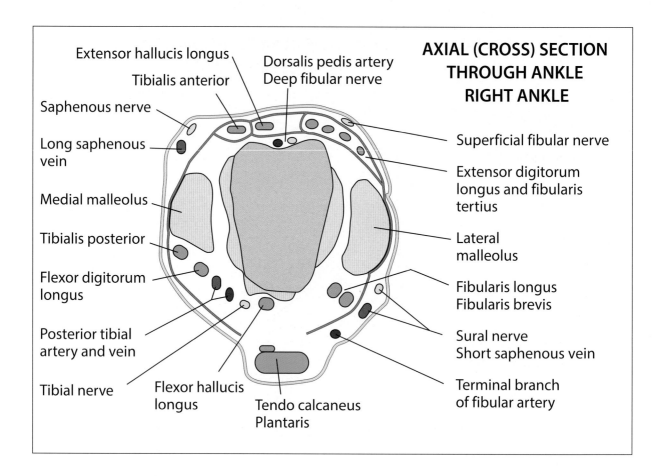

Extensor hallucis longus
Tibialis anterior
Saphenous nerve
Long saphenous vein
Medial malleolus
Tibialis posterior
Flexor digitorum longus
Posterior tibial artery and vein
Tibial nerve
Flexor hallucis longus
Tendo calcaneus Plantaris
Dorsalis pedis artery
Deep fibular nerve

AXIAL (CROSS) SECTION THROUGH ANKLE RIGHT ANKLE

Superficial fibular nerve
Extensor digitorum longus and fibularis tertius
Lateral malleolus
Fibularis longus Fibularis brevis
Sural nerve Short saphenous vein
Terminal branch of fibular artery

COMPARISON OF MUSCLES/TENDONS AND THEIR NERVE SUPPLY IN HAND AND FOOT

HAND MUSCLES (palmar)	NERVE IN HAND	FOOT MUSCLES (plantar)	NERVE IN FOOT
Interossei(ref to middle finger)	Ulnar	Interossei (ref to 2nd toe)	Lateral plantar
Lumbricals 1 and 2	Median	Lumbricals 1	Medial plantar
Lumbricals 3, 4	Ulnar	Lumbricals 2, 3, 4	Lateral plantar
Thenar (abductor pollicis brevis, flexor pollicis brevis, opponens pollicis	Median	To hallux (abductor hallucis flexor hallucis brevis)	Medial plantar
Adductor pollicis	Ulnar	Adductor hallucis	Lateral plantar
Hypothenar (abductor digiti minimi, flexor digiti minimi brevis, opponens digiti minimi)	Ulnar	To 5th toe (abductor digiti minimi, flexor digiti minimi brevis)	Lateral plantar
Flexor digitorum superficialis	Median	Flexor digitorum brevis	Medial plantar

Note: There is no equivalent in the upper limb of **quadratus plantae** (flexor accessorius) which is supplied by the lateral plantar nerve. Easy to remember as this muscle arises on the lateral side of the foot.

This table clearly shows that the lateral plantar nerve is the equivalent to the ulnar nerve and the medial plantar is equivalent to the median nerve.

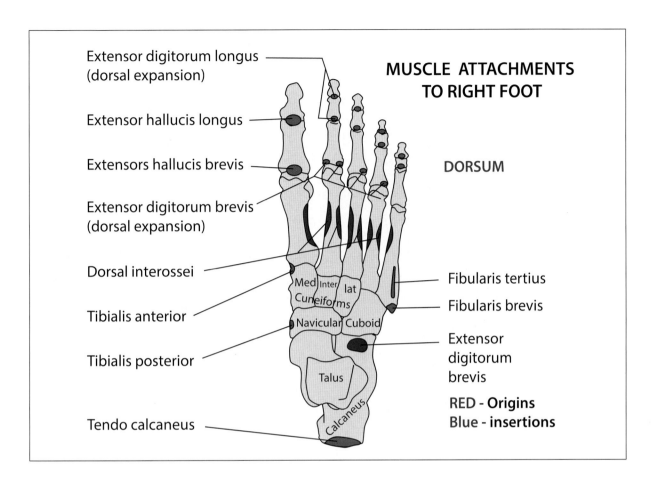

Extensor digitorum longus (dorsal expansion)

Extensor hallucis longus

Extensors hallucis brevis

Extensor digitorum brevis (dorsal expansion)

Dorsal interossei

Tibialis anterior

Tibialis posterior

Tendo calcaneus

MUSCLE ATTACHMENTS TO RIGHT FOOT

DORSUM

Med Inter lat Cuneiforms

Navicular Cuboid

Talus

Calcaneus

Fibularis tertius

Fibularis brevis

Extensor digitorum brevis

RED - Origins
Blue - insertions

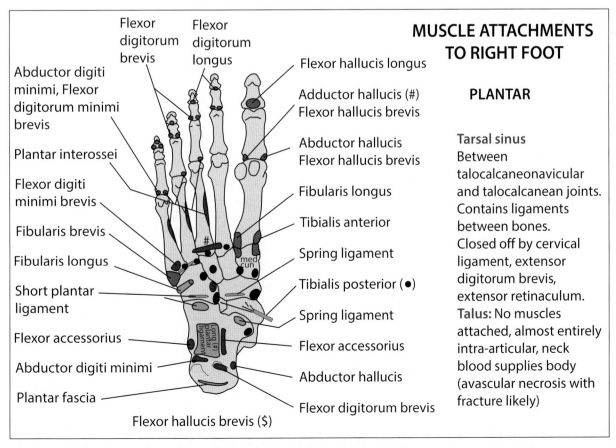

Flexor digitorum brevis

Flexor digitorum longus

Abductor digiti minimi, Flexor digitorum minimi brevis

Plantar interossei

Flexor digiti minimi brevis

Fibularis brevis

Fibularis longus

Short plantar ligament

Flexor accessorius

Abductor digiti minimi

Plantar fascia

Flexor hallucis brevis ($)

Flexor hallucis longus

Adductor hallucis (#)
Flexor hallucis brevis

Abductor hallucis
Flexor hallucis brevis

Fibularis longus

Tibialis anterior

Spring ligament

Tibialis posterior (●)

Spring ligament

Flexor accessorius

Abductor hallucis

Flexor digitorum brevis

med cun

Long (#) plantar ligament

MUSCLE ATTACHMENTS TO RIGHT FOOT

PLANTAR

Tarsal sinus Between talocalcaneonavicular and talocalcanean joints. Contains ligaments between bones. Closed off by cervical ligament, extensor digitorum brevis, extensor retinaculum. **Talus:** No muscles attached, almost entirely intra-articular, neck blood supplies body (avascular necrosis with fracture likely)

ARTERIES IN SOLE OF RIGHT FOOT

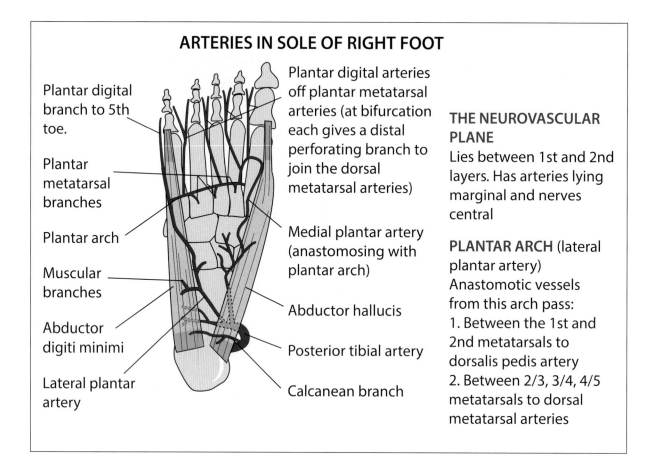

Plantar digital branch to 5th toe.

Plantar metatarsal branches

Plantar arch

Muscular branches

Abductor digiti minimi

Lateral plantar artery

Plantar digital arteries off plantar metatarsal arteries (at bifurcation each gives a distal perforating branch to join the dorsal metatarsal arteries)

Medial plantar artery (anastomosing with plantar arch)

Abductor hallucis

Posterior tibial artery

Calcanean branch

THE NEUROVASCULAR PLANE
Lies between 1st and 2nd layers. Has arteries lying marginal and nerves central

PLANTAR ARCH (lateral plantar artery)
Anastomotic vessels from this arch pass:
1. Between the 1st and 2nd metatarsals to dorsalis pedis artery
2. Between 2/3, 3/4, 4/5 metatarsals to dorsal metatarsal arteries

DORSUM OF LEFT FOOT

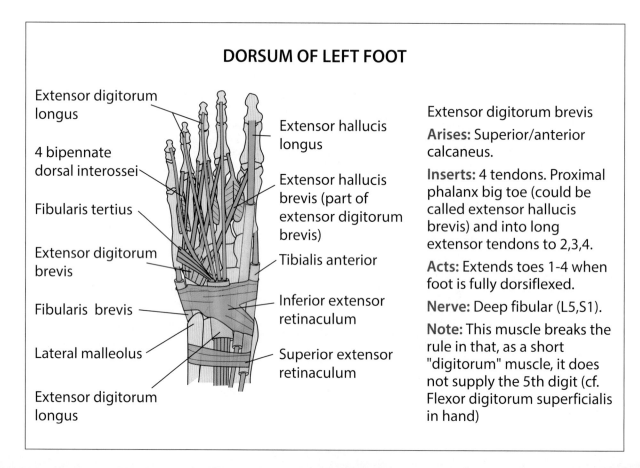

Extensor digitorum longus

4 bipennate dorsal interossei

Fibularis tertius

Extensor digitorum brevis

Fibularis brevis

Lateral malleolus

Extensor digitorum longus

Extensor hallucis longus

Extensor hallucis brevis (part of extensor digitorum brevis)

Tibialis anterior

Inferior extensor retinaculum

Superior extensor retinaculum

Extensor digitorum brevis

Arises: Superior/anterior calcaneus.

Inserts: 4 tendons. Proximal phalanx big toe (could be called extensor hallucis brevis) and into long extensor tendons to 2,3,4.

Acts: Extends toes 1-4 when foot is fully dorsiflexed.

Nerve: Deep fibular (L5,S1).

Note: This muscle breaks the rule in that, as a short "digitorum" muscle, it does not supply the 5th digit (cf. Flexor digitorum superficialis in hand)

LAYERS OF THE SOLE OF FOOT

PLANTAR APONEUROSIS

LAYER 1   3 MUSCLES (ABH, ABDM, FDB)

NEUROVASCULAR PLANE

LAYER 2   2 MUSCLES (LUMBRICALS, ACCESSORIUS)
2 TENDONS (FHL, FDL)

LAYER 3   3 MUSCLES (ADH, FHB, FDMB)
2 LIGAMENTS (SPRING, LONG PLANTAR)

LAYER 4   1 MUSCLE (INTEROSSEI)
1 LIGAMENT (SHORT PLANTAR)
3 TENDONS (FL, TP, TA)

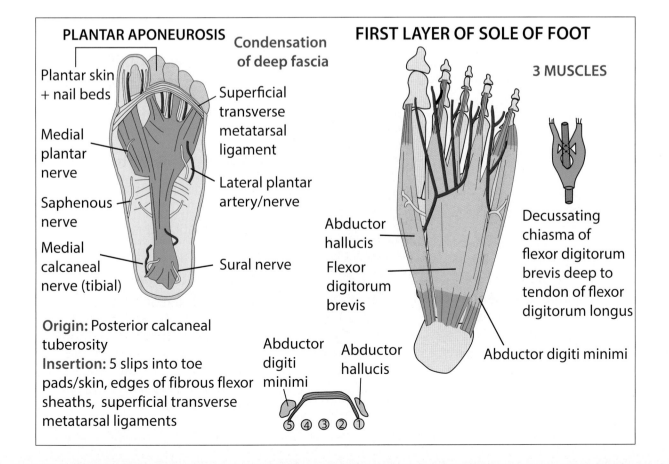

PLANTAR APONEUROSIS Condensation of deep fascia

Plantar skin + nail beds

Medial plantar nerve

Saphenous nerve

Medial calcaneal nerve (tibial)

Superficial transverse metatarsal ligament

Lateral plantar artery/nerve

Sural nerve

Origin: Posterior calcaneal tuberosity
Insertion: 5 slips into toe pads/skin, edges of fibrous flexor sheaths, superficial transverse metatarsal ligaments

Abductor digiti minimi   Abductor hallucis

⑤ ④ ③ ② ①

FIRST LAYER OF SOLE OF FOOT

3 MUSCLES

Abductor hallucis

Flexor digitorum brevis

Decussating chiasma of flexor digitorum brevis deep to tendon of flexor digitorum longus

Abductor digiti minimi

SECOND LAYER OF SOLE OF LEFT FOOT
2 MUSCLES
2 TENDONS

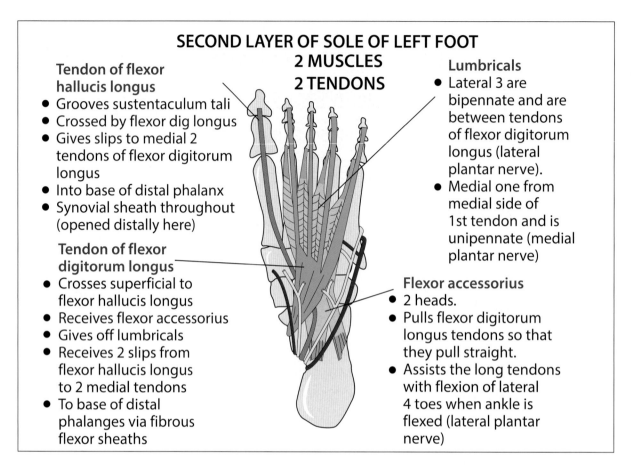

Tendon of flexor hallucis longus
- Grooves sustentaculum tali
- Crossed by flexor dig longus
- Gives slips to medial 2 tendons of flexor digitorum longus
- Into base of distal phalanx
- Synovial sheath throughout (opened distally here)

Tendon of flexor digitorum longus
- Crosses superficial to flexor hallucis longus
- Receives flexor accessorius
- Gives off lumbricals
- Receives 2 slips from flexor hallucis longus to 2 medial tendons
- To base of distal phalanges via fibrous flexor sheaths

Lumbricals
- Lateral 3 are bipennate and are between tendons of flexor digitorum longus (lateral plantar nerve).
- Medial one from medial side of 1st tendon and is unipennate (medial plantar nerve)

Flexor accessorius
- 2 heads.
- Pulls flexor digitorum longus tendons so that they pull straight.
- Assists the long tendons with flexion of lateral 4 toes when ankle is flexed (lateral plantar nerve)

THIRD LAYER OF SOLE OF LEFT FOOT

3 MUSCLES
2 LIGAMENTS

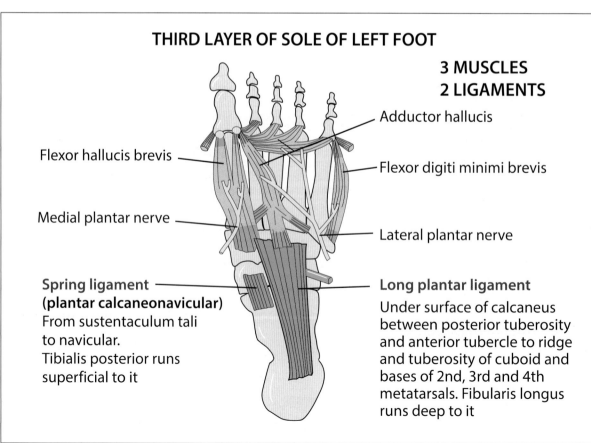

Adductor hallucis

Flexor hallucis brevis

Flexor digiti minimi brevis

Medial plantar nerve

Lateral plantar nerve

Spring ligament (plantar calcaneonavicular)
From sustentaculum tali to navicular.
Tibialis posterior runs superficial to it

Long plantar ligament
Under surface of calcaneus between posterior tuberosity and anterior tubercle to ridge and tuberosity of cuboid and bases of 2nd, 3rd and 4th metatarsals. Fibularis longus runs deep to it

FOURTH LAYER OF SOLE OF LEFT FOOT

**1 MUSCLE
1 LIGAMENT
3 TENDONS**

Unipennate plantar interossei arise medial sides of 3,4,5 metatarsals, insert medial bases of proximal phalanges with slips to dorsal expansion of 3,4,5. Adduct 3,4,5 toes and assists lumbricals to extend interphalangeal joints and flex metatarsophalangeal joints. **Nerve:** deep branch of lateral plantar nerve.

Tibialis anterior tendon (Inserts into medial side of base of 1st metatarsal and medial cuneiform)

Tibialis posterior tendon

Dorsal and plantar interossei

Fibularis longus tendon (In synovial sheath between long and short plantar ligaments. Across cuboid and cuneiforms into lateral base of 1st metatarsal and medial cuneiform)

Short plantar ligament (plantar calcaneocuboid) (Anterior calcaneal tubercle to cuboid)

SECTION 3

Thorax

3.1 Surface Anatomy and Breast

Dermatomes

Nipples in T4 dermatome
Umbilicus in T10 dermatome

VERTEBRAL LEVELS IN THORAX

T2/3 **Suprasternal notch**

T3 Spine of T3; posterior end of oblique fissure of lung

T3-4 Manubrium; vertebral bodies of T3 and T4

T3/4 Top of aortic arch

T4/5 **Manubriosternal junction** (Angle of Louis): under surface of arch of aorta; bifurcation of pulmonary artery; bifurcation of trachea; left recurrent laryngeal nerve; ligamentum arteriosum; rib 2 anteriorly

T5 Thoracic duct crosses midline

T8 **Caval opening in diaphragm:** IVC with right phrenic nerve; left phrenic pierces muscle of diaphragm; hemi-azygos veins cross to right to join azygos vein

T10 **Oesophageal opening in diaphragm:** oesophagus; branches of left gastric vessels; vagus nerves

T12 **Aortic opening in diaphragm:** aorta; azygos and hemi-azygos veins; thoracic duct; origin of coeliac axis

RIB ARTICULATIONS WITH VERTEBRAE

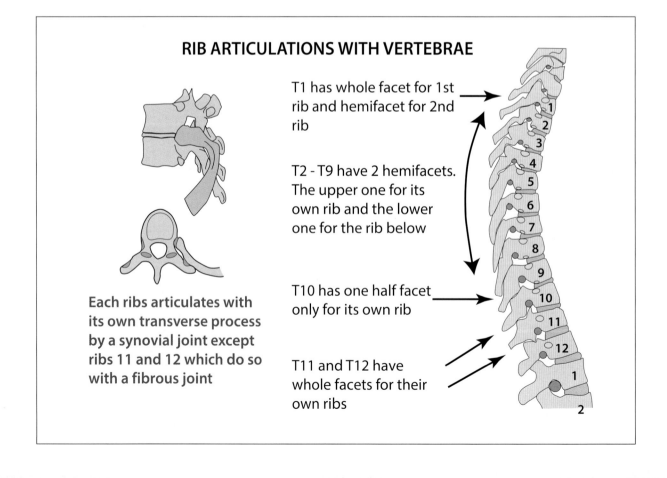

T1 has whole facet for 1st rib and hemifacet for 2nd rib

T2 - T9 have 2 hemifacets. The upper one for its own rib and the lower one for the rib below

T10 has one half facet only for its own rib

T11 and T12 have whole facets for their own ribs

Each ribs articulates with its own transverse process by a synovial joint except ribs 11 and 12 which do so with a fibrous joint

COSTOTRANSVERSE LIGAMENTS

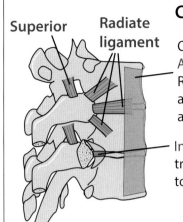

Superior   Radiate ligament

Other ligaments include:
Anterior longitudinal ligament
Runs along anterior bodies and attaches firmly to vertebral body and disc

Intra-articular ligament: From transverse crest of head of rib to intervertebral disc

Radiate ligament (3 parts)
To body above (upper); to own body (lower); hypochordal bow (middle) which lies deep to anterior longitudinal ligament and blends with intervertebral disc and fibres from other side

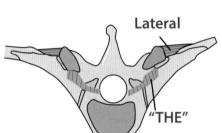

Lateral

"THE"

The costotransverse ligament connects rib to transverse process. It has 3 parts (confusing terminology):
"THE" costotransverse ligament
Fills gap between rib and its own transverse process
LATERAL costotransverse ligament
Lies posteriorly and extends from transverse process to its own rib, just beyond the tubercle
SUPERIOR costotransverse ligament
A 2 layered ligament with fibres at right angles to each other (corresponding and continuous with the intercostal muscles). Passes from upper border of neck of rib to transverse process of vertebra above

SUPRA-11TH OR SUPRA-12TH INCISION

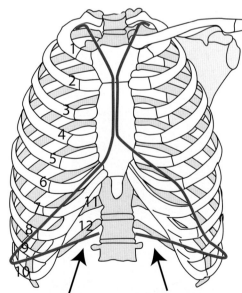

Superior costotransverse ligament

Radiate ligament

PLEURA POSTERIORLY EXTENDS JUST BELOW 12TH RIB

The periosteum of the rib is incised and lifted off the superior aspect. The rib must be mobilised by cutting the **SUPERIOR COSTOTRANSVERSE LIGAMENT** by running a pair of scissors along its superior surface.
Also the last few slips of the diaphragm must be cut to free it and avoid tearing the attached pleura.

STERNUM AND RELATED JOINTS

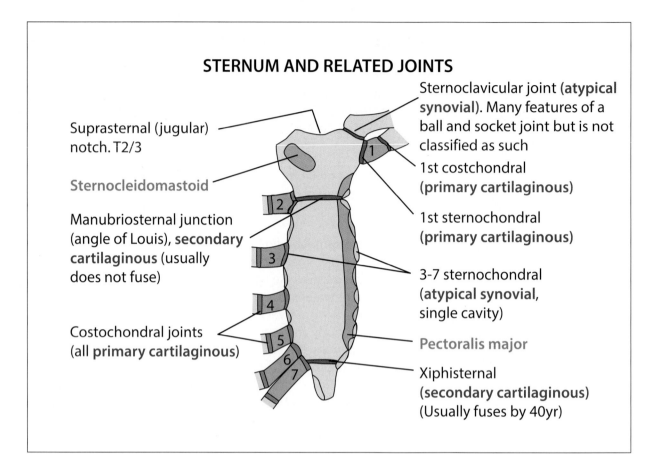

Suprasternal (jugular) notch. T2/3

Sternocleidomastoid

Manubriosternal junction (angle of Louis), **secondary cartilaginous** (usually does not fuse)

Costochondral joints (all **primary cartilaginous**)

Sternoclavicular joint (**atypical synovial**). Many features of a ball and socket joint but is not classified as such

1st costchondral (**primary cartilaginous**)

1st sternochondral (**primary cartilaginous**)

3-7 sternochondral (**atypical synovial, single cavity**)

Pectoralis major

Xiphisternal (**secondary cartilaginous**) (Usually fuses by 40yr)

CHEST WALL

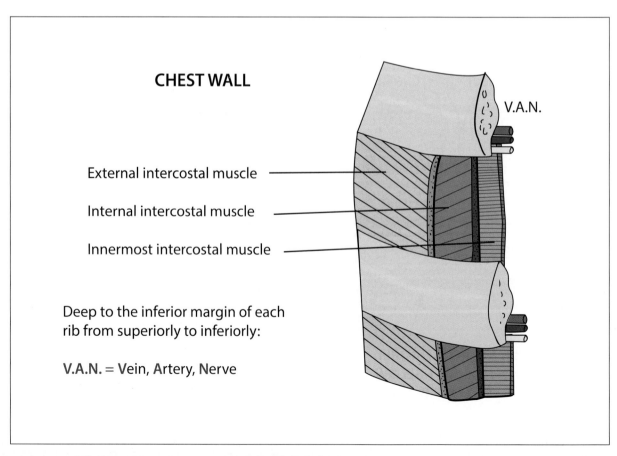

V.A.N.

External intercostal muscle

Internal intercostal muscle

Innermost intercostal muscle

Deep to the inferior margin of each rib from superiorly to inferiorly:

V.A.N. = Vein, Artery, Nerve

LEFT FIRST RIB

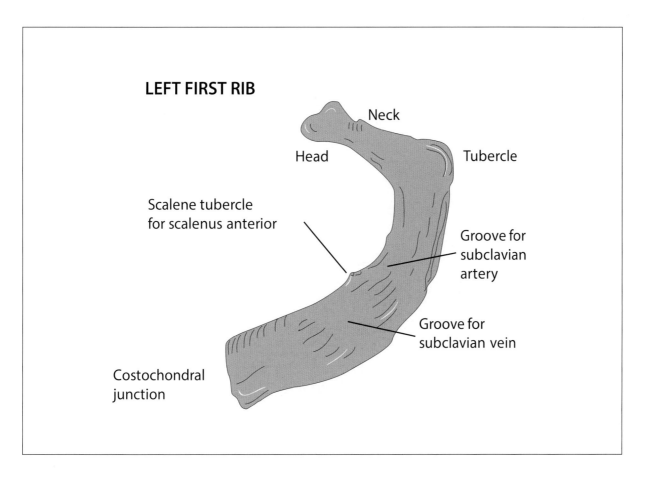

Neck

Head

Tubercle

Scalene tubercle
for scalenus anterior

Groove for
subclavian
artery

Groove for
subclavian vein

Costochondral
junction

RELATIONS AND ATTACHMENTS OF LEFT FIRST RIB

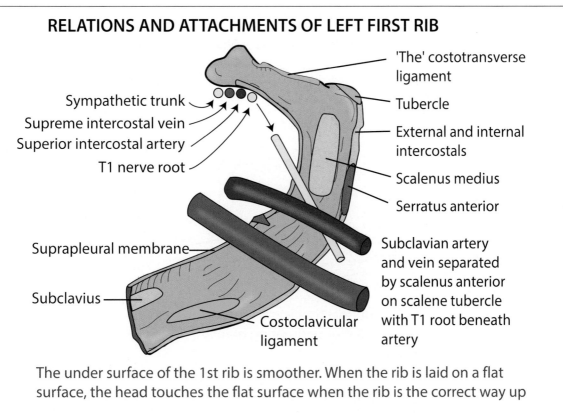

'The' costotransverse
ligament

Sympathetic trunk

Supreme intercostal vein

Superior intercostal artery

T1 nerve root

Tubercle

External and internal
intercostals

Scalenus medius

Serratus anterior

Suprapleural membrane

Subclavius

Costoclavicular
ligament

Subclavian artery
and vein separated
by scalenus anterior
on scalene tubercle
with T1 root beneath
artery

The under surface of the 1st rib is smoother. When the rib is laid on a flat
surface, the head touches the flat surface when the rib is the correct way up

TYPICAL INTERCOSTAL NERVE

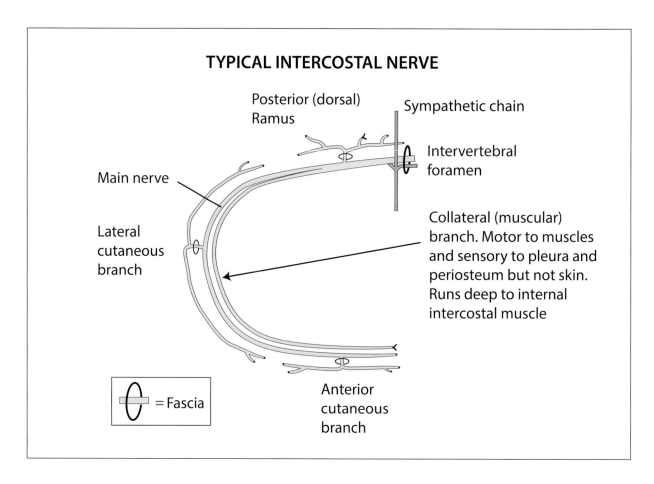

Posterior (dorsal) Ramus

Sympathetic chain

Main nerve

Intervertebral foramen

Lateral cutaneous branch

Collateral (muscular) branch. Motor to muscles and sensory to pleura and periosteum but not skin. Runs deep to internal intercostal muscle

⬭ = Fascia

Anterior cutaneous branch

INTERCOSTAL NERVES AND ARTERIES

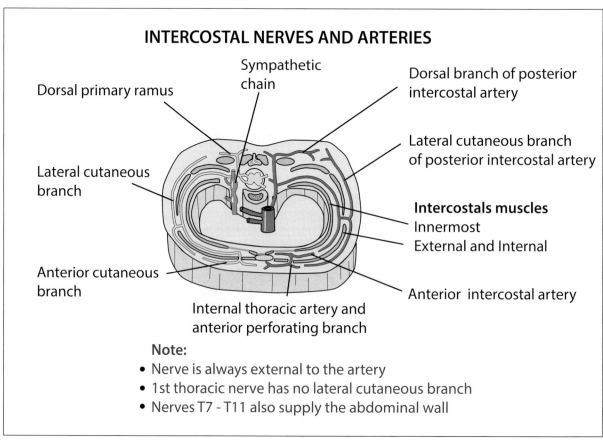

Dorsal primary ramus

Sympathetic chain

Dorsal branch of posterior intercostal artery

Lateral cutaneous branch

Lateral cutaneous branch of posterior intercostal artery

Lateral cutaneous branch

Intercostals muscles
Innermost
External and Internal

Anterior cutaneous branch

Internal thoracic artery and anterior perforating branch

Anterior intercostal artery

Note:
- Nerve is always external to the artery
- 1st thoracic nerve has no lateral cutaneous branch
- Nerves T7 - T11 also supply the abdominal wall

THORAX - SURFACE MARKINGS - CLINICAL IMPLICATIONS

Access to thoracic aorta: Through the left chest (left thoracotomy)
Access to oesophagus: Through right chest (right thoracotomy)
(Both of these are usually through the 5th intercostal space by stripping up the periosteum of the rib below and incising through the rib bed)
Thoraco-abdominal incision:
　For large access to upper abdomen or chest
　Through 9th intercostal space on either side
　9th costal cartilage is usually excised
　The diaphragm is incised radially to avoid damaging its nerve
Pericardial aspiration: Insert needle just to left of xiphoid
Pericardial window: Through left thoracotomy; 5th costal cartilage excised; Pericardial flap cut
Heart transplantation: Via median sternotomy; En bloc - aorta, pulmonary trunk, both atriae; SVC, IVC, SA node are all left in situ
Aspiration of pleural cavity: Siting of drain in 4th space in anterior axillary line

EXTENT OF LIVER IN THORAX

On the right it extends as far as the 4th or 5th rib and extends inferiorly to the 10th ribs

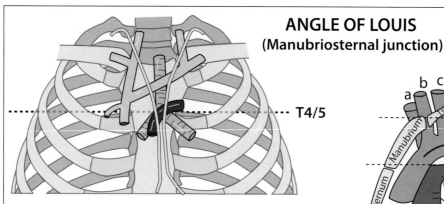

ANGLE OF LOUIS
(Manubriosternal junction)

Vertebral bodies of T3 and T4 lie posterior to the manubrium

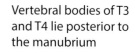
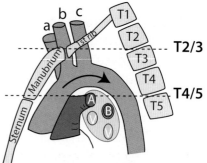

- Manubiosternal junction
- Division of superior and inferior mediastinum
- Second costal cartilage
- Under surface of aortic arch
- Bifurcation of pulmonary artery
- Bifurcation of trachea
- Ligamentum arteriosum
- Left recurrent laryngeal nerve
- Cardiac plexuses
- Azygos arch/vein enters superior vena cava
- Pleura initially meet superiorly

a = Brachiocephalic trunk
b = Left common carotid artery
c = Left subclavian artery
A = Left pulmonary artery
B = Left bronchus
V = Left pulmonary veins
T2/3 = Suprasternal notch
T4/5 = Sternomanubial junction

The direction of the arch is mostly posterior but also to the left

SURFACE MARKINGS OF PLEURA AND LUNGS

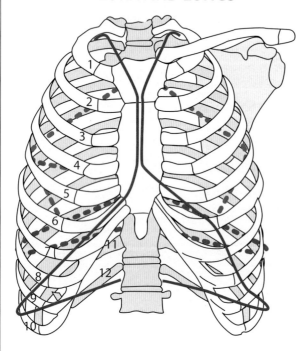

Pleura 2-4-6-8-10-12
Continuous Red line, starting 1" (2.5cm) above mid point of medial 1/3 of clavicle. Meet in midline at rib 2, left side then diverges at rib 4 to make room for the heart, whilst right continues parasternally to rib 6. Both cross rib 8 in the mid-clavicular line, then rib 10 in the mid-axillary line. Both reach posterior chest just below rib 12.

Lungs 2 less than pleura
Blue dotted lines indicate lower extension of lungs in expiration. Below ribs 6, the lungs extend to 2 rib spaces less than the pleura.

Fissures   3-6-4-5
(purple dotted lines)
Oblique: spine of T3 vertebra to rib 6 anteriorly along medial border scapula
Horizontal (on R only): rib/costal cartilage 4 to rib 5 in mid-axillary line.

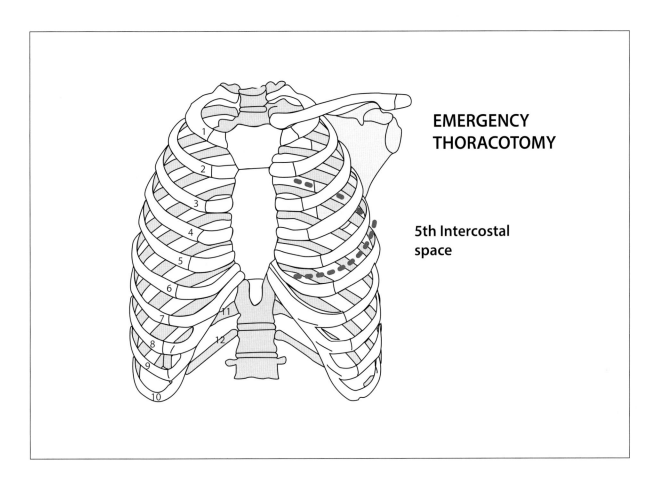

EMERGENCY THORACOTOMY

5th Intercostal space

FLAIL CHEST

Multiple chest wall fractures

During respiration the flail (detached) segment moves paradoxically - inwards when it should be expanding outwards and vice versa

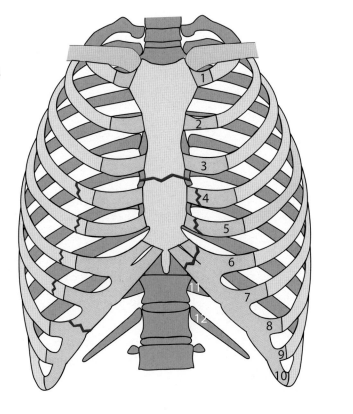

INTERCOSTAL DRAIN SITE

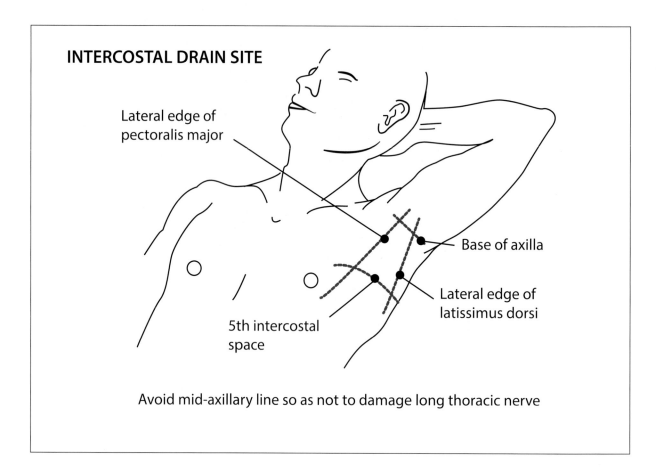

Lateral edge of pectoralis major

Base of axilla

Lateral edge of latissimus dorsi

5th intercostal space

Avoid mid-axillary line so as not to damage long thoracic nerve

MUSCLES OF THE BACK 1

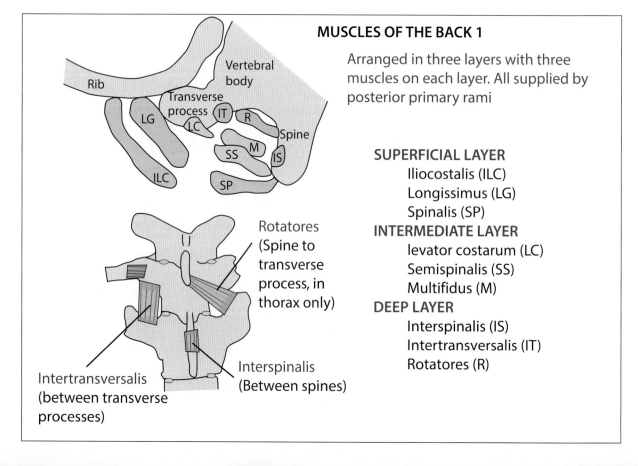

Rib

Vertebral body

Transverse process

LG

LC

IT

R

Spine

SS

M

IS

ILC

SP

Rotatores (Spine to transverse process, in thorax only)

Interspinalis (Between spines)

Intertransversalis (between transverse processes)

Arranged in three layers with three muscles on each layer. All supplied by posterior primary rami

SUPERFICIAL LAYER
 Iliocostalis (ILC)
 Longissimus (LG)
 Spinalis (SP)
INTERMEDIATE LAYER
 levator costarum (LC)
 Semispinalis (SS)
 Multifidus (M)
DEEP LAYER
 Interspinalis (IS)
 Intertransversalis (IT)
 Rotatores (R)

MUSCLES OF THE BACK 2

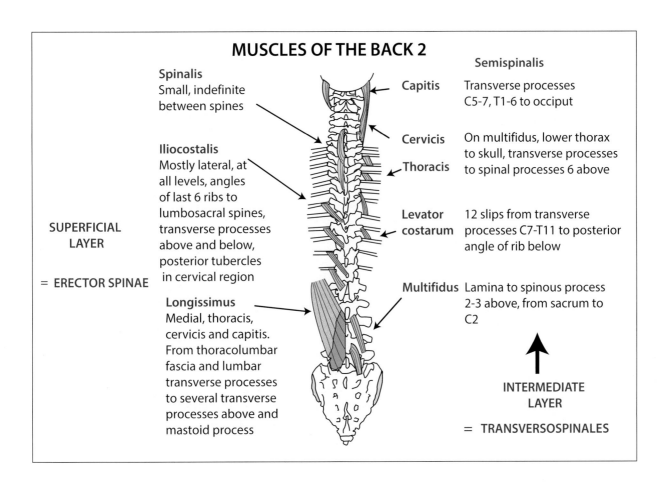

Spinalis
Small, indefinite between spines

Iliocostalis
Mostly lateral, at all levels, angles of last 6 ribs to lumbosacral spines, transverse processes above and below, posterior tubercles in cervical region

Longissimus
Medial, thoracis, cervicis and capitis. From thoracolumbar fascia and lumbar transverse processes to several transverse processes above and mastoid process

SUPERFICIAL LAYER

= ERECTOR SPINAE

Semispinalis

Capitis — Transverse processes C5-7, T1-6 to occiput

Cervicis — On multifidus, lower thorax to skull, transverse processes to spinal processes 6 above

Thoracis

Levator costarum — 12 slips from transverse processes C7-T11 to posterior angle of rib below

Multifidus — Lamina to spinous process 2-3 above, from sacrum to C2

INTERMEDIATE LAYER

= TRANSVERSOSPINALES

MUSCLES OF THE BACK 3

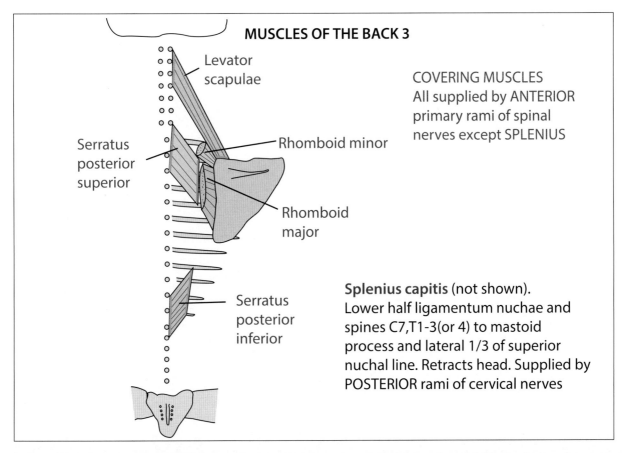

Levator scapulae

Serratus posterior superior

Rhomboid minor

Rhomboid major

Serratus posterior inferior

COVERING MUSCLES
All supplied by ANTERIOR primary rami of spinal nerves except SPLENIUS

Splenius capitis (not shown).
Lower half ligamentum nuchae and spines C7,T1-3(or 4) to mastoid process and lateral 1/3 of superior nuchal line. Retracts head. Supplied by POSTERIOR rami of cervical nerves

THE BREAST
(A modified sweat gland)

Lies on:
- Pectoralis major
- Serratus anterior
- External oblique
  (tail may curl round
  posterior to pectoralis
  minor)

Capsule:
- Posterior to breast
- Thickened Scarpa's fascia

Support:
- Suspensory ligaments
  of Astley Cooper from
  deep fascia to dermis

Structure:
- 15-20 lobes, each with
  15 lactiferous ducts leading
  to ampulla under areola then
  to nipple

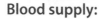

Position:
- On ribs 2-6 in midclavicular line
- Nipple in 4th intercostal space

Lymphatics:
- Run deep to capsule in
  sub-mammary space to-
- Axilla (anterior, apical,
  central nodes)
- Infraclavicular nodes
- Internal thoracic nodes
  (parasternal)
  NB: In disease
  lymph may go to:
  - Other side
  - Deep cervical
  - Into peritoneum
  - Inguinal

Blood supply:
- Internal thoracic (1st part subclavian)
- Lateral thoracic (2nd part axillary)
- Thoraco-acromial (2nd part axillary)
- Intercostal (internal thoracic)

3.2   Mediastinum, Thoracic Inlet, Diaphragm and Lymphatics

DIVISIONS OF THE MEDIASTINUM

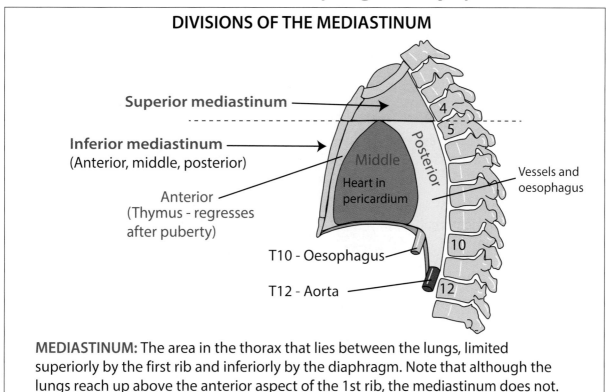

Superior mediastinum

Inferior mediastinum
(Anterior, middle, posterior)

Anterior
(Thymus - regresses
after puberty)

Middle

Heart in
pericardium

Posterior

Vessels and
oesophagus

T10 - Oesophagus

T12 - Aorta

4

5

10

12

MEDIASTINUM: The area in the thorax that lies between the lungs, limited superiorly by the first rib and inferiorly by the diaphragm. Note that although the lungs reach up above the anterior aspect of the 1st rib, the mediastinum does not.

RIGHT LATERAL VIEW OF MEDIASTINUM

LEFT LATERAL VIEW OF MEDIASTINUM

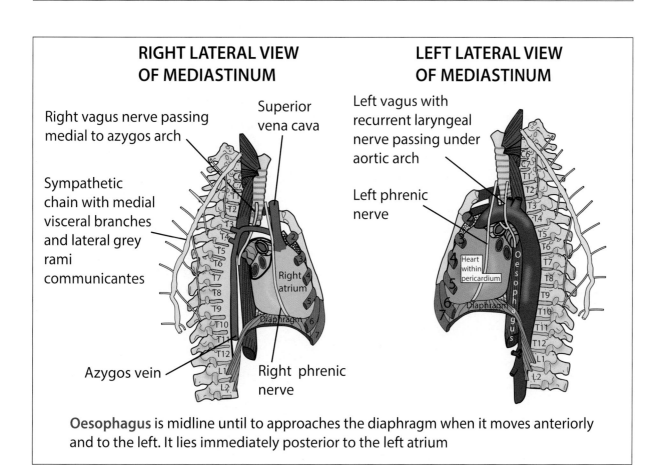

Right vagus nerve passing
medial to azygos arch

Sympathetic
chain with medial
visceral branches
and lateral grey
rami
communicantes

Superior
vena cava

Right
atrium

Diaphragm

Azygos vein

Right phrenic
nerve

Left vagus with
recurrent laryngeal
nerve passing under
aortic arch

Left phrenic
nerve

Heart
within
pericardium

Oesophagus

Diaphragm

Oesophagus is midline until to approaches the diaphragm when it moves anteriorly and to the left. It lies immediately posterior to the left atrium

MEDIASTINUM

The area in the thorax that lies between the lungs BUT does not extend above the first rib

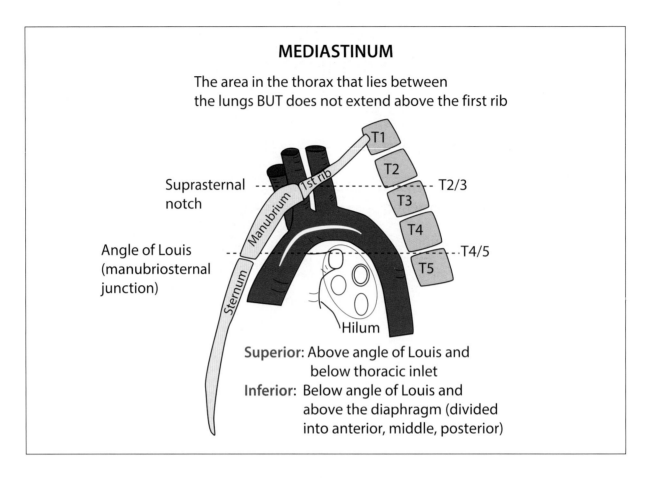

Suprasternal notch

Angle of Louis (manubriosternal junction)

Hilum

Superior: Above angle of Louis and below thoracic inlet

Inferior: Below angle of Louis and above the diaphragm (divided into anterior, middle, posterior)

THORACIC INLET

Note: T1 root comes up out of the thorax

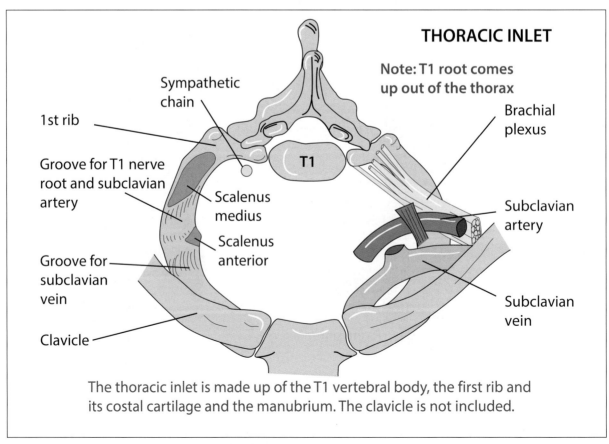

Sympathetic chain

1st rib

Groove for T1 nerve root and subclavian artery

Scalenus medius

Scalenus anterior

Groove for subclavian vein

Clavicle

Brachial plexus

Subclavian artery

Subclavian vein

The thoracic inlet is made up of the T1 vertebral body, the first rib and its costal cartilage and the manubrium. The clavicle is not included.

THORACIC INLET

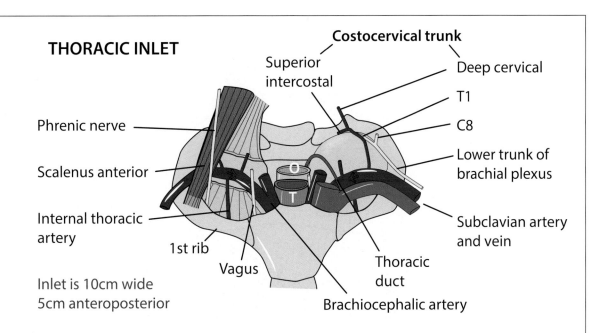

Costocervical trunk
Superior intercostal
Deep cervical
T1
C8
Phrenic nerve
Lower trunk of brachial plexus
Scalenus anterior
Internal thoracic artery
Subclavian artery and vein
1st rib
Vagus
Thoracic duct
Brachiocephalic artery

Inlet is 10cm wide
5cm anteroposterior

Dome of pleura is covered by suprapleural membrane (Sibson's fascia). Held up by scalenus minimis (pleuralis) from transverse process of C7 vertebra.
It extends 4cm above middle of medial third of clavicle and first rib, BUT NOT above neck of first rib

DIAPHRAGM - OPENINGS AND RELATIONS

OPENINGS
Caval (T8): Inferior vena cava and right phrenic nerve
Left muscular dome (T8): Left phrenic nerve
Anterior hiatus (T9): Superior epigastric artery and vein
Oesophageal (T10): Oesophagus, left and right vagus nerves, oesophageal branches of left gastric artery and vein, lymphatics
Aortic (T12) (Strictly posterior to diaphragm): Aorta, azygos vein and hemiazygos vein (may pass through left crus), thoracic duct
Crura (T12): Greater, lesser and least splanchnic nerves
Posterior to medial arcuate ligament: Sympathetic chain
Posterior to lateral arcuate ligament: Subcostal nerve (T12), artery and vein

RELATIONS
Right dome: Reaches 4th costal space (nipple) in expiration
Left dome: Reaches 5th rib in expiration
Superior: - Pericardium, basal lung segments
Inferior: - Right - liver, suprarenal, kidney
                    Left - stomach, suprarenal, kidney and spleen
Posterior: - Aorta, azygos veins, oesophagus, vagi, pleural folds

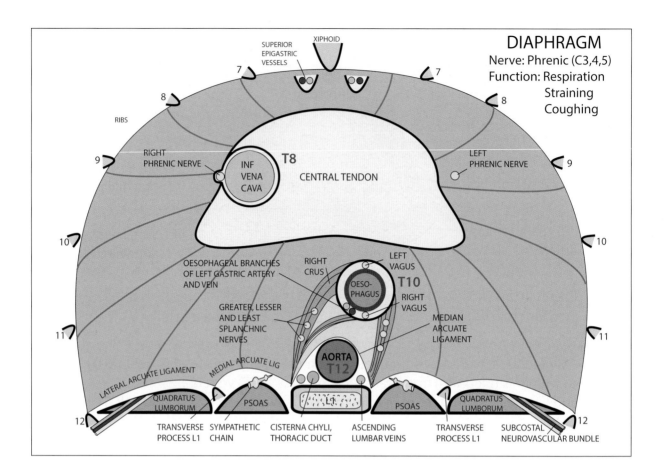

DIAPHRAGM
Nerve: Phrenic (C3,4,5)
Function: Respiration
Straining
Coughing

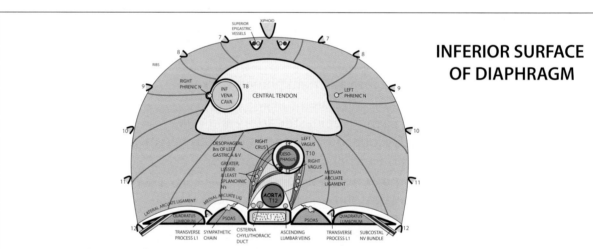

INFERIOR SURFACE
OF DIAPHRAGM

Origin: Vertebral - Right crus (L1,2,3), left crus (L1,2), 5 arcuate ligaments
Sternal - Xiphoid, Costal - Ribs and costal cartilages 7-12
Insertion: Central tendon (trefoil-1 anterior and 2 posterior, fused with pericardium)
Action: Inspiration - 70% at rest (5cm of movement). Less % on exertion (10cm movement)
Straining - Outlet of chest is fixed and larynx closed to raise intra-abdominal pressure
Nerve supply: Phrenic nerves - C3,4,5. 1/3 sensory, 2/3 motor. Diaphragm has no other
motor supply
Blood supply: Outer - lower 5 intercostals and subcostal arteries. Inner - Inferior phrenic
from aorta, musculophrenic/pericardiacophrenic from internal thoracic

CONGENITAL DIAPHRAGMATIC HERNIAS

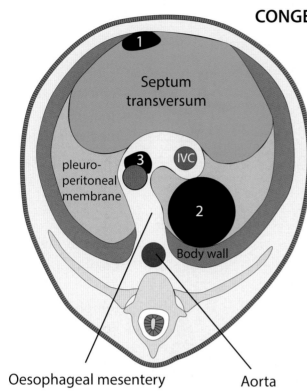

Septum transversum

pleuro-peritoneal membrane

IVC

Body wall

Oesophageal mesentery

Aorta

Development of diaphragm from:
1. Septum transversum
2. Pleuroperitoneal membrane
3. Oesophageal mesentery
4. Body wall

Sites of hernias:
1. Foramen of **M**orgagni (Parasternal - nearly "**m**idline")

2. Foramen of **B**ochdalek (at "**b**ack") (Pleuroperitoneal hernia)

3. Oesophageal hiatus

4. Dome of diaphragm (not shown)

LYMPHATICS IN THE THORAX

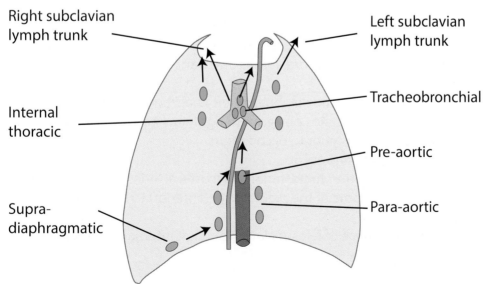

Right subclavian lymph trunk

Left subclavian lymph trunk

Internal thoracic

Tracheobronchial

Pre-aortic

Para-aortic

Supra-diaphragmatic

Normal drainage from the breast is to anterior and posterior axillary, infraclavicular and internal thoracic groups of nodes. With pathological blockage from disease, the spread can to be to opposite side, cervical, peritoneal cavity, liver and occasionally to inguinal nodes.

LYMPHATIC DRAINAGE

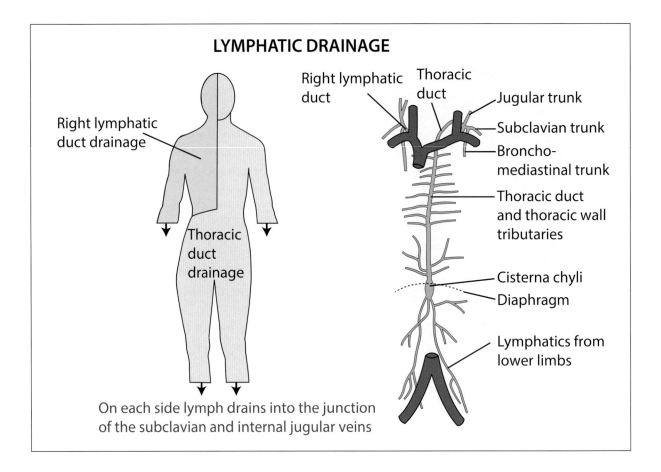

Right lymphatic duct

Thoracic duct

Right lymphatic duct drainage

Jugular trunk

Subclavian trunk

Broncho-mediastinal trunk

Thoracic duct and thoracic wall tributaries

Thoracic duct drainage

Cisterna chyli

Diaphragm

Lymphatics from lower limbs

On each side lymph drains into the junction of the subclavian and internal jugular veins

THORACIC DUCT

1. 45cm long (see also spinal cord, femur, vas, transverse colon, teeth to cardia)
2. Many valves in system
3. Drains all lymph below the diaphragm, left head/neck and left thorax
4. Commences at T12, ascends posterior to right crus; to right of aorta and oesophagus, then posterior to oesophagus
5. Crosses to left of midline at T5
6. Lies superficial (anterior) to posterior intercostal arteries and the crossing azygos systems; over the dome of the pleura; over (anterior) to left vertebral and left subclavian arteries
7. Enters into confluence of left subclavian and left internal jugular veins

THORACIC DUCT 1

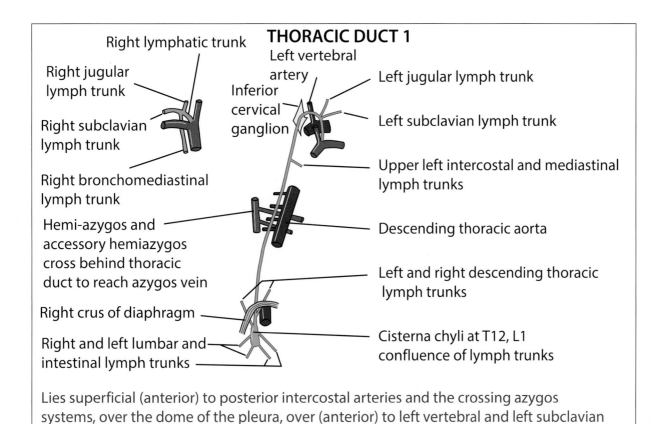

Right lymphatic trunk

Right jugular lymph trunk

Right subclavian lymph trunk

Right bronchomediastinal lymph trunk

Hemi-azygos and accessory hemiazygos cross behind thoracic duct to reach azygos vein

Right crus of diaphragm

Right and left lumbar and intestinal lymph trunks

Left vertebral artery

Inferior cervical ganglion

Left jugular lymph trunk

Left subclavian lymph trunk

Upper left intercostal and mediastinal lymph trunks

Descending thoracic aorta

Left and right descending thoracic lymph trunks

Cisterna chyli at T12, L1 confluence of lymph trunks

Lies superficial (anterior) to posterior intercostal arteries and the crossing azygos systems, over the dome of the pleura, over (anterior) to left vertebral and left subclavian arteries, into confluence of left subclavian and left internal jugular veins.

THORACIC DUCT 2

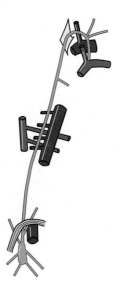

Several terminal branches. Many valves in the system

↑

Drains all lymph below diaphragm, left head/neck and left thorax

↑

45cm long (similar in length to the spinal cord, femur, vas, transverse colon and distance between teeth and oesophagogastric junction)

↑

Commences at T12, ascends behind right crus, to right of aorta and oesophagus. Then crosses the midline behind the oesophagus at T5

3.3 Heart and Pericardium

HEART

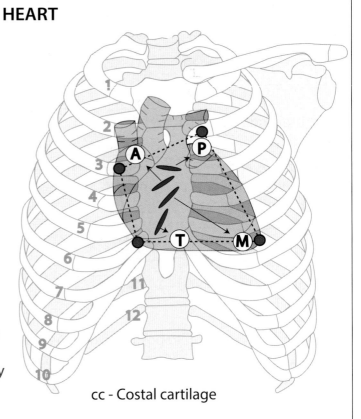

BORDERS: ●------●

2cc - 3cc - 6cc - 5 1/2

VALVES:

P - A - M - T

AUSCULTATION:
P - 2L (parasternal space)
A - 2R (parasternal space)
M - 5L (mid clavicular line)
T - Lower left sternal border

As the valves open and close they produce sounds that appear to be transmitted in the direction of the flow of blood. Thus, by picturing the heart and the positions of the four valves it is easy to work out the likely points for maximal audibility of the sounds.

cc - Costal cartilage

HEART, HEART VALVES AND SITES OF AUSCULTATION

Surface anatomy: Normal sized heart in thorax. **Borders:** Anticlockwise starting from upper left: Left 2nd costal cartilage to right 3rd costal cartilage to right 6th costal cartilage to left 5th intercostal space in the mid-clavicular line (summary 2-3-6-51/2)
Auscultation: As the valves open and close they produce sounds that are transmitted in the direction of blood flow. The 4 valves lie behind the sternum. Sounds are transmitted as follows:
PULMONARY - 2nd left intercostal space, parasternally.
AORTIC - 2nd right intercostal space, parasternally.
MITRAL - 5th left intercostal space, midclavicular line (apex).
TRICUSPID - To right or over lower sternum

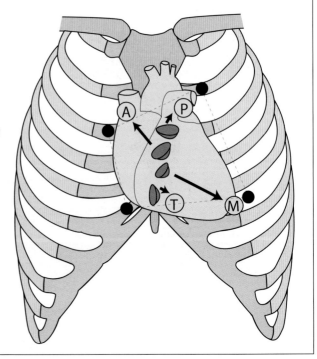

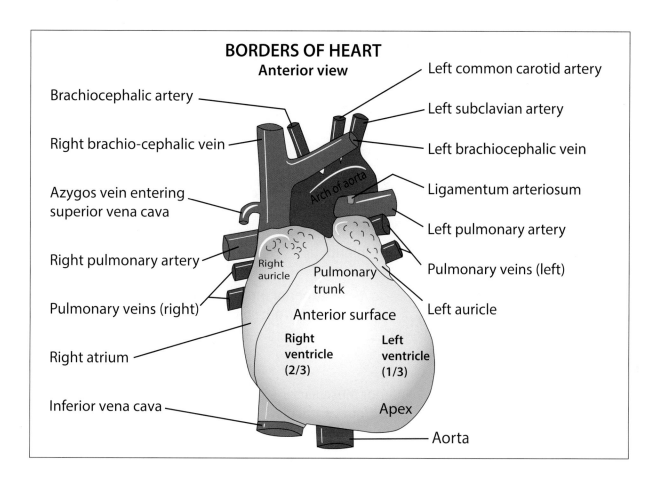

BORDERS OF HEART
Anterior view

- Brachiocephalic artery
- Right brachio-cephalic vein
- Azygos vein entering superior vena cava
- Right pulmonary artery
- Pulmonary veins (right)
- Right atrium
- Inferior vena cava
- Left common carotid artery
- Left subclavian artery
- Left brachiocephalic vein
- Ligamentum arteriosum
- Left pulmonary artery
- Pulmonary veins (left)
- Left auricle
- Arch of aorta
- Right auricle
- Pulmonary trunk
- Anterior surface
- **Right ventricle (2/3)**
- **Left ventricle (1/3)**
- Apex
- Aorta

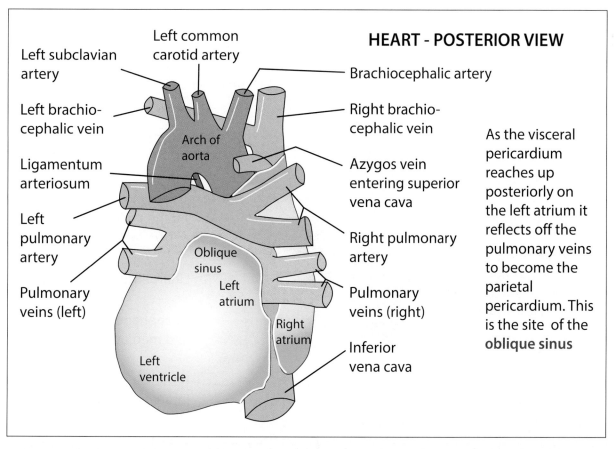

HEART - POSTERIOR VIEW

- Left subclavian artery
- Left common carotid artery
- Brachiocephalic artery
- Left brachio-cephalic vein
- Right brachio-cephalic vein
- Ligamentum arteriosum
- Azygos vein entering superior vena cava
- Left pulmonary artery
- Right pulmonary artery
- Pulmonary veins (left)
- Pulmonary veins (right)
- Arch of aorta
- Oblique sinus
- Left atrium
- Right atrium
- Left ventricle
- Inferior vena cava

As the visceral pericardium reaches up posteriorly on the left atrium it reflects off the pulmonary veins to become the parietal pericardium. This is the site of the **oblique sinus**

HEART - SURFACES AND SEPTUM

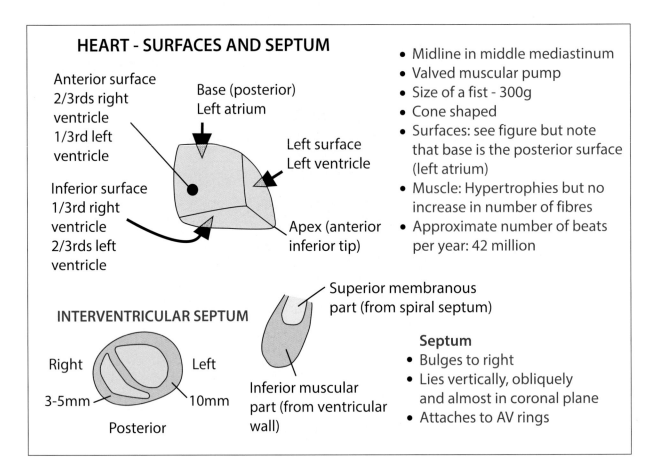

Anterior surface
2/3rds right ventricle
1/3rd left ventricle

Base (posterior)
Left atrium

Left surface
Left ventricle

Inferior surface
1/3rd right ventricle
2/3rds left ventricle

Apex (anterior inferior tip)

- Midline in middle mediastinum
- Valved muscular pump
- Size of a fist - 300g
- Cone shaped
- Surfaces: see figure but note that base is the posterior surface (left atrium)
- Muscle: Hypertrophies but no increase in number of fibres
- Approximate number of beats per year: 42 million

INTERVENTRICULAR SEPTUM

Right

Left

3-5mm

10mm

Posterior

Superior membranous part (from spiral septum)

Inferior muscular part (from ventricular wall)

Septum
- Bulges to right
- Lies vertically, obliquely and almost in coronal plane
- Attaches to AV rings

AORTIC ARCH AND ARTERIAL BRANCHES

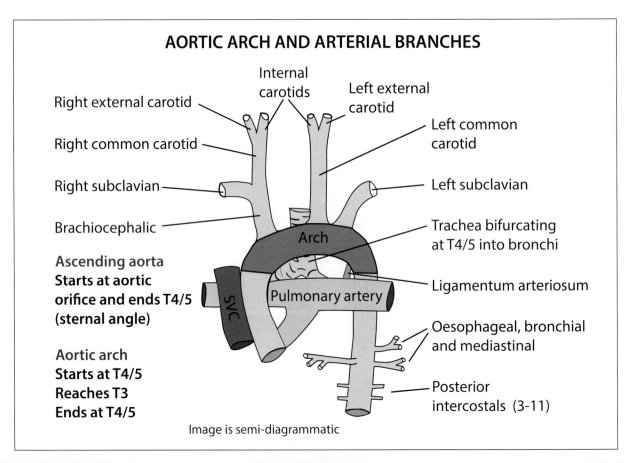

Right external carotid

Internal carotids

Left external carotid

Left common carotid

Right common carotid

Right subclavian

Left subclavian

Brachiocephalic

Arch

Trachea bifurcating at T4/5 into bronchi

Ascending aorta
Starts at aortic orifice and ends T4/5 (sternal angle)

SVC

Pulmonary artery

Ligamentum arteriosum

Oesophageal, bronchial and mediastinal

Aortic arch
Starts at T4/5
Reaches T3
Ends at T4/5

Posterior intercostals (3-11)

Image is semi-diagrammatic

HEART - PERICARDIUM

PERICARDIUM
- Outer layer - Fibrous
  Blends with adventitia of aorta, pulmonary trunk, superior
  vena cava (not inferior vena cava) and central tendon of diaphragm
- Inner layer - Serous
  - Visceral
  - Parietal
- **Blood:** pericardiacophrenic and internal thoracic
- **Nerve:** Phrenic to fibrous and parietal serous layers
  Sympathetic for pain and muscles and vessels of heart
  General visceral afferents (or maybe nil) to visceral layer

PERICARDIUM

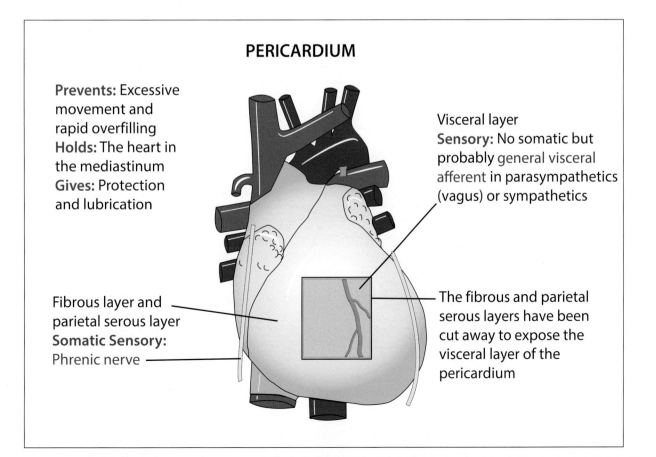

Prevents: Excessive movement and rapid overfilling
Holds: The heart in the mediastinum
Gives: Protection and lubrication

Visceral layer
Sensory: No somatic but probably general visceral afferent in parasympathetics (vagus) or sympathetics

Fibrous layer and parietal serous layer
Somatic Sensory:
Phrenic nerve

The fibrous and parietal serous layers have been cut away to expose the visceral layer of the pericardium

PERICARDIUM - HEART REMOVED WITH VISCERAL LAYER

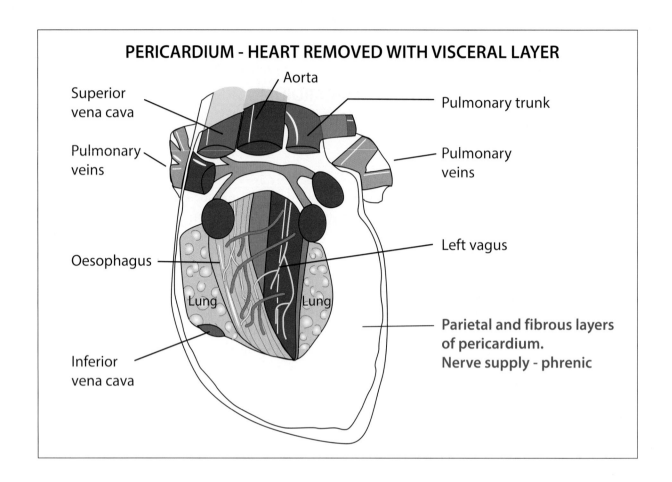

Superior vena cava

Aorta

Pulmonary trunk

Pulmonary veins

Pulmonary veins

Oesophagus

Left vagus

Lung

Lung

Parietal and fibrous layers of pericardium.
Nerve supply - phrenic

Inferior vena cava

PERICARDIAL SINUSES

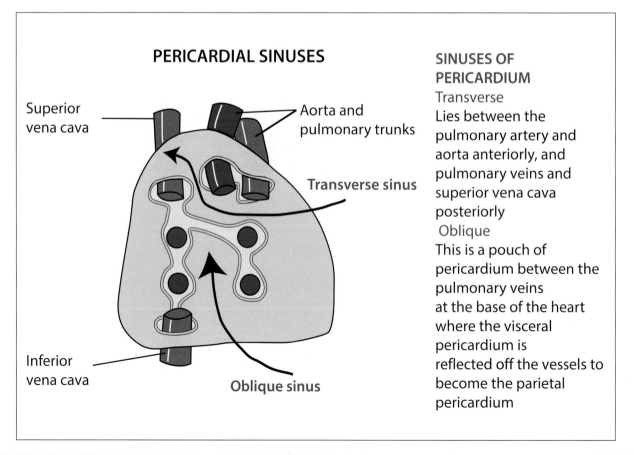

Superior vena cava

Aorta and pulmonary trunks

Transverse sinus

Inferior vena cava

Oblique sinus

SINUSES OF PERICARDIUM

Transverse
Lies between the pulmonary artery and aorta anteriorly, and pulmonary veins and superior vena cava posteriorly

Oblique
This is a pouch of pericardium between the pulmonary veins at the base of the heart where the visceral pericardium is reflected off the vessels to become the parietal pericardium

ASPIRATION OF PERICARDIAL EFFUSION

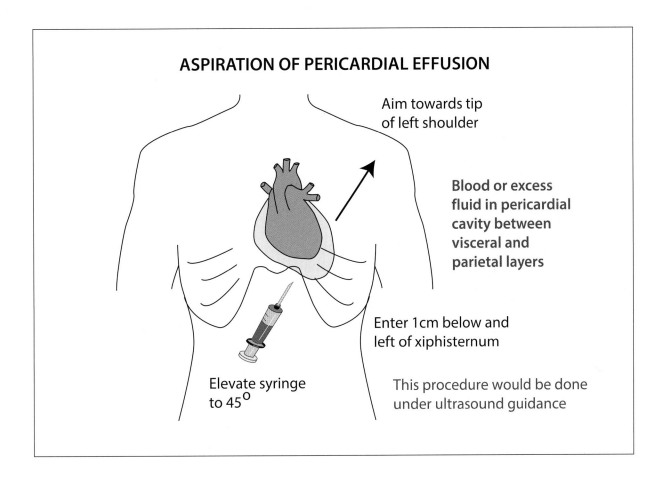

Aim towards tip of left shoulder

Blood or excess fluid in pericardial cavity between visceral and parietal layers

Enter 1cm below and left of xiphisternum

This procedure would be done under ultrasound guidance

Elevate syringe to 45°

RIGHT ATRIUM

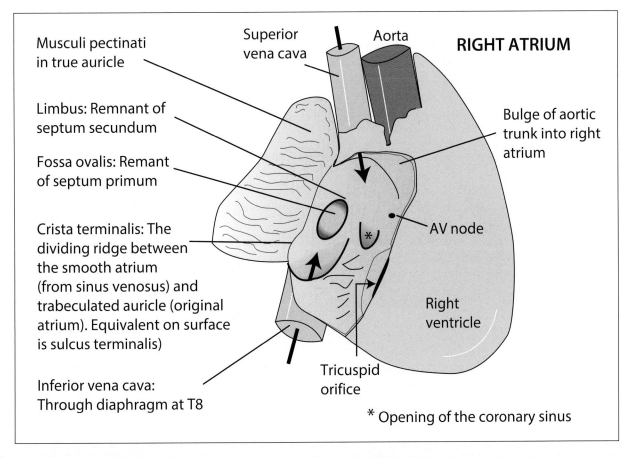

Musculi pectinati in true auricle

Limbus: Remnant of septum secundum

Fossa ovalis: Remant of septum primum

Crista terminalis: The dividing ridge between the smooth atrium (from sinus venosus) and trabeculated auricle (original atrium). Equivalent on surface is sulcus terminalis)

Inferior vena cava: Through diaphragm at T8

Superior vena cava

Aorta

Bulge of aortic trunk into right atrium

AV node

Right ventricle

Tricuspid orifice

* Opening of the coronary sinus

FETAL SHUNTING

In the fetus oxygenated blood passing up the inferior vena cava (IVC) is diverted by the **"valve of the IVC" (V)** into the foramen ovale and hence to the left atrium. Blood returning via the superior vena cava (SVC) passes down into the right ventricle

Opening of the coronary sinus (*)
Lies between the opening of the inferior vena cava and the atrioventricular orifice. Protected by a small valve which prevents regurgitation during atrial contraction. Between this orifice and the septal cusp of the tricuspid valve lies the atrioventricular node (AV)

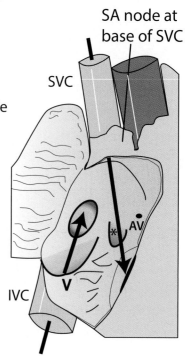

SA node at base of SVC

SVC

IVC

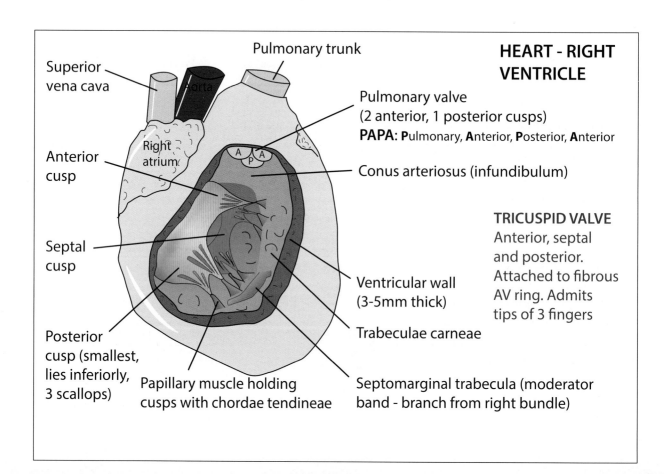

HEART - RIGHT VENTRICLE

Pulmonary trunk

Superior vena cava

Aorta

Right atrium

Anterior cusp

Septal cusp

Posterior cusp (smallest, lies inferiorly, 3 scallops)

Papillary muscle holding cusps with chordae tendineae

Pulmonary valve (2 anterior, 1 posterior cusps)
PAPA: Pulmonary, **A**nterior, **P**osterior, **A**nterior

Conus arteriosus (infundibulum)

TRICUSPID VALVE
Anterior, septal and posterior. Attached to fibrous AV ring. Admits tips of 3 fingers

Ventricular wall (3-5mm thick)

Trabeculae carneae

Septomarginal trabecula (moderator band - branch from right bundle)

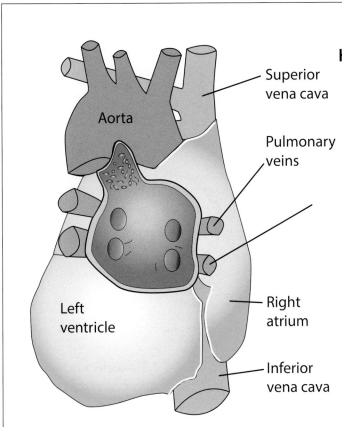

HEART - LEFT ATRIUM

Superior vena cava

Aorta

Pulmonary veins

Left ventricle

Right atrium

Inferior vena cava

Base of heart(posterior surface). The left atrium is opened to show its smooth walled interior, apart from the musculi pectinati of the auricle. Four large, valveless pulmonary veins drain into it. On the interatrial wall there is a oval, thin area which is the left side of the fossa ovalis of the right atrium

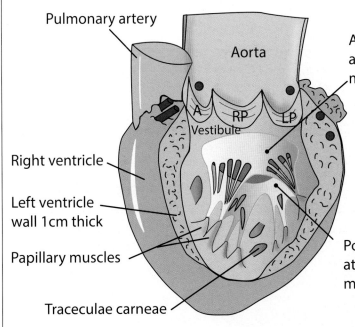

HEART - LEFT VENTRICLE

Pulmonary artery

Aorta

A RP LP
Vestibule

Right ventricle

Left ventricle wall 1cm thick

Papillary muscles

Traceculae carneae

Anterior cusp of mitral valve attached to anterior papillary muscle via chordae tendineae

MITRAL VALVE (Bishop's mitre)
- Anterior cusp is larger, septal and thicker
- Posterior is smaller and has 3 scallops
- Admits the tips of 2 fingers
- Attached to fibrous AV ring

Posterior cusp of mitral valve attached to posterior papillary muscle via chordae tendineae

A: Anterior cusp and sinus (opening of right coronary artery)

RP: Right posterior (non-coronary) cusp and sinus

LP: Left posterior cusp and sinus (orifice of left coronary artery)

HEART - LOOKING DOWN ON SUPERIOR SURFACE

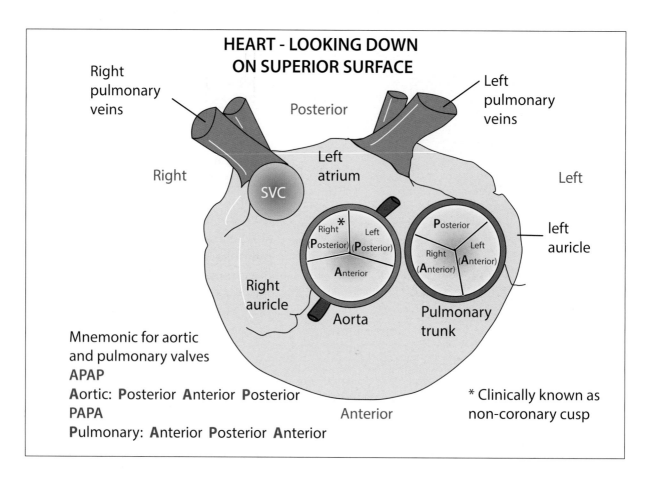

Right pulmonary veins

Left pulmonary veins

Posterior

Right

Left

Left atrium

SVC

left auricle

Right (Posterior) *

Left (Posterior)

Posterior

Anterior

Right (Anterior)

Left (Anterior)

Right auricle

Aorta

Pulmonary trunk

Mnemonic for aortic and pulmonary valves
APAP
Aortic: Posterior Anterior Posterior
PAPA
Pulmonary: Anterior Posterior Anterior

Anterior

* Clinically known as non-coronary cusp

HEART - ELECTRICAL SYSTEM 1

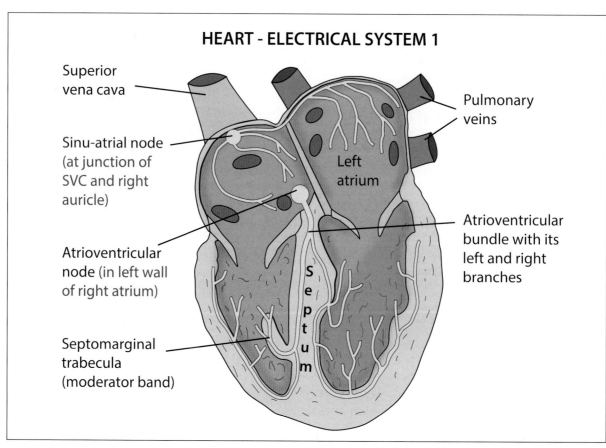

Superior vena cava

Pulmonary veins

Sinu-atrial node (at junction of SVC and right auricle)

Left atrium

Atrioventricular node (in left wall of right atrium)

Atrioventricular bundle with its left and right branches

Septum

Septomarginal trabecula (moderator band)

HEART - ELECTRICAL SYSTEM 2

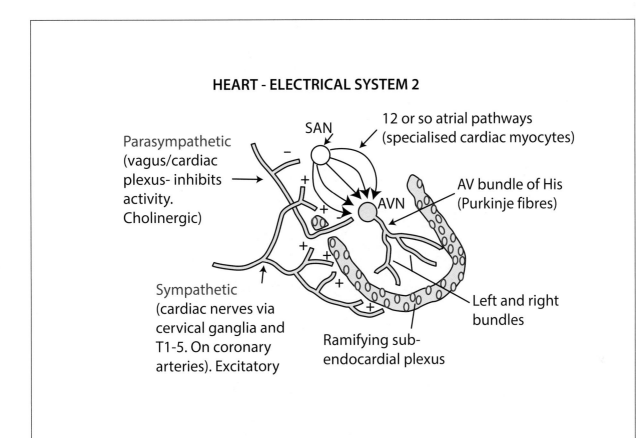

SAN

12 or so atrial pathways (specialised cardiac myocytes)

Parasympathetic (vagus/cardiac plexus- inhibits activity. Cholinergic)

AVN

AV bundle of His (Purkinje fibres)

Sympathetic (cardiac nerves via cervical ganglia and T1-5. On coronary arteries). Excitatory

Ramifying sub-endocardial plexus

Left and right bundles

BUNDLE OF HIS AND MODERATOR BAND

Branch of right bundle that enters the moderator band and then into the papillary muscle that extends from it

Left bundle running just beneath the endothelium of ventricle to start excitation from inferior aspect of chamber.

Right bundle running just beneath the endothelium of ventricle to start excitation from inferior aspect of chamber.

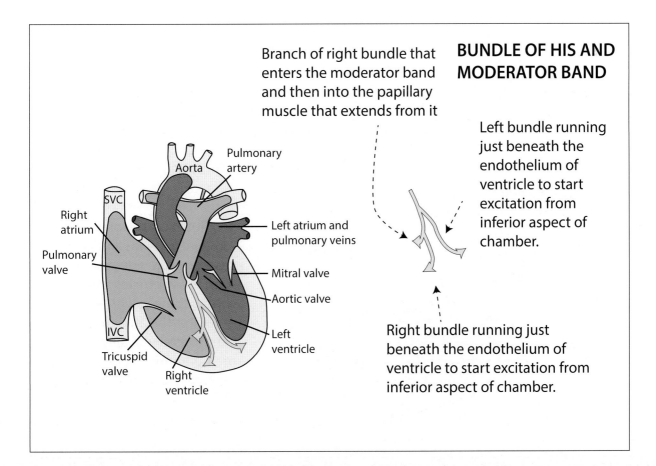

Pulmonary artery

Aorta

SVC

Right atrium

Left atrium and pulmonary veins

Pulmonary valve

Mitral valve

Aortic valve

IVC

Left ventricle

Tricuspid valve

Right ventricle

AUTONOMIC NERVE SUPPLY TO HEART

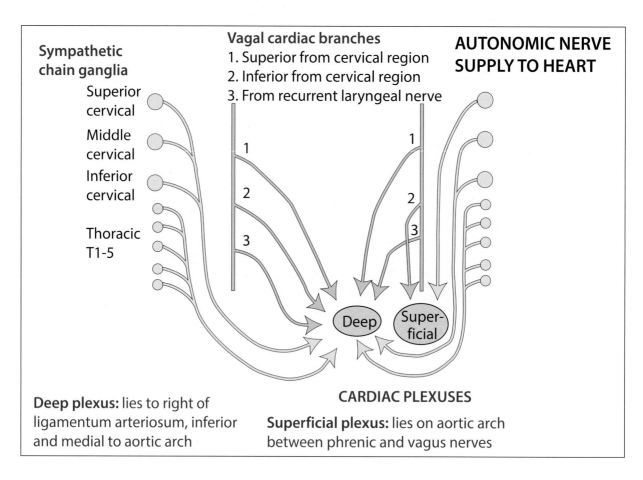

Sympathetic chain ganglia
- Superior cervical
- Middle cervical
- Inferior cervical
- Thoracic T1-5

Vagal cardiac branches
1. Superior from cervical region
2. Inferior from cervical region
3. From recurrent laryngeal nerve

Deep

Super-ficial

CARDIAC PLEXUSES

Deep plexus: lies to right of ligamentum arteriosum, inferior and medial to aortic arch

Superficial plexus: lies on aortic arch between phrenic and vagus nerves

HEART - FIBROUS SKELETON

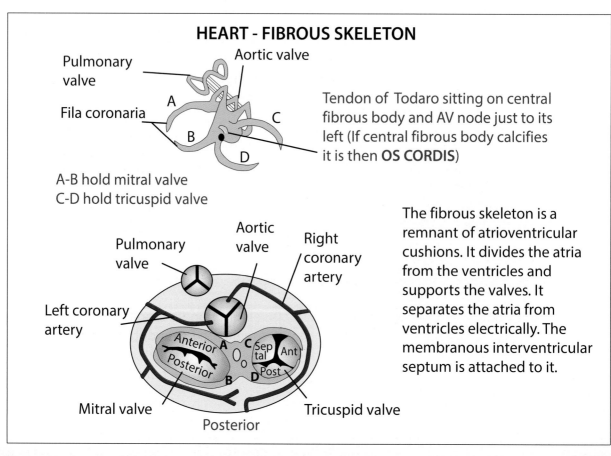

Pulmonary valve

Aortic valve

Fila coronaria

A

B

C

D

A-B hold mitral valve
C-D hold tricuspid valve

Tendon of Todaro sitting on central fibrous body and AV node just to its left (If central fibrous body calcifies it is then **OS CORDIS**)

Pulmonary valve

Aortic valve

Right coronary artery

Left coronary artery

Anterior
Posterior

A

C Sep tal Ant

B

D Post

Mitral valve

Tricuspid valve

Posterior

The fibrous skeleton is a remnant of atrioventricular cushions. It divides the atria from the ventricles and supports the valves. It separates the atria from ventricles electrically. The membranous interventricular septum is attached to it.

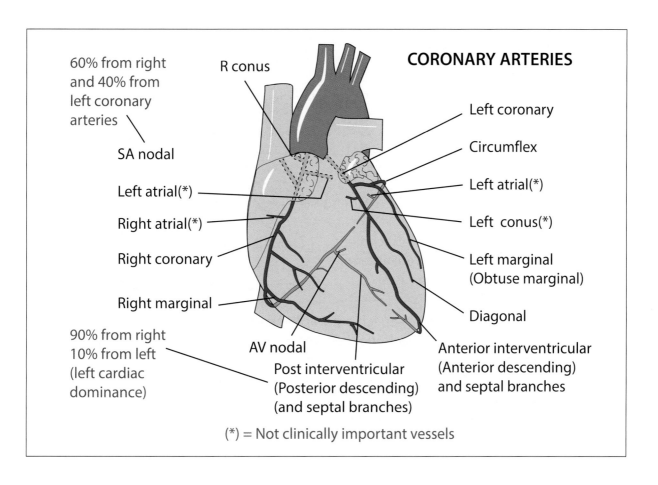

CORONARY ARTERIES

60% from right and 40% from left coronary arteries

SA nodal

R conus

Left coronary

Circumflex

Left atrial(*)

Right atrial(*)

Left atrial(*)

Right coronary

Left conus(*)

Right marginal

Left marginal (Obtuse marginal)

90% from right 10% from left (left cardiac dominance)

AV nodal

Diagonal

Post interventricular (Posterior descending) (and septal branches)

Anterior interventricular (Anterior descending) and septal branches

(*) = Not clinically important vessels

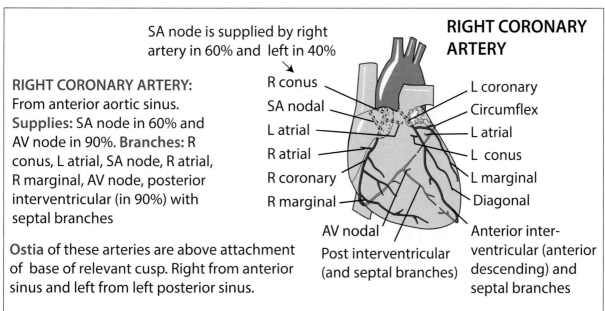

RIGHT CORONARY ARTERY

SA node is supplied by right artery in 60% and left in 40%

RIGHT CORONARY ARTERY:
From anterior aortic sinus.
Supplies: SA node in 60% and AV node in 90%. **Branches:** R conus, L atrial, SA node, R atrial, R marginal, AV node, posterior interventricular (in 90%) with septal branches

R conus

SA nodal

L atrial

R atrial

R coronary

R marginal

L coronary

Circumflex

L atrial

L conus

L marginal

Diagonal

AV nodal

Ostia of these arteries are above attachment of base of relevant cusp. Right from anterior sinus and left from left posterior sinus.

Post interventricular (and septal branches)

Anterior inter-ventricular (anterior descending) and septal branches

Right artery passes anteriorly between right atrial appendage and pulmonary trunk into right anterior atrioventricular (AV) groove and then right posterior AV groove where it anastomoses with circumflex branch of left coronary artery. In 90% of people it gives the posterior interventricular artery which anastomoses with termination of anterior interventricular artery (left coronary) in this groove. The AV node is supplied by right coronary artery in 90% of people

LEFT CORONARY ARTERY

LEFT CORONARY ARTERY: From left posterior aortic sinus. Supplies: SA node in 40% and AV in 10%. Branches: Circumflex, L atrial, L conus, anterior interventricular, diagonal and posterior ventricular (in 10%) with septal branches.

Ostia of these arteries are above attachment of base of relevant cusp. Right from anterior sinus and left from left posterior sinus.

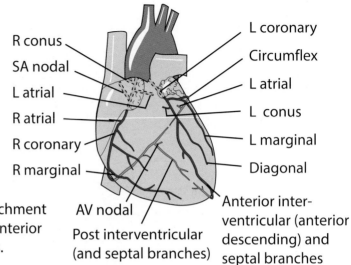

R conus
SA nodal
L atrial
R atrial
R coronary
R marginal
AV nodal
Post interventricular (and septal branches)
L coronary
Circumflex
L atrial
L conus
L marginal
Diagonal
Anterior inter-ventricular (anterior descending) and septal branches

Left artery passes anteriorly between left atrial appendage and pulmonary trunk into left anterior AV groove. It divides into anterior interventricular and circumflex arteries. The latter artery continues first in anterior and then in posterior AV groove. It anastomoses with terminal branches of right coronary artery. In 10% of people it gives posterior interventricular artery (left dominence) and also supplies AV node. Anterior interventricular (anterior descending) passes down and around apex of heart to anastomose with terminal branches of posterior interventricular artery.

DOMINANCE
In 10% of people the left coronary artery gives the posterior interventricular artery. This is **left cardiac dominance** and means that both ventricles and septum are supplied by the single left coronary artery. Left cardiac dominance is associated with the presence of a bicuspid aortic valve

CARDIAC DOMINANCE

SA node is supplied by right artery in 60% and left artery in 40%

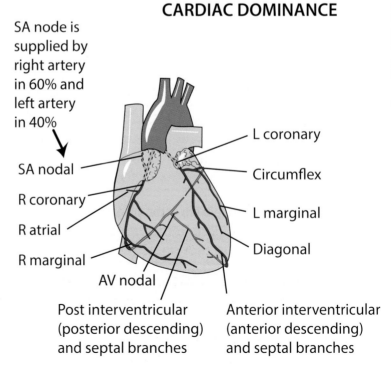

SA nodal
R coronary
R atrial
R marginal
AV nodal
L coronary
Circumflex
L marginal
Diagonal
Post interventricular (posterior descending) and septal branches
Anterior interventricular (anterior descending) and septal branches

CORONARY ARTERIES AS SEEN ON A CORONARY ANGIOGRAM

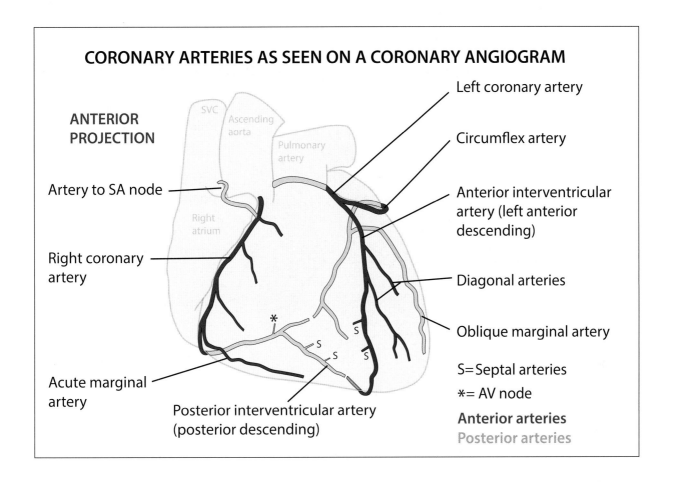

ANTERIOR PROJECTION

Left coronary artery

Circumflex artery

Anterior interventricular artery (left anterior descending)

Artery to SA node

Right coronary artery

Diagonal arteries

Oblique marginal artery

S=Septal arteries

*= AV node

Acute marginal artery

Posterior interventricular artery (posterior descending)

Anterior arteries
Posterior arteries

CARDIAC VEINS

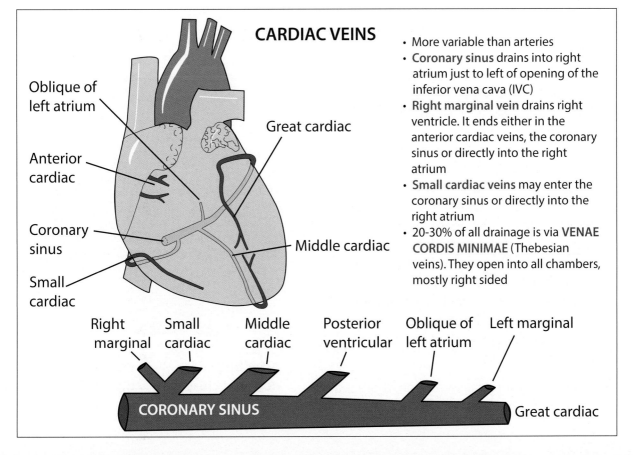

Oblique of left atrium

Anterior cardiac

Great cardiac

Coronary sinus

Small cardiac

Middle cardiac

Right marginal

Small cardiac

Middle cardiac

Posterior ventricular

Oblique of left atrium

Left marginal

CORONARY SINUS

Great cardiac

- More variable than arteries
- **Coronary sinus** drains into right atrium just to left of opening of the inferior vena cava (IVC)
- **Right marginal vein** drains right ventricle. It ends either in the anterior cardiac veins, the coronary sinus or directly into the right atrium
- **Small cardiac veins** may enter the coronary sinus or directly into the right atrium
- 20-30% of all drainage is via **VENAE CORDIS MINIMAE** (Thebesian veins). They open into all chambers, mostly right sided

NORMAL CIRCULATION IN THE HEART

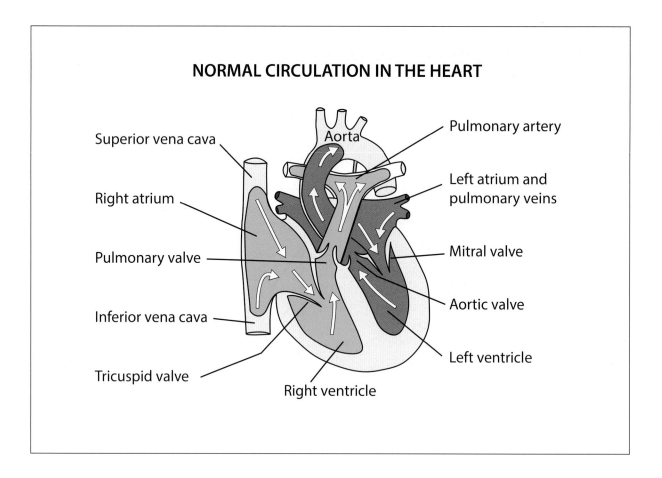

Superior vena cava

Right atrium

Pulmonary valve

Inferior vena cava

Tricuspid valve

Aorta

Pulmonary artery

Left atrium and pulmonary veins

Mitral valve

Aortic valve

Left ventricle

Right ventricle

PATENT DUCTUS ARTERIOSUS

Embryologically the ductus arteriosus is the distal part of the left 6th aortic arch.
In fetal life blood shunts from the higher pressure pulmonary artery to the aorta as a means of bypassing the fetal lungs.
After birth it closes due to the lack of **maternal prostaglandins** and the production of **bradykinin** from the fetal lungs to become the ligamentum arteriosum. If it does not close then high pressure aortic blood raises the pressure in the pulmonary circulation.
It may be an isolated finding or part of a complex congenital heart problem.
It can be closed surgically or by giving antiprostaglandins.

Note: During surgical correction, there is a risk of damaging the left recurrent laryngeal nerve

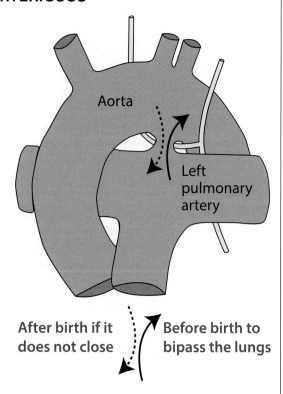

Aorta

Left pulmonary artery

After birth if it does not close

Before birth to bipass the lungs

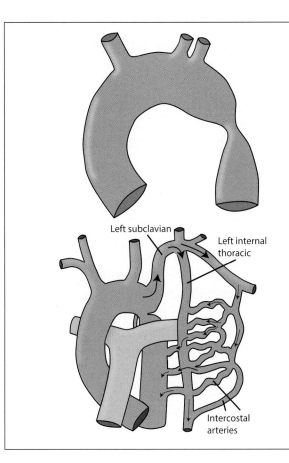

COARCTATION OF AORTA

A congenital narrowing of aorta at or near site of ligamentum arteriosum caused by hypoplasia of the 4th arterial arch with post-stenotic dilatation. Maybe due to spread of ductus tissue into the aorta, narrowing it when the ductus arteriosus closes off.

Enlarged collateral circulations in internal thoracic, subclavian and posterior intercostal arteries. Erosion of ribs with "notching".
Poor femoral pulses in both limbs.
Treatment is surgical.

NORMAL FETAL CIRCULATION

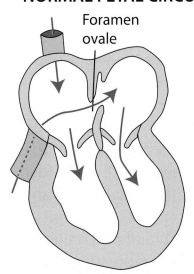

ATRIAL SEPTAL DEFECT

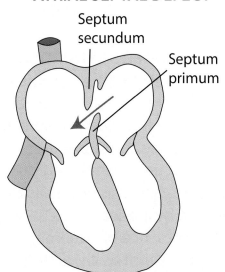

Atrial septal defect: Often associated with a ventricular septal defect. Treatment for septum secundum is a surgical graft. For septum primum it is more difficult surgery. Often associated with VSD.
Note: Blood flows from the higher pressured left atrium to the right atrium and only when there is a temporary rise in right atrial pressure will there be the possibility of cyanosis

INTERVENTRICULAR SEPTAL DEFECT (VSD)

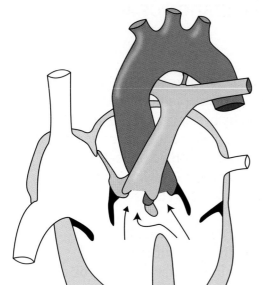

The upper membraneous part, which is formed by the inferior end of the spiral septum, is missing

Note: Risk of Eisenmenger Syndrome where the left to right shunt is reversed due to right ventricular hypertrophy and resulting increasing right sided pressure. This risk is lessened by early corrective surgery

EISENMENGER'S SYNDROME

EISENMENGER'S SYNDROME occurs when there is reversal of a left-to-right shunt to become a right-to-left shunt, such as in a ventricular septal defect or Fallot's tetralogy where there is an increase in flow and pressure in the right heart. There is right ventricle hypertrophy and subsequent rise in pulmonary artery pressure. The shunt occurs when the right sided pressure exceeds the left sided pressure. Cyanosis occurs as the blood becomes desaturated and this leads to dyspnoea.

In the presence of Eisenmenger's Syndrome, it might be unwise to close the shunt as it is acting as a means of decompressing the pulmonary circulation.

Eisenmenger's syndrome is now less common due to earlier corrective surgery.

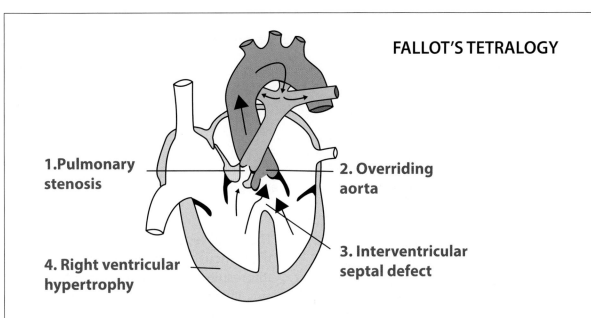

FALLOT'S TETRALOGY

1. Pulmonary stenosis

2. Overriding aorta

3. Interventricular septal defect

4. Right ventricular hypertrophy

The spiral septum (neural crest cells) divides the truncus arteriosus asymmetrically giving a narrow pulmonary trunk and a wider aorta. Failure of the lowest part of the spiral septum to form the membraneous part of the interventriculum leaves a septal defect. As blood cannot reach the lungs by the pulmonary trunk, the ductus arteriosus needs to be kept open. This is a primarily cyanotic condition that requires major surgery.

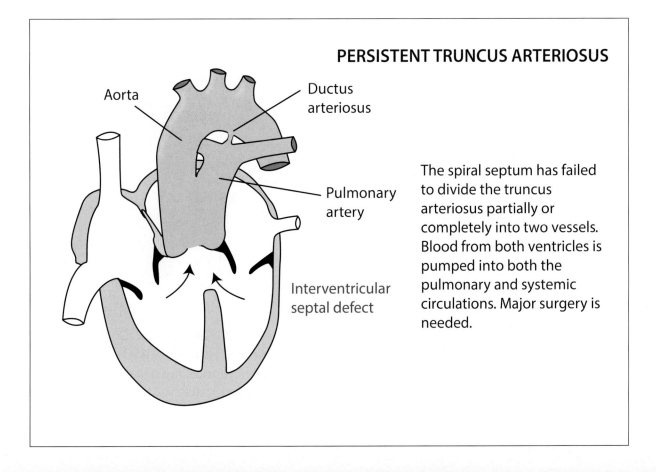

PERSISTENT TRUNCUS ARTERIOSUS

Aorta

Ductus arteriosus

Pulmonary artery

Interventricular septal defect

The spiral septum has failed to divide the truncus arteriosus partially or completely into two vessels. Blood from both ventricles is pumped into both the pulmonary and systemic circulations. Major surgery is needed.

TRANSPOSITION OF GREAT VESSELS

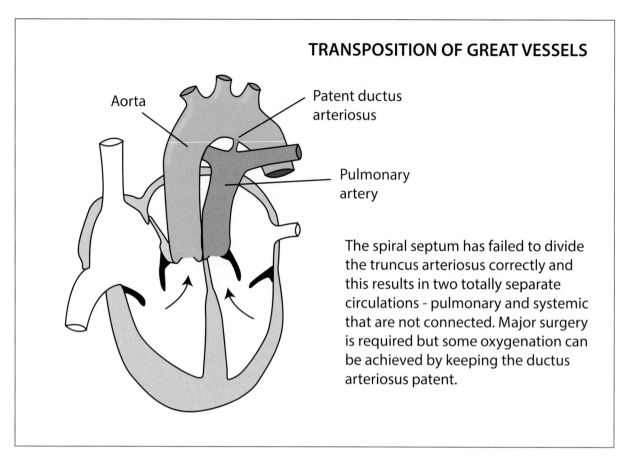

Aorta

Patent ductus arteriosus

Pulmonary artery

The spiral septum has failed to divide the truncus arteriosus correctly and this results in two totally separate circulations - pulmonary and systemic that are not connected. Major surgery is required but some oxygenation can be achieved by keeping the ductus arteriosus patent.

OTHER CONGENITAL ANOMALIES OF HEART

RETRO-OESOPHAGEAL RIGHT SUBCLAVIAN ARTERY
Gives dysphagia lusoria

DOUBLE AORTIC ARCH
Vascular ring enclosing trachea and oesophagus

See also:
PERSISTENT RIGHT DORSAL AORTA

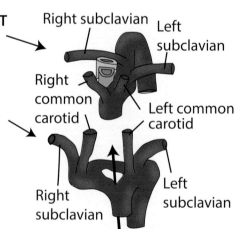

Right subclavian   Left subclavian

Right common carotid

Left common carotid

Right subclavian   Left subclavian

CYANOTIC CONDITIONS
- Persistent truncus with VSD
- Transposition of aorta with patent ductus and VSD
- Fallot's tetralogy
- Pumonary atresia with patent ductus
- Tricuspid atresia with ASD

ACYANOTIC CONDITIONS
- Primary/secondary ASD
- Membranous/muscular VSD
- Patent ductus

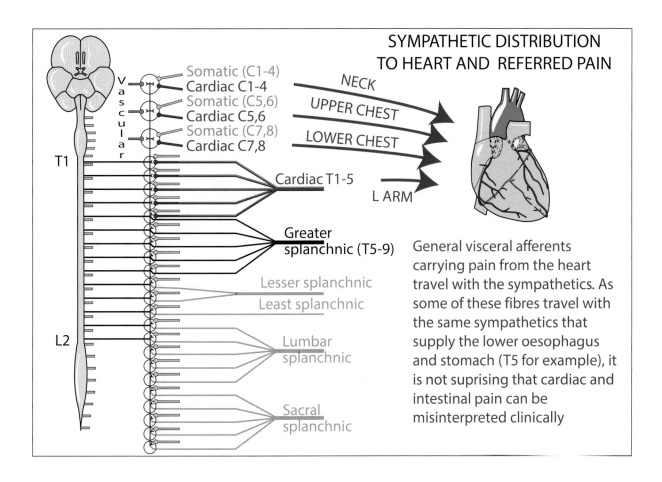

SYMPATHETIC DISTRIBUTION TO HEART AND REFERRED PAIN

Vascular

Somatic (C1-4)
Cardiac C1-4
Somatic (C5,6)
Cardiac C5,6
Somatic (C7,8)
Cardiac C7,8

NECK
UPPER CHEST
LOWER CHEST

T1

Cardiac T1-5

L ARM

Greater splanchnic (T5-9)

Lesser splanchnic
Least splanchnic

L2

Lumbar splanchnic

Sacral splanchnic

General visceral afferents carrying pain from the heart travel with the sympathetics. As some of these fibres travel with the same sympathetics that supply the lower oesophagus and stomach (T5 for example), it is not suprising that cardiac and intestinal pain can be misinterpreted clinically

AUTONOMIC REFERRED PAIN

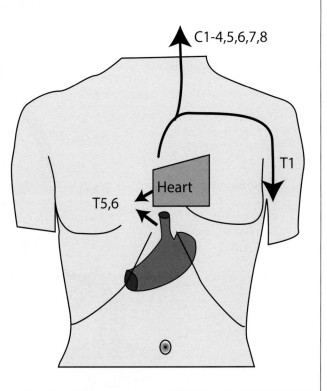

General visceral afferents from the heart (via sympathetics) refer pain to:
Neck
Left arm
Epigastrium

Note that the T5,6 sympathetics not only supply the **heart** but also the lower **oesophagus and stomach** so the body can confuse indigestion with coronary pain.

Note: See also details on referred pain in abdominal section

C1-4,5,6,7,8

T1

Heart

T5,6

LOOPING OF HEART

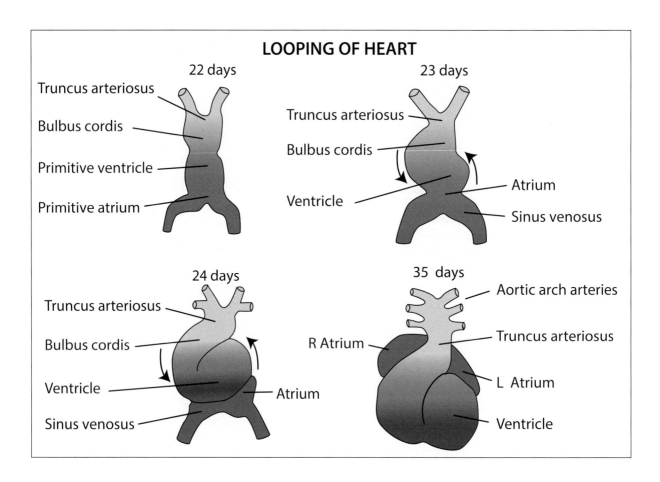

22 days

Truncus arteriosus

Bulbus cordis

Primitive ventricle

Primitive atrium

23 days

Truncus arteriosus

Bulbus cordis

Ventricle

Atrium

Sinus venosus

24 days

Truncus arteriosus

Bulbus cordis

Ventricle

Sinus venosus

Atrium

35 days

Aortic arch arteries

R Atrium

Truncus arteriosus

L Atrium

Ventricle

PERCENTAGES OF OXYGEN IN FETAL CIRCULATION

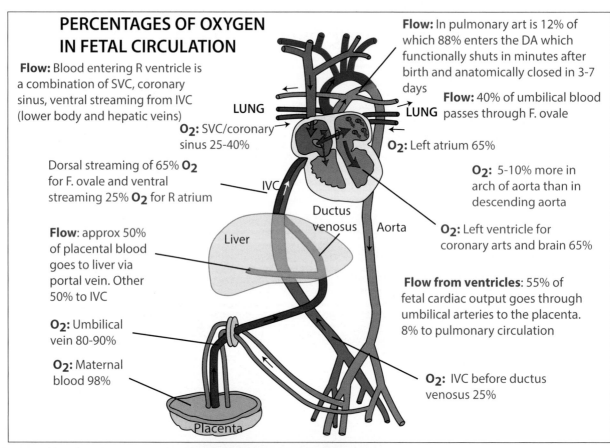

Flow: Blood entering R ventricle is a combination of SVC, coronary sinus, ventral streaming from IVC (lower body and hepatic veins)

O₂: SVC/coronary sinus 25-40%

Dorsal streaming of 65% **O₂** for F. ovale and ventral streaming 25% **O₂** for R atrium

Flow: approx 50% of placental blood goes to liver via portal vein. Other 50% to IVC

O₂: Umbilical vein 80-90%

O₂: Maternal blood 98%

LUNG

IVC

Liver

Ductus venosus

Aorta

Placenta

Flow: In pulmonary art is 12% of which 88% enters the DA which functionally shuts in minutes after birth and anatomically closed in 3-7 days

Flow: 40% of umbilical blood passes through F. ovale

LUNG

O₂: Left atrium 65%

O₂: 5-10% more in arch of aorta than in descending aorta

O₂: Left ventricle for coronary arts and brain 65%

Flow from ventricles: 55% of fetal cardiac output goes through umbilical arteries to the placenta. 8% to pulmonary circulation

O₂: IVC before ductus venosus 25%

3.4 Trachea, Lungs and Oesophagus

RELATIONS OF TRACHEA & BRONCHI

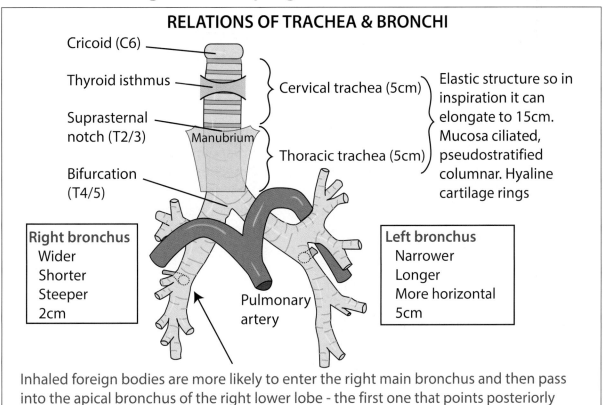

Cricoid (C6)

Thyroid isthmus

Suprasternal notch (T2/3)

Manubrium

Bifurcation (T4/5)

Cervical trachea (5cm)

Thoracic trachea (5cm)

Elastic structure so in inspiration it can elongate to 15cm. Mucosa ciliated, pseudostratified columnar. Hyaline cartilage rings

Right bronchus
Wider
Shorter
Steeper
2cm

Left bronchus
Narrower
Longer
More horizontal
5cm

Pulmonary artery

Inhaled foreign bodies are more likely to enter the right main bronchus and then pass into the apical bronchus of the right lower lobe - the first one that points posteriorly

BRONCHOPULMONARY SEGMENTS

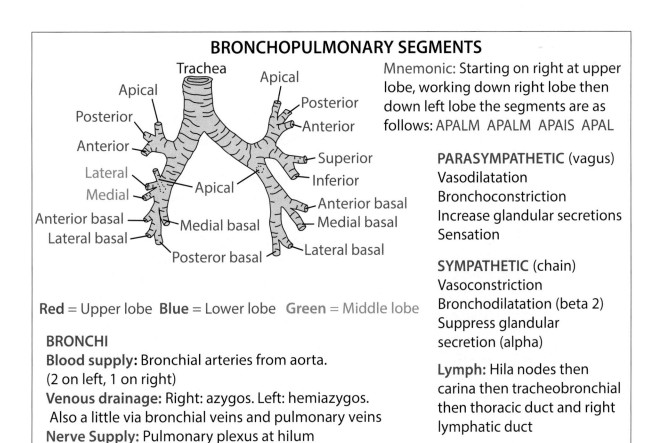

Trachea

Apical
Posterior
Anterior
Lateral
Medial
Anterior basal
Lateral basal
Apical
Medial basal
Posteror basal

Apical
Posterior
Anterior
Superior
Inferior
Anterior basal
Medial basal
Lateral basal

Red = Upper lobe **Blue** = Lower lobe **Green** = Middle lobe

Mnemonic: Starting on right at upper lobe, working down right lobe then down left lobe the segments are as follows: APALM APALM APAIS APAL

PARASYMPATHETIC (vagus)
Vasodilatation
Bronchoconstriction
Increase glandular secretions
Sensation

SYMPATHETIC (chain)
Vasoconstriction
Bronchodilatation (beta 2)
Suppress glandular secretion (alpha)

Lymph: Hila nodes then carina then tracheobronchial then thoracic duct and right lymphatic duct

BRONCHI
Blood supply: Bronchial arteries from aorta.
(2 on left, 1 on right)
Venous drainage: Right: azygos. Left: hemiazygos.
Also a little via bronchial veins and pulmonary veins
Nerve Supply: Pulmonary plexus at hilum

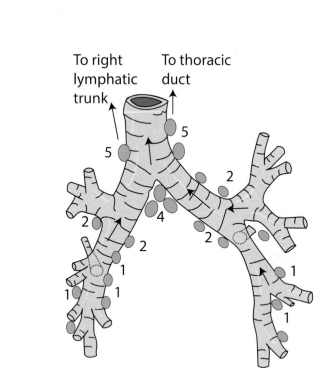

LYMPHATIC DRAINAGE OF LUNGS AND BRONCHI

To right lymphatic trunk

To thoracic duct

NODES
1. Intrapulmonary
2. Bronchopulmonary (hilar)
3. Superior tracheobronchial
4. Inferior tracheobronchial (carinal)
5. Paratracheal

RIB MOVEMENTS IN RESPIRATION

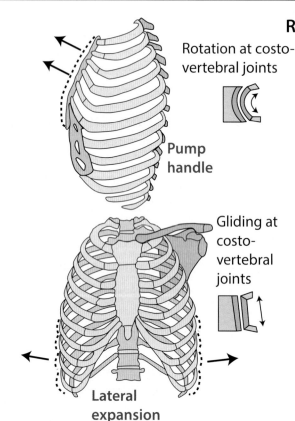

Rotation at costo-vertebral joints

Pump handle

Gliding at costo-vertebral joints

Lateral expansion

Upper thorax (ribs 1-6)
There is **pump handle** movement on inspiration. Mostly anteroposterior expansion - minimal lateral expansion

Lower thorax (ribs 7-10)
In quiet inspiration the costal margins separate producing lateral and slight upwards movement of the whole lower thorax.
In forced inspiration there is an additional eversion of the last few ribs by the diaphragm pulling on them. This is likened to the lifting of a **bucket handle** (not illustrated)

MUSCLE ACTION IN RESPIRATION

3 INTERCOSTAL MUSCLES
Lift ribs and increase in activity the deeper the inspiration. Minimal activity in quiet respiration

DIAPHRAGM (C3,4,5)
70% of quiet inspiration (5cm downwards movement of domes). 10cm movement in deeper inspirations

ACCESSORY MUSCLES OF RESPIRATION (some need fixation of arms to work effectively)
Abdominal wall muscles, 3 scalene muscles, pectoralis major and minor, trapezius, sternocleidomastoid, serratus anterior, latissimus dorsi, erector spinae, quadratus lumborum

MUSCLES ATTACHED TO COSTAL CARTILAGES
- Internal oblique abdominis
- Transversus abdominis
- Rectus abdominis
- Transversus thoracis (sternocostalis)
- Pectoralis major (1-7)
- Diaphragm

PLEURAL AND LUNG SURFACE MARKINGS

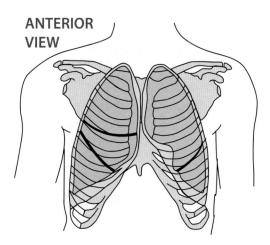

ANTERIOR VIEW

Lung is purple
Pleura is yellow

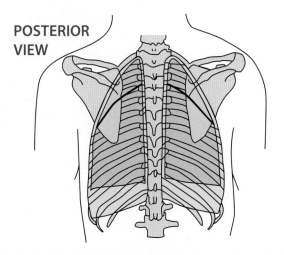

POSTERIOR VIEW

Note that the pleura extends just below the 12th rib posteriorly. This is important in approaching the kidney surgically from behind

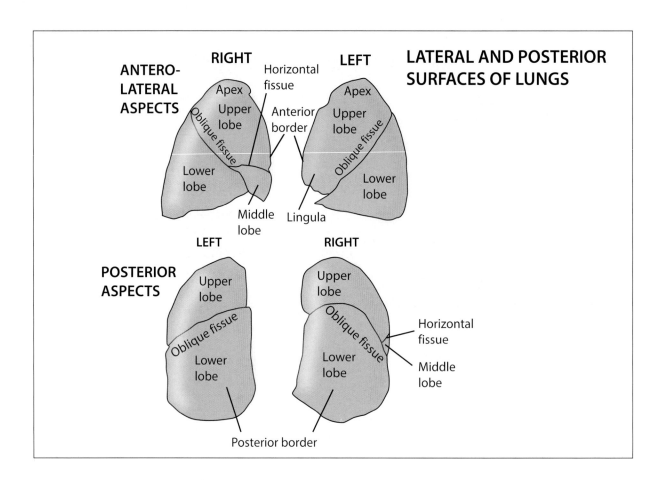

ANTERO-LATERAL ASPECTS

RIGHT

LEFT

LATERAL AND POSTERIOR SURFACES OF LUNGS

Apex
Horizontal fissue
Upper lobe
Anterior border
Oblique fissue
Lower lobe
Middle lobe

Apex
Upper lobe
Oblique fissue
Lower lobe
Lingula

POSTERIOR ASPECTS

LEFT

RIGHT

Upper lobe
Oblique fissue
Lower lobe

Upper lobe
Oblique fissue
Horizontal fissue
Lower lobe
Middle lobe

Posterior border

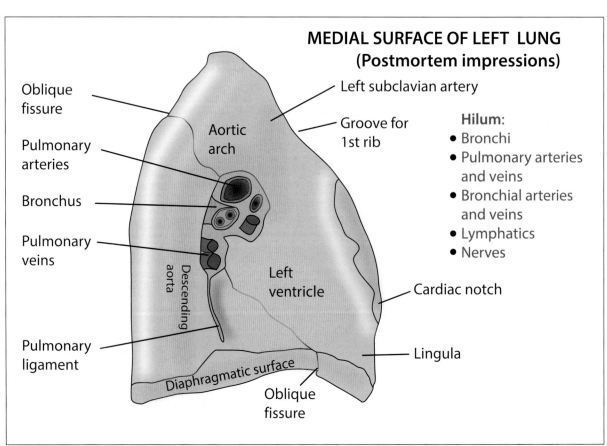

MEDIAL SURFACE OF LEFT LUNG (Postmortem impressions)

Oblique fissure

Pulmonary arteries

Bronchus

Pulmonary veins

Pulmonary ligament

Aortic arch

Descending aorta

Left ventricle

Diaphragmatic surface

Oblique fissure

Left subclavian artery

Groove for 1st rib

Hilum:
- Bronchi
- Pulmonary arteries and veins
- Bronchial arteries and veins
- Lymphatics
- Nerves

Cardiac notch

Lingula

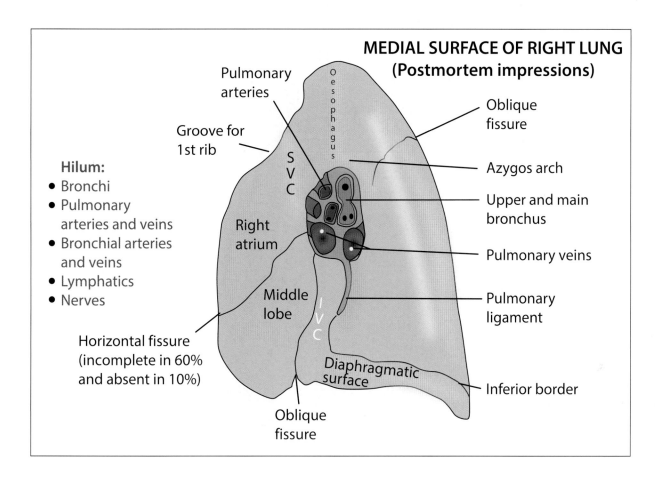

MEDIAL SURFACE OF RIGHT LUNG
(Postmortem impressions)

Pulmonary arteries

Groove for 1st rib

Hilum:
- Bronchi
- Pulmonary arteries and veins
- Bronchial arteries and veins
- Lymphatics
- Nerves

Horizontal fissure (incomplete in 60% and absent in 10%)

Oesophagus

S V C

Right atrium

Middle lobe

I V C

Oblique fissure

Diaphragmatic surface

Oblique fissure

Azygos arch

Upper and main bronchus

Pulmonary veins

Pulmonary ligament

Inferior border

AZYGOS LOBE OF RIGHT LUNG

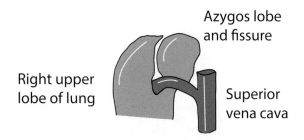

Right upper lobe of lung

Azygos lobe and fissure

Superior vena cava

Occasionally the azygos vein reaches the superior vena cava by passing through the substance of the right lobe trapping a segment of upper right lobe and creating an azygos fissure

Other notes:
- The lingula of the left lobe arises from the upper bronchus
- Incomplete segmentation is common
- Left lung is longer and lower but lighter

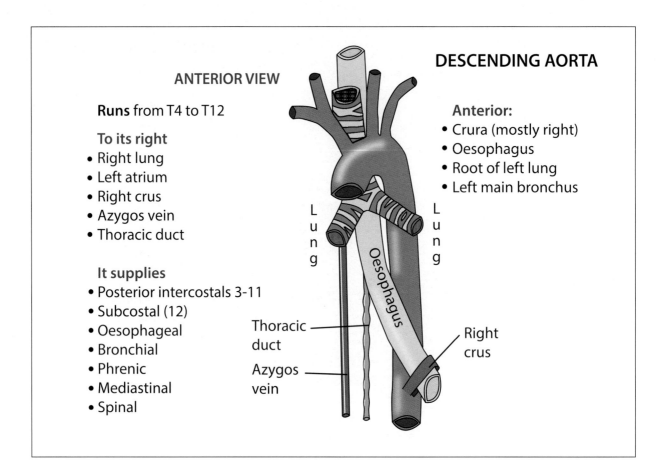

ANTERIOR VIEW

DESCENDING AORTA

Runs from T4 to T12

To its right
- Right lung
- Left atrium
- Right crus
- Azygos vein
- Thoracic duct

It supplies
- Posterior intercostals 3-11
- Subcostal (12)
- Oesophageal
- Bronchial
- Phrenic
- Mediastinal
- Spinal

Anterior:
- Crura (mostly right)
- Oesophagus
- Root of left lung
- Left main bronchus

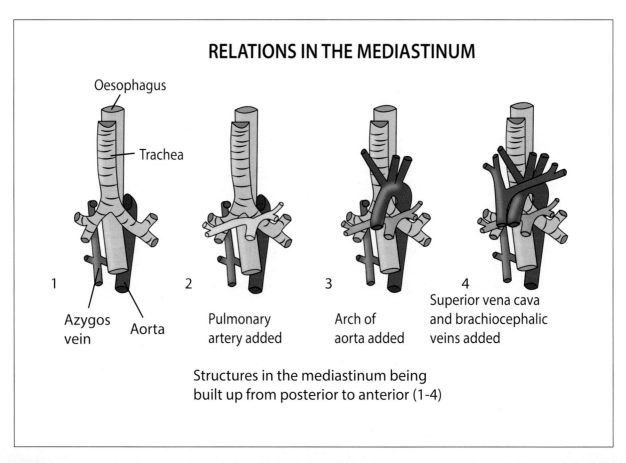

RELATIONS IN THE MEDIASTINUM

1 — Azygos vein, Aorta

2 — Pulmonary artery added

3 — Arch of aorta added

4 — Superior vena cava and brachiocephalic veins added

Structures in the mediastinum being built up from posterior to anterior (1-4)

AORTIC ARCH AND ARTERIAL BRANCHES

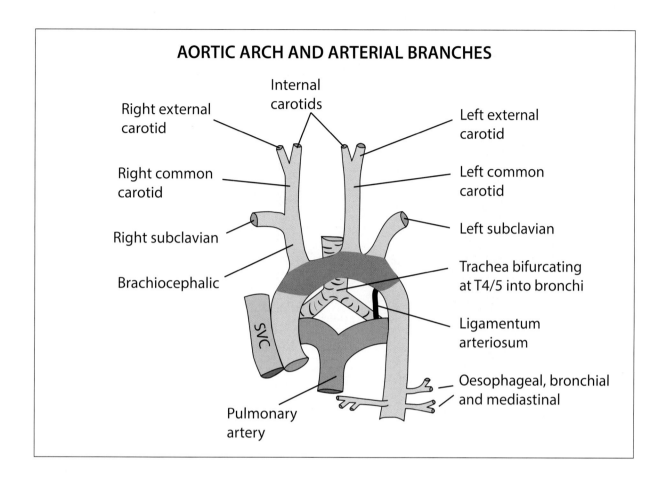

Internal carotids

Right external carotid

Left external carotid

Right common carotid

Left common carotid

Right subclavian

Left subclavian

Brachiocephalic

Trachea bifurcating at T4/5 into bronchi

SVC

Ligamentum arteriosum

Oesophageal, bronchial and mediastinal

Pulmonary artery

SUPERIOR MEDIASTINAL RELATIONS

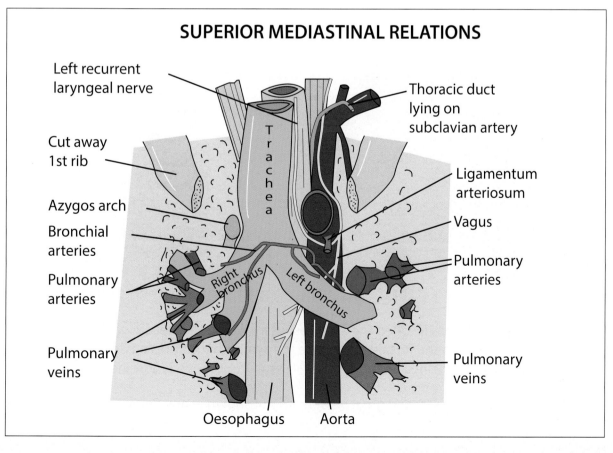

Left recurrent laryngeal nerve

Thoracic duct lying on subclavian artery

Cut away 1st rib

Trachea

Azygos arch

Ligamentum arteriosum

Bronchial arteries

Vagus

Pulmonary arteries

Pulmonary arteries

Right bronchus

Left bronchus

Pulmonary arteries

Pulmonary veins

Pulmonary veins

Oesophagus

Aorta

PLEURAL NERVE SUPPLY

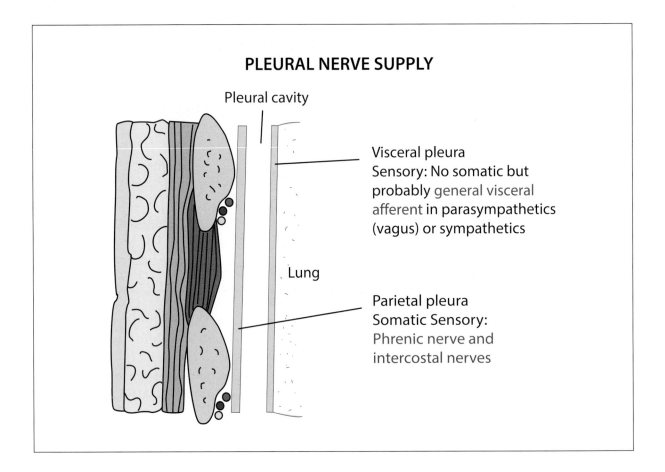

Pleural cavity

Visceral pleura
Sensory: No somatic but
probably general visceral
afferent in parasympathetics
(vagus) or sympathetics

Lung

Parietal pleura
Somatic Sensory:
Phrenic nerve and
intercostal nerves

APICAL TUMOUR OF THE LEFT LUNG (PANCOAST'S TUMOUR)

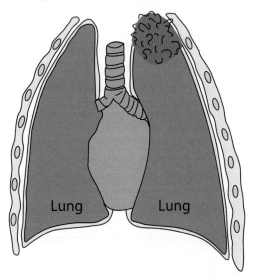

Lung   Lung

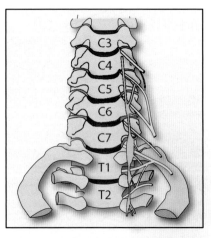

C3
C4
C5
C6
C7
T1
T2

The tumour has invaded the local tissues including the stellate ganglion
by the neck of the first rib and hence the sympathetic fibres passing up
the chain to the head region. This will result in Horner's Syndrome

The heart and great vessels are not shown in any detail

RIGHT SIMPLE NON- TENSION PNEUMOTHORAX

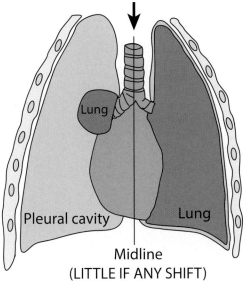

Lung

Lung

Pleural cavity

Midline
(LITTLE IF ANY SHIFT)

Air has entered the pleural cavity by a defect in the lung (e.g. ruptured bulla) or trauma and the right lung has completely collapsed. The mediastinum has not shifted to the left but there is disappearance of lung markings on the right on an X-ray

The heart and great vessels are not shown in detail

LEFT TENSION PNEUMOTHORAX

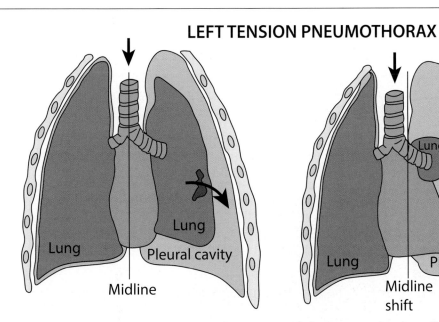
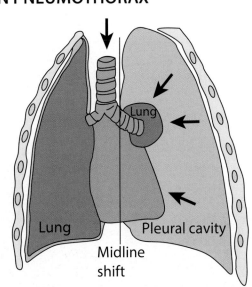

Lung

Lung

Pleural cavity

Lung

Midline

Lung

Lung

Pleural cavity

Midline
shift

A valvular leak into the pleural cavity from the lung due to tearing of the lung

Left lung completely collapsed, mediastinum shifted to right and disappearance of lung markings on left on X-ray

The heart and great vessels are not shown in detail

LEFT PLEURAL EFFUSION

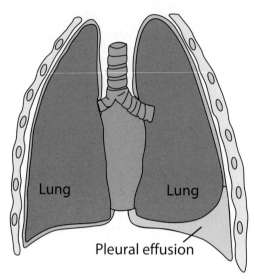

Lung

Lung

Pleural effusion

Fluid has entered the pleural cavity on the left side and accumulated inferior to the lung.

The heart and great vessels are not shown in detail

ANAESTHETISING CHEST WALL TISSUES FOR INSERTION OF CHEST DRAIN

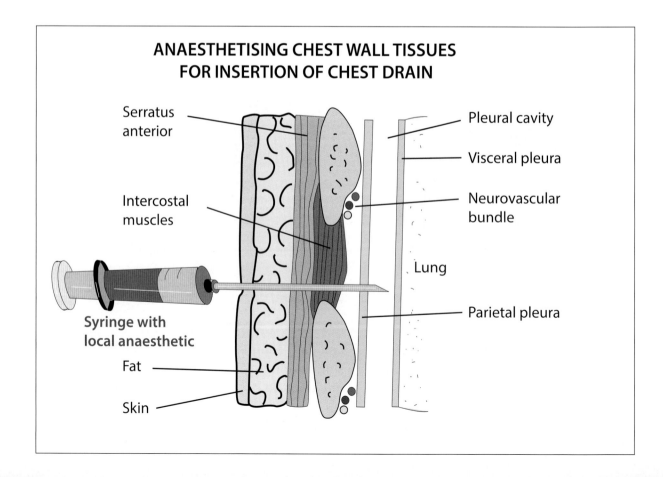

Serratus anterior

Intercostal muscles

Syringe with local anaesthetic

Fat

Skin

Pleural cavity

Visceral pleura

Neurovascular bundle

Lung

Parietal pleura

INTERCOSTAL DRAIN INSERTION

Aim upwards for air and downwards for fluid. 4th or 5th space in anterior axillary line (to avoid long thoracic nerve), posterior to pectoralis major. Oblique tract to avoid leakage on removal.

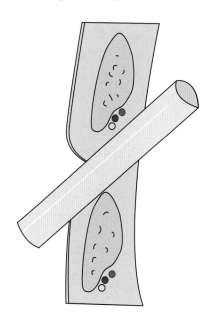
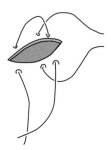

Suture in place and ready to be tied rapidly to avoid air entering the chest when drain is removed

DRAINING A PLEURAL EFFUSION

Chest drain draining air or fluids from the pleural cavity is connected to an underwater seal

Air is forced down this tube (chest drain) during expiration

Air is allowed to escape through this tube

The end of this tube is below the surface of the fluid in the bottle to prevent air returning in the chest tube during inspiration

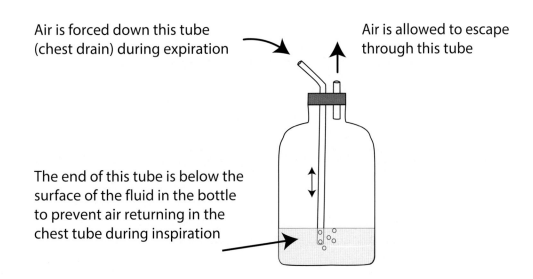

OESOPHAGUS (27cm long)
C6 - T10

Nerves: Sensation and motor via vagus nerves
Lining: Stratified squamous (non-keratinising) becoming columnar at stomach
Thick muscularis mucosae ++
Mucous glands in mucosa and submucosa

1/3rds	MUSCLE	ARTERY	VEIN	LYMPH	LENGTH (27cm)
Upper	**Striated**	Inferior thyroid	Inferior thyroid	**Deep cervical**	9cm
Middle	**Striated/ smooth**	Aortic branches	Azygos branches	**Mediastinal**	9cm
Lower	**Smooth**	Left gastric	Left gastric	**Gastric**	9cm

RELATIONS OF OESOPHAGUS

Slight compression (endoscopic narrowings) distance from teeth) from:

Cricoid   15cm
cartilage

Aorta   27cm
Left bronchus
left atrium

Diaphragmatic 40cm
hiatus

Posterior: vertebrae, thoracic duct crosses to left at T5, hemiazygos/ accessory hemiazygos cross to right at T8/9, descending aorta, first 2 intercostal arteries from aorta

Anterior: trachea to T4/5, recurrent laryngeal nerves, left bronchus, left atrium, diaphragm

Left: thoracic duct, aorta, left subclavian artery, lung

Right: lung, azygos vein (hence good side to approach the oesophagus surgically)

Note: 40-45cm is also the length of thoracic duct, vas, femur, spinal cord and transverse colon

THE ROLE OF CRICOPHARYNGEUS IN THE MALLORY WEISS AND BOERHAAVE'S SYNDROMES

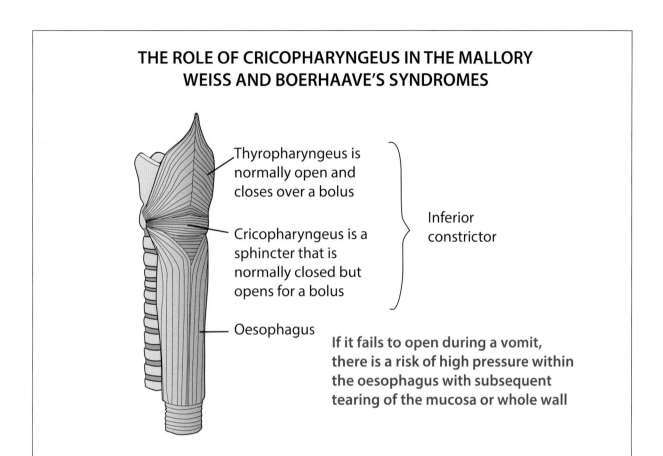

Thyropharyngeus is normally open and closes over a bolus

Cricopharyngeus is a sphincter that is normally closed but opens for a bolus

Inferior constrictor

Oesophagus

If it fails to open during a vomit, there is a risk of high pressure within the oesophagus with subsequent tearing of the mucosa or whole wall

PORTOSYSTEMIC ANASTOMOSIS IN LOWER OESOPHAGUS

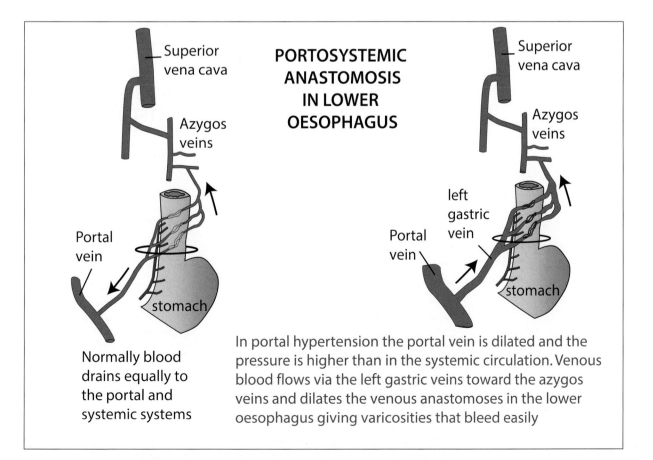

Superior vena cava

Azygos veins

Portal vein

stomach

Normally blood drains equally to the portal and systemic systems

Superior vena cava

Azygos veins

left gastric vein

Portal vein

stomach

In portal hypertension the portal vein is dilated and the pressure is higher than in the systemic circulation. Venous blood flows via the left gastric veins toward the azygos veins and dilates the venous anastomoses in the lower oesophagus giving varicosities that bleed easily

3.5 Vessels and Nerves

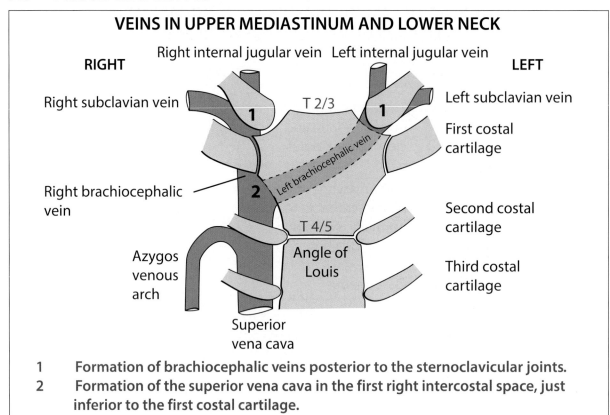

VEINS IN UPPER MEDIASTINUM AND LOWER NECK

Right internal jugular vein   Left internal jugular vein

RIGHT

LEFT

Right subclavian vein

T 2/3

1   **1**

Left subclavian vein

First costal cartilage

Left brachiocephalic vein

Right brachiocephalic vein

2

Second costal cartilage

T 4/5

Azygos venous arch

Angle of Louis

Third costal cartilage

Superior vena cava

1   Formation of brachiocephalic veins posterior to the sternoclavicular joints.
2   Formation of the superior vena cava in the first right intercostal space, just inferior to the first costal cartilage.

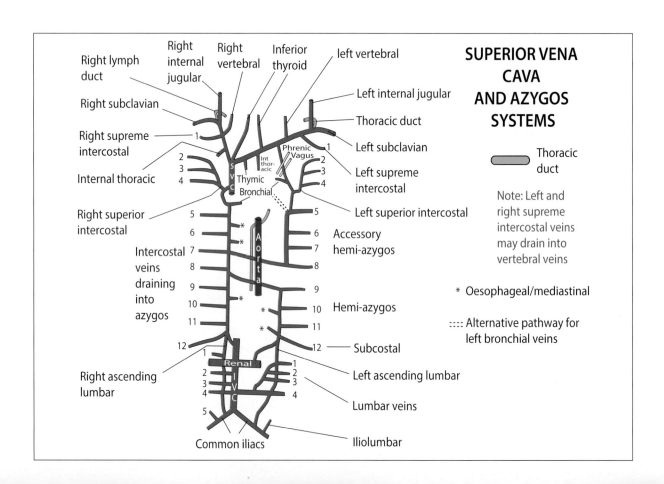

Right lymph duct

Right internal jugular

Right vertebral

Inferior thyroid

left vertebral

Right subclavian

Left internal jugular

Thoracic duct

Right supreme intercostal

1

Phrenic Vagus

1

Left subclavian

2
3
4

Int thor-acic

2
3
4

Left supreme intercostal

Internal thoracic

Thymic
Bronchial

Right superior intercostal

5

5

Left superior intercostal

6

6

Accessory hemi-azygos

Intercostal veins draining into azygos

7

*

Aorta

7

8

8

9

9

10

*

10

Hemi-azygos

11

*

11

12

12

Subcostal

Right ascending lumbar

1
Renal
2
3
IVC
4
5

1
2
3
4

Left ascending lumbar

Lumbar veins

Common iliacs

Iliolumbar

SUPERIOR VENA CAVA AND AZYGOS SYSTEMS

Thoracic duct

Note: Left and right supreme intercostal veins may drain into vertebral veins

* Oesophageal/mediastinal

:::: Alternative pathway for left bronchial veins

VENOUS DRAINAGE OF INTERCOSTAL SPACES

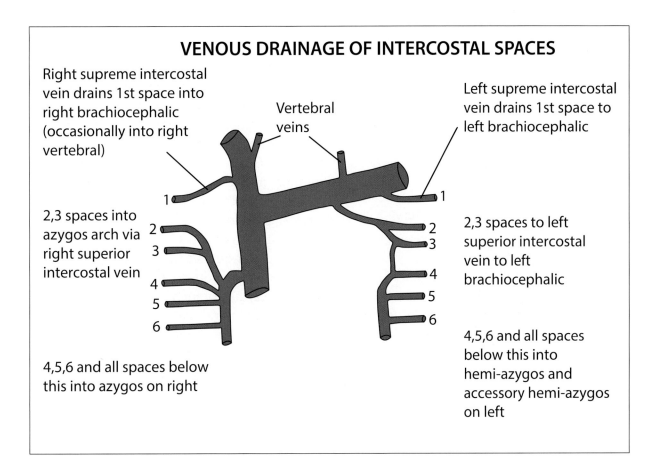

Right supreme intercostal vein drains 1st space into right brachiocephalic (occasionally into right vertebral)

Vertebral veins

Left supreme intercostal vein drains 1st space to left brachiocephalic

2,3 spaces into azygos arch via right superior intercostal vein

2,3 spaces to left superior intercostal vein to left brachiocephalic

4,5,6 and all spaces below this into azygos on right

4,5,6 and all spaces below this into hemi-azygos and accessory hemi-azygos on left

MAJOR VESSELS AND RECURRENT LARYNGEAL NERVES

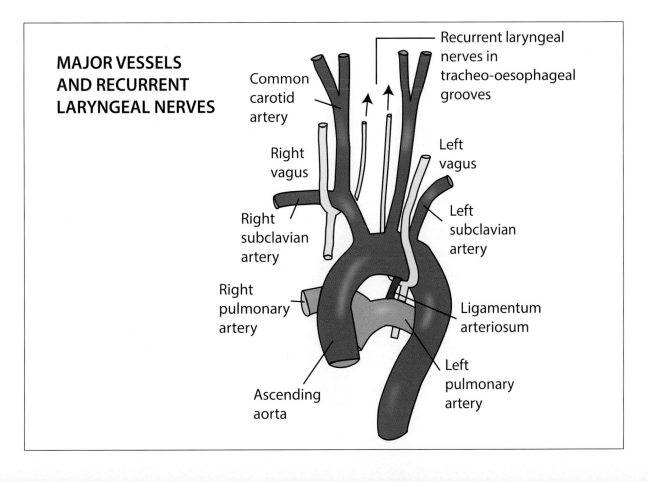

Recurrent laryngeal nerves in tracheo-oesophageal grooves

Common carotid artery

Right vagus

Left vagus

Right subclavian artery

Left subclavian artery

Right pulmonary artery

Ligamentum arteriosum

Ascending aorta

Left pulmonary artery

AORTIC ARCH

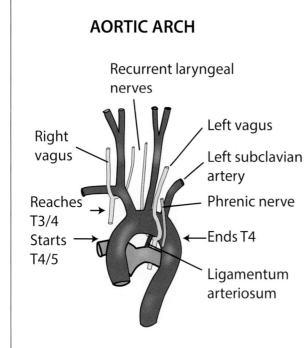

Recurrent laryngeal nerves

Right vagus

Reaches T3/4

Starts T4/5

Left vagus

Left subclavian artery

Phrenic nerve

Ends T4

Ligamentum arteriosum

Relations:
Left: Pleura, vagus, left phrenic nerve
Right: Trachea, oesophagus, thoracic duct, left recurrent laryngeal nerve, superior vena cava, right phrenic nerve
Anterior: Thymus, superficial cardiac plexus, (Inferior cardiac branch of left vagus and left cardiac sympathetic branch from superior cervical ganglion)
Inferior: Ligamentum arteriosum, left recurrent laryngeal nerve, bifurcation of pulmonary trunk, deep cardiac plexus (superior cardiac branch of left vagus, superior and inferior cardiac branches from right vagus, left and right recurrent laryngeal nerves, left cardiac sympathetic branch from middle and inferior cervical ganglion, right cardiac sympathetic branch from all 3 cervical ganglia)

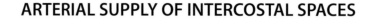

ARTERIAL SUPPLY OF INTERCOSTAL SPACES

SUPERIOR INTERCOSTAL ARTERY (2nd part of subclavian via costocervical artery)
Upper 2 spaces

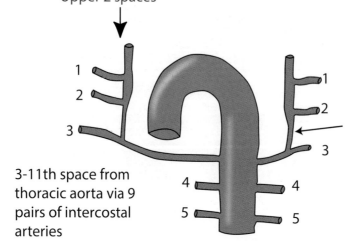

3-11th space from thoracic aorta via 9 pairs of intercostal arteries

If superior intercostal artery is missing (usually on left) the first 2 spaces are supplied by branches from the aorta

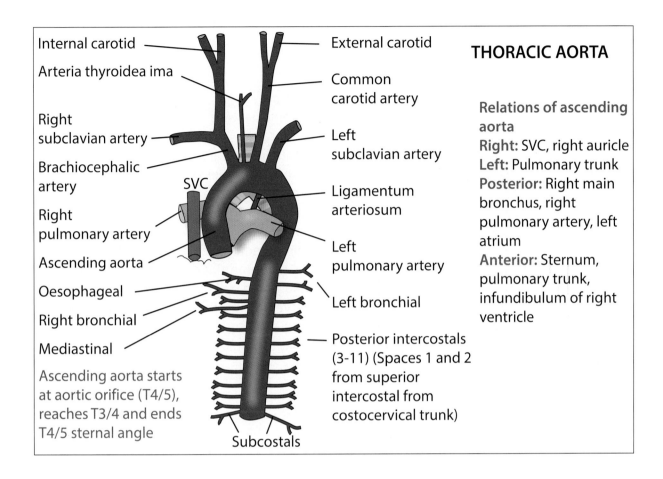

Internal carotid

Arteria thyroidea ima

Right subclavian artery

Brachiocephalic artery

SVC

Right pulmonary artery

Ascending aorta

Oesophageal

Right bronchial

Mediastinal

Ascending aorta starts at aortic orifice (T4/5), reaches T3/4 and ends T4/5 sternal angle

External carotid

Common carotid artery

Left subclavian artery

Ligamentum arteriosum

Left pulmonary artery

Left bronchial

Posterior intercostals (3-11) (Spaces 1 and 2 from superior intercostal from costocervical trunk)

Subcostals

THORACIC AORTA

Relations of ascending aorta
Right: SVC, right auricle
Left: Pulmonary trunk
Posterior: Right main bronchus, right pulmonary artery, left atrium
Anterior: Sternum, pulmonary trunk, infundibulum of right ventricle

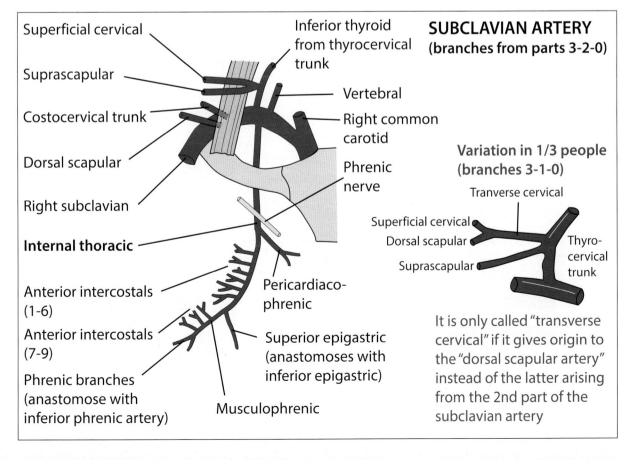

Superficial cervical

Suprascapular

Costocervical trunk

Dorsal scapular

Right subclavian

Internal thoracic

Anterior intercostals (1-6)

Anterior intercostals (7-9)

Phrenic branches (anastomose with inferior phrenic artery)

Inferior thyroid from thyrocervical trunk

Vertebral

Right common carotid

Phrenic nerve

Pericardiaco-phrenic

Superior epigastric (anastomoses with inferior epigastric)

Musculophrenic

SUBCLAVIAN ARTERY
(branches from parts 3-2-0)

Variation in 1/3 people (branches 3-1-0)

Tranverse cervical
Superficial cervical
Dorsal scapular
Suprascapular
Thyro-cervical trunk

It is only called "transverse cervical" if it gives origin to the "dorsal scapular artery" instead of the latter arising from the 2nd part of the subclavian artery

THE PHRENIC NERVE

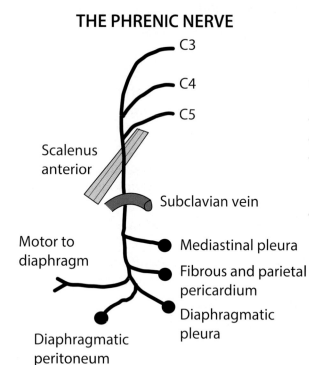

C3
C4
C5
Scalenus anterior
Subclavian vein
Motor to diaphragm
Mediastinal pleura
Fibrous and parietal pericardium
Diaphragmatic pleura
Diaphragmatic peritoneum

Notes:
- Phrenic nerve is the only motor supply to diaphragm.
- A third of its fibres are sensory.
- In the neck it lies on scalenus anterior.
- It passes into the thorax with the large veins anterior to it and the large arteries posterior to it.
- Pain detected by the phrenic nerve from the diaphragmatic peritoneum from an inflammed gall bladder is referred to C4 nerve distribution to the right shoulder tip via the supraclavicular nerves. There is no autonomic component to this type of referred pain.

VAGUS AND PHRENIC NERVES IN NECK

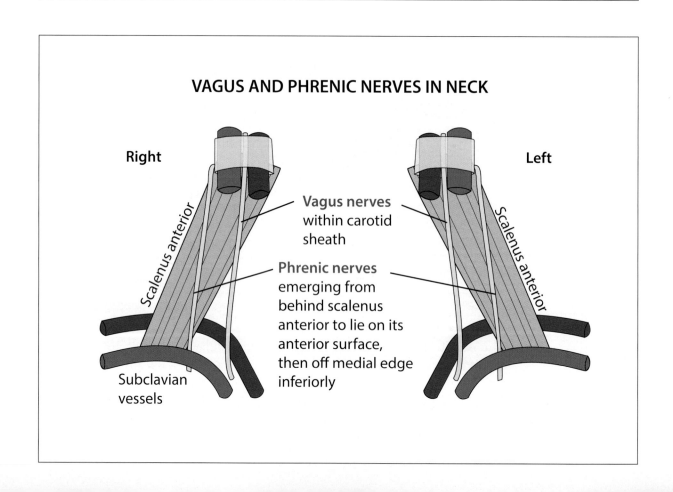

Right

Left

Scalenus anterior

Scalenus anterior

Vagus nerves within carotid sheath

Phrenic nerves emerging from behind scalenus anterior to lie on its anterior surface, then off medial edge inferiorly

Subclavian vessels

PHRENIC AND VAGUS NERVES ENTERING THE THORAX

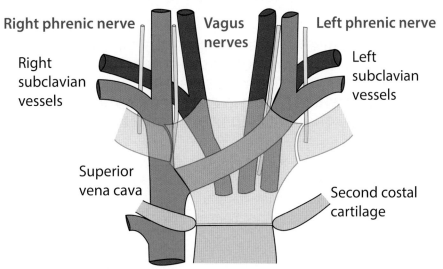

Left and right internal jugular veins and common carotid arteries

Right phrenic nerve

Vagus nerves

Left phrenic nerve

Right subclavian vessels

Left subclavian vessels

Superior vena cava

Second costal cartilage

At the level of the thoracic inlet, both vagus and phrenic nerves enter the thorax between the veins anteriorly and the arteries posteriorly

RELATIONS OF PHRENIC AND VAGUS NERVES TO HILA OF LUNGS

Right vagus medial to azygos arch then **POSTERIOR** to hilum to reach oesophagus

Left vagus over arch of aorta then **POSTERIOR** to hilum to reach oesophagus

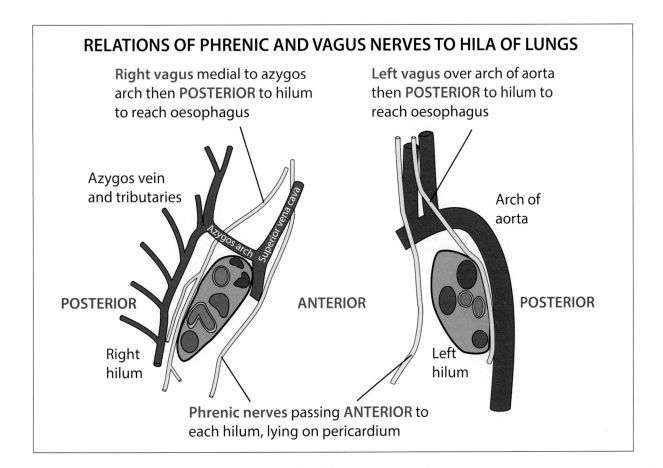

Azygos vein and tributaries

Azygos arch

Superior vena cava

Arch of aorta

POSTERIOR

ANTERIOR

POSTERIOR

Right hilum

Left hilum

Phrenic nerves passing **ANTERIOR** to each hilum, lying on pericardium

THORACIC SYMPATHETICS

ALL SYMPATHETIC FIBRES ENTERING THE CHAIN FROM THE SPINAL CORD AS WHITE RAMI COMMUNICANTES SYNAPSE IN THE GANGLION FROM WHICH THEY LEAVE FOR DISTRIBUTION EXCEPT THOSE TO "GUT" AND ADRENAL GLAND.

In practice this means that the splanchnic nerves (greater, lesser, least, lumbar and sacral) do not synapse until they reach their peripheral ganglia, whilst all others synapse in the chain ganglia.

3.6   Cross Sections

CROSS-SECTIONS OF THE THORAX BETWEEN T1 AND T10 VERTEBRAL LEVELS

Key to abbreviations

AscA   Ascending aorta
AV   Azygos vein
BA   Brachiocephalic artery
CS   Coronary sinus
CT   Crista terminalis
DscA   Descending aorta
IAS   Interatrial septum
LA   Left atrium/auricle
LB   Left bronchus
LBV   Left brachiocephalic vein
LCCA   Left common carotid artery
LPA   Left pulmonary artery
LSA   Left subclavian artery
LSV   Left subclavian vein
LV   Left ventricle
MB   Moderator band

MV   Mitral valve
O   Oesophagus
PT   Pulmonary trunk
PV   Pulmonary veins
RA   Right atrium/auricle
RB   Right bronchus
RBV   Right brachiocephalic vein
RPA   Right pulmonary artery
RSV   Right subclavian vein
RV   Right ventricle
SVC   Superior vena cava
T   Trachea
TD   Thoracic duct
TV   Tricuspid valve
TY   Thymus
V   Valve of IVC

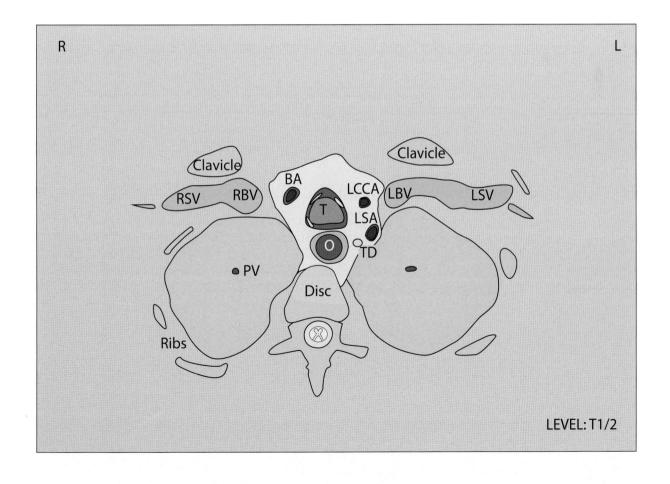

LEVEL: T1/2

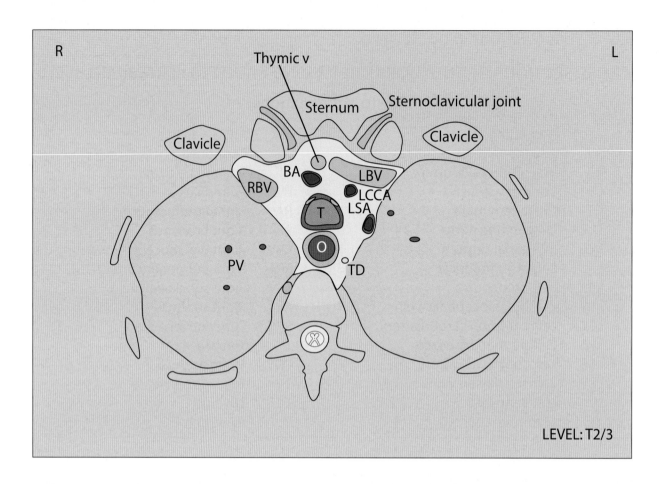

R
L
Thymic v
Sternum
Sternoclavicular joint
Clavicle
Clavicle
BA
LBV
RBV
LCCA
LSA
T
O
PV
TD
LEVEL: T2/3

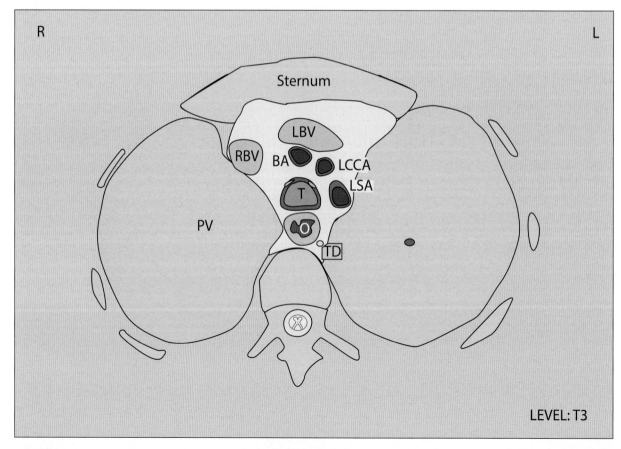

R
L
Sternum
LBV
RBV
BA
LCCA
LSA
T
O
PV
TD
LEVEL: T3

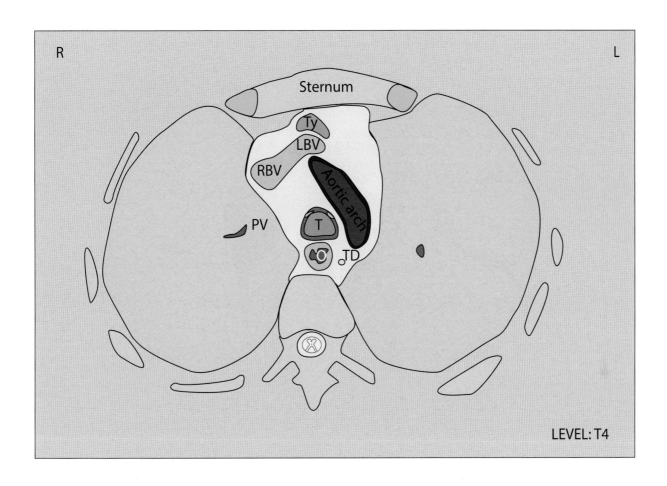

LEVEL: T4

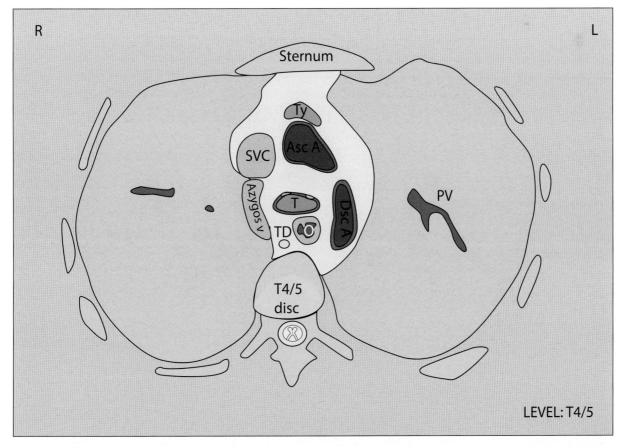

LEVEL: T4/5

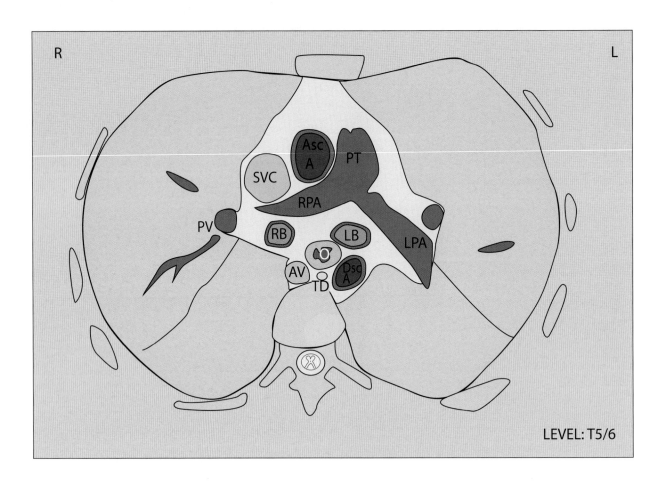

LEVEL: T5/6

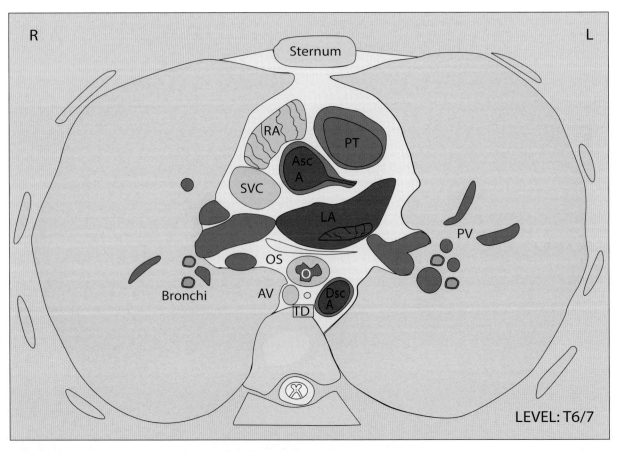

LEVEL: T6/7

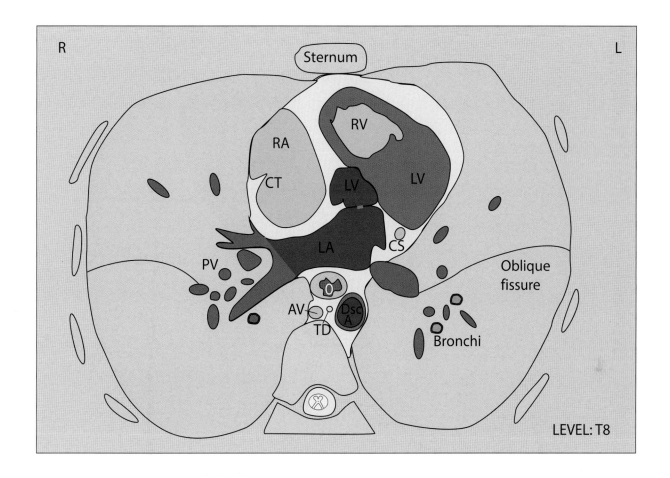

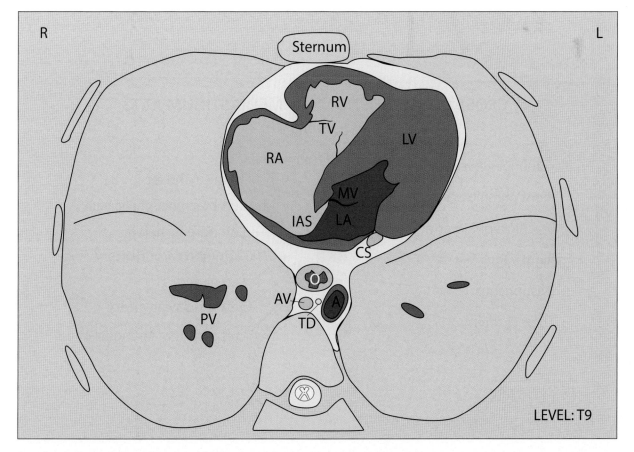

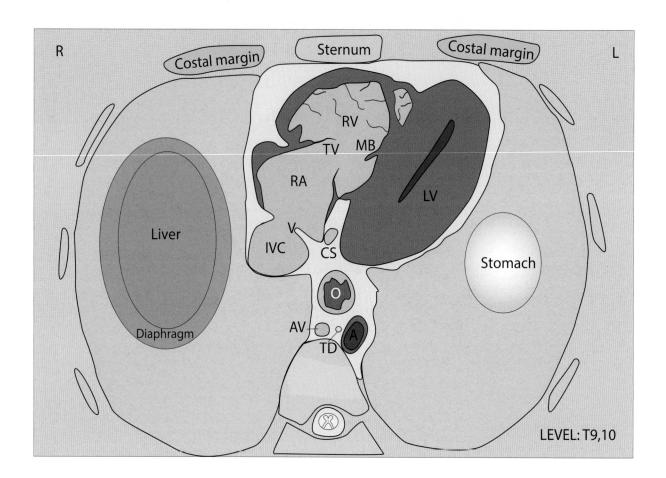

R   Costal margin   Sternum   Costal margin   L

RV

TV   MB

RA

LV

Liver

V

IVC   CS

Stomach

O

Diaphragm

AV

TD

A

LEVEL: T9,10

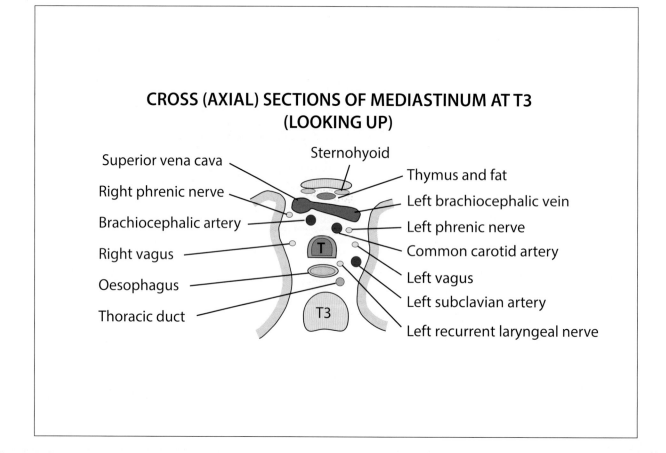

CROSS (AXIAL) SECTIONS OF MEDIASTINUM AT T3 (LOOKING UP)

Superior vena cava

Sternohyoid

Right phrenic nerve

Thymus and fat

Brachiocephalic artery

Left brachiocephalic vein

Right vagus

Left phrenic nerve

Oesophagus

Common carotid artery

Thoracic duct

Left vagus

Left subclavian artery

Left recurrent laryngeal nerve

T

T3

CROSS (AXIAL) SECTIONS OF MEDIASTINUM AT T4
(LOOKING UP)

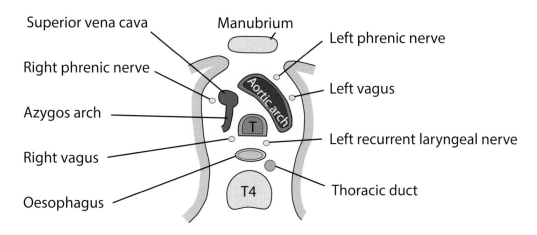

Superior vena cava

Manubrium

Left phrenic nerve

Right phrenic nerve

Aortic arch

Left vagus

Azygos arch

T

Right vagus

Left recurrent laryngeal nerve

Oesophagus

T4

Thoracic duct

CROSS (AXIAL) SECTIONS OF MEDIASTINUM AT T5
(LOOKING UP)

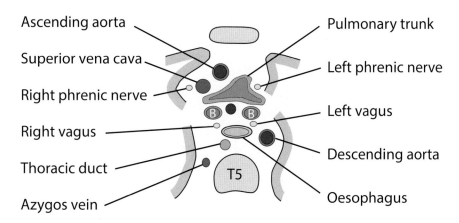

Ascending aorta

Pulmonary trunk

Superior vena cava

Left phrenic nerve

Right phrenic nerve

B   B

Left vagus

Right vagus

Descending aorta

Thoracic duct

Oesophagus

Azygos vein

T5

SECTION 4

Abdomen and Pelvis

4.1 Surface Anatomy and Hernia

SURFACE ANATOMY OF POSTERIOR ABDOMINAL WALL

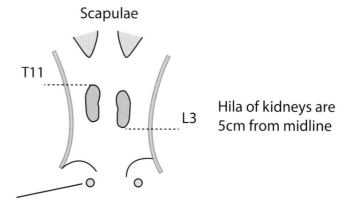

Scapulae

T11

L3

Hila of kidneys are 5cm from midline

Sacral dimples (S2)
- Mid point of sacro-iliac joints
- End of dural sac
- Posterior superior iliac spine

VERTEBRAL LEVELS

T8

T10

T12

L1

L2

L3

L4

L5

S2

S3

T8   Caval opening (diaphragm); right phrenic nerve

T10 Oesophageal opening (diaphragm); branches of left gastric vessels to lower oesophagus; vagus nerves)

T12 Aortic opening (diaphragm); aorta; ascending lumbar veins becoming azygos veins; cisterna chyli becoming thoracic duct; coeliac axis/trunk

L1   Transpyloric plane; superior mesenteric artery

L1/2 Spinal cord ends; renal arteries

L2   Subcostal plane; gonadal arteries

L3   Inferior mesenteric artery

L3/4 Umbilicus

L4   Bifurcation of aorta; supracristal plane

L5   Formation of vena cava

S2   Sacral dimple; mid point of sacroiliac joint; end of dural sac: lower attachment of small bowel mesentery

S3   Start of rectum

TRANSPYLORIC PLANE

(Horizontal line half way between suprasternal notch and pubic symphysis)

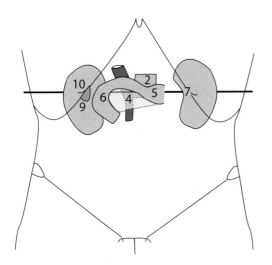

Structures approximately on this line:
1. End of spinal cord
2. L1 vertebral body
3. Origin of superior mesenteric artery
4. Origin of portal vein and neck of pancreas
5. Pylorus of the stomach
6. Second part of duodenum and Sphincter of Oddi
7. Hilum of each kidney
8. Duodenojejunal flexure
9. Fundus of gall bladder
10. Tips of ninth costal cartilages

REGIONS OF ABDOMEN

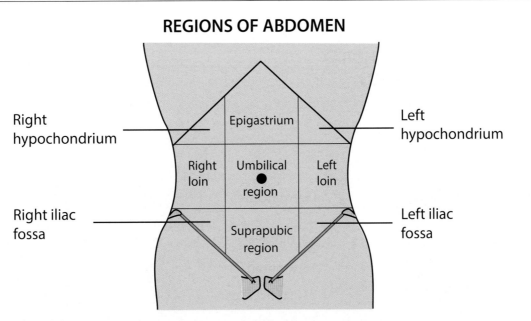

For descriptive purposes, both anatomically and clinically, the abdomen is divided into 9 regions by 2 horizontal and 2 vertical lines. Books tend to define these lines but, in reality and because of human variation in shape and size, the lines are arbitrary.
An alternative method, often used clinically, is simply to divide the abdomen into 4 quadrants, upper, lower, left and right, with 2 loins posteriorly

SURFACE MARKINGS ON ABDOMINAL WALL

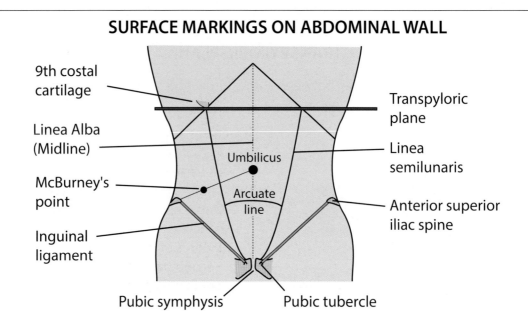

9th costal cartilage

Linea Alba (Midline)

McBurney's point

Inguinal ligament

Transpyloric plane

Linea semilunaris

Anterior superior iliac spine

Umbilicus

Arcuate line

Pubic symphysis

Pubic tubercle

Transpyloric plane: Half way between suprasternal notch and symphysis pubis
Inguinal ligament: Anterior superior iliac spine to pubic tubercle
Arcuate line: 3-5cm inferior to umbilicus
Linea semilunaris: Lateral edge of rectus sheath
McBurney's point: One third along a line from ASIS to umbilicus. Incision site for appendicectomy

DERMATOMES OF THORAX AND ABDOMEN

DERMATOMES OF ABDOMEN

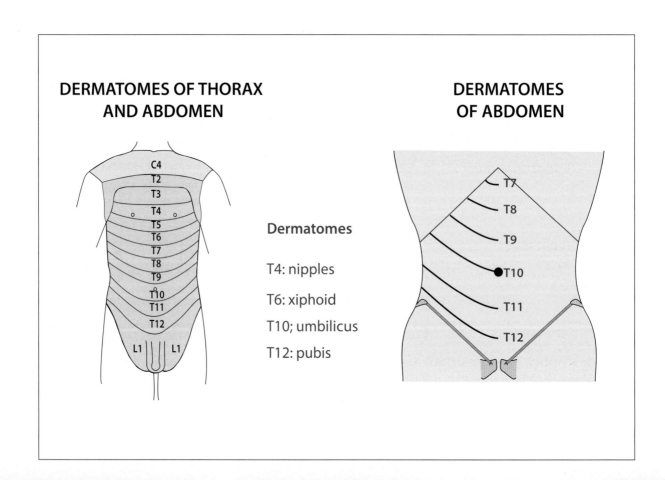

C4
T2
T3
T4
T5
T6
T7
T8
T9
T10
T11
T12
L1   L1

T7
T8
T9
T10
T11
T12

Dermatomes

T4: nipples

T6: xiphoid

T10; umbilicus

T12: pubis

LAYERS OF THE ABDOMINAL WALL

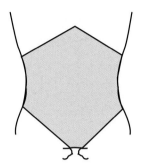

1   Skin
2   Fat
3   Camper's fascia (superficial layer of superficial fascia - thin)
4   Fat
5   Scarpa's fascia (deep layer of superficial fascia - thick)
6   Fat
7   Aponeurosis
8   Three muscles
9   Transversalis fascia
10 Peritoneum

ABDOMINAL WALL MUSCLES 1

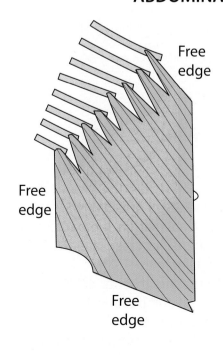

Free edge

Free edge

Free edge

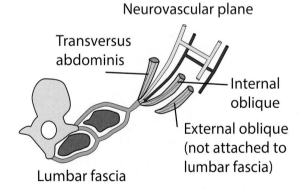

Neurovascular plane

Transversus abdominis

Internal oblique

External oblique (not attached to lumbar fascia)

Lumbar fascia

EXTERNAL OBLIQUE
From: Anterior angles last 8 ribs.
To: Xiphisternum, linea alba, pubic symphysis and crest, inguinal ligament, anterior 1/2 iliac crest.
Fibres: Run down/medial
Nerves: T7-12

LAYERS OF THORACOLUMBAR FASCIA

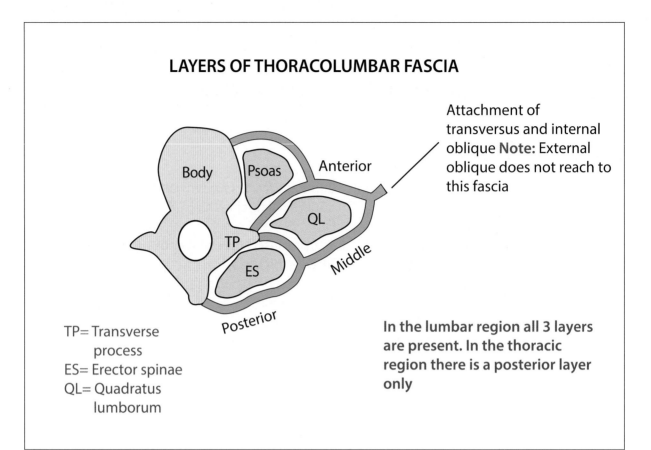

Attachment of transversus and internal oblique **Note:** External oblique does not reach to this fascia

Anterior

Body

Psoas

QL

TP

ES

Middle

Posterior

TP= Transverse process
ES= Erector spinae
QL= Quadratus lumborum

In the lumbar region all 3 layers are present. In the thoracic region there is a posterior layer only

ABDOMINAL WALL MUSCLES 2

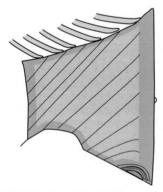

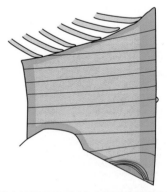

INTERNAL OBLIQUE
From: Anterior 2/3 iliac crest, lateral 2/3 inguinal ligament, lumbar fascia
To: Costal margin, rectus sheath. Conjoint tendon (CT) on pubic crest and pectineal line.
Fibres: Run upward/medial
Nerves: T7-12, ilioinguinal to CT

TRANSVERSUS ABDOMINIS
From: Costal margin, lumbar fascia, anterior 2/3 iliac crest, lateral 1/2 inguinal ligament
To: Rectus sheath, linea alba, CT to pubic crest and pectineal line
Fibres: Transverse
Nerves: T7-12, ilioinguinal to CT

ABDOMINAL WALL MUSCLES
RECTUS ABDOMINIS

RECTUS ABDOMINIS
From: Pubic crest, tubercle and symphysis pubis
To: Costal cartilages 5,6,7 and costal margin
of rib 7, sternum and diaphragm
Nerve: T7-12
(Note: 3 morphological layers)

Diaphragm

5
6
7

Xiphoid

3 Tendinous
intersections
(rarely 4)
Fusion to
anterior sheath

PYRAMIDALIS
From: Anterior of body
of pubic symphysis
To: Linea alba
Nerve: T12 (subcostal)

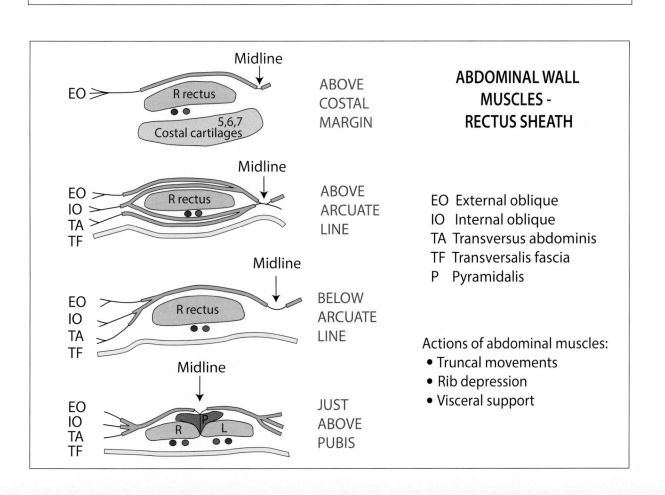

ABDOMINAL WALL
MUSCLES -
RECTUS SHEATH

Midline

EO
R rectus

ABOVE
COSTAL
MARGIN

5,6,7
Costal cartilages

Midline

EO
IO
TA
TF
R rectus

ABOVE
ARCUATE
LINE

Midline

EO
IO
TA
TF
R rectus

BELOW
ARCUATE
LINE

Midline

EO
IO
TA
TF
R   L
P

JUST
ABOVE
PUBIS

EO External oblique
IO Internal oblique
TA Transversus abdominis
TF Transversalis fascia
P   Pyramidalis

Actions of abdominal muscles:
• Truncal movements
• Rib depression
• Visceral support

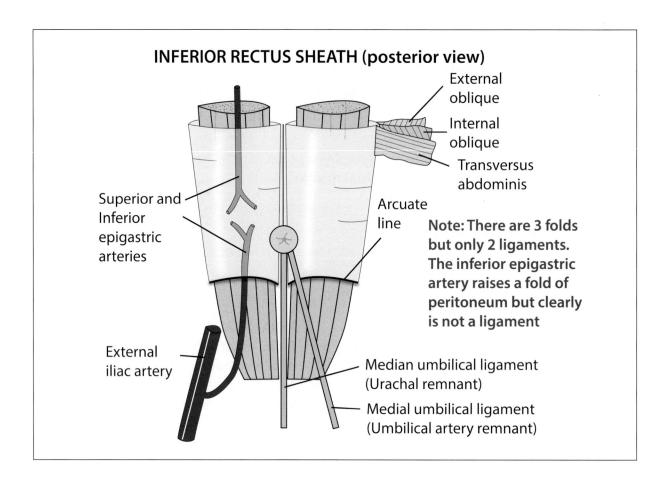

INFERIOR RECTUS SHEATH (posterior view)

External oblique

Internal oblique

Transversus abdominis

Superior and Inferior epigastric arteries

Arcuate line

Note: There are 3 folds but only 2 ligaments. The inferior epigastric artery raises a fold of peritoneum but clearly is not a ligament

External iliac artery

Median umbilical ligament (Urachal remnant)

Medial umbilical ligament (Umbilical artery remnant)

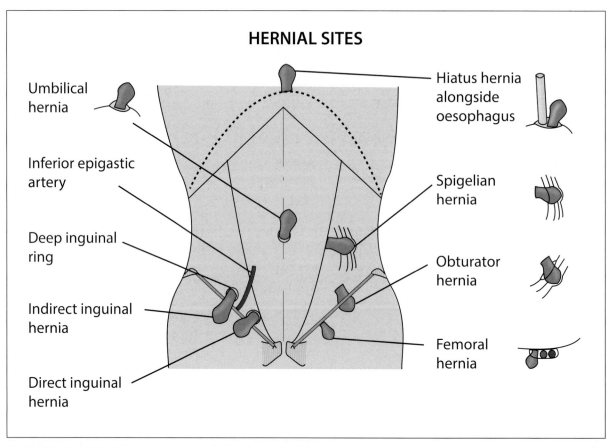

HERNIAL SITES

Umbilical hernia

Inferior epigastic artery

Deep inguinal ring

Indirect inguinal hernia

Direct inguinal hernia

Hiatus hernia alongside oesophagus

Spigelian hernia

Obturator hernia

Femoral hernia

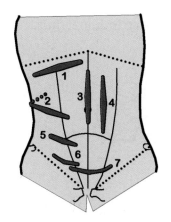

ABDOMINAL INCISIONS

Surgical Access
The more anterior the incision the poorer the blood supply and the worse the healing, but the less nerve and muscle damage. Vice versa for more posterior incisions

1	Subcostal	Muscle cutting	Gall bladder
2	Loin	Muscle cutting	Kidney/ureter
3	Midline	Between rectus sheaths	Upper/lower abdomen
4	Paramedian	Rectus sheath cutting	General
5	Grid iron	Muscle splitting	Appendix
6	Inguinal	Rectus sheath splitting	Hernia
7	Suprapubic	Sheath/muscle cutting	Pelvic organs

RIGHT INGUINAL LIGAMENT

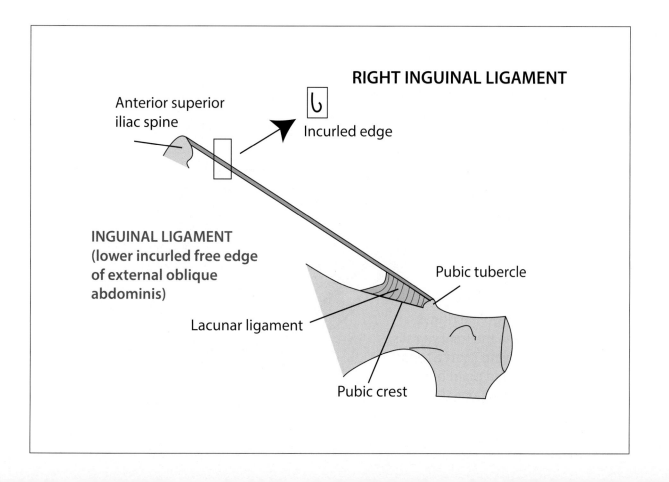

Anterior superior iliac spine

Incurled edge

INGUINAL LIGAMENT (lower incurled free edge of external oblique abdominis)

Pubic tubercle

Lacunar ligament

Pubic crest

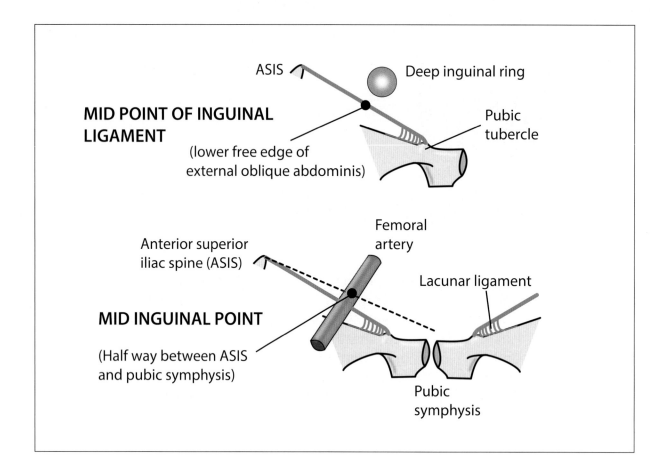

ASIS

Deep inguinal ring

MID POINT OF INGUINAL LIGAMENT

(lower free edge of external oblique abdominis)

Pubic tubercle

Anterior superior iliac spine (ASIS)

Femoral artery

Lacunar ligament

MID INGUINAL POINT

(Half way between ASIS and pubic symphysis)

Pubic symphysis

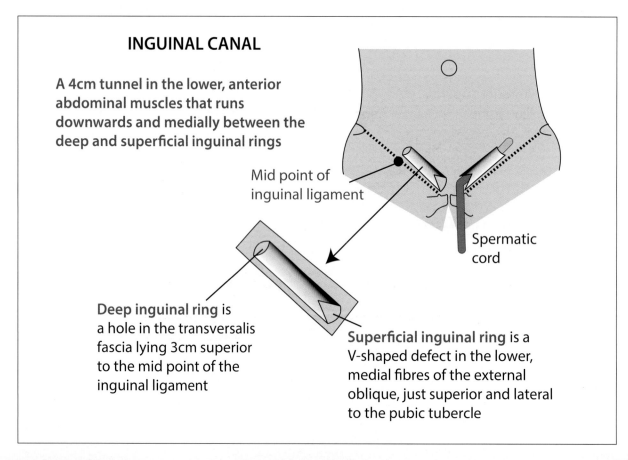

INGUINAL CANAL

A 4cm tunnel in the lower, anterior abdominal muscles that runs downwards and medially between the deep and superficial inguinal rings

Mid point of inguinal ligament

Spermatic cord

Deep inguinal ring is a hole in the transversalis fascia lying 3cm superior to the mid point of the inguinal ligament

Superficial inguinal ring is a V-shaped defect in the lower, medial fibres of the external oblique, just superior and lateral to the pubic tubercle

RIGHT INGUINAL CANAL

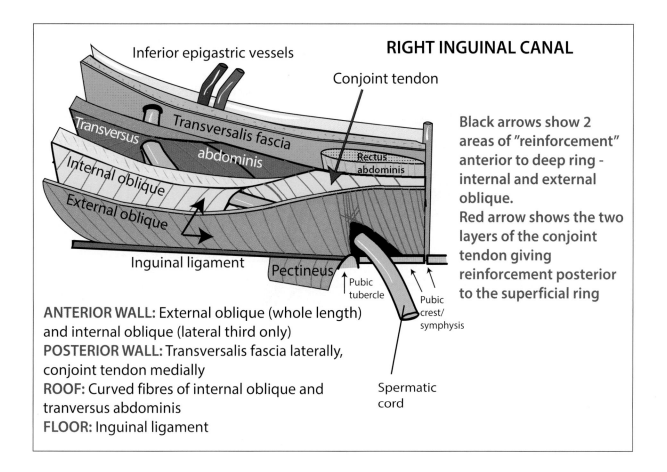

Inferior epigastric vessels

Conjoint tendon

Transversus

Transversalis fascia

abdominis

Internal oblique

External oblique

Rectus abdominis

Inguinal ligament

Pectineus

Pubic tubercle

Pubic crest/ symphysis

Spermatic cord

Black arrows show 2 areas of "reinforcement" anterior to deep ring - internal and external oblique.
Red arrow shows the two layers of the conjoint tendon giving reinforcement posterior to the superficial ring

ANTERIOR WALL: External oblique (whole length) and internal oblique (lateral third only)
POSTERIOR WALL: Transversalis fascia laterally, conjoint tendon medially
ROOF: Curved fibres of internal oblique and tranversus abdominis
FLOOR: Inguinal ligament

INGUINAL HERNIAS AND SPERMATIC CORD

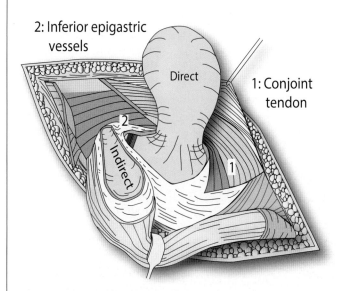

2: Inferior epigastric vessels

Direct

1: Conjoint tendon

Indirect

2

1

SPERMATIC CORD. Contents:
1. **3 arteries** (testicular, cremasteric, artery to vas)
2. **3 veins** (as above)
3. **3 fascia** (internal, spermatic, external)
4. **3 nerves** (ilio-inguinal, genital branch of genitofemoral, sympathetics)
5. **3 others** (vas, processus vaginalis, lymphatics)

INDIRECT hernia though deep ring, lateral to inferior epigastric vessels. **DIRECT** hernia through transversalis fascia and conjoint tendon, medial to inferior epigastric vessels

"EXPLODED" RIGHT INGUINAL CANAL

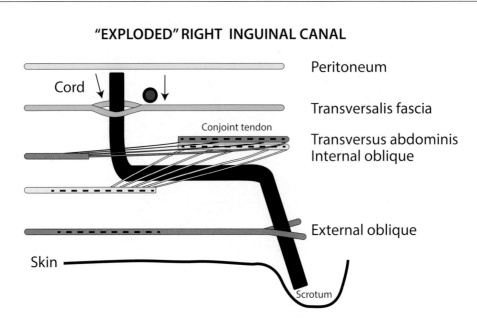

- Arrows indicate sites of weakness at deep ring (indirect hernia) and at transversalis fascia lateral to conjoint tendon (direct hernia).
- Dotted lines indicate the 2 layers that support both the deep and superficial inguinal rings.

ABDOMINAL WALL
RIGHT DEEP INGUINAL RING FROM INSIDE

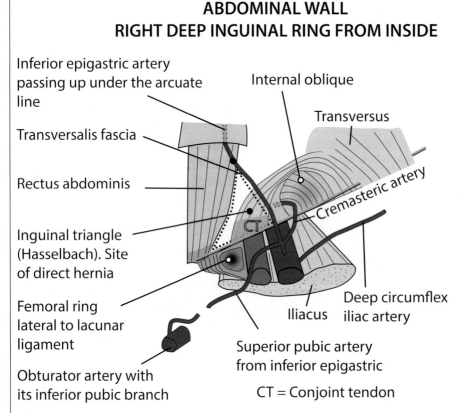

Note: If the obturator artery is missing then the superior pubic branch of the inferior epigastric takes over. This artery is then called an abnormal (aberrant) obturator artery. Whether or not an abnormal obturator artery is present, the superior pubic branch of the inferior epigastric may run anteromedial to the sac of a femoral hernia in the femoral ring. If so, it can easily be damaged during a hernia repair. In this illustration it runs posterolateral and is thus not a hazard

CT = Conjoint tendon

ABDOMINAL WALL -
FASCIA OVER INGUINAL REGION

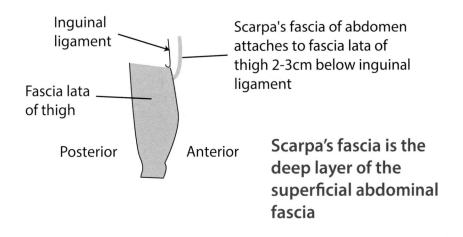

Inguinal ligament

Scarpa's fascia of abdomen attaches to fascia lata of thigh 2-3cm below inguinal ligament

Fascia lata of thigh

Posterior   Anterior

Scarpa's fascia is the deep layer of the superficial abdominal fascia

FEMORAL SHEATH AND CANAL

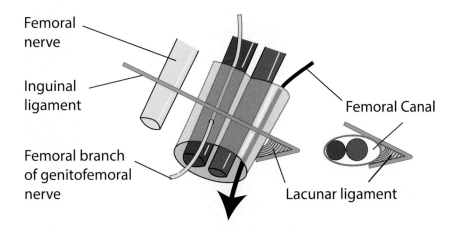

Femoral nerve

Inguinal ligament

Femoral branch of genitofemoral nerve

Femoral Canal

Lacunar ligament

FEMORAL CANAL lies within the femoral sheath between the lacunal ligament (medial), femoral vein (lateral), pubic ramus (posterior) and inguinal ligament (anterior). It transmits all the lower limb lymphatics and allows expansion of the femoral vein during high venous return. **A FEMORAL HERNIA** passes downwards through the canal and can be released by cutting the lacunar ligament.

FEMORAL HERNIA

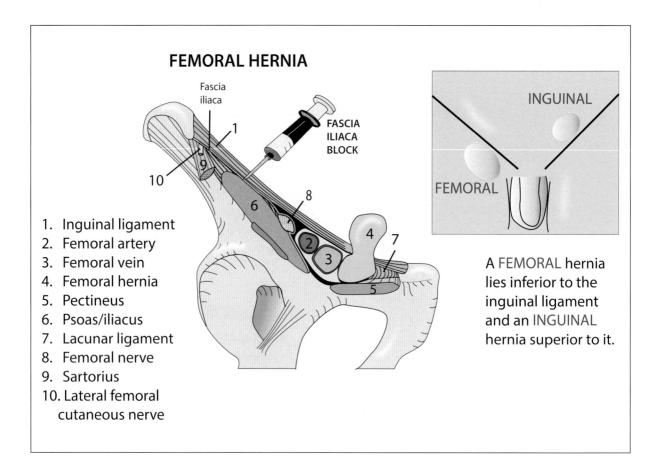

Fascia iliaca

FASCIA ILIACA BLOCK

1. Inguinal ligament
2. Femoral artery
3. Femoral vein
4. Femoral hernia
5. Pectineus
6. Psoas/iliacus
7. Lacunar ligament
8. Femoral nerve
9. Sartorius
10. Lateral femoral cutaneous nerve

INGUINAL

FEMORAL

A FEMORAL hernia lies inferior to the inguinal ligament and an INGUINAL hernia superior to it.

STRANGULATED BOWEL IN A HERNIA

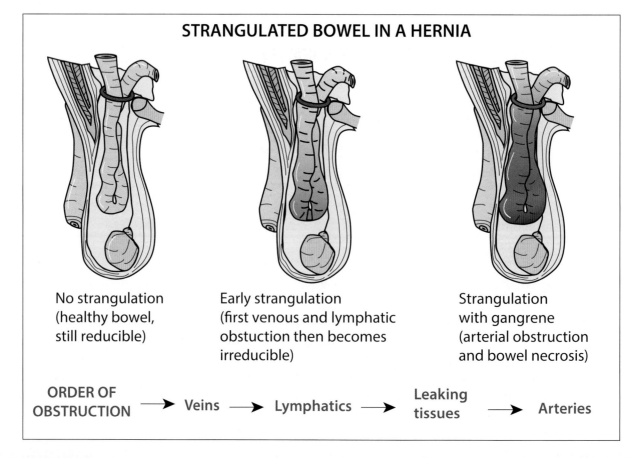

No strangulation (healthy bowel, still reducible)

Early strangulation (first venous and lymphatic obstuction then becomes irreducible)

Strangulation with gangrene (arterial obstruction and bowel necrosis)

ORDER OF OBSTRUCTION → Veins → Lymphatics → Leaking tissues → Arteries

ALTERNATIVE VENOUS DRAINAGE WHEN THE INFERIOR VENA CAVA IS BLOCKED

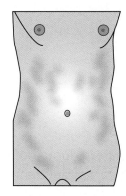

When the IVC is blocked there are two main alternative pathways for the return of blood to the heart. Via the epigastric veins, giving diffuse venous dilatation on the abdominal wall, or via the vertebral plexuses of **valveless** veins

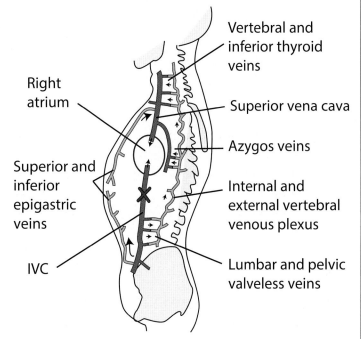

Right atrium

Superior and inferior epigastric veins

IVC

Vertebral and inferior thyroid veins

Superior vena cava

Azygos veins

Internal and external vertebral venous plexus

Lumbar and pelvic valveless veins

4.2 Peritoneum, Vessels and Nerves

RETROPERITONEAL	ON A MESENTERY
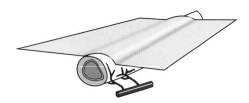	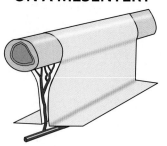

RETROPERITONEAL

- Most of duodenum
- Ascending colon
- Descending colon
- Rectum
- Pancreas
- Kidneys

ON A MESENTERY

- Stomach
- 1st half of 1st part of duodenum
- 2nd half of 4th part of duodenum
- All small bowel
- Caecum (size dependent)
- Appendix
- Transverse colon
- Sigmoid colon

The only items that are intraperitoneal are: A small amount of peritoneal fluid, the surface of the ovary and the end of the Fallopian tube. All other organs are intra-abdominal but not intraperitoneal

---

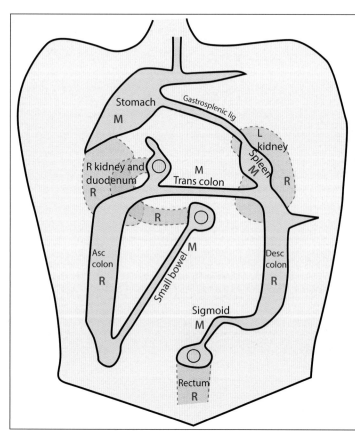

MESENTERY

All the intestines have been removed as far posterior as possible leaving the cut edges of the peritoneum. If the area of denuded peritoneum is narrow then the piece of bowel is on a mesentery. If it is wide then it was retroperitoneal, the exception being the stomach

M = On a mesentery

R = Retroperitoneal

ORGANS
Adrenals(*)
Kidneys
Ureters
Aorta and branches
IVC and branches
Rectum
Lumbar plexus
Duodenum
Pancreas

DISEASES
Pancreatitis
Trauma
Aneurysms
Iatrogenic

OTHER STRUCTURES
Muscles
Diaphragm
Nerves

RETROPERITONEUM

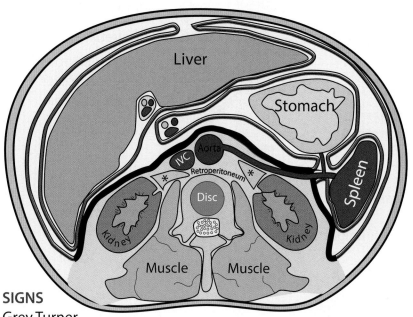

SIGNS
Grey Turner
(Flank bruising in
retroperitoneal bleeding)

Note: Right adrenal lies
partially posterior to IVC

RETROPERITONEUM

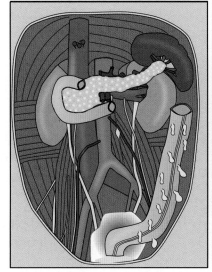

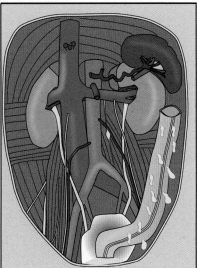

Pancreas present   **Pancreas removed**

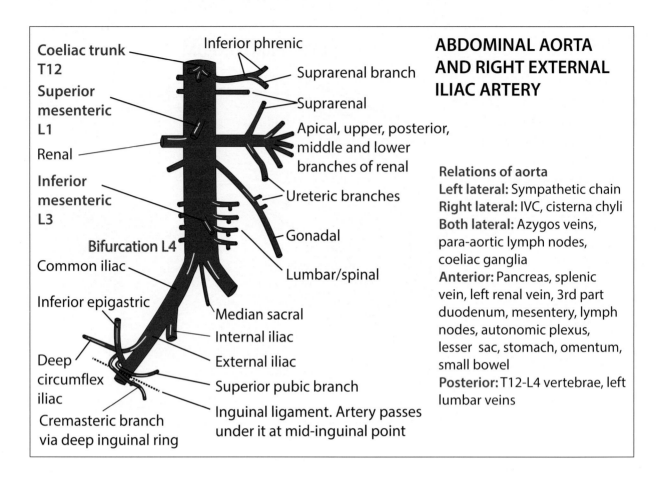

Coeliac trunk
T12

Superior
mesenteric
L1

Renal

Inferior
mesenteric
L3

Bifurcation L4

Common iliac

Inferior epigastric

Deep
circumflex
iliac

Cremasteric branch
via deep inguinal ring

Inferior phrenic

Suprarenal branch

Suprarenal

Apical, upper, posterior,
middle and lower
branches of renal

Ureteric branches

Gonadal

Lumbar/spinal

Median sacral

Internal iliac

External iliac

Superior pubic branch

Inguinal ligament. Artery passes
under it at mid-inguinal point

ABDOMINAL AORTA AND RIGHT EXTERNAL ILIAC ARTERY

Relations of aorta
Left lateral: Sympathetic chain
Right lateral: IVC, cisterna chyli
Both lateral: Azygos veins, para-aortic lymph nodes, coeliac ganglia
Anterior: Pancreas, splenic vein, left renal vein, 3rd part duodenum, mesentery, lymph nodes, autonomic plexus, lesser sac, stomach, omentum, small bowel
Posterior: T12-L4 vertebrae, left lumbar veins

LONGITUDINAL SECTION VIEWED FROM RIGHT

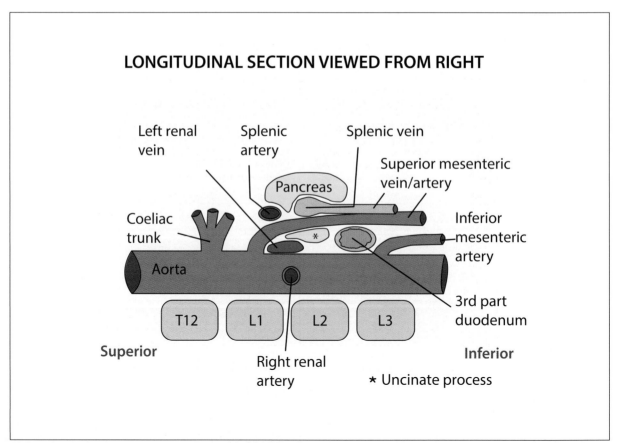

Left renal vein

Splenic artery

Splenic vein

Superior mesenteric vein/artery

Pancreas

Coeliac trunk

Inferior mesenteric artery

Aorta

3rd part duodenum

T12 L1 L2 L3

Superior

Right renal artery

Inferior

* Uncinate process

AXIAL (CROSS) SECTION AT L1 LOOKING UP

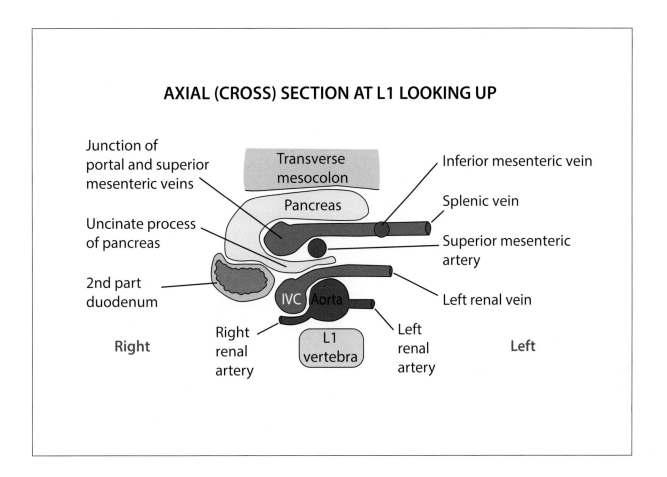

Junction of portal and superior mesenteric veins

Uncinate process of pancreas

2nd part duodenum

Transverse mesocolon

Pancreas

Inferior mesenteric vein

Splenic vein

Superior mesenteric artery

Left renal vein

Right renal artery

IVC Aorta

Left renal artery

L1 vertebra

Right

Left

LYMPHATIC DRAINAGE IN ABDOMEN

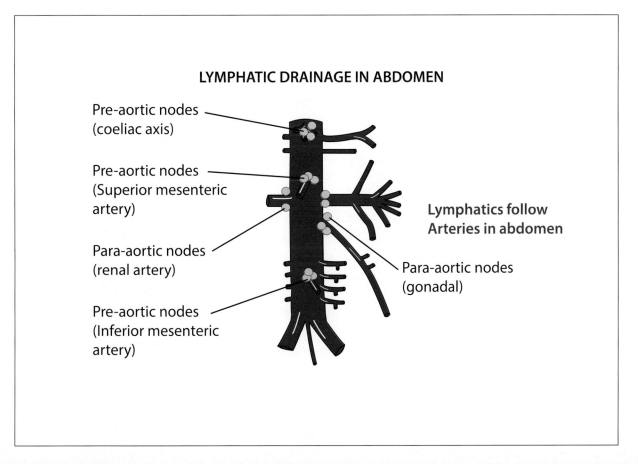

Pre-aortic nodes (coeliac axis)

Pre-aortic nodes (Superior mesenteric artery)

Para-aortic nodes (renal artery)

Pre-aortic nodes (Inferior mesenteric artery)

Lymphatics follow Arteries in abdomen

Para-aortic nodes (gonadal)

ABDOMINOPELVIC LYMPHATICS

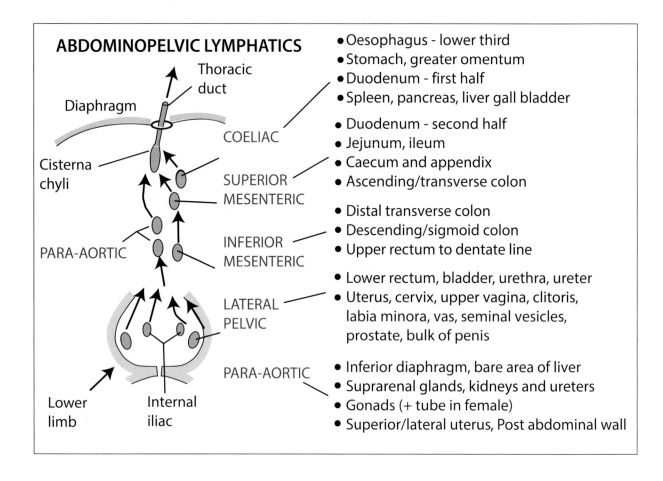

- Oesophagus - lower third
- Stomach, greater omentum
- Duodenum - first half
- Spleen, pancreas, liver gall bladder

COELIAC

- Duodenum - second half
- Jejunum, ileum
- Caecum and appendix
- Ascending/transverse colon

SUPERIOR MESENTERIC

- Distal transverse colon
- Descending/sigmoid colon
- Upper rectum to dentate line

INFERIOR MESENTERIC

- Lower rectum, bladder, urethra, ureter
- Uterus, cervix, upper vagina, clitoris, labia minora, vas, seminal vesicles, prostate, bulk of penis

LATERAL PELVIC

- Inferior diaphragm, bare area of liver
- Suprarenal glands, kidneys and ureters
- Gonads (+ tube in female)
- Superior/lateral uterus, Post abdominal wall

PARA-AORTIC

(Diagram labels: Thoracic duct, Diaphragm, Cisterna chyli, PARA-AORTIC, Lower limb, Internal iliac)

INFERIOR VENA CAVA

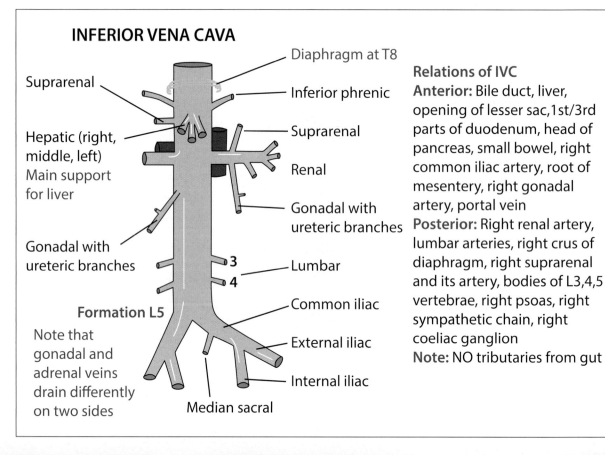

(Diagram labels: Suprarenal, Hepatic (right, middle, left) Main support for liver, Gonadal with ureteric branches, Formation L5, Note that gonadal and adrenal veins drain differently on two sides, Median sacral, Diaphragm at T8, Inferior phrenic, Suprarenal, Renal, Gonadal with ureteric branches, 3, 4, Lumbar, Common iliac, External iliac, Internal iliac)

Relations of IVC
Anterior: Bile duct, liver, opening of lesser sac, 1st/3rd parts of duodenum, head of pancreas, small bowel, right common iliac artery, root of mesentery, right gonadal artery, portal vein
Posterior: Right renal artery, lumbar arteries, right crus of diaphragm, right suprarenal and its artery, bodies of L3,4,5 vertebrae, right psoas, right sympathetic chain, right coeliac ganglion
Note: NO tributaries from gut

CUTANEOUS NERVE SUPPLY OF BUTTOCKS

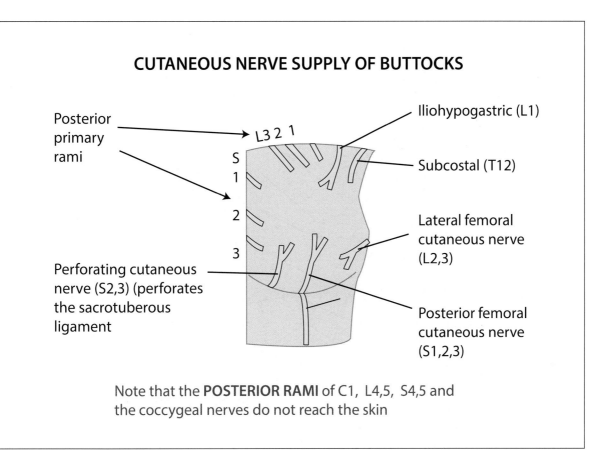

Posterior primary rami

L3 2 1

S
1

2

3

Iliohypogastric (L1)

Subcostal (T12)

Lateral femoral cutaneous nerve (L2,3)

Perforating cutaneous nerve (S2,3) (perforates the sacrotuberous ligament

Posterior femoral cutaneous nerve (S1,2,3)

Note that the **POSTERIOR RAMI** of C1, L4,5, S4,5 and the coccygeal nerves do not reach the skin

LUMBAR PLEXUS
L1,2,3,4,5

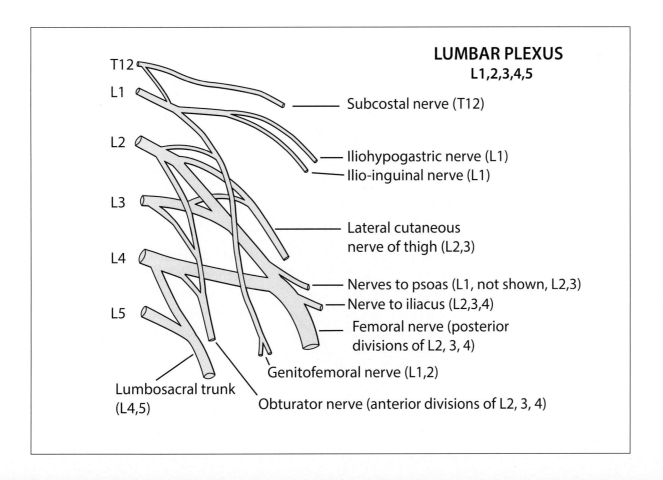

T12

L1

L2

L3

L4

L5

Subcostal nerve (T12)

Iliohypogastric nerve (L1)
Ilio-inguinal nerve (L1)

Lateral cutaneous nerve of thigh (L2,3)

Nerves to psoas (L1, not shown, L2,3)
Nerve to iliacus (L2,3,4)
Femoral nerve (posterior divisions of L2, 3, 4)

Genitofemoral nerve (L1,2)

Lumbosacral trunk (L4,5)

Obturator nerve (anterior divisions of L2, 3, 4)

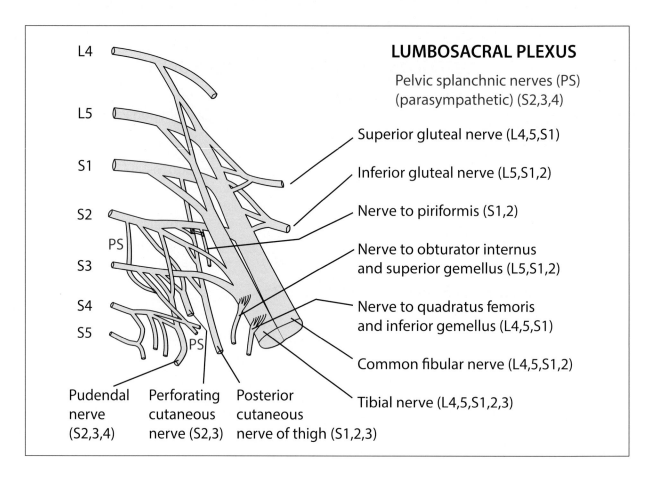

LUMBOSACRAL PLEXUS

L4
L5
S1
S2
PS
S3
S4
S5
PS

Pelvic splanchnic nerves (PS)
(parasympathetic) (S2,3,4)

Superior gluteal nerve (L4,5,S1)

Inferior gluteal nerve (L5,S1,2)

Nerve to piriformis (S1,2)

Nerve to obturator internus
and superior gemellus (L5,S1,2)

Nerve to quadratus femoris
and inferior gemellus (L4,5,S1)

Common fibular nerve (L4,5,S1,2)

Tibial nerve (L4,5,S1,2,3)

Pudendal
nerve
(S2,3,4)

Perforating
cutaneous
nerve (S2,3)

Posterior
cutaneous
nerve of thigh (S1,2,3)

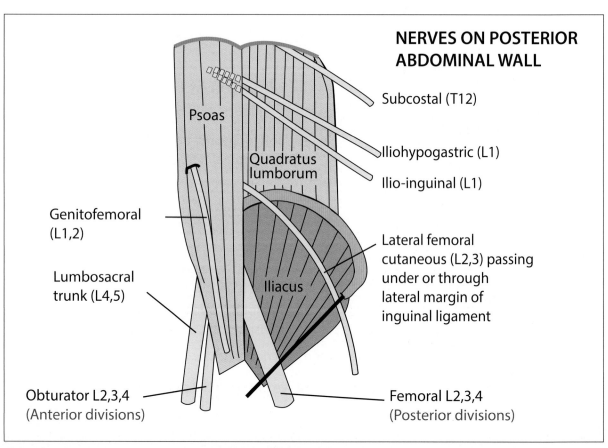

NERVES ON POSTERIOR ABDOMINAL WALL

Psoas

Quadratus
lumborum

Iliacus

Subcostal (T12)

Iliohypogastric (L1)

Ilio-inguinal (L1)

Genitofemoral
(L1,2)

Lateral femoral
cutaneous (L2,3) passing
under or through
lateral margin of
inguinal ligament

Lumbosacral
trunk (L4,5)

Obturator L2,3,4
(Anterior divisions)

Femoral L2,3,4
(Posterior divisions)

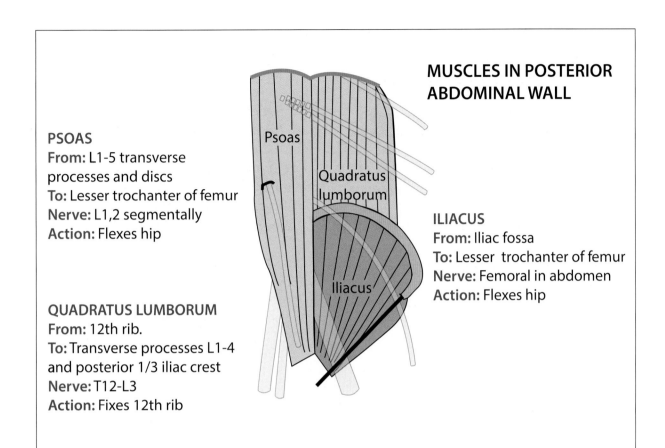

MUSCLES IN POSTERIOR ABDOMINAL WALL

PSOAS
From: L1-5 transverse processes and discs
To: Lesser trochanter of femur
Nerve: L1,2 segmentally
Action: Flexes hip

QUADRATUS LUMBORUM
From: 12th rib.
To: Transverse processes L1-4 and posterior 1/3 iliac crest
Nerve: T12-L3
Action: Fixes 12th rib

ILIACUS
From: Iliac fossa
To: Lesser trochanter of femur
Nerve: Femoral in abdomen
Action: Flexes hip

ILIOHYPOGASTRIC, ILIO-INGUINAL AND GENITOFEMORAL NERVES

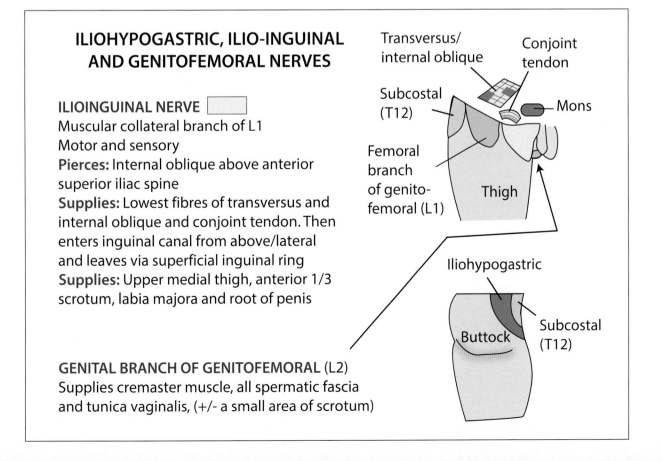

ILIOINGUINAL NERVE
Muscular collateral branch of L1
Motor and sensory
Pierces: Internal oblique above anterior superior iliac spine
Supplies: Lowest fibres of transversus and internal oblique and conjoint tendon. Then enters inguinal canal from above/lateral and leaves via superficial inguinal ring
Supplies: Upper medial thigh, anterior 1/3 scrotum, labia majora and root of penis

GENITAL BRANCH OF GENITOFEMORAL (L2)
Supplies cremaster muscle, all spermatic fascia and tunica vaginalis, (+/- a small area of scrotum)

ILIOHYPOGASTRIC, ILIO-INGUINAL AND GENITOFEMORAL NERVES

ILIOHYPOGASTRIC NERVE
Main branch of L1
Sensory and motor
Pierces: Internal oblique above anterior superior iliac spine
Pierces: External oblique above superficial inguinal ring
Supplies: Upper buttock (lateral cutaneous branch); Lowest fibres of transversus and internal oblique; skin of mons pubis

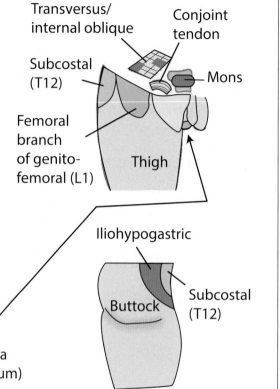

GENITAL BRANCH OF GENITOFEMORAL (L2)
Supplies cremaster muscle, all spermatic fascia and tunica vaginalis, (+/- a small area of scrotum)

4.3 General Bowel Anatomy and Foregut

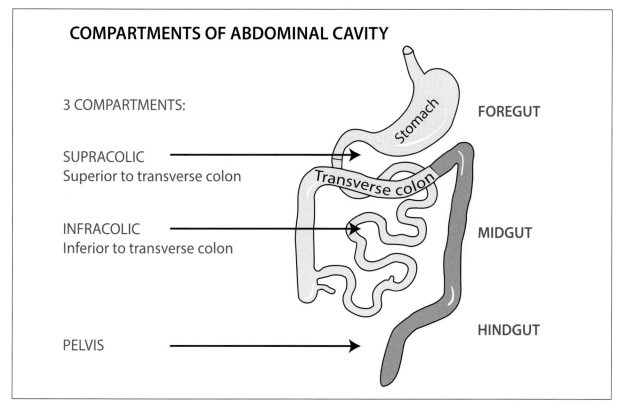

COMPARTMENTS OF ABDOMINAL CAVITY

3 COMPARTMENTS:

SUPRACOLIC
Superior to transverse colon

INFRACOLIC
Inferior to transverse colon

PELVIS

Stomach

Transverse colon

FOREGUT

MIDGUT

HINDGUT

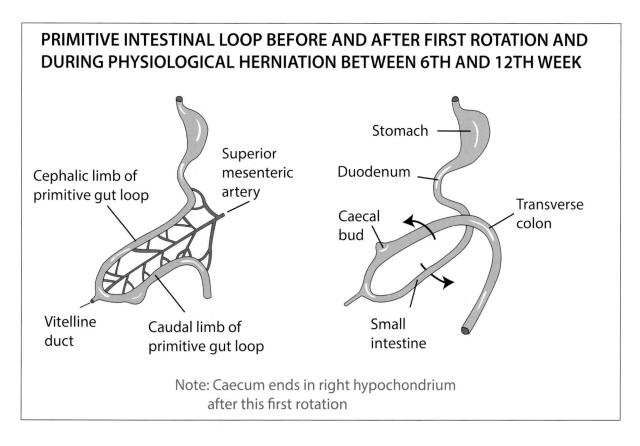

PRIMITIVE INTESTINAL LOOP BEFORE AND AFTER FIRST ROTATION AND DURING PHYSIOLOGICAL HERNIATION BETWEEN 6TH AND 12TH WEEK

Cephalic limb of
primitive gut loop

Superior
mesenteric
artery

Vitelline
duct

Caudal limb of
primitive gut loop

Stomach

Duodenum

Caecal
bud

Transverse
colon

Small
intestine

Note: Caecum ends in right hypochondrium
after this first rotation

DEVELOPING INTESTINE
BEFORE AND AFTER SECOND ROTATION

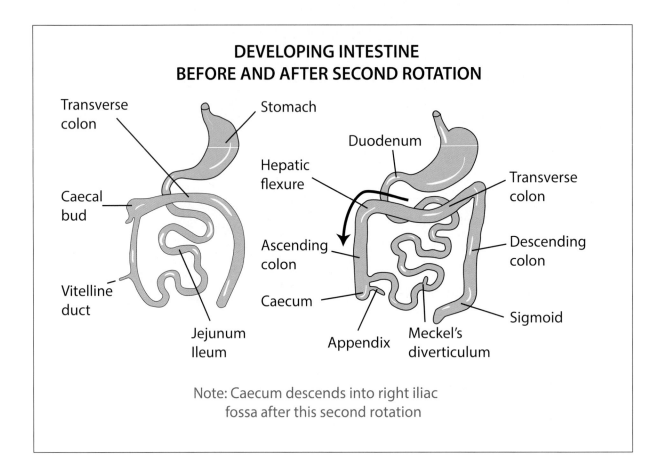

Note: Caecum descends into right iliac
fossa after this second rotation

PRINCIPLES OF MESENTERY DEVELOPMENT

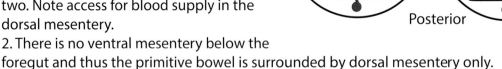

1. At the level of the developing foregut which includes the stomach there are two peritoneal cavities separated by a dorsal and ventral mesentery. The stomach is covered by, and suspended between the two. Note access for blood supply in the dorsal mesentery.

2. There is no ventral mesentery below the foregut and thus the primitive bowel is surrounded by dorsal mesentery only.

3. This dorsal mesentery can do one of three things. It can regress posteriorly so that the bowel is then retroperitoneal (A), (e.g. majority of duodenum). Or the bowel can fall on its side and the mesentery is absorbed (B), such as ascending and descending colons. This can be called a pseudo-mesentery. The third alternative is that the mesentery persists (C), such as with the small bowel, and this is described as being "on a mesentery". The length of the mesentery varies throughout the intestine.

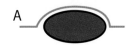

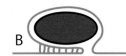

GREATER OMENTUM

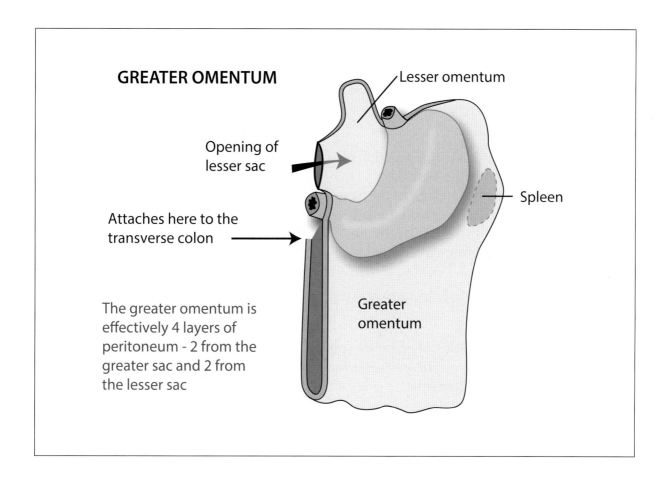

Opening of lesser sac

Lesser omentum

Spleen

Attaches here to the transverse colon

Greater omentum

The greater omentum is effectively 4 layers of peritoneum - 2 from the greater sac and 2 from the lesser sac

GREATER OMENTUM

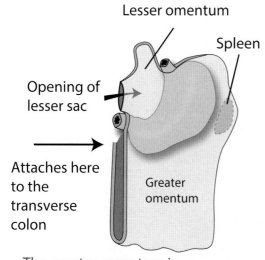

Lesser omentum

Spleen

Opening of lesser sac

Attaches here to the transverse colon

Greater omentum

The greater omentum is effectively 4 layers of peritoneum - 2 from the greater sac and 2 from the lesser sac

The lesser sac (omental bursa) is an unpaired diverticulum from the general peritoneal cavity that lies posterior to the stomach and lesser omentum. It is accessed via the foramen of Winslow. It is lined by peritoneum that was invaginated from the right side of the stomach as the stomach rotated. It contains nothing apart from a little peritoneal fluid.

Its peritoneum covers:

1: Inferior and posterior surface of the liver. 2: Lesser omentum. 3: Body and fundus of stomach and first 2.5cm of duodenum. 4: Inside of greater omentum. 5: Superior aspect of transverse colon 6: Upper body of pancreas. 7: Left adrenal gland. 8: Upper pole of left kidney. 9: Right side of the spleen, gastrosplenic and lienorenal ligaments. 10: Posterior to the floor are: inferior vena cava, aorta, coeliac trunk and its branches. 11: In its free right edge are the portal vein, hepatic artery and bile duct.

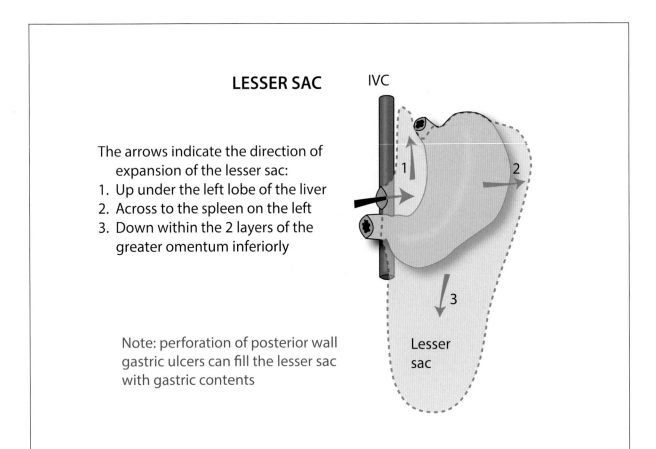

LESSER SAC

IVC

The arrows indicate the direction of expansion of the lesser sac:
1. Up under the left lobe of the liver
2. Across to the spleen on the left
3. Down within the 2 layers of the greater omentum inferiorly

Note: perforation of posterior wall gastric ulcers can fill the lesser sac with gastric contents

Lesser sac

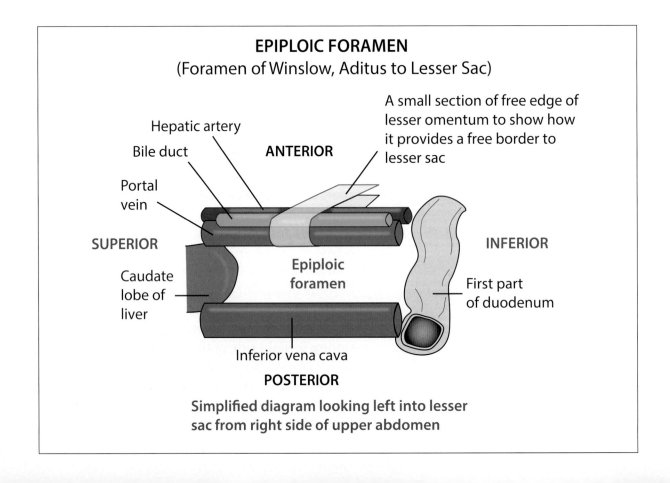

EPIPLOIC FORAMEN
(Foramen of Winslow, Aditus to Lesser Sac)

Hepatic artery

Bile duct

ANTERIOR

A small section of free edge of lesser omentum to show how it provides a free border to lesser sac

Portal vein

SUPERIOR

INFERIOR

Caudate lobe of liver

Epiploic foramen

First part of duodenum

Inferior vena cava

POSTERIOR

Simplified diagram looking left into lesser sac from right side of upper abdomen

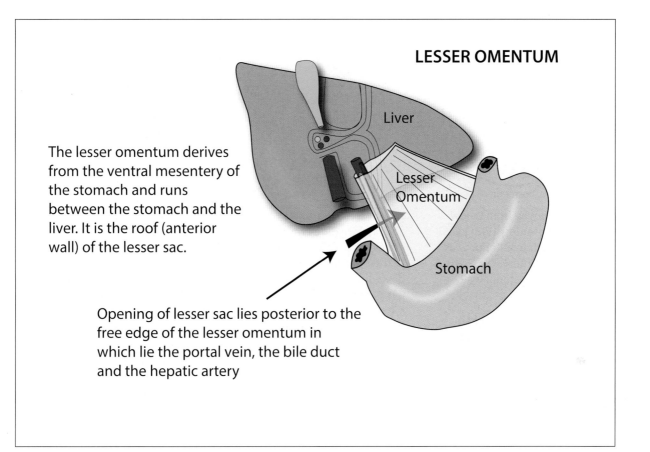

LESSER OMENTUM

The lesser omentum derives from the ventral mesentery of the stomach and runs between the stomach and the liver. It is the roof (anterior wall) of the lesser sac.

Opening of lesser sac lies posterior to the free edge of the lesser omentum in which lie the portal vein, the bile duct and the hepatic artery

AXIAL SECTION ACROSS FAR LEFT SIDE OF LESSER SAC

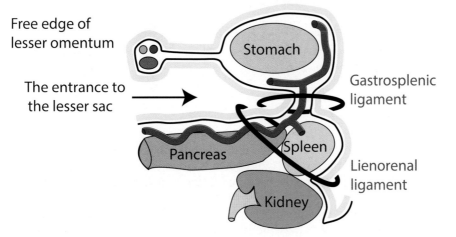

Free edge of lesser omentum

The entrance to the lesser sac

Gastrosplenic ligament

Lienorenal ligament

The gastrosplenic ligament **contains the short gastric and left gastro-epiploic vessels**
The lienorenal ligament **contains the tail of pancreas and splenic vessels.**

The two ligments are the **remnants of the the DORSAL mesentery** of the stomach. **The ventral mesentery** is the **lesser omentum and the falciform ligament**

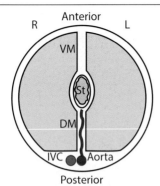

1. Fetus viewed from below. Ventral mesentery (VM) joins the stomach to anterior wall. Dorsal mesentery (DM) joins stomach to posterior wall

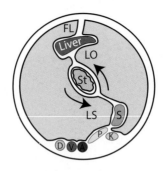

2. The stomach rotates anticlockwise. VM with developing liver in it is thrown to the right and DM with developing spleen in it to the left. Duodenum (D) is pushed retroperitoneally and pancreas (P) is formed posterior to the developing lesser sac (LS) alongside the IVC (V) and the aorta (A). The left kidney (K) lies just posterior to the spleen

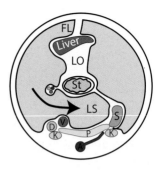

3. As the liver enlarges the remnant of the VM between it and the stomach widens to give the lesser omentum (LO) with its free edge holding the bile duct, portal veins and hepatic artery. The anterior remnant of the VM becomes the falciform ligament (FL). The stomach completes its rotation dragging the peritoneum posteriorly to give the lining of the LS. The IVC moves anteriorly to narrow the opening of the lesser sac.

ROTATION OF THE STOMACH AND THE FORMATION OF THE LESSER SAC

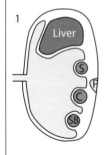 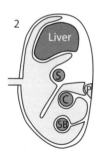 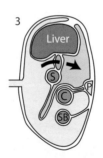   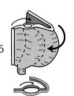

PERITONEAL DEVELOPMENT

This description is a useful way at looking at peritoneal development but it is NOT the way that it actually happens. Imagine that a large, soft balloon is inserted through the umbilicus and blown up within the abdominal cavity so that it covers all the organs (1,2). It extends around the liver as far as it can but is limited by the attachments of the IVC posteriorly and the bare area. It covers stomach (S), colon (C), small bowel (SB) and pancreas (P).

Between stomach and colon there is a prolapse of peritoneum - the greater omentum. As the SB moves anterior, its peritoneal covering becomes its mesentery. The stomach rotates so that its right side is now facing posteriorly (4 -7). The peritoneum that was on its right side expands posterior to the stomach to become the lesser sac and continues to expand up behind the liver, over the posterior wall of the stomach, onto the superior wall of the transverse colon and half the pancreas. Finally it pushes down between the two layers of the greater omentum to give it four layers. As the stomach also rotates in a coronal plane (7), the opening of the lesser sac (3) becomes a small hole posterior to the lesser omentum (LO) which is called the aditus (opening) of the lesser sac (foramen of Winslow or epiploic foramen).

The LO is the remnant of the ventral mesentery, joining the stomach to the liver (3) which has developed in this mesentery. Note that the spleen develops in the dorsal mesentery of the stomach and thus must finally be in the far left wall of the lesser sac.

PALPABLE ORGANS AND AORTIC BIFURCATION

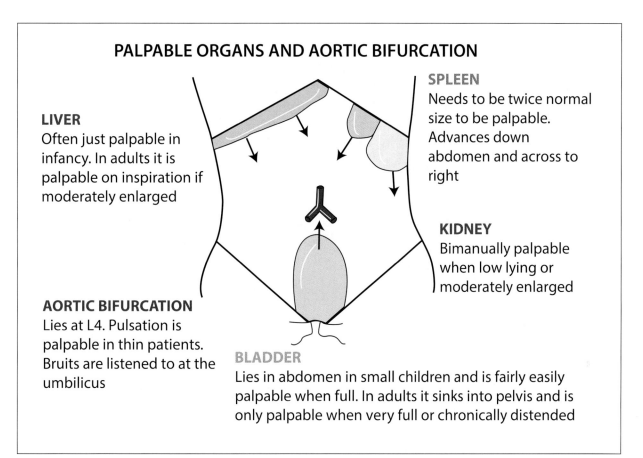

LIVER
Often just palpable in infancy. In adults it is palpable on inspiration if moderately enlarged

SPLEEN
Needs to be twice normal size to be palpable. Advances down abdomen and across to right

KIDNEY
Bimanually palpable when low lying or moderately enlarged

AORTIC BIFURCATION
Lies at L4. Pulsation is palpable in thin patients. Bruits are listened to at the umbilicus

BLADDER
Lies in abdomen in small children and is fairly easily palpable when full. In adults it sinks into pelvis and is only palpable when very full or chronically distended

STOMACH AND GREATER OMENTUM

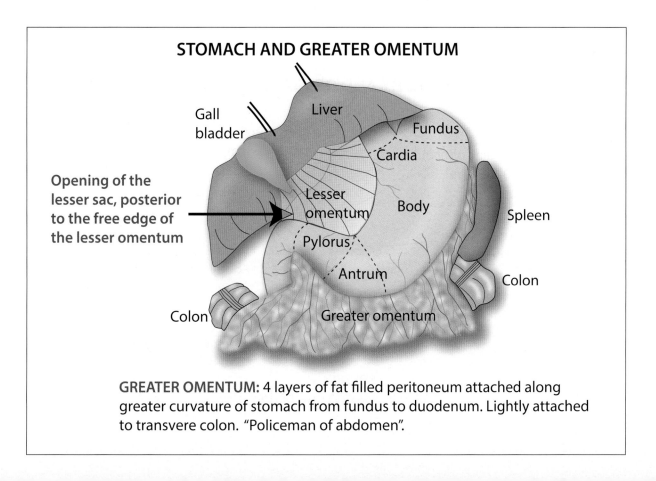

Gall bladder

Liver

Fundus

Cardia

Opening of the lesser sac, posterior to the free edge of the lesser omentum

Lesser omentum

Body

Spleen

Pylorus

Antrum

Colon

Colon

Greater omentum

GREATER OMENTUM: 4 layers of fat filled peritoneum attached along greater curvature of stomach from fundus to duodenum. Lightly attached to transvere colon. "Policeman of abdomen".

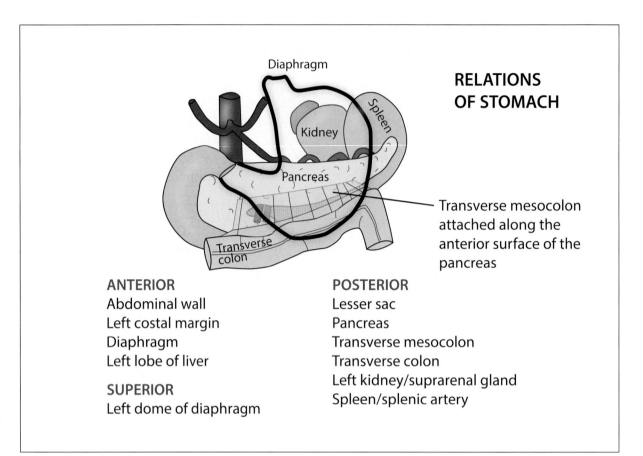

RELATIONS OF STOMACH

Transverse mesocolon attached along the anterior surface of the pancreas

ANTERIOR
Abdominal wall
Left costal margin
Diaphragm
Left lobe of liver

SUPERIOR
Left dome of diaphragm

POSTERIOR
Lesser sac
Pancreas
Transverse mesocolon
Transverse colon
Left kidney/suprarenal gland
Spleen/splenic artery

STOMACH - TOPOGRAPHY AND OESOPHAGOGASTRIC JUNCTION

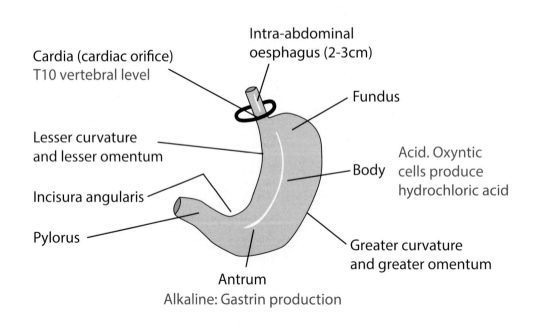

Cardia (cardiac orifice)
T10 vertebral level

Intra-abdominal oesphagus (2-3cm)

Fundus

Lesser curvature and lesser omentum

Incisura angularis

Pylorus

Body

Acid. Oxyntic cells produce hydrochloric acid

Greater curvature and greater omentum

Antrum
Alkaline: Gastrin production

FACTORS PREVENTING GASTRO-OESOPHAGEAL REFLUX

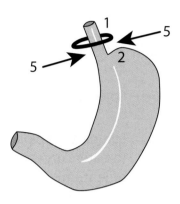

1. Crura. Mostly right but together giving effectively a circle of muscle

2. Angle of oesophagogastric junction

3. Apposition of mucosal folds

4. Phrenico-oesophageal ligament (a fold of connective tissue)

5. Intra-abdominal pressure acting laterally on small section of intra-abdominal oesophagus

STOMACH - MUSCLE COATS AND CELLS

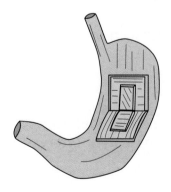

- Outer longitudinal
- Inner circular
- Incomplete oblique innermost
- Mucosal rugae caused by muscle fibres

Note: The following are produced from the cells of the stomach; Pepsin, hydrochloric acid, gastrin, intrinsic factor, somatostatin, serotonin and endomorphin

BLOOD SUPPLY OF STOMACH FROM COELIAC AXIS

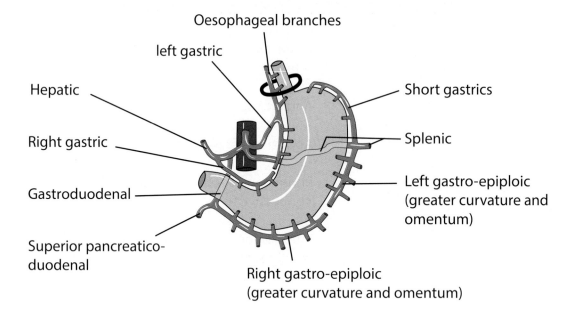

Oesophageal branches

left gastric

Hepatic

Right gastric

Gastroduodenal

Superior pancreatico-duodenal

Short gastrics

Splenic

Left gastro-epiploic (greater curvature and omentum)

Right gastro-epiploic (greater curvature and omentum)

VASCULAR WATERSHED BETWEEN FOREGUT AND MIDGUT

Superior pancreaticoduodenal (**Coeliac trunk**)

Inferior pancreaticoduodenal (**Superior mesenteric artery**)

2nd part of duodenum

VENOUS DRAINAGE OF STOMACH

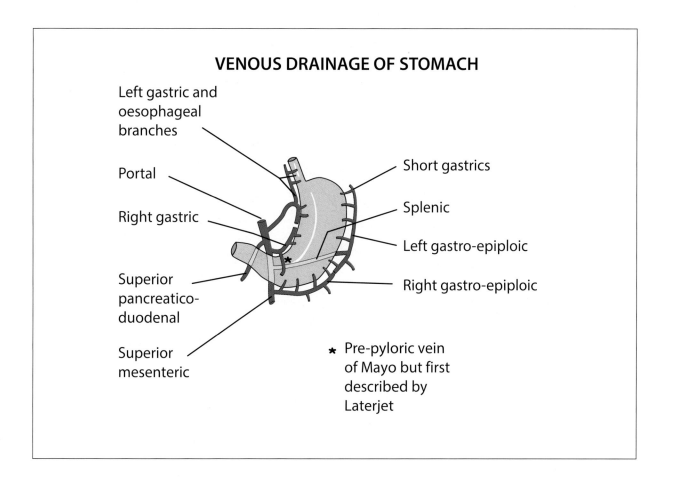

Left gastric and oesophageal branches

Portal

Right gastric

Superior pancreatico-duodenal

Superior mesenteric

Short gastrics

Splenic

Left gastro-epiploic

Right gastro-epiploic

* Pre-pyloric vein of Mayo but first described by Laterjet

STOMACH - LYMPHATIC DRAINAGE

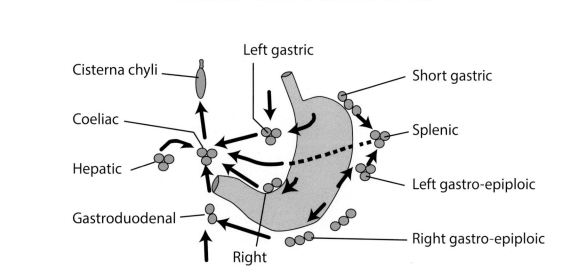

Cisterna chyli

Left gastric

Short gastric

Coeliac

Hepatic

Splenic

Left gastro-epiploic

Gastroduodenal

Right gastro-epiploic

Right gastric

STOMACH NERVE SUPPLY

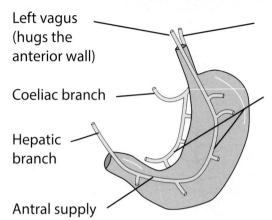

Left vagus (hugs the anterior wall)

Right vagus (a little away from posterior wall)

Coeliac branch

Anterior/posterior nerves of Laterjet

Hepatic branch

Referred pain via general visceral afferents in greater splanchnic nerves (visceral sympathetics to T5-9) to epigastrium and lower chest

Antral supply

Vagus nerves are 80% sensory. 20% motor for increasing motility, opening pylorus and initiating secretions

Sympathetics
Greater splanchnic nerves (T5-9) for decreasing motility, vasoconstriction, closing pylorus and sensation

Note: Highly selective vagotomy destroys vagus to fundus and body but preserves nerve to antral pump

4.4   Midgut and Hindgut

DUODENUM - GENERAL

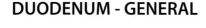

SECOND PART (3" or 8cm)
- Retroperitoneal
- On transpyloric plane
- Over hilum of right kidney

FIRST PART (2" or 5cm)
- 1st 1/2 with mesentery
- Passes to right, upwards, backwards

Arteries: Superior and inferior pancreatico-duodenal arteries, right gastric artery, right gastro-epiploic artery
Veins: To portal

THIRD PART (4" or 10cm)
- Retroperitoneal
- Superior mesenteric artery and vein pass between body and uncinate process

FOURTH PART (1" or 2.5cm)
- Mesentery begins
- Ends as duodenojejunal junction

DUODENUM - MAIN RELATIONS

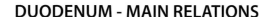

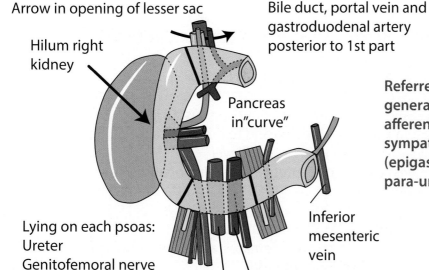

Arrow in opening of lesser sac

Hilum right kidney

Bile duct, portal vein and gastroduodenal artery posterior to 1st part

Pancreas in"curve"

Referred pain via general visceral afferents in sympathetics to T5-11 (epigastrium and para-umbilical)

Lying on each psoas:
Ureter
Genitofemoral nerve
Gonadal vessels

Inferior mesenteric vein

IVC

Aorta and inferior mesenteric artery

DUODENUM - HISTOLOGY

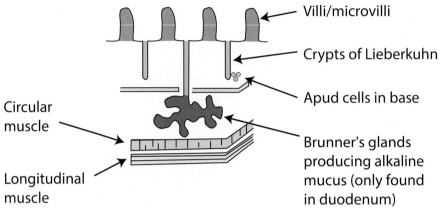

Villi/microvilli

Crypts of Lieberkuhn

Apud cells in base

Circular muscle

Brunner's glands producing alkaline mucus (only found in duodenum)

Longitudinal muscle

Note: Mucosa is thrown into folds called plicae circulares or valvulae conniventes

SMALL BOWEL MESENTERY AND SECRETIONS

ORIGIN OF SMALL BOWEL MESENTERY
- 6 inches (15cm) long
- Starts at the duodenojejunal junction, just to left of L2 vertebra and extends down and to the right to reach the right sacro-iliac joint at S2 sacral level
- Contains superior mesenteric vessels, lymphatics and autonomic nerves

SECRETIONS FROM SMALL BOWEL
- Mucus, lysozyme, secretin, somatostatin, cholecystokinin, serotonin and endomorphin, VIP, GIP, etc

SMALL BOWEL MESENTERY

SMALL BOWEL MESENTERY
15cm (6") long. Bowel average length 6m (2-10m)
Starts at the duodenojejunal junction, just to left of L2 vertebra and extends down and to the right to right sacro-iliac joint at S2 sacral level. Contains superior mesenteric vessels, lymphatics and autonomic nerves.

JEJUNUM
2/5, red, wide
bore, thick wall

Valvulae conniventes, plicae circulares ++, sparce arcades

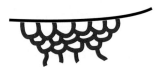

ILEUM
3/5, pink, narrow
bore, thin wall

Smooth wall, Peyer's patches, multiple arcades

BLOOD: Ileal and jejunal branches of superior mesenteric artery.
NERVES: General visceral afferents in lesser splanchnics (sympathetic) referred to T10/11 (para-umbilical)

MECKEL'S DIVERTICULUM

- Remnant of the vitello-intestinal duct which normally closes off early in development.
- Approximately: 2-3% of people, 2-3 inches long and 2-3 feet from the ileocaecal valve.
- May contain gastric, pancreatic, liver, carcinoid or lymph tissue.
- May remain attached to umbilicus as persistent vitello-intestinal tract which may leak or cause intestinal obstruction as the bowel wraps around it.
- Symptoms very similar to appendicitis. Erosion by acid producing cells can lead to haemorrhage within the bowel.
- Lies on antimesenteric border of ileum.

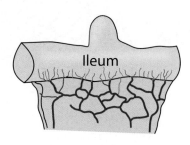

Ileum

UMBILICUS
Problems associated with Meckel's diverticulum

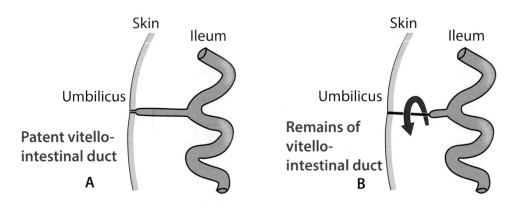

Skin
Ileum
Umbilicus
**Patent vitello-
intestinal duct**
A

Skin
Ileum
Umbilicus
**Remains of
vitello-
intestinal duct**
B

Meckel's diverticulum is the remnant of the vitello-intestinal duct. It may remain open to give a fistula to the surface at the umbilicus (A) with leakage of intestinal content. Or it can remain as a strand of tissue around which the small bowel can rotate and become obstructed.

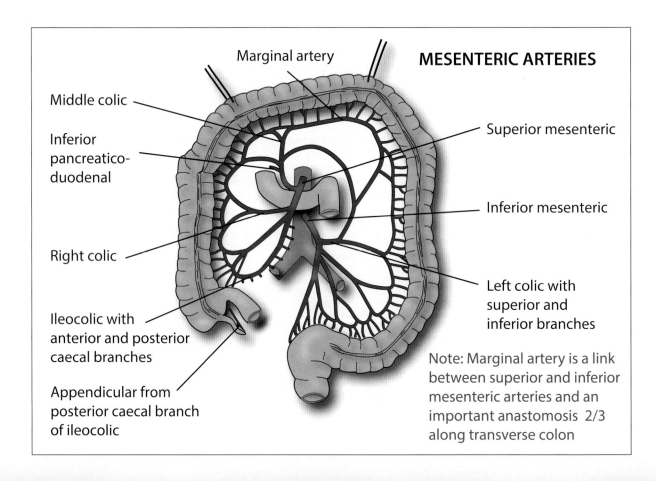

MESENTERIC ARTERIES

Marginal artery

Middle colic

Inferior pancreatico-duodenal

Right colic

Ileocolic with anterior and posterior caecal branches

Appendicular from posterior caecal branch of ileocolic

Superior mesenteric

Inferior mesenteric

Left colic with superior and inferior branches

Note: Marginal artery is a link between superior and inferior mesenteric arteries and an important anastomosis 2/3 along transverse colon

COLON

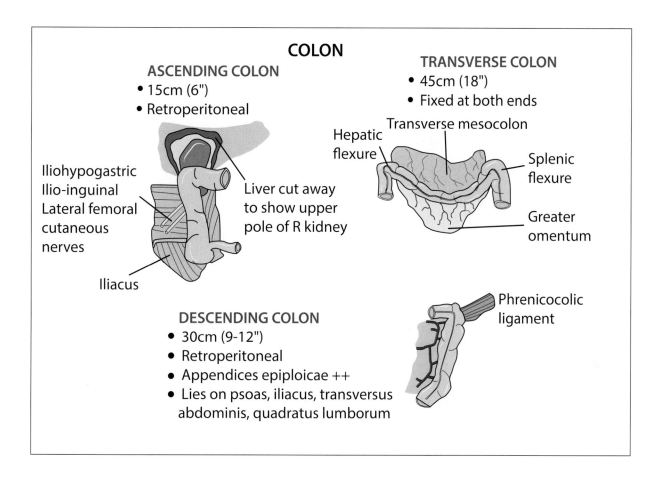

ASCENDING COLON
- 15cm (6")
- Retroperitoneal

Iliohypogastric
Ilio-inguinal
Lateral femoral
cutaneous
nerves

Liver cut away
to show upper
pole of R kidney

Iliacus

TRANSVERSE COLON
- 45cm (18")
- Fixed at both ends

Hepatic
flexure

Transverse mesocolon

Splenic
flexure

Greater
omentum

Phrenicocolic
ligament

DESCENDING COLON
- 30cm (9-12")
- Retroperitoneal
- Appendices epiploicae ++
- Lies on psoas, iliacus, transversus abdominis, quadratus lumborum

CAECUM AND APPENDIX 1

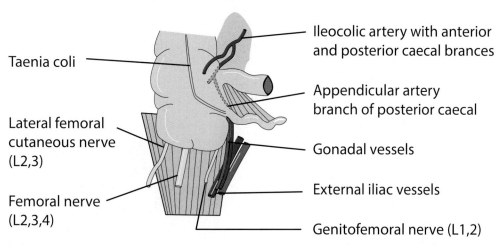

Taenia coli

Ileocolic artery with anterior
and posterior caecal brances

Appendicular artery
branch of posterior caecal

Lateral femoral
cutaneous nerve
(L2,3)

Gonadal vessels

External iliac vessels

Femoral nerve
(L2,3,4)

Genitofemoral nerve (L1,2)

CAECUM
- On mesentery; Below ileocaecal valve
- Retrocaecal fossa behind it
- 3 taenia coli meet at base of appendix
- Ileocaecal valve is a double fold of mucosa and circular muscle of ileum which acts as an anti-reflux mechanism

CAECUM AND APPENDIX 2

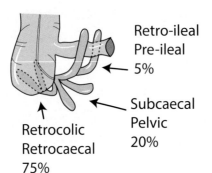

Retro-ileal
Pre-ileal
5%

Subcaecal
Pelvic
20%

Retrocolic
Retrocaecal
75%

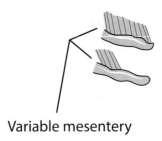

Variable mesentery

APPENDIX
- At McBurney's point
- 2-25cm (1/2"-9") average 7-8cm
- Fully coated diverticulum
- Appendicular artery usually from posterior caecal artery. It is an end artery hence appendix can easily become gangrenous. Appendix moves posterior and medial with caecal expansion

PERITONEAL RECESSES

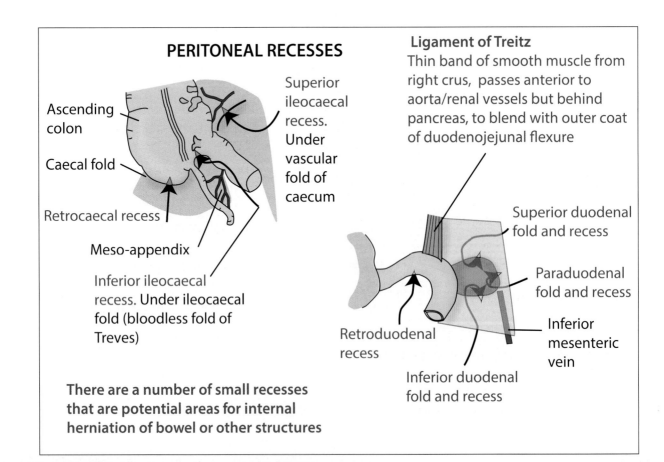

Ascending colon

Caecal fold

Retrocaecal recess

Meso-appendix

Inferior ileocaecal recess. Under ileocaecal fold (bloodless fold of Treves)

Superior ileocaecal recess. Under vascular fold of caecum

Ligament of Treitz
Thin band of smooth muscle from right crus, passes anterior to aorta/renal vessels but behind pancreas, to blend with outer coat of duodenojejunal flexure

Superior duodenal fold and recess

Paraduodenal fold and recess

Inferior mesenteric vein

Retroduodenal recess

Inferior duodenal fold and recess

There are a number of small recesses that are potential areas for internal herniation of bowel or other structures

COLON
(Approximately 5 foot -1.4m)

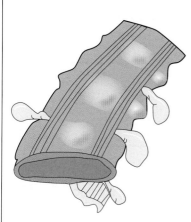

Colon
Appendices epiploicae: Little tags of fat on the mesentery border of the bowel.
Taenia coli: Outer longitudinal muscle in three flat bands. Not in appendix
Sacculations and Haustrations/valvulae conniventes: Due to shortness of taenia coli
Mesentery: Transverse and sigmoid only
THEY ALL STOP BEFORE THE RECTUM BEGINS

Lymphatics: Alongside superior/inferior mesenteric vessels to para-aortics to coeliac and on upwards to thoracic duct.
Nerves: Parasympathetic - vagus to 2/3 along transverse colon then S2,3,4 to rest of bowel.
Sympathetics T10-L2 for vasoconstriction and to carry general visceral afferents (GVA's) for pain. For organs of cloacal origin GVAs may be carried in the parasympathetics

SIGMOID COLON

Base of mesentery crosses:
- Common iliac artery bifurcation
- Left ureter
- left sacro-iliac joint

Descending colon

Peritoneum

Sigmoid mesentery

Cut edge of peritoneum

External iliac artery

Ureter

Rectum

- 5-45cm (5-30")
- From pelvic brim to S3 midline
- On mesentery
- Appendices epiploicae +++
- Taenia become progressively more as a longitudinal coat

RECTUM
(length and peritoneal covering)

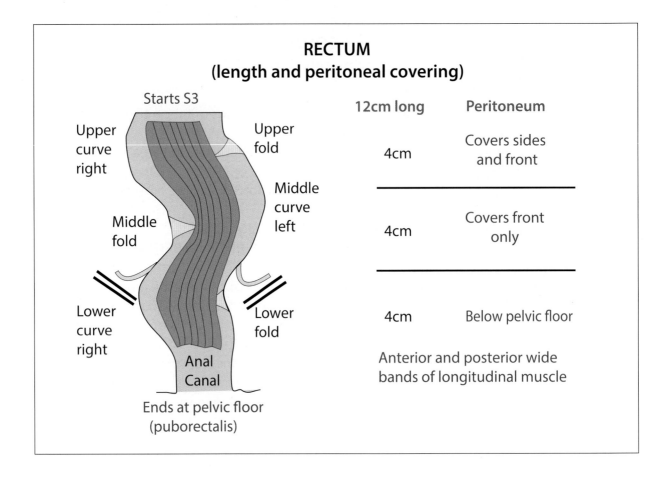

Starts S3

Upper curve right

Upper fold

Middle curve left

Middle fold

Lower curve right

Lower fold

Anal Canal

Ends at pelvic floor (puborectalis)

12cm long

	Peritoneum
4cm	Covers sides and front
4cm	Covers front only
4cm	Below pelvic floor

Anterior and posterior wide bands of longitudinal muscle

RECTUM: DETAILS

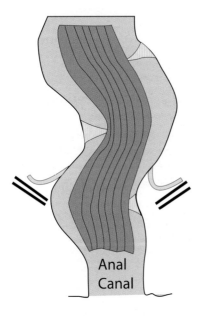

Anal Canal

- No mesentery

- Folds (shelves) are mucosa and circular muscle = valves of Houston

- The rectum is normally empty but fills before and during defaecation

- Upper 2/3 is distensible into abdominal cavity and may store faeces in constipation

- Lower 1/3 can distend laterally into the ischio-anal fossa during defaecation

- Note: longitudinal muscle is two wide bands anteriorly and posteriorly

ANAL SPHINCTERS

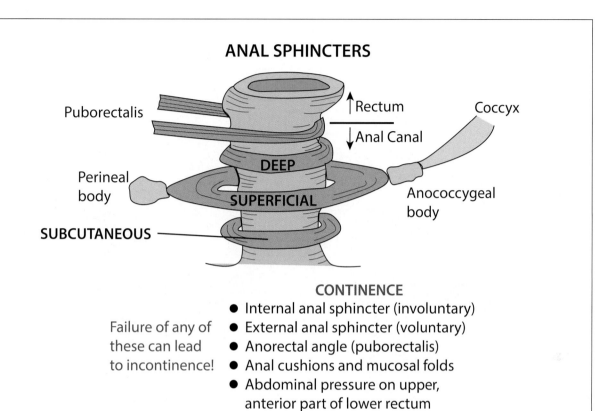

Puborectalis

↑ Rectum

↓ Anal Canal

Coccyx

Perineal body

DEEP

SUPERFICIAL

Anococcygeal body

SUBCUTANEOUS

CONTINENCE

Failure of any of these can lead to incontinence!

- Internal anal sphincter (involuntary)
- External anal sphincter (voluntary)
- Anorectal angle (puborectalis)
- Anal cushions and mucosal folds
- Abdominal pressure on upper, anterior part of lower rectum

INTERNAL AND EXTERNAL ANAL SPHINCTERS

Circular muscle becomes the "involuntary internal anal sphincter" which relaxes with moderate pressure from above

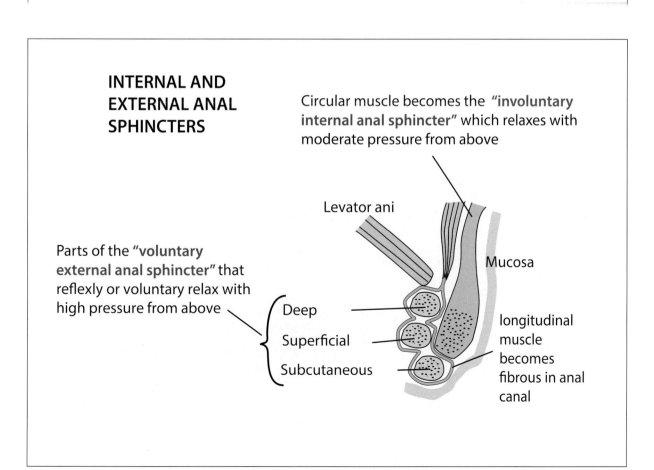

Levator ani

Mucosa

Parts of the "voluntary external anal sphincter" that reflexly or voluntary relax with high pressure from above

Deep

Superficial

Subcutaneous

longitudinal muscle becomes fibrous in anal canal

PUBORECTALIS SLING

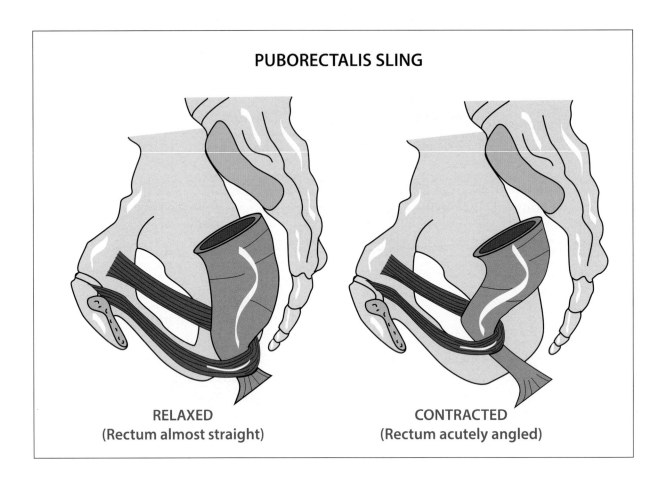

RELAXED
(Rectum almost straight)

CONTRACTED
(Rectum acutely angled)

ISCHIOANAL FOSSA AND RECTAL MUSCLES

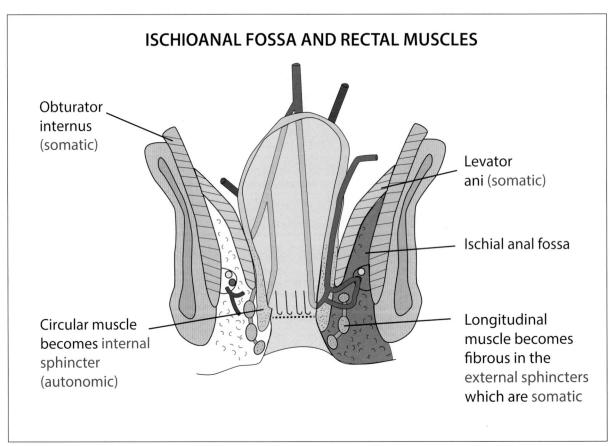

Obturator internus (somatic)

Levator ani (somatic)

Ischial anal fossa

Circular muscle becomes internal sphincter (autonomic)

Longitudinal muscle becomes fibrous in the external sphincters which are somatic

RECTAL BLOOD SUPPLY

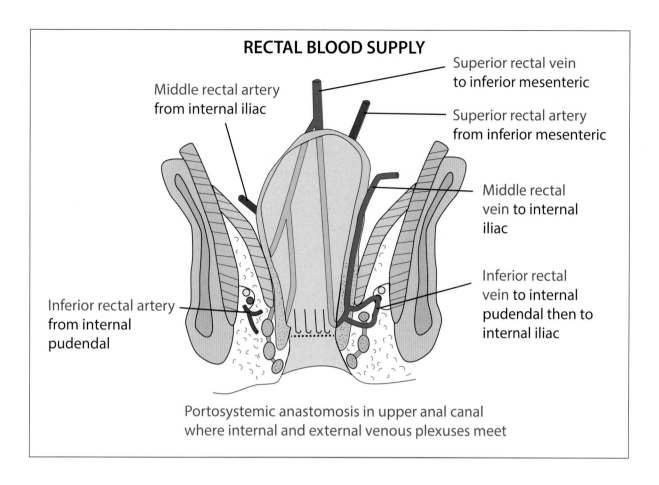

Middle rectal artery from internal iliac

Superior rectal vein to inferior mesenteric

Superior rectal artery from inferior mesenteric

Middle rectal vein to internal iliac

Inferior rectal vein to internal pudendal then to internal iliac

Inferior rectal artery from internal pudendal

Portosystemic anastomosis in upper anal canal where internal and external venous plexuses meet

RECTAL LYMPHATICS

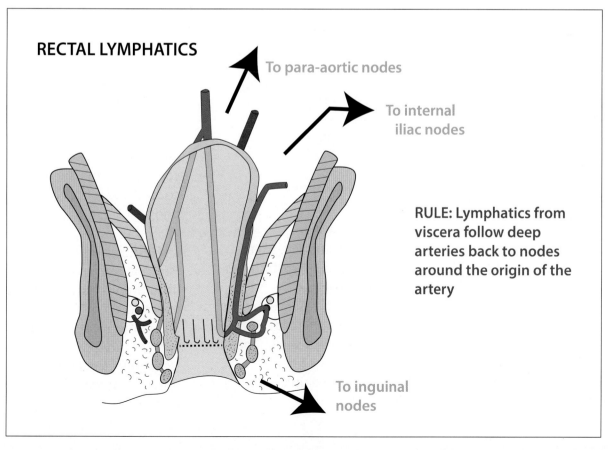

To para-aortic nodes

To internal iliac nodes

RULE: Lymphatics from viscera follow deep arteries back to nodes around the origin of the artery

To inguinal nodes

RECTAL NERVE SUPPLY - AUTONOMIC

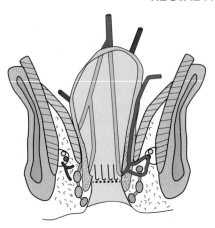

Sympathetic:
Contract smooth muscle sphincters, relax bowel, transmit pain

Parasympathetic:
Relax smooth muscle sphincters, contract bowel, transmit fullness

Anocutaneous reflex
Lightly stroking the buttock skin near the anal canal should cause a reflex contraction of the voluntary external anal sphincters

Note: Rectum is capable of distinguishing between AIR, WATER AND FAECES

RELATIONS OF RECTUM

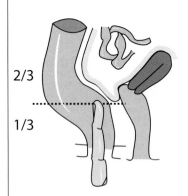

2/3

1/3

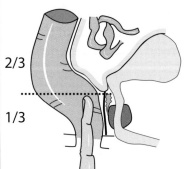

2/3

1/3

FEMALE - anterior
Recto-uterine pouch (of Douglas), Small bowel, posterior fornix/vagina, uterus and bladder

MALE - anterior
Rectovesical pouch, small bowel, bladder, prostate, vas, seminal vesicles, Denonvillier's fascia (which is probably a double layer of peritoneum acting as a major factor in preventing the spread of cancer in either direction)

POSTERIOR - both
Fascia, median sacral and rectal vessels, sympathetic trunk, pelvic splanchnic nerves, piriformis, sacral and coccygeal roots, sacrum, coccyx, anococcygeal body

LATERAL - both
Peritoneum, fat, nodes, obturator internus and its fascia, Alcock's canal and contents, levator ani and coccygeus, ischio-anal fossa, lateral (fascial) ligaments of rectum

ANAL CANAL
4cm long. Pelvic floor (puborectalis) to outside

Anocutaneous reflex: Touching the skin near the anus (S2,3,4) gives a reflex contraction of the external anal sphincters

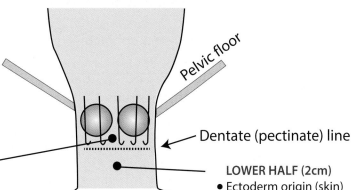

Pelvic floor

← Dentate (pectinate) line

UPPER HALF (2cm)
- Endoderm origin (bowel)
- Columnar mucosa
- 12 columns/valves and 3 cushions
- Autonomic nerves
- Insensitive to touch
- Superior, middle, inferior rectal arteries
- Mixed portal and systemic venous drainage
- Lymphatics to para-aortic lymph nodes
- Potential for adenocarcinoma
- Site of haemorrhoids

LOWER HALF (2cm)
- Ectoderm origin (skin)
- Squamous mucosa
- Somatic nerves
- Sensitive to touch
- Mainly inferior rectal artery
- Systemic venous drainage
- Lymphatics to superficial inguinal nodes
- Potential for squamous carcinoma
- No haemorrhoids

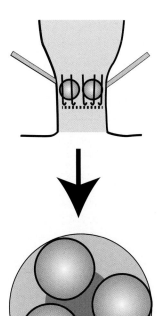

ANAL CANAL - UPPER HALF

3 spongy muscosal cushions are in the upper half, at 3, 7 and 11 o'clock. They contain bright red capillary blood.
They help with continence , air tightness and mucus production.
Enlargement leads to haemorrhoids (piles).

NOTE: Although they are at the same level as the venous plexuses (which can enlarge in a portosystemic anastomosis) they are quite separate from them

INVESTIGATION OF FAECAL INCONTINENCE

Digital anorectal examination, wearing a well lubricated glove

Assess:
- Puborectalis and external sphincters
- Evidence of constipation
- Pressure on rectum from other organs
- Tumours in prostate or rectum

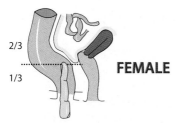

FEMALE

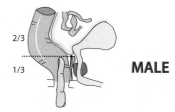

MALE

Anterior: Recto-uterine pouch, small bowel, posterior fornix/vagina, uterus

Anterior: Rectovesical pouch, small bowel, bladder, prostate, vas, seminal vesicles, Denonvillier's fascia

Consider a central prolapsed disc!

4.5   Biliary System, Portal System, Pancreas and Spleen

BILIARY DUCTS

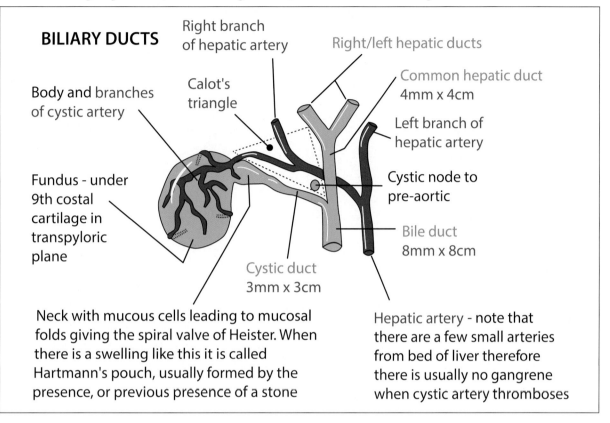

Right branch of hepatic artery

Right/left hepatic ducts

Common hepatic duct
4mm x 4cm

Calot's triangle

Body and branches of cystic artery

Left branch of hepatic artery

Cystic node to pre-aortic

Fundus - under 9th costal cartilage in transpyloric plane

Bile duct
8mm x 8cm

Cystic duct
3mm x 3cm

Neck with mucous cells leading to mucosal folds giving the spiral valve of Heister. When there is a swelling like this it is called Hartmann's pouch, usually formed by the presence, or previous presence of a stone

Hepatic artery - note that there are a few small arteries from bed of liver therefore there is usually no gangrene when cystic artery thromboses

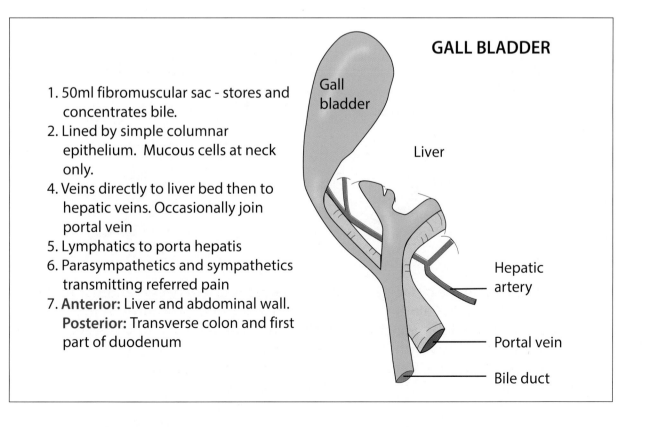

GALL BLADDER

1. 50ml fibromuscular sac - stores and concentrates bile.
2. Lined by simple columnar epithelium. Mucous cells at neck only.
4. Veins directly to liver bed then to hepatic veins. Occasionally join portal vein
5. Lymphatics to porta hepatis
6. Parasympathetics and sympathetics transmitting referred pain
7. **Anterior:** Liver and abdominal wall. **Posterior:** Transverse colon and first part of duodenum

Gall bladder

Liver

Hepatic artery

Portal vein

Bile duct

GALL BLADDER VARIATIONS

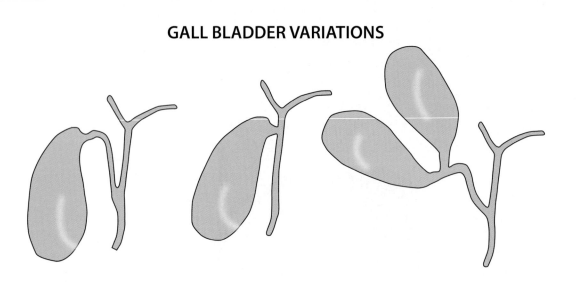

A long cystic duct joining the hepatic duct low, even behind the duodenum

Absent cystic duct. The gall bladder opens directly into the common hepatic duct

A rare double gall bladder resulting from a bifid embryonic diverticulum from the hepatic duct

VARIATIONS IN CYSTIC ARTERY

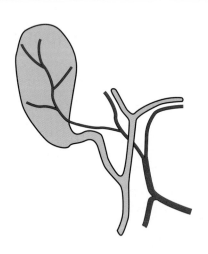

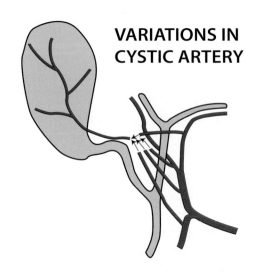

In 75% of people the cystic artery is given off in Calot's triangle from the right branch of the hepatic artery which lies posterior to the common hepatic duct

In 25% the cystic artery passes anterior to the common hepatic duct and arises from
1. Right branch of hepatic artery (14%)
2. Left branch of hepatic artery (6%)
3. Gastroduodenal artery (3%)
4. Main hepatic artery (2%)

PRINGLE'S MANOEUVRE

Pressure is applied to both the portal vein and the hepatic artery to prevent bleeding from the liver

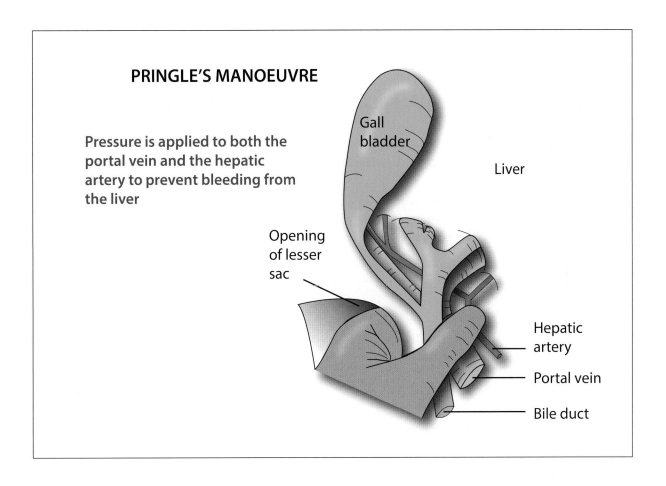

Gall bladder

Liver

Opening of lesser sac

Hepatic artery

Portal vein

Bile duct

BILE DUCT
(8CM LONG 8MM WIDE)

Ampulla of Vater opens into 2nd part of duodenum on posteromedial wall, 10cm from pylorus

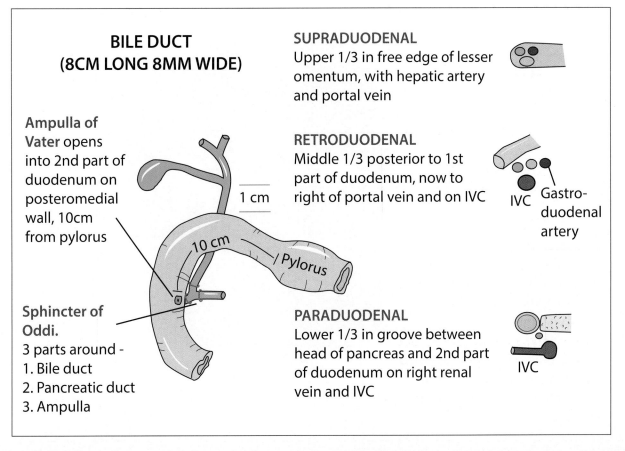

Sphincter of Oddi.
3 parts around -
1. Bile duct
2. Pancreatic duct
3. Ampulla

SUPRADUODENAL
Upper 1/3 in free edge of lesser omentum, with hepatic artery and portal vein

RETRODUODENAL
Middle 1/3 posterior to 1st part of duodenum, now to right of portal vein and on IVC

IVC Gastro-duodenal artery

PARADUODENAL
Lower 1/3 in groove between head of pancreas and 2nd part of duodenum on right renal vein and IVC

IVC

BILIARY DUCTS AND GALLBLADDER

Blood:
Cystic, hepatic, gastroduodenal arteries
Nerves:
Parasympathetic - anterior vagus for contraction of gallbladder, relaxation of sphincter of Oddi (+ cholecystokinin from small bowel)
Sympathetic - coeliac ganglion, relaxes gallbladder
Sensation: General visceral afferent with sympathetics and somatic via phrenic referred to right shoulder tip

SPHINCTER OF ODDI

3 sphincters make up this sphincter of Oddi. Biliary is always present - others may be missing

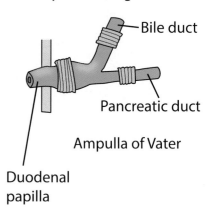

Bile duct

Pancreatic duct

Ampulla of Vater

Duodenal papilla

PORTAL VEIN & TRIBUTARIES

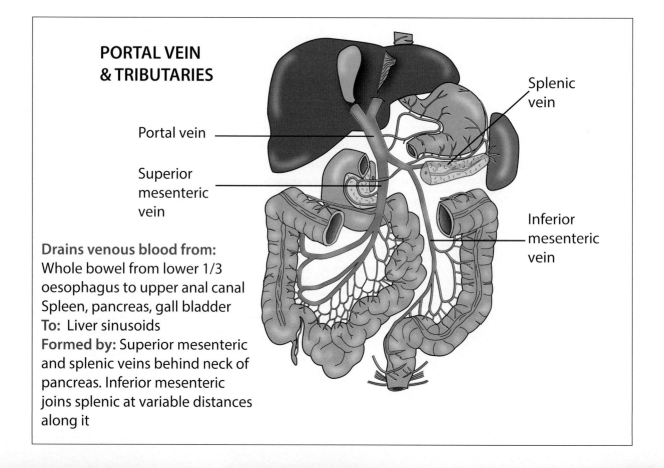

Portal vein

Superior mesenteric vein

Splenic vein

Inferior mesenteric vein

Drains venous blood from:
Whole bowel from lower 1/3 oesophagus to upper anal canal
Spleen, pancreas, gall bladder
To: Liver sinusoids
Formed by: Superior mesenteric and splenic veins behind neck of pancreas. Inferior mesenteric joins splenic at variable distances along it

HEPATIC PORTAL SYSTEM

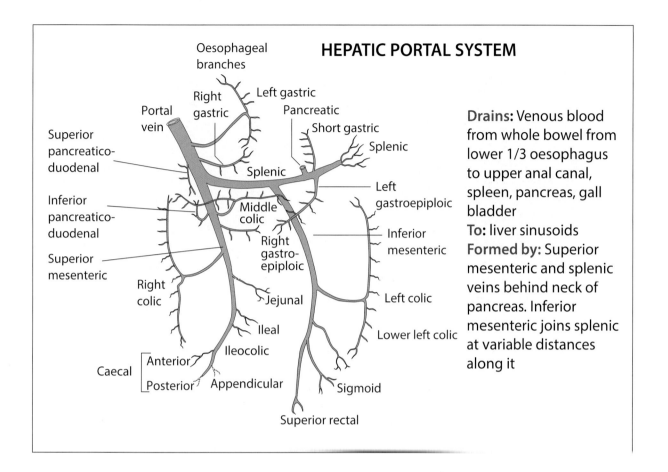

Oesophageal branches
Left gastric
Right gastric
Portal vein
Pancreatic
Short gastric
Splenic
Superior pancreatico-duodenal
Splenic
Left gastroepiploic
Inferior pancreatico-duodenal
Middle colic
Superior mesenteric
Right gastro-epiploic
Inferior mesenteric
Right colic
Jejunal
Left colic
Ileal
Lower left colic
Ileocolic
Caecal
Anterior
Posterior
Appendicular
Sigmoid
Superior rectal

Drains: Venous blood from whole bowel from lower 1/3 oesophagus to upper anal canal, spleen, pancreas, gall bladder
To: liver sinusoids
Formed by: Superior mesenteric and splenic veins behind neck of pancreas. Inferior mesenteric joins splenic at variable distances along it

LIVER - GENERAL DESCRIPTION

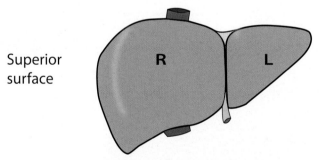

Superior surface

R   L

Wedge shaped, largest organ in body, weight 1500g
1500ml blood flow per minute (30% of cardiac output)
Lies: Right - 6-10 ribs/costal cartilages; Left - 6-7 costal cartilages
Surfaces: Anterior, superior, posteror, right - all smooth/convex. Postero-inferior (visceral) concave and many features
Supports: IVC and hepatic veins (+ ligamentum teres and peritoneum)
Nerve supply: Right vagus via coeliac ganglia, left directly to porta hepatis. Sympathetics on vessels
Reaches: T5 vertebra, nipples (4th intercostal space on right), xiphisternal joint

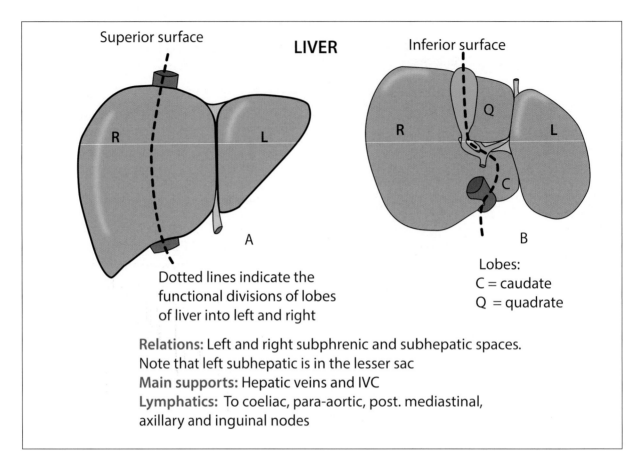

LIVER

Superior surface

Inferior surface

R   L

R   Q   L

A

B

Dotted lines indicate the
functional divisions of lobes
of liver into left and right

Lobes:
C = caudate
Q = quadrate

Relations: Left and right subphrenic and subhepatic spaces.
Note that left subhepatic is in the lesser sac
Main supports: Hepatic veins and IVC
Lymphatics: To coeliac, para-aortic, post. mediastinal,
axillary and inguinal nodes

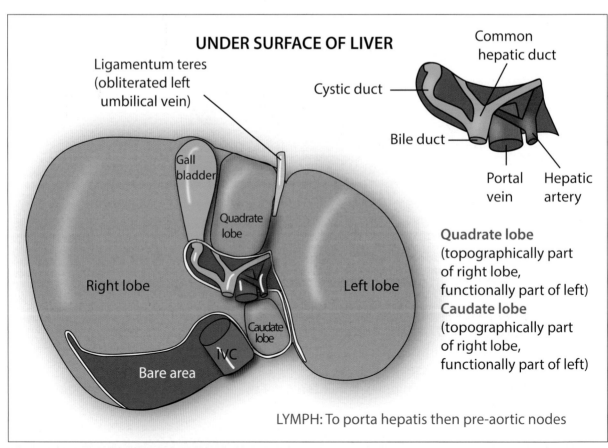

UNDER SURFACE OF LIVER

Common
hepatic duct

Ligamentum teres
(obliterated left
umbilical vein)

Cystic duct

Bile duct

Gall
bladder

Quadrate
lobe

Right lobe

Left lobe

Caudate
lobe

IVC

Bare area

Portal   Hepatic
vein   artery

Quadrate lobe
(topographically part
of right lobe,
functionally part of left)
Caudate lobe
(topographically part
of right lobe,
functionally part of left)

LYMPH: To porta hepatis then pre-aortic nodes

LIVER - PORTA HEPATIS

The **porta hepatis** is the area on the under surface of the liver at which the structures in the free edge of the lesser omentum enter/leave the liver. Peritoneum is reflected around it.
It contains the following structures:

- Portal vein
- Left/right branches of hepatic artery
- Left/right hepatic ducts
- Lymphatics and lymph nodes
- Autonomic nerves

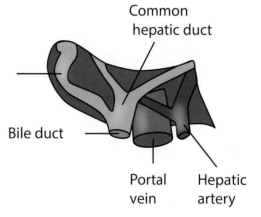

Cystic duct

Common hepatic duct

Bile duct

Portal vein

Hepatic artery

LIVER

LOBULES

HISTOLOGY

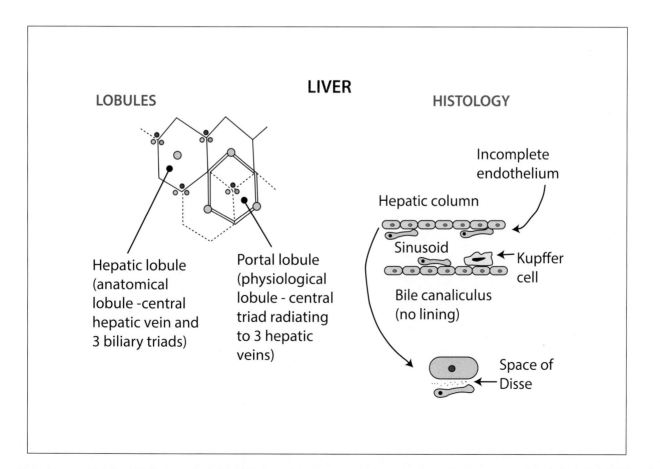

Hepatic lobule (anatomical lobule -central hepatic vein and 3 biliary triads)

Portal lobule (physiological lobule - central triad radiating to 3 hepatic veins)

Incomplete endothelium

Hepatic column

Sinusoid

Kupffer cell

Bile canaliculus (no lining)

Space of Disse

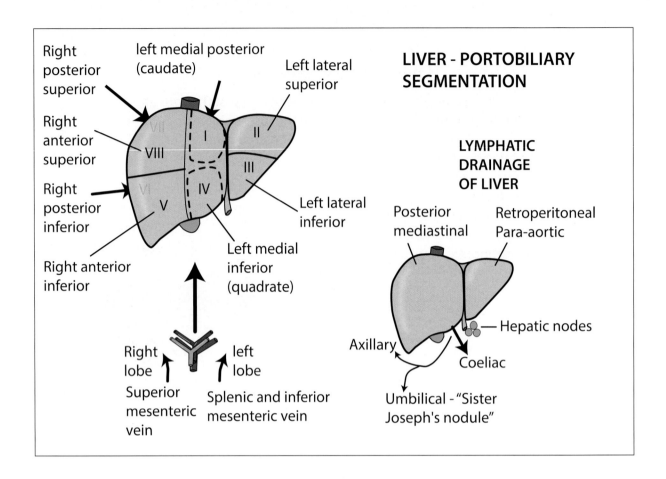

Right posterior superior

left medial posterior (caudate)

Left lateral superior

LIVER - PORTOBILIARY SEGMENTATION

Right anterior superior

Right posterior inferior

Right anterior inferior

Left lateral inferior

Left medial inferior (quadrate)

Right lobe

left lobe

Superior mesenteric vein

Splenic and inferior mesenteric vein

LYMPHATIC DRAINAGE OF LIVER

Posterior mediastinal

Retroperitoneal Para-aortic

Axillary

Hepatic nodes

Coeliac

Umbilical - "Sister Joseph's nodule"

HEPATIC VEINS

These veins drain the "cleansed" blood back into the systemic circulation from the liver. They do not follow the portobiliary segmentation. The veins suspend the liver from the inferior vena cava and are helped by the peritoneal reflections

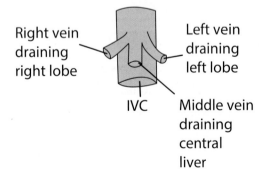

Right vein draining right lobe

Left vein draining left lobe

IVC

Middle vein draining central liver

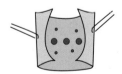

Accessory veins drain the liver directly into the (opened) IVC

PORTOSYSTEMIC ANASTOMOSES 1

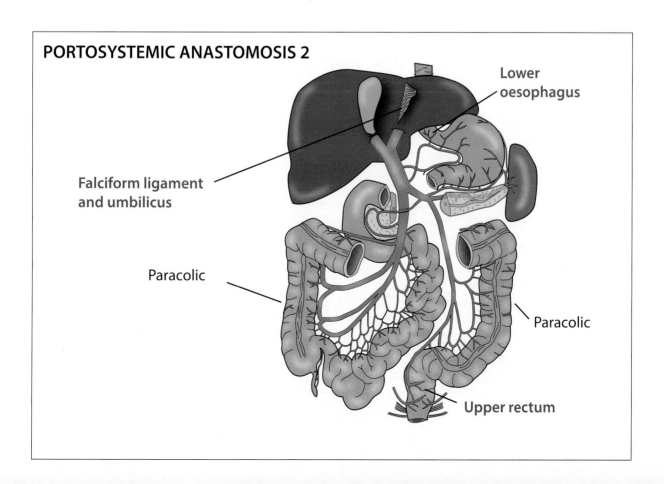

1 **Lower oesophagus**
Portal: Oesophageal branches of left gastric veins
Systemic: Azygos veins

2 **Upper anal canal**
Portal: Superior rectal vein
Systemic: Middle/inferior rectal veins

3 **Umbilical**
Portal: Veins of ligamentum teres
Systemic: Superior/inferior epigastic veins

4 **Bare area of liver**
Portal: Hepatic/portal veins
Systemic: Inferior phrenic veins

5 **Patent ductus venosus (rare)**
Portal: Left branch of portal vein
Systemic: Inferior vena cava

6 **Retroperitoneal**
Portal: Colonic veins
Systemic: Body wall veins

PORTOSYSTEMIC ANASTOMOSIS 2

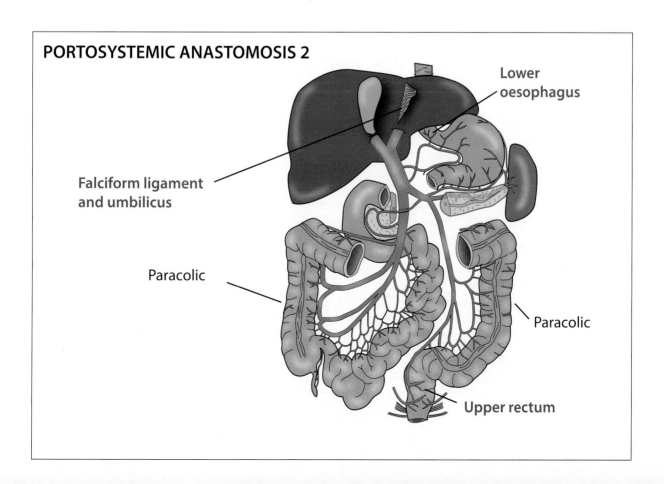

PANCREAS 1

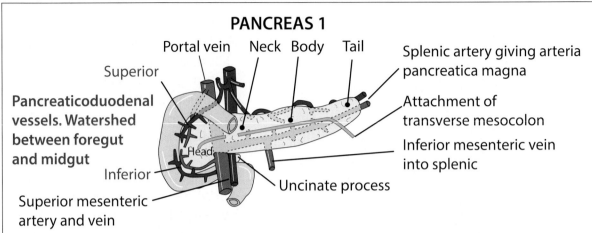

Retroperitoneal, Neck in the transpyloric plane, 15cm long, lobulated with fine capsule. Islets of Langerhans between alveoli. Exocrine volume much greater than endocrine
Main duct (Wirsung) leads to ampulla of Vater. Accessory duct (**Santorini**) from uncinate process opens proximally, may be absent, often communicates with main duct
Secretion: Alveoli of serous secretory cells lead to ductules then to principal ducts. Amylase. Secretin causes juice rich in bicarbonate; cholecystokinin causes juices rich in enzymes - trypsinogen, chymotrypsinogen anc pancreatic lipase. Alpha islet cells give glucogon, beta cells give insulin, delta give somatostatin which inhibits secretion of pancreatic hormones including glucogon and insulin. Pancreatic polypeptide is produced by the tail of the pancreas.

PANCREAS 2

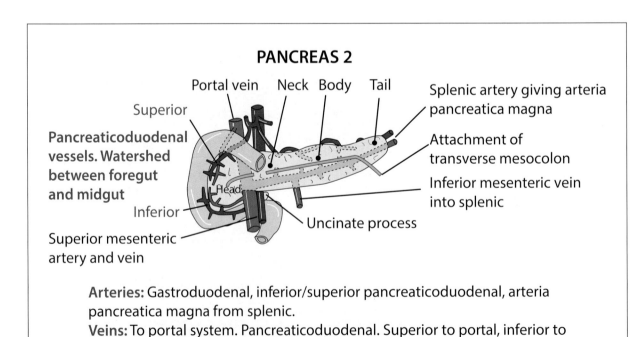

Arteries: Gastroduodenal, inferior/superior pancreaticoduodenal, arteria pancreatica magna from splenic.
Veins: To portal system. Pancreaticoduodenal. Superior to portal, inferior to superior mesenteric
Lymphatics: In groove between head and duodenum and root of arteries
Nerves: Parasympathetic (posterior vagus) to stimulate exocrine secretion. Sympathetic for vasoconstriction and pain (T6-10)

PANCREAS: RELATIONS

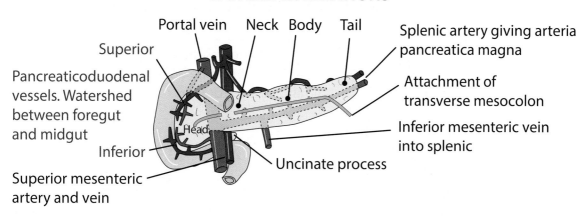

Anterior: Lesser sac, pylorus, 1st part of duodenum, transverse mesocolon, stomach; superior mesenteric artery and vein lying between body and uncinate process
Superior: Splenic artery
Lateral on right: 2nd part of duodenum, ampulla of Vater
Lateral on left: Hilum of spleen
Posterior: Left crus of diaphragm, psoas, right renal vein, inferior vena cava, bile duct, spleen, left renal vessels, left kidney, left suprarenal gland, coeliac plexus, inferior mesenteric vein, splenic vein, portal vein, aorta; superior mesenteric artery and vein

SPLEEN GENERAL

- Size of a fist. 200g
- 2.5cm x 8cm x 13cm (1 x 3 x 5")
- Part of the reticuloendothelial system
- Becomes palpable when it is twice normal size
- Thin capsule, has notch and moves on respiration (cf. kidney)

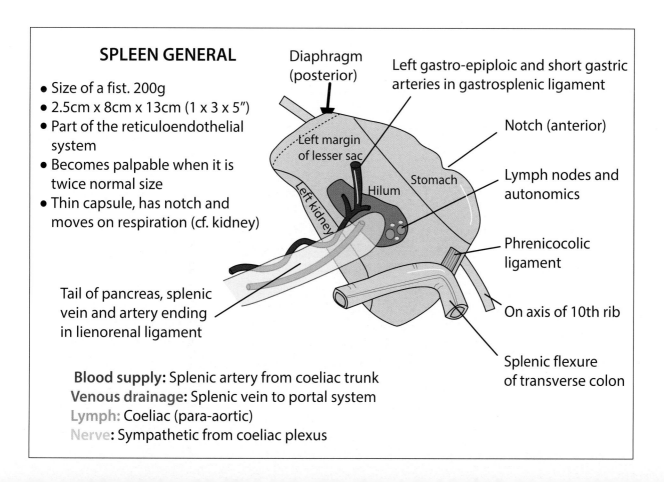

Blood supply: Splenic artery from coeliac trunk
Venous drainage: Splenic vein to portal system
Lymph: Coeliac (para-aortic)
Nerve: Sympathetic from coeliac plexus

SPLEEN - RELATIONS, FUNCTION AND DEVELOPMENT

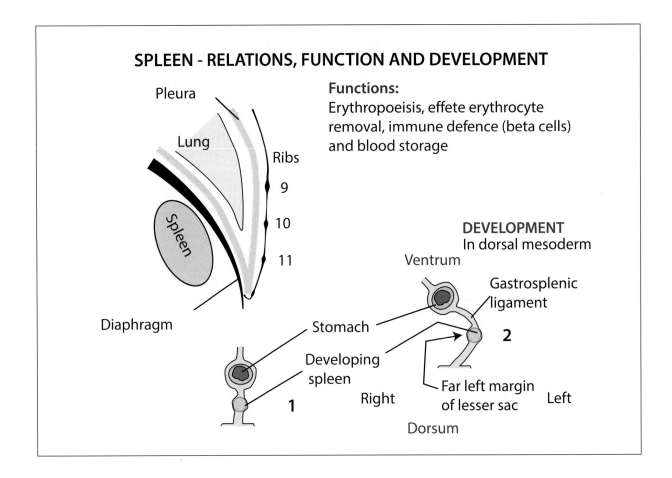

Pleura

Lung

Ribs

9

10

11

Spleen

Diaphragm

Functions:
Erythropoeisis, effete erythrocyte removal, immune defence (beta cells) and blood storage

DEVELOPMENT
In dorsal mesoderm

Ventrum

Gastrosplenic ligament

Stomach

Developing spleen

Far left margin of lesser sac

Right

Left

Dorsum

1

2

4.6   Female and Male Genitourinary and Renal Tracts

UTERUS AND BROAD LIGAMENT

BROAD LIGAMENT: A double layer of peritoneum draped over uterus and tubes. Between the two layers are arteries, veins, round ligament, ligament of ovary and lymphatics. The ovary is partially covered by a separate posterior fold of the broad ligament (mesovarium) but the surface of the ovary is devoid of peritoneum to allow exit of the ova.

FALLOPIAN TUBES: Lie in the upper edge of the broad ligament (mesosalpinx). they are 10cm long. Outer longitudinal and inner circular muscle and a ciliated columnar lining. Their distal ends protrude out of the posterior layer of the broad ligament and lie free in the peritoneal cavity.

LIGAMENT OF THE OVARY: Extends between the ovary and the side wall of the uterus.

ROUND LIGAMENTS OF UTERUS: Extend from the side wall of the uterus to the labia majora via the inguinal canal. The ligament of the ovary and the round ligament are in continuity and represent the homologue of the gubernaculum in the male.

THE URETERS: Pass through the base of the broad ligament in close relationship to the uterine artery, level with the uterine os.

UTERINE ARTERY: Supplies the uterus, vagina and anastomoses with ovarian artery.

NERVES: Sensory: General visceral afferents via pelvic plexus. In parasympathetics from cervix and in sympathetics for rest of uterus and tube. Parasympathetics motor to uterus and tube. No parasympathetics to ovary.

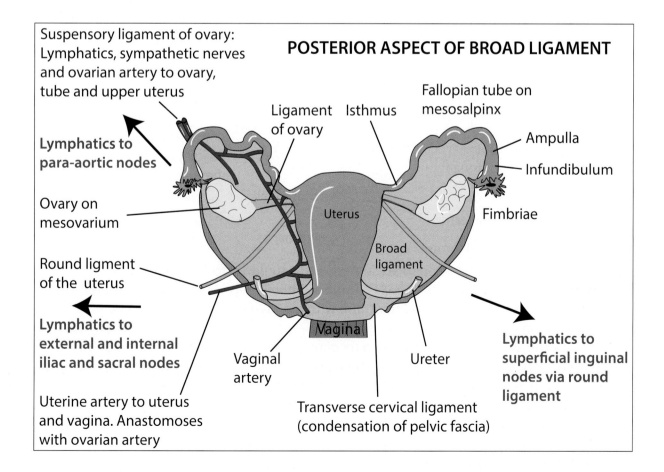

POSTERIOR ASPECT OF BROAD LIGAMENT

Suspensory ligament of ovary: Lymphatics, sympathetic nerves and ovarian artery to ovary, tube and upper uterus

Lymphatics to para-aortic nodes

Ligament of ovary

Isthmus

Fallopian tube on mesosalpinx

Ampulla

Infundibulum

Ovary on mesovarium

Uterus

Fimbriae

Broad ligament

Round ligment of the uterus

Lymphatics to external and internal iliac and sacral nodes

Vagina

Lymphatics to superficial inguinal nodes via round ligament

Vaginal artery

Ureter

Uterine artery to uterus and vagina. Anastomoses with ovarian artery

Transverse cervical ligament (condensation of pelvic fascia)

ANTERIOR VIEW OF LEFT SIDE OF BROAD LIGAMENT

Suspensory ligament of the ovary is a double fold of peritoneum at the lateral end of the broad ligament where the ovarian neurovascular bundle leaves the posterolateral abdominal wall to enter the broad ligament

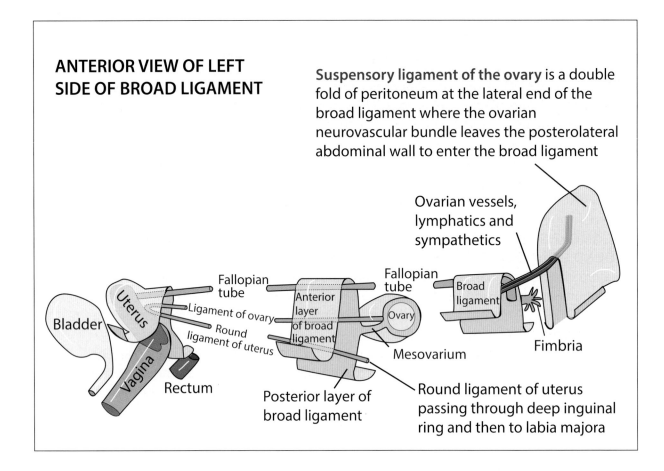

Ovarian vessels, lymphatics and sympathetics

Fallopian tube

Anterior layer of broad ligament

Fallopian tube

Broad ligament

Ovary

Uterus

Bladder

Ligament of ovary

Round ligament of uterus

Vagina

Rectum

Mesovarium

Fimbria

Posterior layer of broad ligament

Round ligament of uterus passing through deep inguinal ring and then to labia majora

UTERUS

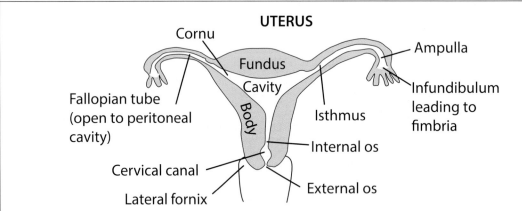

Cornu

Fundus

Cavity

Ampulla

Infundibulum leading to fimbria

Fallopian tube (open to peritoneal cavity)

Body

Isthmus

Internal os

Cervical canal

Lateral fornix

External os

Pear shaped. Usually anteverted to 90 degrees and anteflexed to 170 degrees
Histology: No submucosa. Cervix: Tall columnar epithelium becoming squamous outside, alkaline mucus. Rest of uterus: Endometrium with glands, arterioles, smooth whorls of muscle, columnar epithelium.
Nerves: Motor: Smooth muscle activated by parasympathetic, relaxed by sympathetic. Both from pelvic plexus. Sensory: Sympathetic for uterus. Parasympathetic cervix only.
Blood supply: Uterine artery with some anastomosis from ovarian artery.
Venous drainage: Highly plexiform to vesical and rectal plexuses.
Relations: Anterior - vesicouterine pouch, posterior/superior bladder anterior fornix, small bowel. **Posterior** - Pouch of Douglas, ileum, sigmoid. **Lateral** - Uterine vessels, ureter, lateral fornix, broad ligament

VAGINA

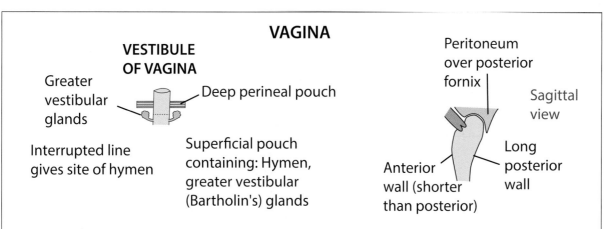

VESTIBULE OF VAGINA

Greater vestibular glands

Deep perineal pouch

Interrupted line gives site of hymen

Superficial pouch containing: Hymen, greater vestibular (Bartholin's) glands

Peritoneum over posterior fornix

Sagittal view

Anterior wall (shorter than posterior)

Long posterior wall

10cm long, potential space apart from posterior fornix which is real space
Fornices: Anterior, lateral and posterior
Artery: Vaginal branch of uterine, middle rectal, inferior vesical
Veins: Pelvic floor plexus to internal iliac
Nerves: Autonomic from pelvic plexus for vasoconstriction, smooth muscle action, stretch sensation.
Somatic: Perineal branches of pudendal, ilio-inguinal
Lymphatics: External/internal iliac, sacral, superficial inguinal
Support: levator ani (pubovaginalis) and perineal body
Structure: Non-keratinising stratified squamous epithelium, smooth muscle, sweat glands, no mucous glands
Relations: Anterior: Bladder, urethra. **Posterior:** Recto-uterine pouch, rectum, perineal body, anal canal.
Lateral: Ureter, uterine artery, levator ani, urogenital diaphragm

COMPARISONS OF PELVIC PERITONEUM IN THE MALE AND FEMALE PELVIS

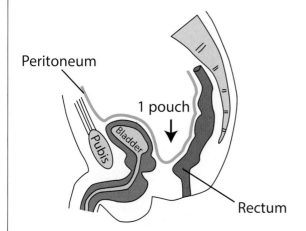

Peritoneum

1 pouch

Pubis

Bladder

Rectum

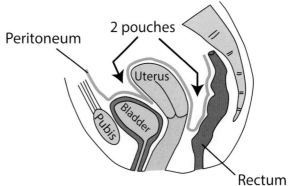

Peritoneum

2 pouches

Uterus

Pubis

Bladder

Rectum

MALE: In males the peritoneum passes from the posterior surface of the bladder to the lower third of the rectum, giving a single - **rectovesical pouch**

FEMALE: In females the uterus protrudes into the pelvis between the bladder and rectum giving two pouches. The **vesicouterine pouch** anteriorly and the **rectouterine pouch** (of Douglas) posteriorly.

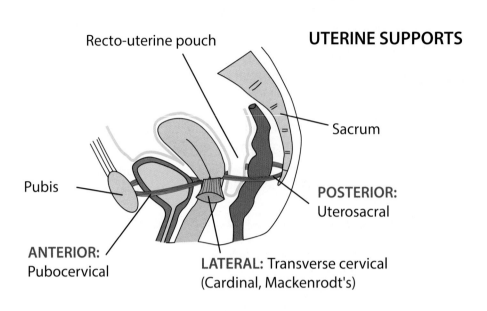

UTERINE SUPPORTS

Recto-uterine pouch

Sacrum

Pubis

POSTERIOR: Uterosacral

ANTERIOR: Pubocervical

LATERAL: Transverse cervical (Cardinal, Mackenrodt's)

These ligaments/Supports are condensations of fascia known as parametrium.

NOTE: Suspensory ligament of ovary, round ligament and broad ligament are **NOT** primarily supportive

UTERINE PROLAPSE AND PROCIDENTIA

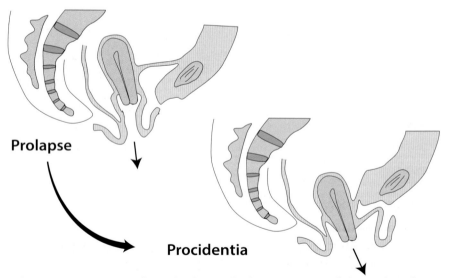

Prolapse

Procidentia

As the uterus passes inferiorly through the opening of the pelvic floor there is a substantial risk of the ureters lying alongside it becoming obstructed and leading to acute bilateral hydroureteronephrosis and acute renal impairment.

GONADAL VESSELS

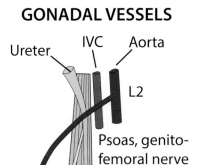

Ureter IVC Aorta

L2

Psoas, genito-
femoral nerve

Gonadal artery enters
suspensory ligament of
ovary at pelvic brim

Tube   Sagittal section
of broad ligament

Ovary with
low columnar
epithelium but
NO peritoneum

OVARY RELATIONS

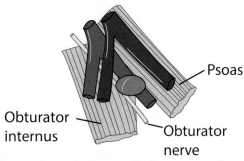

Psoas

Obturator
internus

Obturator
nerve

Ovary lies in fossa between bifurcation of common
iliac artery, on obturator nerve and external iliac
vein. Overlaid by ileum and sigmoid colon

Almond shaped - 4cm x 2cm
Attached to posterior aspect of broad
ligament by mesovarium
Attached to uterus by ligament of ovary
Artery: Ovarian from aorta at L2
Vein: Left to left renal. Right to IVC
Lymphatics: Para-aortics. (Inguinal via round
ligament and to opposite ovary in disease)

GONADAL VESSELS

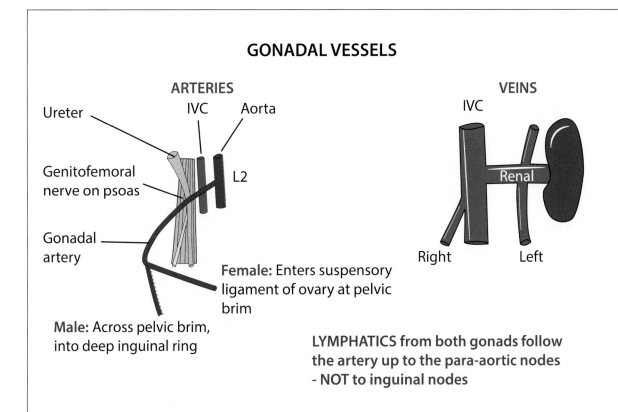

ARTERIES

Ureter

IVC Aorta

Genitofemoral
nerve on psoas

L2

Gonadal
artery

VEINS

IVC

Renal

Right   Left

Female: Enters suspensory
ligament of ovary at pelvic
brim

Male: Across pelvic brim,
into deep inguinal ring

**LYMPHATICS from both gonads follow
the artery up to the para-aortic nodes
- NOT to inguinal nodes**

MALE URETHRA

Prostatic approximately 2.5cm and **membranous** 2cm together make the posterior urethra.
Bulbous and **pendulous** make the anterior urethra. Approximately 20cm.
Blood: Artery to bulb to both glans and corpus spongiosum; Deep artery of penis to corpus cavernosum; Dorsal artery of penis to skin, fascia, glans; Urethral artery from dorsal artery
Veins: Superficial and deep dorsal veins of penis
Lymph: Skin to superficial inguinal nodes. Glans, corpora, urethra to deep inguinal nodes
Nerves: Posterior scrotal to skin and glans. Pudendal gives dorsal nerve of penis. Sympathetics for ejaculation, Parasympathetics to corpora for erection.
Receives: Ejaculatory ducts, bulbourethral glands, urethral glands

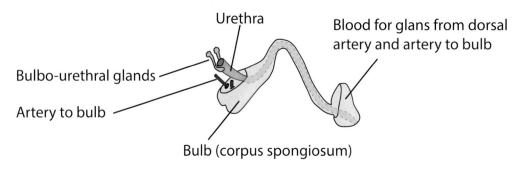

PENIS - CONSTITUENT PARTS

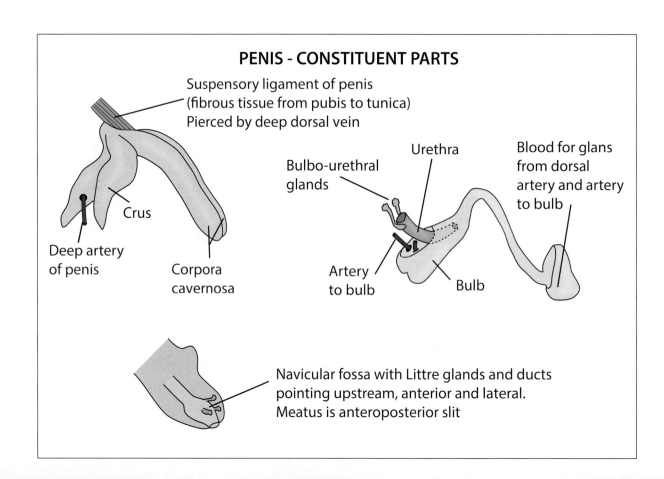

PENIS - CORONAL SECTION AT PUBIS

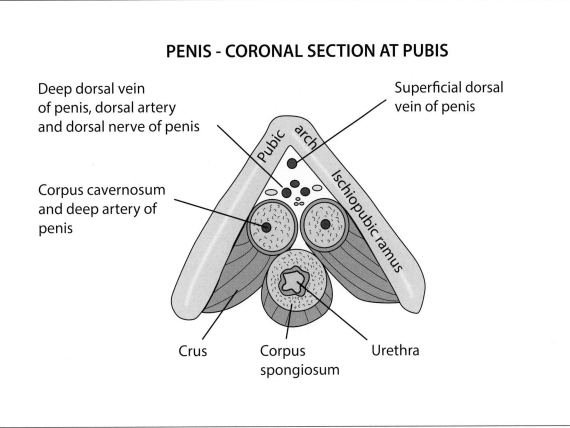

Deep dorsal vein of penis, dorsal artery and dorsal nerve of penis

Superficial dorsal vein of penis

Corpus cavernosum and deep artery of penis

Pubic arch

Ischiopubic ramus

Crus

Corpus spongiosum

Urethra

CROSS SECTION OF MID SHAFT PENIS

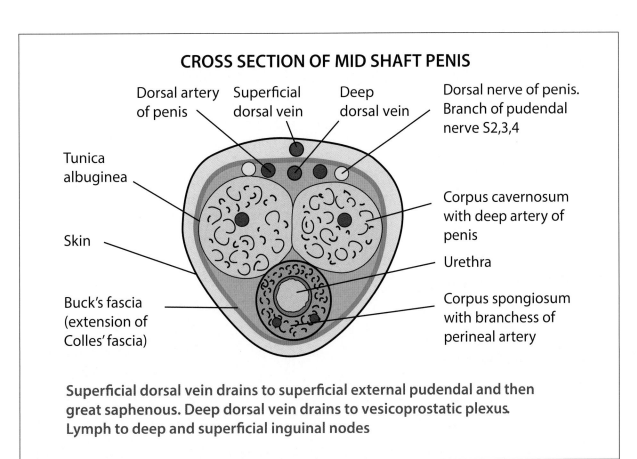

Dorsal artery of penis

Superficial dorsal vein

Deep dorsal vein

Dorsal nerve of penis. Branch of pudendal nerve S2,3,4

Tunica albuginea

Skin

Buck's fascia (extension of Colles' fascia)

Corpus cavernosum with deep artery of penis

Urethra

Corpus spongiosum with branchess of perineal artery

Superficial dorsal vein drains to superficial external pudendal and then great saphenous. Deep dorsal vein drains to vesicoprostatic plexus. Lymph to deep and superficial inguinal nodes

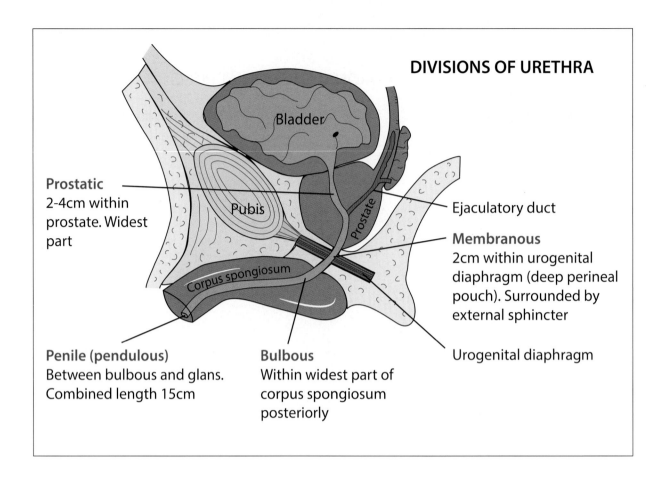

DIVISIONS OF URETHRA

Prostatic
2-4cm within prostate. Widest part

Bladder

Pubis

Prostate

Corpus spongiosum

Ejaculatory duct

Membranous
2cm within urogenital diaphragm (deep perineal pouch). Surrounded by external sphincter

Urogenital diaphragm

Penile (pendulous)
Between bulbous and glans. Combined length 15cm

Bulbous
Within widest part of corpus spongiosum posteriorly

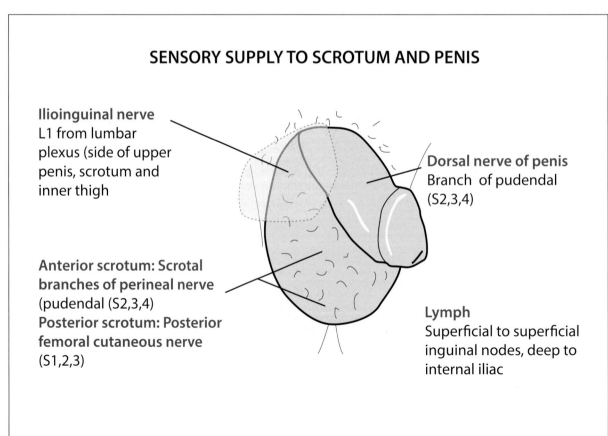

SENSORY SUPPLY TO SCROTUM AND PENIS

Ilioinguinal nerve
L1 from lumbar plexus (side of upper penis, scrotum and inner thigh)

Dorsal nerve of penis
Branch of pudendal (S2,3,4)

**Anterior scrotum: Scrotal branches of perineal nerve (pudendal (S2,3,4)
Posterior scrotum: Posterior femoral cutaneous nerve (S1,2,3)**

Lymph
Superficial to superficial inguinal nodes, deep to internal iliac

PROSTATE

- Pyramidal shape
- Posterior groove
- Size of chestnut (2 x 3 x 4cm)
- Sits on urogenital diaphragm
- Intrinsic urethral mechanism around it
- Gives nutrients for sperm
- 30% ejaculate volume
- Urethra runs through it
- True and false capsules
- Ejaculatory ducts and prostatic utricle (paramesonephric remnant) open onto verumontanum in floor of prostatic urethra
- **Veins:** Preprostatic plexus - valveless (to vertebral plexuses)
- **Arteries:** Inferior vesical, middle rectal, internal pudendal
- **Nerves:** Sympathetic for ejaculation and smooth muscle contraction. Parasympathetic for erection and secretomotor of acini
- **Lymph:** Iliac nodes

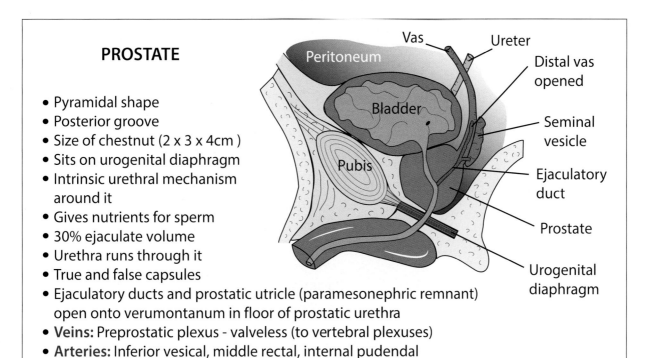

AXIAL PROSTATE TO SHOW "ZONAL" LOBES

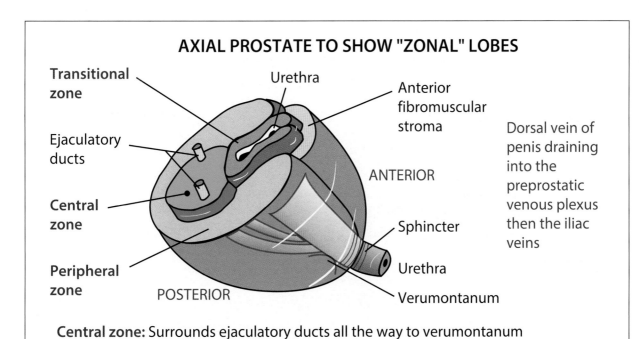

Dorsal vein of penis draining into the preprostatic venous plexus then the iliac veins

Central zone: Surrounds ejaculatory ducts all the way to verumontanum

Transitional zone: Surrounds the urethra. Liable to nodular benign enlargement (stroma and glandular) from 40 yrs onwards. Causes: ageing, circulating androgens

Peripheral zone: Surrounds the other two zones. 70% of cancers start here. It is pushed peripherally by benign enlargement and compressed

PROSTATIC DUCTS

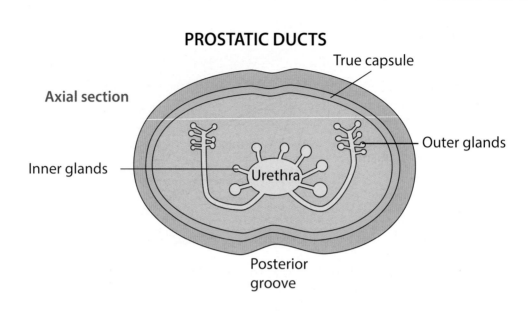

Axial section

True capsule

Outer glands

Inner glands

Urethra

Posterior groove

- Prostatic ducts open into urethra as two groups: inner and outer
- True fibrous capsule, but a false "capsule" develops when hypertrophic prostatic tissue compresses the posterior lobe (peripheral zone)

PROSTATIC LIGAMENTS AND SUPPORTS

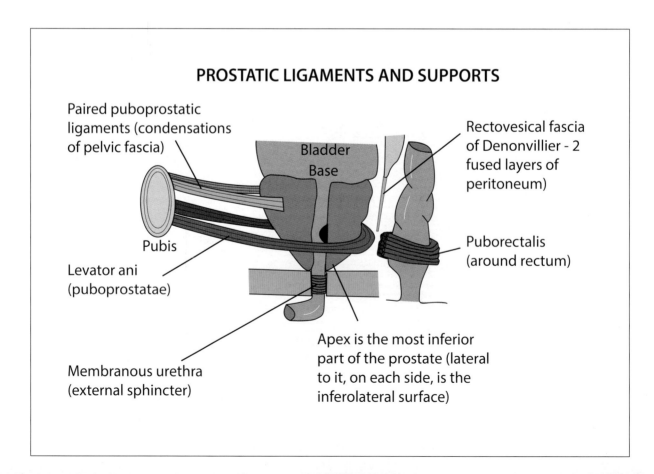

Paired puboprostatic ligaments (condensations of pelvic fascia)

Bladder Base

Rectovesical fascia of Denonvillier - 2 fused layers of peritoneum)

Pubis

Puborectalis (around rectum)

Levator ani (puboprostatae)

Membranous urethra (external sphincter)

Apex is the most inferior part of the prostate (lateral to it, on each side, is the inferolateral surface)

SEMINAL VESICLES

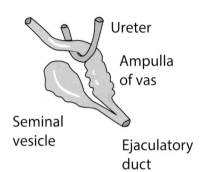

Ureter

Ampulla
of vas

Seminal
vesicle

Ejaculatory
duct

The seminal vesicles are thin walled sacs lying posterior to the bladder and prostate, producing 70% of the ejaculate but **containing NO sperm**. The remaining 30% is produced by the prostate. They produce fructose with medicolegal importance in identifying seminal fluid. They are covered posteriorly by Denonvillier's fascia.
Arterial supply: Vesical or middle rectal arteries.
Nerve supply: Post-ganglionic sympathetic fibres.
Structure: The lining is outer longitudinal and inner circular smooth muscle - needed for ejaculation. The ejaculatory ducts are formed by the distal vas and the seminal vesicle duct and enter the posterior urethra at the verumontanum.

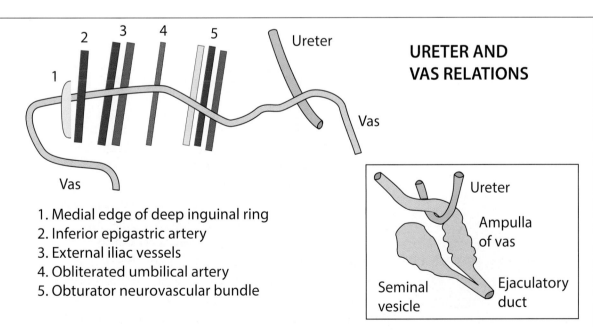

URETER AND VAS RELATIONS

Ureter

Vas

Vas

1. Medial edge of deep inguinal ring
2. Inferior epigastric artery
3. External iliac vessels
4. Obliterated umbilical artery
5. Obturator neurovascular bundle

Ureter

Ampulla
of vas

Seminal
vesicle

Ejaculatory
duct

The ductus (vas) deferens is about 45cm long and is a highly muscular (smooth muscle) tube. It starts at the lower pole of the epididymis and ends at the ejaculatory duct. It lies just beneath the peritoneum for most of its intra-abdominal course. It is supplied by a branch of either the superior or inferior vesical artery. Motor activity during ejaculation is controlled by post-ganglionic sympathetic fibres

TESTIS

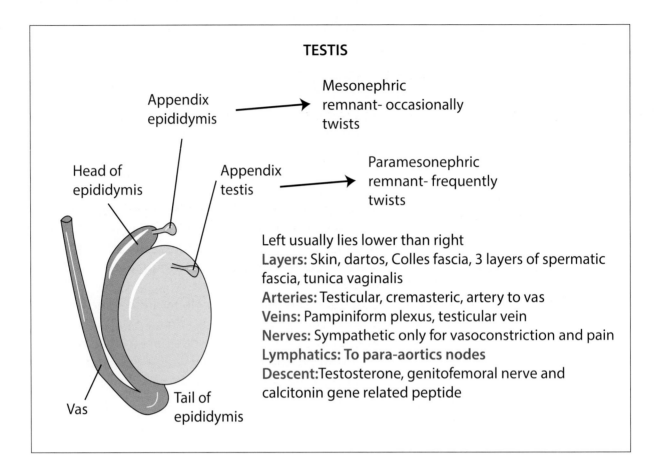

Appendix epididymis → Mesonephric remnant- occasionally twists

Appendix testis → Paramesonephric remnant- frequently twists

Head of epididymis

Vas

Tail of epididymis

Left usually lies lower than right
Layers: Skin, dartos, Colles fascia, 3 layers of spermatic fascia, tunica vaginalis
Arteries: Testicular, cremasteric, artery to vas
Veins: Pampiniform plexus, testicular vein
Nerves: Sympathetic only for vasoconstriction and pain
Lymphatics: To para-aortics nodes
Descent: Testosterone, genitofemoral nerve and calcitonin gene related peptide

TORSION OF TESTIS

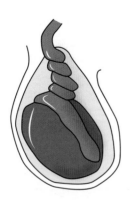

When the attachments of the testis within the tunica vaginalis is less than normal the testis hangs like a clapper in a bell and this allows it to twist. The blood supply is cut off and there is strangulation of the testis. This is then a surgical emergency to save the testis. When the delay is over 12 hours, the testis is usually lost. Such torsion is common around puberty, but can occur at any age. It is frequently associated with subsequent infertility.

In neonates, the torsion is characteristically outside the tunica vaginalis and the twist involves the whole spermatic cord. The testis is usually not viable.

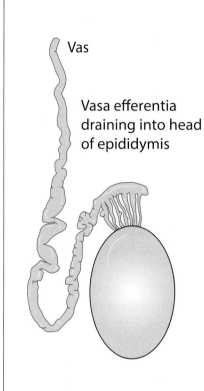

Vas

Vasa efferentia draining into head of epididymis

VAS DEFERENS

- 45cm long from epididymis to ejaculatory duct
- Has own artery from superior or inferior vesical artery
- Mesonephric (Wolffian) origin
- Ciliated epithelium
- **Nerve supply:** To testis and epididymis. Sympathetics from chain at L2 for vasoconstriction and carrying general visceral afferents for pain to T10 dermatome. NO parasympathetic

PATENT PROCESSUS VAGINALIS IN CHILDREN

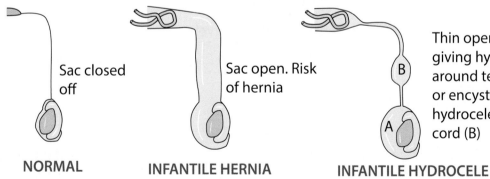

Sac closed off

Sac open. Risk of hernia

Thin open tract giving hydrocele around testis (A) or encysted hydrocele of cord (B)

NORMAL　　　**INFANTILE HERNIA**　　　**INFANTILE HYDROCELE**

DESCENT OF THE TESTIS

FIRST 7 MONTHS:
Under hormonal control
LAST 2 MONTHS:
Controlled by genitofemoral nerve

Cell bodies of genitofemoral nerve in males contain Calitonin Gene Related Peptide (CGRP) which acts on the gubernaculum to give rhythmic contraction in baby mice. If the genitofemoral nerve is cut then there is no descent.

SPERMATIC CORD
(Cross section just beyond external inguinal ring)

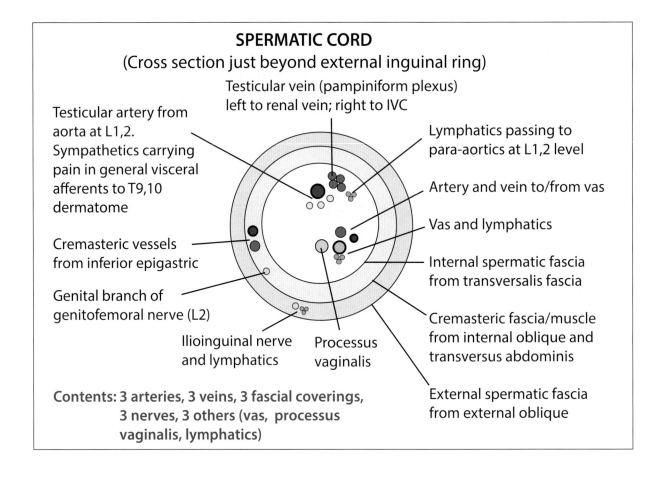

Testicular vein (pampiniform plexus) left to renal vein; right to IVC

Testicular artery from aorta at L1,2. Sympathetics carrying pain in general visceral afferents to T9,10 dermatome

Lymphatics passing to para-aortics at L1,2 level

Artery and vein to/from vas

Vas and lymphatics

Cremasteric vessels from inferior epigastric

Internal spermatic fascia from transversalis fascia

Genital branch of genitofemoral nerve (L2)

Cremasteric fascia/muscle from internal oblique and transversus abdominis

Ilioinguinal nerve and lymphatics

Processus vaginalis

External spermatic fascia from external oblique

Contents: 3 arteries, 3 veins, 3 fascial coverings, 3 nerves, 3 others (vas, processus vaginalis, lymphatics)

SPERMATIC CORD

Contents of cord at 3 levels

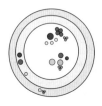

VIA THE DEEP INGUINAL RING
- Vas
- Artery to vas (from superior or inferior vesical artery)
- Testicular artery (direct from aorta)
- Cremasteric artery (from inferior epigastric) artery
- Cremasteric vein (to inferior epigastric vein)
- Testicular vein (to IVC and left renal vein)
- Obliterated processus vaginalis
- Lymphatics
- Sympathetics
- Genital branch of genitofemoral nerve (L2). Motor to cremaster, sensory to fascia, tunica, scrotal skin, round ligament and labia majus

IN CANAL
- All these plus
- Internal spermatic fascia
- Cremasteric fascia
- Cremaster muscle
- Ilio-inguinal nerve

OUTSIDE SUPERFICIAL RING
- All these plus
- External spermatic fascia from external oblique

RENAL VESSELS

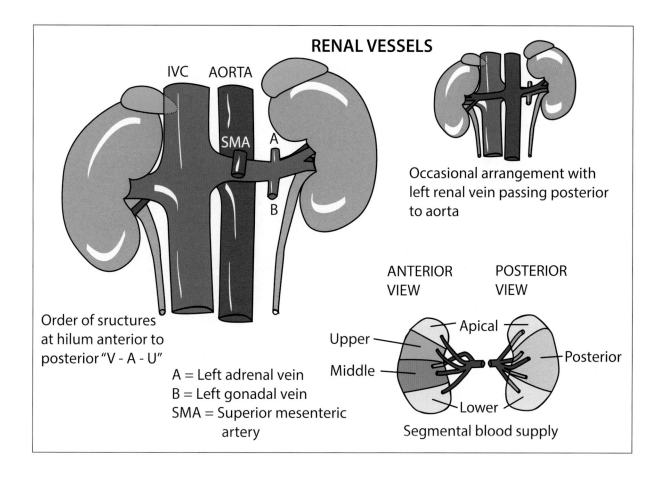

Occasional arrangement with left renal vein passing posterior to aorta

Order of sructures at hilum anterior to posterior "V - A - U"

A = Left adrenal vein
B = Left gonadal vein
SMA = Superior mesenteric artery

ANTERIOR VIEW   POSTERIOR VIEW

Apical
Upper
Middle
Posterior
Lower

Segmental blood supply

KIDNEY - GENERAL

- 135g in female; 150g in male
- 11x6x3cm in adults
- 1200ml of blood per minute
- 1 million nephrons per kidney
- Lies retroperitoneal
- Moves 3 - 4cm on respiration
- Palpable lower pole in thin or young person
- Pelvis faces anteromedially
- Lymphatics to para-aortic nodes
- Sympathetics from T12-L1 for pain and vasoconstriction
- Parasympathetics from vagus. Function unknown
- Fetal kidney is lobulated
- Thin capsule. Easy to strip off in normal kidney
- Hila lie on transpyloric plane

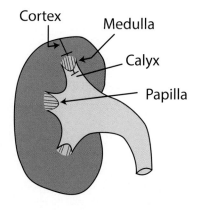

Cortex
Medulla
Calyx
Papilla

Blood from renal artery

↓

Segmental arteries

↓

Lobar arteries
(to each pyramid)

↓

3 interlobar arteries
(junction of cortex and medulla)

↓

Arcuate arteries
(running at right angles)

↓

Efferent arterioles
(to the cortex and glomeruli)

ARTERIAL SUPPLY OF KIDNEY

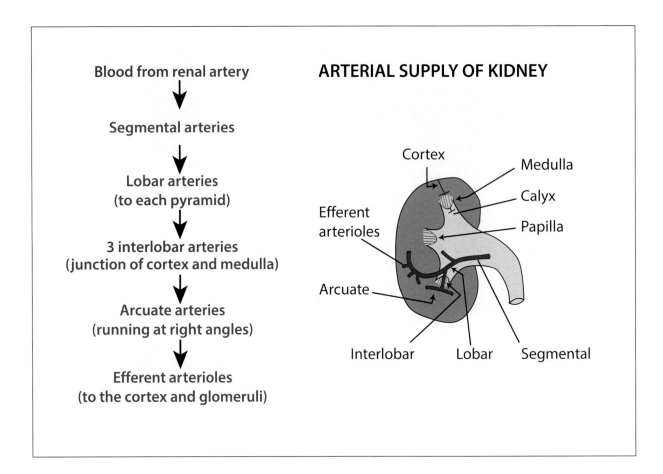

Cortex

Medulla

Calyx

Papilla

Efferent arterioles

Arcuate

Interlobar   Lobar   Segmental

ANTERIOR RELATIONS OF KIDNEYS

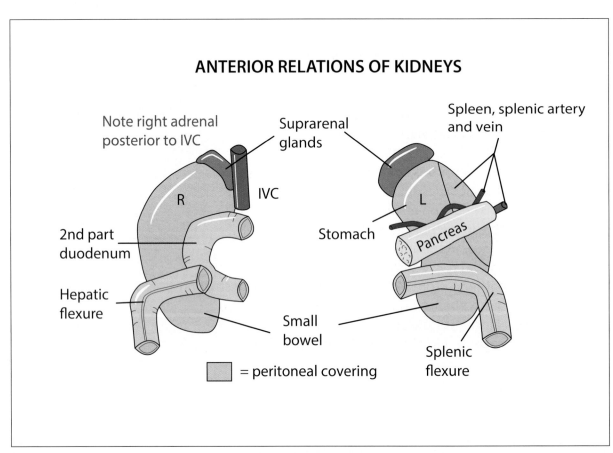

Note right adrenal posterior to IVC

Suprarenal glands

Spleen, splenic artery and vein

R

IVC

L

Pancreas

2nd part duodenum

Stomach

Hepatic flexure

Small bowel

Splenic flexure

▢ = peritoneal covering

KIDNEY - RELATIONS

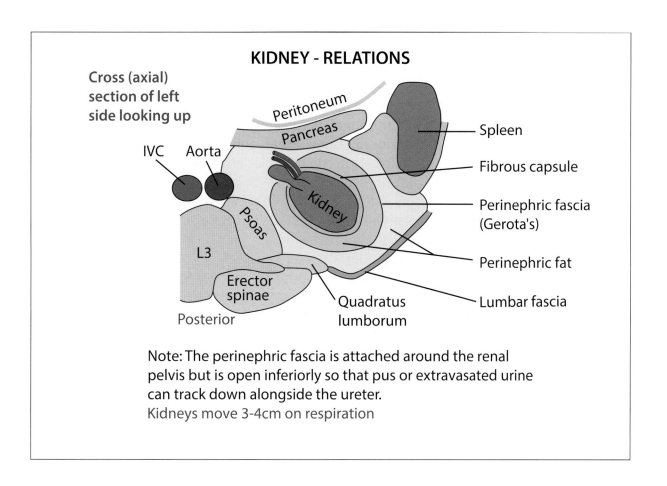

Cross (axial) section of left side looking up

Labels: Peritoneum, Pancreas, IVC, Aorta, Psoas, L3, Erector spinae, Posterior, Quadratus lumborum, Kidney, Spleen, Fibrous capsule, Perinephric fascia (Gerota's), Perinephric fat, Lumbar fascia

Note: The perinephric fascia is attached around the renal pelvis but is open inferiorly so that pus or extravasated urine can track down alongside the ureter.

Kidneys move 3-4cm on respiration

POSTERIOR RENAL RELATIONS

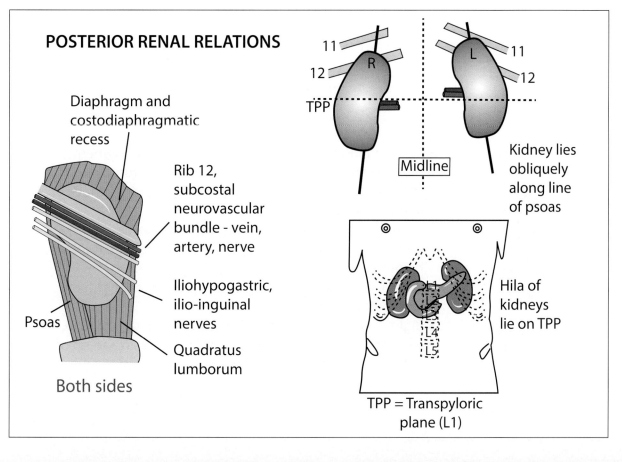

Diaphragm and costodiaphragmatic recess

Rib 12, subcostal neurovascular bundle - vein, artery, nerve

Iliohypogastric, ilio-inguinal nerves

Quadratus lumborum

Psoas

Both sides

Kidney lies obliquely along line of psoas

Hila of kidneys lie on TPP

Midline

TPP = Transpyloric plane (L1)

URETER 1

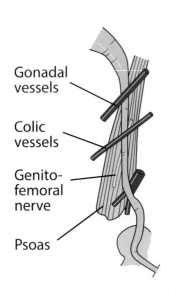

Gonadal vessels

Colic vessels

Genito-femoral nerve

Psoas

25cm long. From renal pelvis to bladder. Smooth muscle and transitional urothelium

Posterior relations: Psoas, genitofemoral nerve, sacroiliac joint, common iliac artery bifurcation

Anterior relations: Right- Duodenum, right gonadal artery, right colic artery, ileal mesentery, superior mesenteric artery. **Left**- Left gonadal artery, left colic artery, sigmoid mesentery

Passes under: Vas, uterine artery

Related to: Lateral fornix of vagina in females

Blood supply: Renal, gonadal, vesical. Smaller branches from aorta, common iliac and vaginal arteries

Nerves: General visceral afferents for pain and sympathetics probably for vasoconstriction only

Points of potential hold up: Pelviureteric junction, pelvic brim, ureterovesical junction

URETER 2

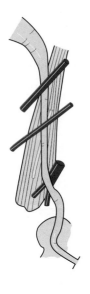

- The ureter is recognisable as it shows peristalsis when pinched and is the most superficial retroperitonal structure in the pelvis adhering to the posterior surface of the peritoneum
- It crosses the bifurcation of the iliac arteries and then passes around the pelvis to 1cm short of the ischial spine before swinging medially
- On a plain abdominal X-ray it enters the bladder at the level of the pubic tubercle
- Right ureter may be irritated by an inflamed appendix
- Pain is referred progressively from loin to groin and tip of penis as a stone progresses down the ureter

URETEROVESICAL JUNCTION

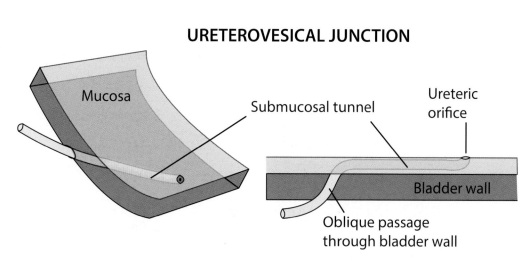

The ureter passes obliquely through the bladder wall then runs sub-mucosally for a distance that is 5 times the diameter of the ureter. This prevents vesico-ureteric reflux of urine

BLADDER - GENERAL

Epithelium: Transitional - watertight, stretchy, no glands. No peritoneum on anterior wall
Muscle: Detrusor, smooth muscle - 3 layers- inner/outer longitudinal, middle circular
Arteries: Superior/inferior vesical
Veins: Converge to vesicoprostatic plexus in males. Converge to plexus at base of broad ligament in female. Then to internal iliac veins
Lymphatics: Internal and external iliac nodes
Nerves: Sympathetic: Motor to bladder neck for closure at ejaculation, in males only. Inhibitory, vasomotor, pain in both sexes. Parasympathetic - motor to detrusor, sensory for full bladder, some pain

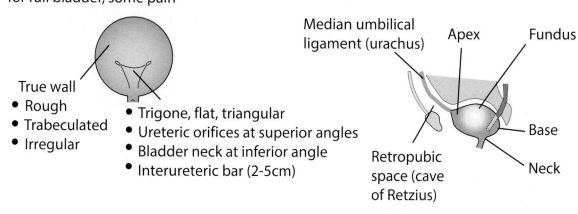

True wall
- Rough
- Trabeculated
- Irregular

- Trigone, flat, triangular
- Ureteric orifices at superior angles
- Bladder neck at inferior angle
- Interureteric bar (2-5cm)

Median umbilical ligament (urachus)

Apex

Fundus

Base

Neck

Retropubic space (cave of Retzius)

BLADDER - RELATIONS

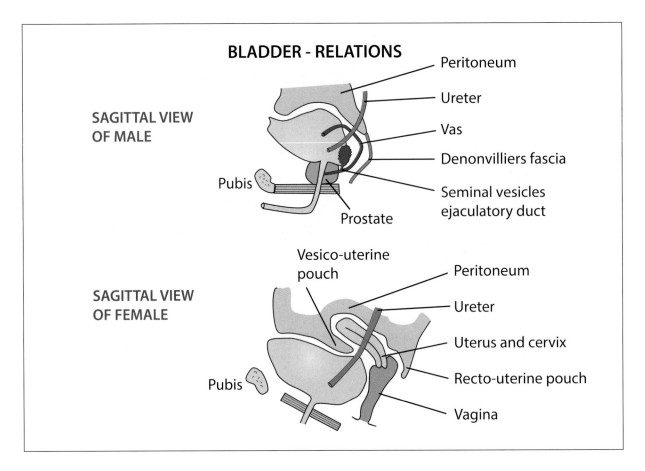

SAGITTAL VIEW OF MALE

- Peritoneum
- Ureter
- Vas
- Denonvilliers fascia
- Seminal vesicles ejaculatory duct
- Pubis
- Prostate

SAGITTAL VIEW OF FEMALE

- Vesico-uterine pouch
- Peritoneum
- Ureter
- Uterus and cervix
- Recto-uterine pouch
- Vagina
- Pubis

BLADDER AND SPHINCTER MUSCLES

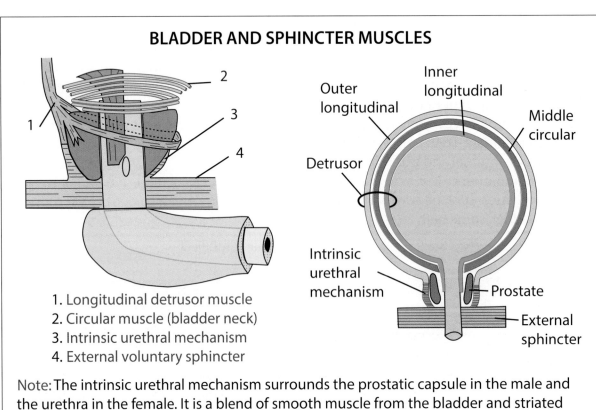

1. Longitudinal detrusor muscle
2. Circular muscle (bladder neck)
3. Intrinsic urethral mechanism
4. External voluntary sphincter

Outer longitudinal • Inner longitudinal • Middle circular • Detrusor • Intrinsic urethral mechanism • Prostate • External sphincter

Note: The intrinsic urethral mechanism surrounds the prostatic capsule in the male and the urethra in the female. It is a blend of smooth muscle from the bladder and striated muscle from the external sphincter

URACHAL DEFECTS

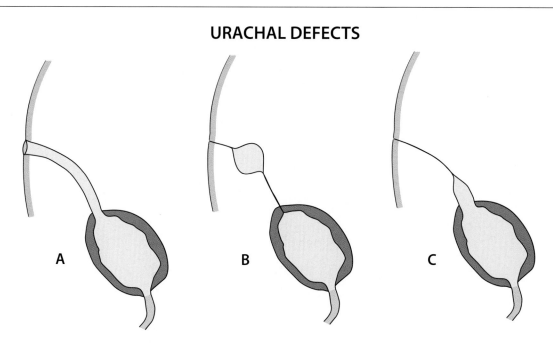

The urachus, which is a remnant of the allantois, may not close off correctly and it can either remain open with urine leakage (A) or form a cyst along it tract (B) or remain as a diverticulum of the bladder (C).

4.7   Pelvis and Perineum

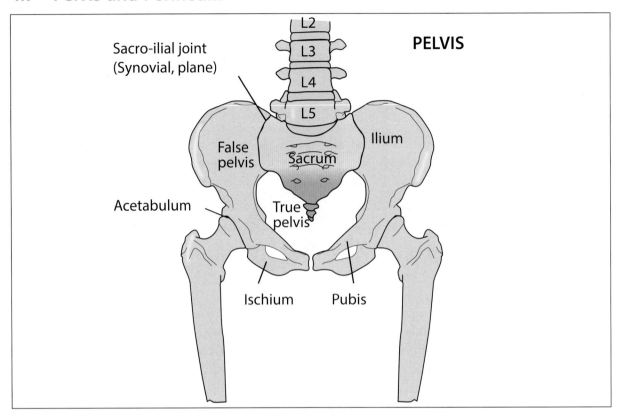

PELVIS

L2
L3
L4
L5

Sacro-ilial joint
(Synovial, plane)

False pelvis

Sacrum

Ilium

Acetabulum

True pelvis

Ischium   Pubis

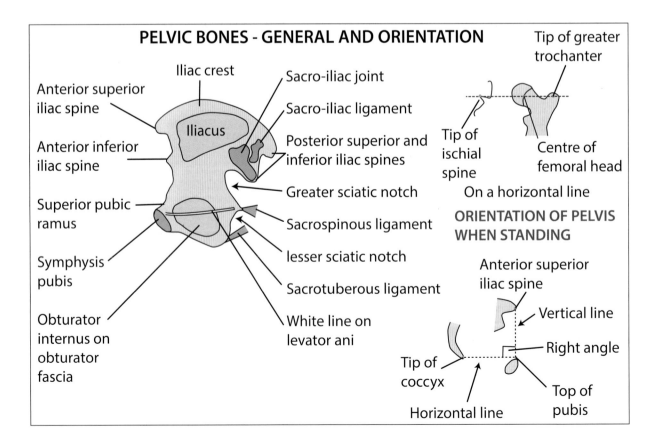

PELVIC BONES - GENERAL AND ORIENTATION

Iliac crest

Anterior superior iliac spine

Iliacus

Anterior inferior iliac spine

Superior pubic ramus

Symphysis pubis

Obturator internus on obturator fascia

Sacro-iliac joint

Sacro-iliac ligament

Posterior superior and inferior iliac spines

Greater sciatic notch

Sacrospinous ligament

lesser sciatic notch

Sacrotuberous ligament

White line on levator ani

Tip of greater trochanter

Tip of ischial spine

Centre of femoral head

On a horizontal line

ORIENTATION OF PELVIS WHEN STANDING

Anterior superior iliac spine

Vertical line

Right angle

Tip of coccyx

Top of pubis

Horizontal line

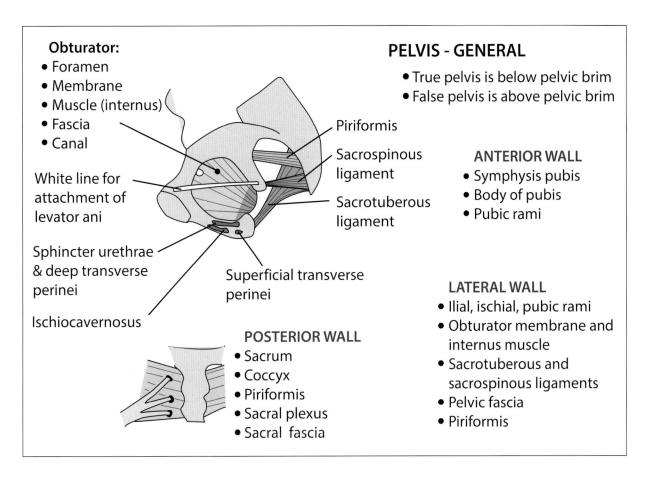

Obturator:
- Foramen
- Membrane
- Muscle (internus)
- Fascia
- Canal

White line for attachment of levator ani

Sphincter urethrae & deep transverse perinei

Ischiocavernosus

Superficial transverse perinei

Piriformis

Sacrospinous ligament

Sacrotuberous ligament

PELVIS - GENERAL
- True pelvis is below pelvic brim
- False pelvis is above pelvic brim

ANTERIOR WALL
- Symphysis pubis
- Body of pubis
- Pubic rami

LATERAL WALL
- Ilial, ischial, pubic rami
- Obturator membrane and internus muscle
- Sacrotuberous and sacrospinous ligaments
- Pelvic fascia
- Piriformis

POSTERIOR WALL
- Sacrum
- Coccyx
- Piriformis
- Sacral plexus
- Sacral fascia

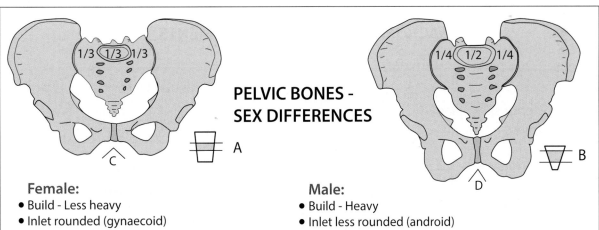

PELVIC BONES - SEX DIFFERENCES

Female:
- Build - Less heavy
- Inlet rounded (gynaecoid)
- Short segment of long cone (A)
- Subpubic angle - >90 degrees (C)
- Obturator foramen - elongated/triangular
- Muscle markings +
- Wider between ischial spines
- Ratio between vertebral facet of sacrum and ala of sacrum 1/3, 1/3, 1/3
- Greater sciatic notch - nearly a right angle
- Ischiopubic ramus - smooth
- Pubic tubercle to acetabular margin V diameter of acetabulum - greater

Male:
- Build - Heavy
- Inlet less rounded (android)
- Long segment of short cone (B)
- Subpubic angle - <90 degrees (D)
- Obturator fossa - rounded/oval
- Muscle markings +++
- Narrower between ischial spines
- Ratio between vertebral facet of sacrum and ala of sacrum 1/4, 1/2, 1/4
- Greater sciatic notch - less than a right angle (J shape)
- Ischiopubic ramus - rough (crura)
- Pubic tubercle to acetabular margin V diameter of acetabulum - equal or less

ANTERIOR SACRUM

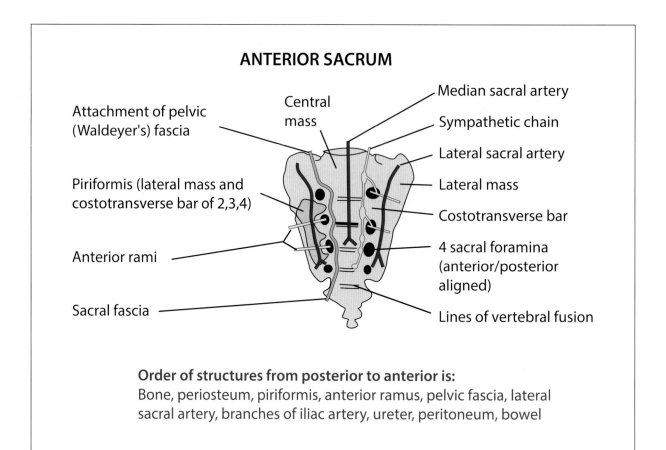

Attachment of pelvic (Waldeyer's) fascia

Central mass

Median sacral artery

Sympathetic chain

Lateral sacral artery

Piriformis (lateral mass and costotransverse bar of 2,3,4)

Lateral mass

Costotransverse bar

Anterior rami

4 sacral foramina (anterior/posterior aligned)

Sacral fascia

Lines of vertebral fusion

Order of structures from posterior to anterior is:
Bone, periosteum, piriformis, anterior ramus, pelvic fascia, lateral sacral artery, branches of iliac artery, ureter, peritoneum, bowel

SACRUM - POSTERIOR ATTACHMENTS

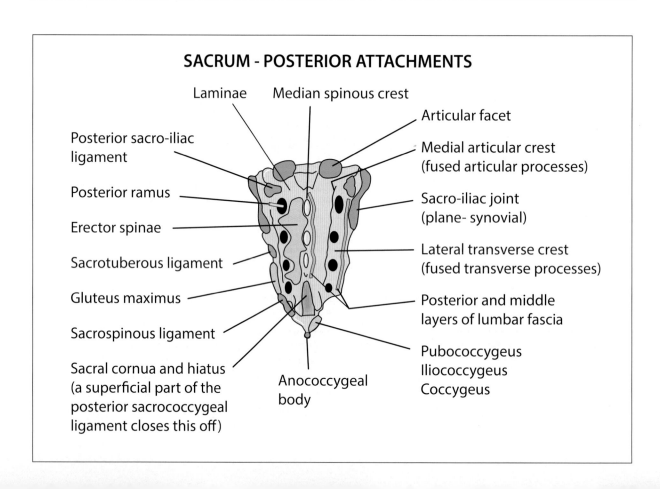

Laminae

Median spinous crest

Articular facet

Posterior sacro-iliac ligament

Medial articular crest (fused articular processes)

Posterior ramus

Sacro-iliac joint (plane- synovial)

Erector spinae

Sacrotuberous ligament

Lateral transverse crest (fused transverse processes)

Gluteus maximus

Sacrospinous ligament

Posterior and middle layers of lumbar fascia

Sacral cornua and hiatus (a superficial part of the posterior sacrococcygeal ligament closes this off)

Anococcygeal body

Pubococcygeus
Iliococcygeus
Coccygeus

LATERAL SACRUM

Dural sac (subarachnoid space). It contains CSF, nerve roots and filum terminale (pia that extends to the coccyx)

Spinal cord ends at lower border of L1

T12
L1
L2
L3
L4
L5
S1
S2
S3
S4
S5

End of dural sac (S2)

Extradural space below S2 with loose fat and veins. Used for caudal anaesthetic

SACRAL DIMPLE INDICATES
- S2
- End of dural sac
- Posterior inferior iliac spine
  Mid sacro-iliac joint

SACRUM - GENERAL AND SACRO-ILIAC JOINT
- 5 fused vertebrae (may be 6 or 7)
- L5 may be sacralised
- Spina bifida occulta common
- Iliolumbar ligament from iliac crest to tip of 5th lumbar transverse process

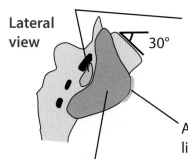

Lateral view

30°

Posterior sacro- iliac ligament. strong ++

Sacroiliac joint jagged surfaces minimal movement but synovial

Anterior sacro- iliac ligament (thickening of joint capsule). Weakest of the ligaments

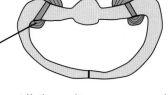

Viewed from above

All these ligament need to be strong to prevent sacrum sliding forwards

POSTERIOR ABDOMINAL WALL

- 5 vertebrae
- Transverse process of L3 is largest
- Transverse process of L5 is conical

PSOAS MAJOR
Origin: Intervertebral discs T12/L1 to L4/5, bodies of T12-L5, transverse processes L1-5
Inserts: Lesser trochanter
Nerve: L1,2
Action: Flexes hip

PSOAS MINOR (not shown)
Origin: Bodies T12, L1
Inserts: Fascia over psoas major behind inguinal ligament
Nerve: L1
Action: Weak spine flexor

ILIACUS
Origin: Hollow of iliac fossa
Inserts: Psoas tendon and lesser trochanter
Nerve: Femoral (L2,3)
Action: Flexes hip

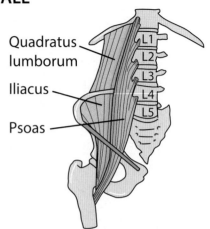

Quadratus lumborum
Iliacus
Psoas
L1
L2
L3
L4
L5

QUADRATUS LUMBORUM
Origin: Inferior border of rib 12
Inserts: Transverse processes L1-4, iliolumbar ligament and posterior 1/3 iliac crest
Nerve: T12-L3
Action: Holds down 12th rib and aids lateral flexion of trunk

SACRAL PLEXUS
L4,5,S1,2,3,4,5

Lies on piriformis on posterior wall of pelvis, deep to the vessels
and covered by parietal pelvic fascia

6 BRANCHES OFF THE SACRAL ROOTS BEFORE THEY DIVIDE INTO ANTERIOR AND POSTERIOR DIVISIONS
They all begin with the letter "P"
1. Posterior femoral cutaneous nerve (S1,2,3)
2. Pudendal nerve (S2,3,4)
    (1 and 2 - leave via greater sciatic foramen)
3. Perforating cutaneous nerve (S2,3)
    (3 - perforates sacrotuberous ligament)
4. Nerve to piriformis (S1,2)
5. Perineal branch of S4 (to levator ani)
6. Pelvic splanchnics (S2,3,4)
    Parasympathetic motor to bladder, hind gut, erection.
    Sensory for distension and pain from bladder, lower uterus,
    lower colon and rectum
    (4,5,6 - all remain in pelvis)

FROM ANTERIOR DIVISONS
- Nerve to quadratus femoris (L4,5,S1)
- Nerve to obturator internus (L5,S1,2)
- Tibial portion of sciatic nerve (L4,5,S1,2,3)
  (see sciatic nerve in lower limb section)

FROM POSTERIOR DIVISIONS
- Superior gluteal (L4,5,S1)
- Inferior gluteal (L5,S1,2)
- Common fibular portion of sciatic nerve (L4,5,S1,2)
  (see sciatic nerve in lower limb section)

PELVIC FLOOR FROM ABOVE

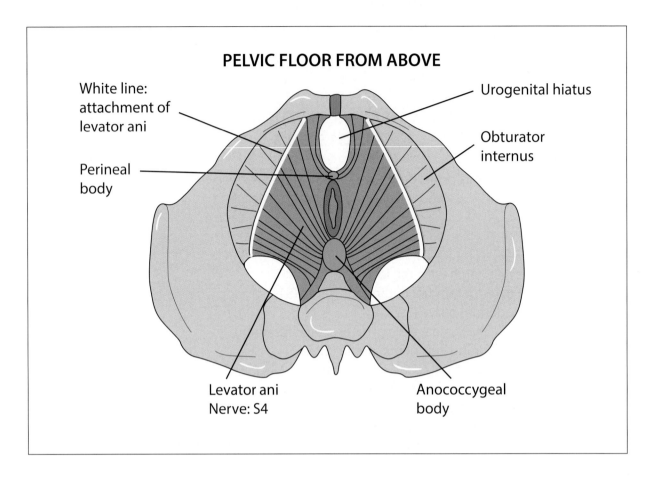

White line: attachment of levator ani

Perineal body

Urogenital hiatus

Obturator internus

Levator ani
Nerve: S4

Anococcygeal body

PELVIC FLOOR FROM BELOW

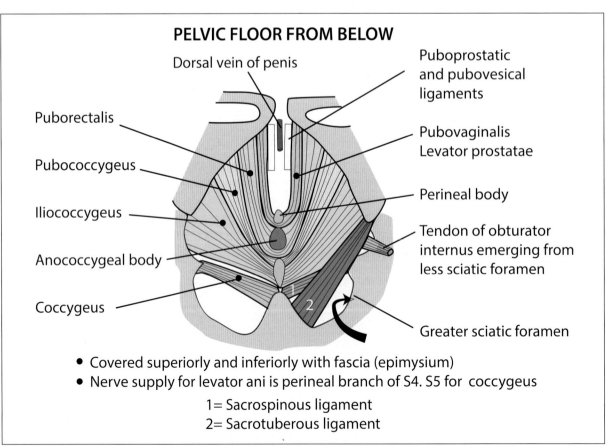

Dorsal vein of penis

Puboprostatic and pubovesical ligaments

Puborectalis

Pubococcygeus

Iliococcygeus

Anococcygeal body

Coccygeus

Pubovaginalis
Levator prostatae

Perineal body

Tendon of obturator internus emerging from less sciatic foramen

Greater sciatic foramen

- Covered superiorly and inferiorly with fascia (epimysium)
- Nerve supply for levator ani is perineal branch of S4. S5 for coccygeus

1= Sacrospinous ligament
2= Sacrotuberous ligament

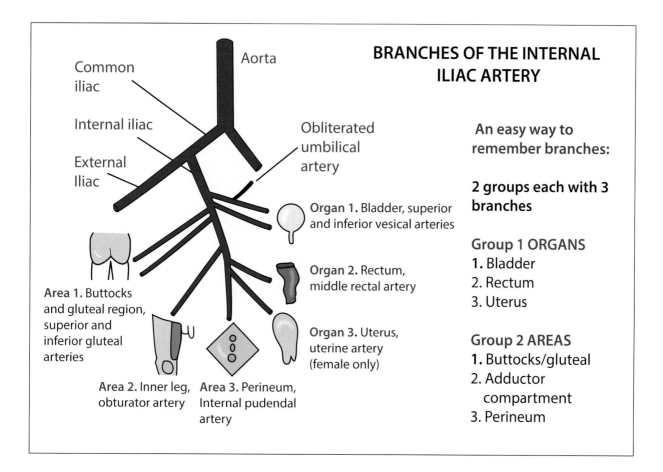

BRANCHES OF THE INTERNAL ILIAC ARTERY

Aorta

Common iliac

Internal iliac

External Iliac

Obliterated umbilical artery

Organ 1. Bladder, superior and inferior vesical arteries

Organ 2. Rectum, middle rectal artery

Organ 3. Uterus, uterine artery (female only)

Area 1. Buttocks and gluteal region, superior and inferior gluteal arteries

Area 2. Inner leg, obturator artery

Area 3. Perineum, Internal pudendal artery

An easy way to remember branches:

2 groups each with 3 branches

Group 1 ORGANS
1. Bladder
2. Rectum
3. Uterus

Group 2 AREAS
1. Buttocks/gluteal
2. Adductor compartment
3. Perineum

DEFINITION OF THE PERINEUM

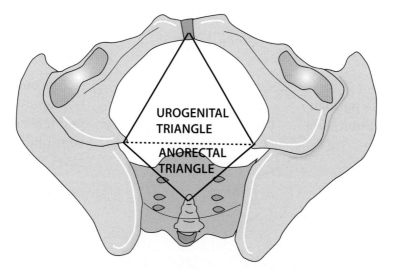

UROGENITAL TRIANGLE

ANORECTAL TRIANGLE

The perineum is that part of the trunk distal to the pelvic diaphragm.
It is 2 triangles lying at nearly a right angle to each other:
Urogenital - covered in below with urogenital diaphragm
Anal - covered only with skin, fascia and gluteus maximus when standing up

SACROTUBEROUS AND SACROSPINOUS LIGAMENTS AND UROGENITAL DIAPHRAGM

Pudendal nerve exiting via greater sciatic foramen, passing over sacrospinous ligament, entering lesser sciatic foramen, then into Alcock's canal to reach urogenital diaphragm

Internal pudendal artery exiting from greater sciatic foramen, over ischial spine and entering lesser sciatic foramen. Then running in Alcock's canal to reach urogenital diaphragm

AC

Sacrospinous ligament

Sacrotuberous ligament

Nerve and artery give off inferior rectal branches in Alcock's canal (AC)

MALE PERINEUM

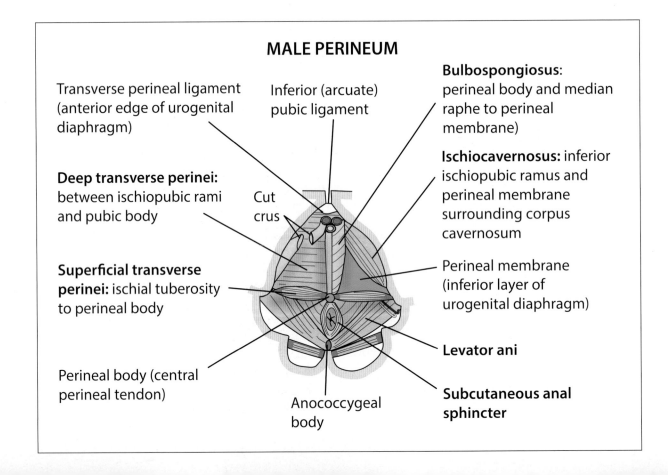

Transverse perineal ligament (anterior edge of urogenital diaphragm)

Inferior (arcuate) pubic ligament

Bulbospongiosus: perineal body and median raphe to perineal membrane)

Deep transverse perinei: between ischiopubic rami and pubic body

Cut crus

Ischiocavernosus: inferior ischiopubic ramus and perineal membrane surrounding corpus cavernosum

Superficial transverse perinei: ischial tuberosity to perineal body

Perineal membrane (inferior layer of urogenital diaphragm)

Levator ani

Perineal body (central perineal tendon)

Anococcygeal body

Subcutaneous anal sphincter

MALE PERINEUM - DEEP PERINEAL POUCH

Deep perineal pouch (between perineal membrane and superior fascia of urogenital diaphragm).

Contains: Membranous urethra, deep transverse perinei, external urethral sphincter, bulbourethral (Cowper's) glands which drain into urethra below the perineal membrane, internal pudendal vessels, dorsal nerve of penis

Note: The external sphincter has striated muscle extensions around lower prostatic urethra, above the urogenital diaphragm, that mix with smooth bladder wall muscle and are called the **intrinsic urethral mechanism**

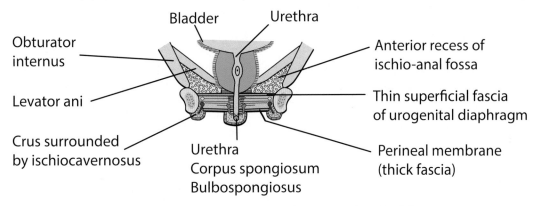

Coronal section through urogenital diaphragm at level of the prostate

MALE SUPERFICIAL PERINEAL POUCH

Scarpa's fascia is fused to the pubis then extends into the scrotum as Colles' fascia and around the penis as Buck's fascia

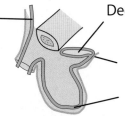

Deep perineal pouch

Colles' fascia (superficial perineal fascia) attached posteriorly to ischiopubic ramus and posterior part of perineal membrane

Superficial perineal pouch: Contains all perineal structures below perineal membrane: 2 crura with ischiocavernosus muscles around them. Distal urethra with corpus spongiosum around it. Bulbospongiosus muscle around bulb. Superficial transverse perinei muscles, perineal body, perineal branches of internal pudendal artery, pudendal nerve and branches, Colles' fascia, ducts of Cowper's glands, deep and superficial external pudendal arteries, spermatic cords, testes, penis, dartos muscle (panniculus carnosus of animals), branches of ilio-inguinal and genitofemoral nerves

Scrotal blood supply: Deep and superficial external pudendal arteries, branches of internal pudendal arteries. Veins to external pudendal

Nerves to scrotum: Anterior 1/3 - ilio-inguinal; posterior 2/3 - posterior scrotal branches of perineal nerve and perineal branches of posterior femoral cutaneous nerve

Lymph: Superficial inguinal glands

ATTACHMENTS OF PENIS

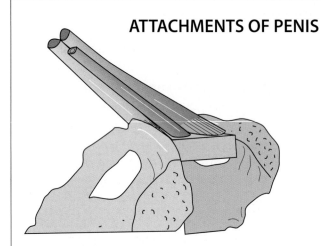

This inferior view of the urogenital diaphragm (purple) in a male shows attachments of crura of penis to ischiopubic rami on each side and urethra joining them to complete the structure of penis (right).

CROSS SECTION

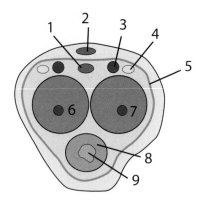

1 Deep dorsal vein of penis
2 Superficial dorsal vein of penis
3 Dorsal artery of penis
4 Dorsal nerve of penis
5 Buck's fascia
6 Corpus cavernosum
7 Deep artery of penis
8 Corpus spongiosum
9 Urethra

FEMALE PERINEUM

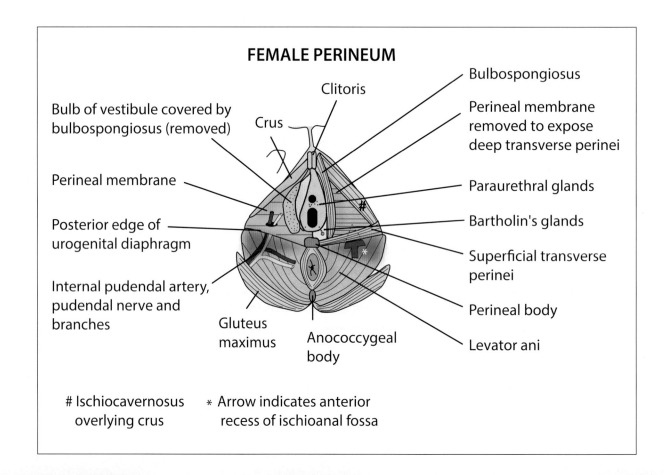

Clitoris

Bulbospongiosus

Bulb of vestibule covered by bulbospongiosus (removed)

Crus

Perineal membrane removed to expose deep transverse perinei

Perineal membrane

Paraurethral glands

Posterior edge of urogenital diaphragm

Bartholin's glands

Superficial transverse perinei

Internal pudendal artery, pudendal nerve and branches

Gluteus maximus

Anococcygeal body

Perineal body

Levator ani

Ischiocavernosus overlying crus

* Arrow indicates anterior recess of ischioanal fossa

FEMALE PERINEUM - GENERAL

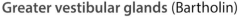

Greater vestibular glands (Bartholin)
Round (<1cm) glands at 4 and 8 o'clock behind bulb. 2cm duct into posterolateral vaginal orifice. In superficial perineal pouch. Homologues of Cowper's glands in males. Cysts and infection possible
Paraurethral glands (Skene)
Mucous glands opening just inside urethra. Homologue of prostate
Lesser vestibular glands
Not shown. Multiple small mucous glands opening between vagina and urethra
Labia majora - joined back and front by anterior and posterior commissures. Round ligament of uterus ends anterior end of each.
labia minora give clitoral prepuce. **Clitoris** - 2 small corpora cavernosa. **Bulb** - spongy erectile tissue in labia minora

FEMALE PERINEUM VESSELS AND POUCHES

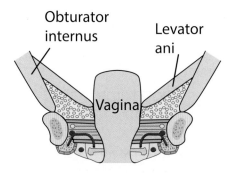

Obturator internus

Levator ani

Vagina

Coronal section through urogenital diaphragm at level of vagina

Deep perineal pouch (between perineal membrane inferiorly and the superior fascia of urogenital diaphragm superiorly)
- Vagina
- Urethra
- Sphincter urethrae
- Deep tranverse perinei
- Dorsal nerve of clitoris
- Dorsal/deep clitoral arteries

Superficial perineal pouch
(everything inferior to perineal membrane)
- 2 crura of clitoris
- Bulb and bulbospongiosus
- Superficial transverse perinei
- Perineal body
- Perineal artery/nerve/branches
- Vestibular glands

ISCHIOANAL (ISCHIORECTAL) FOSSA

Wedge shaped space filled with fat; Crossed by inferior rectal nerve and artery; Alcock's canal in its lateral wall; **Base:** Perineal skin; **Medial:** Anal canal, levator ani; **Lateral:** Ischial tuberosity, obturator internus; **Apex:** White line; **Anterior:** Perineal body, urogenital diaphragm, anterior recess; **Posterior:** Posterior recess, gluteus maximus, sacrotuberous ligament, anococcygeal body, horseshoe connection; **Contains:** Fat, Alcock's (pudendal) canal, internal pudendal artery, pudendal nerve, inferior rectal artery/nerve, perineal branch of S4, perforating cutaneous nerve

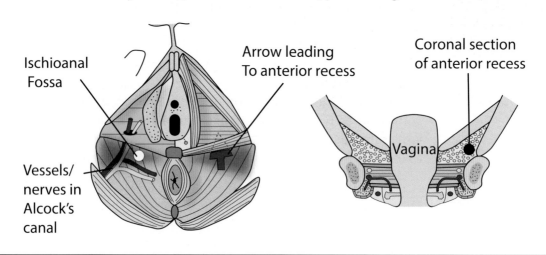

VESSELS AND NERVES OF THE PERINEUM

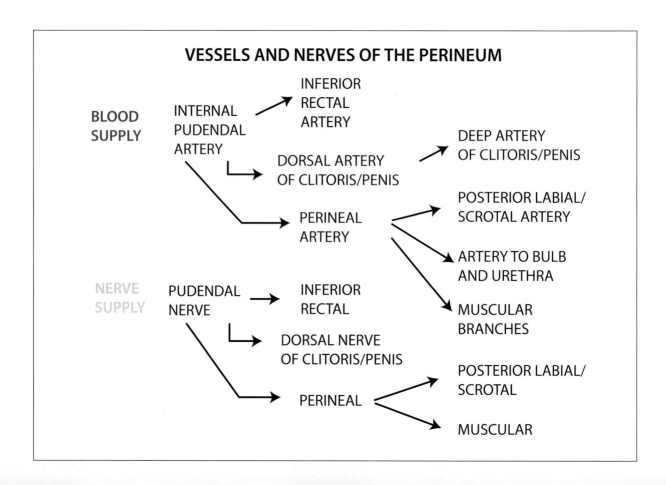

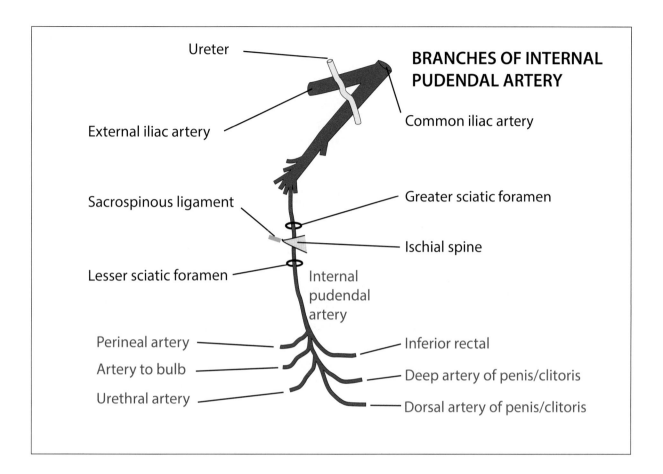

BRANCHES OF INTERNAL PUDENDAL ARTERY

Ureter

Common iliac artery

External iliac artery

Greater sciatic foramen

Sacrospinous ligament

Ischial spine

Lesser sciatic foramen

Internal pudendal artery

Perineal artery

Inferior rectal

Artery to bulb

Deep artery of penis/clitoris

Urethral artery

Dorsal artery of penis/clitoris

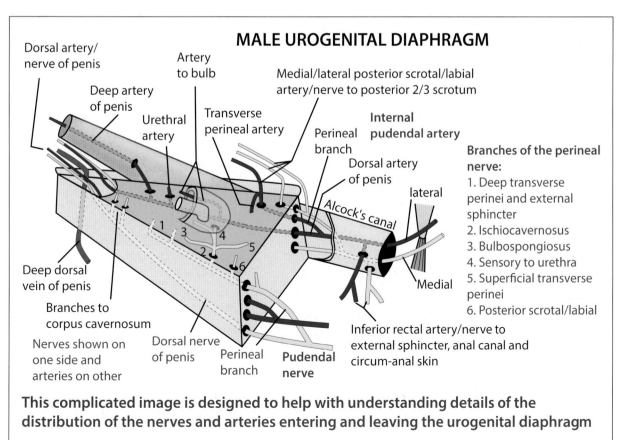

MALE UROGENITAL DIAPHRAGM

Dorsal artery/nerve of penis

Artery to bulb

Medial/lateral posterior scrotal/labial artery/nerve to posterior 2/3 scrotum

Deep artery of penis

Urethral artery

Transverse perineal artery

Perineal branch

Internal pudendal artery

Dorsal artery of penis

lateral

Alcock's canal

Branches of the perineal nerve:
1. Deep transverse perinei and external sphincter
2. Ischiocavernosus
3. Bulbospongiosus
4. Sensory to urethra
5. Superficial transverse perinei
6. Posterior scrotal/labial

Deep dorsal vein of penis

Branches to corpus cavernosum

Nerves shown on one side and arteries on other

Dorsal nerve of penis

Perineal branch

Pudendal nerve

Medial

Inferior rectal artery/nerve to external sphincter, anal canal and circum-anal skin

This complicated image is designed to help with understanding details of the distribution of the nerves and arteries entering and leaving the urogenital diaphragm

4.8   Referred Pain and Autonomics

REFERRED PAIN

Pain generated in one site
and felt in another

TYPES OF REFERRED PAIN

1. SOMATIC TO SOMATIC
Involving somatic nerves only with no autonomic involvement.
2. PRESSURE OR TRAUMA TO NERVES
Involving somatic nerves only with no autonomic involvement.
3. GENERAL VISCERAL AFFERENT (GVA)
Pain from visceral organs (intestine, heart, etc.). GVAs detect ischaemia, distension and inflammation and travel mostly in sympathetic nerves throughout the thorax and abdomen and probably with parasympathetics from organs of cloacal origin (bladder, rectum, lower vagina)

SOMATIC TO SOMATIC REFERRED PAIN

Example 1
Somatic pain detected by the phrenic nerve (C3,4,5) supplying the peritoneum on the under surface of the diaphragm from, say, an inflammed gallbladder, refers the pain to the dermatomes C3,4,5 (mostly C4) which supply the skin over the shoulder in the same side via the supraclavicular nerves from the cervical plexus.
This is explained by the descent of the septum transversum from a cephalad position to form the diaphragm and taking its nerve supply with it.

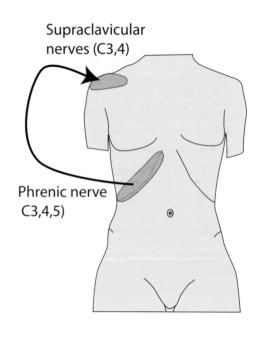

Supraclavicular nerves (C3,4)

Phrenic nerve C3,4,5)

SOMATIC TO SOMATIC REFERRED PAIN

TONSIL
Glossopharyngeal (IX)
in oropharynx

MIDDLE EAR
Glossopharyngeal (IX)
tympanic branch

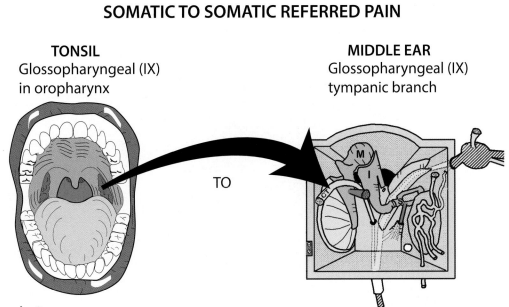

TO

Example 2

The oropharynx and the palatine tonsil within it is supplied by the glossopharyngeal nerve (IX). Pain from the tonsil or tonsillar bed, for instance after a tonsillectomy, is referred to the middle ear which is also supplied by the glossopharyngeal nerve via its tympanic branch. There is no autonomic involvement.

SOMATIC TO SOMATIC REFERRED PAIN

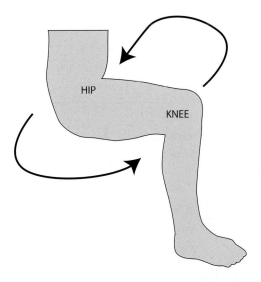

HIP

KNEE

Example 3

Hilton's Law states that the sensory nerve supply of a joint is the same as the nerve supply of the muscles that move it. The obturator nerve thus supplies both the hip and the knee. In small children who stop weight bearing the pain could be arising in either joint and the clinician should be aware of this.

DIRECT PRESSURE ON A NERVE

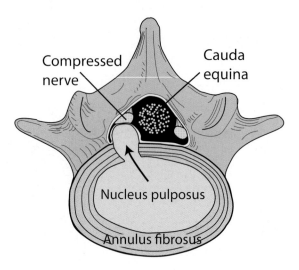

Example

Pressure from a prolapsed disc in the lumbar region gives local pain but also referred pain to the lower limb. Another example is pressure on a nerve in the cervical region giving pain in the upper limb. The autonomic nerves are not involved.

AUTONOMIC SUPPLY OF GASTRO-INTESTINAL TRACT

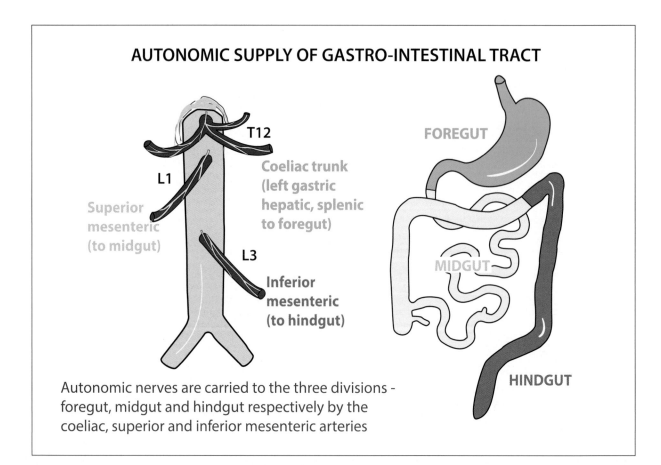

Autonomic nerves are carried to the three divisions - foregut, midgut and hindgut respectively by the coeliac, superior and inferior mesenteric arteries

REFERRED PAIN IN GENERAL VISCERAL AFFERENT NERVES

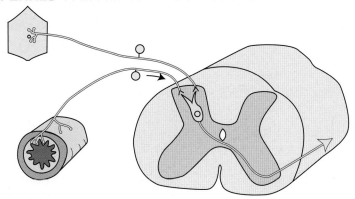

Pain from an internal organ is referred to a relevant dermatome. **General Visceral Afferents (GVA)** detect pain such as ischaemia from the heart or inflammation or distension of the intestine and these fibres return to the spinal cord mostly with the sympathetic nerves. These GVA relay with the receptor cells in the dorsal horn of the spinal cord which are also receiving sensory input from distant somatic structures, including dermatomes. The central nervous system seemingly cannot accurately distinguish these incoming signals from viscera and incorrectly assigns the visceral pain to a somatic area - a relevant dermatome. In the example shown here the pain from the inflammed appendix is being referred to the peri-umbilical region (T10,11).

AUTONOMIC SUPPLY TO FOREGUT, MIDGUT AND HINDGUT

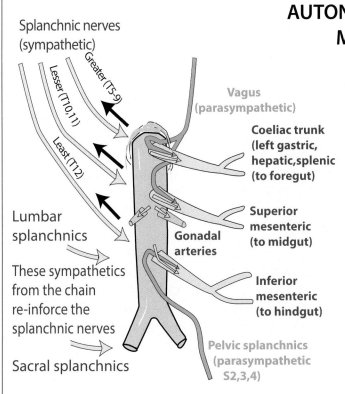

Splanchnic nerves (sympathetic)

Greater (T5-9)

Lesser (T10,11)

Least (T12)

Vagus (parasympathetic)

Coeliac trunk (left gastric, hepatic, splenic (to foregut)

Superior mesenteric (to midgut)

Gonadal arteries

Inferior mesenteric (to hindgut)

Lumbar splanchnics

These sympathetics from the chain re-inforce the splanchnic nerves

Sacral splanchnics

Pelvic splanchnics (parasympathetic S2,3,4)

Autonomics are an internal adjustment system controlling the activity of the abdominal and pelvic organs. Largely autonomous but influenced by environment and thought processes (e.g. stress leading to diarrhoea or urinary frequency)

Referred pain is carried by **general visceral afferents** in the sympathetic splanchnic nerves to the dermatomes as indicated by the origins of these nerves. Shown here by black arrows

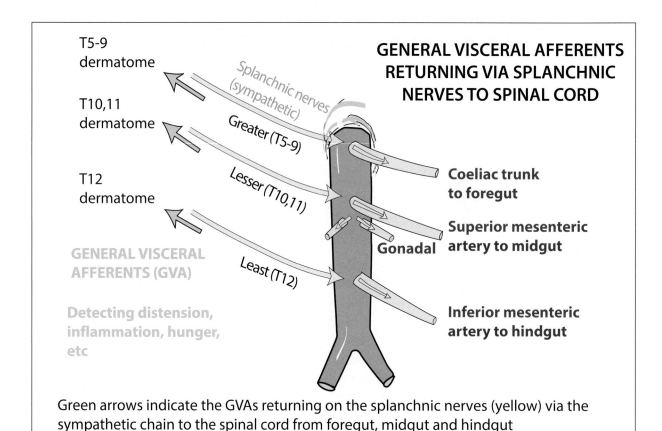

T5-9
dermatome

T10,11
dermatome

T12
dermatome

**GENERAL VISCERAL
AFFERENTS (GVA)**

**Detecting distension,
inflammation, hunger,
etc**

Splanchnic nerves
(sympathetic)

Greater (T5-9)

Lesser (T10,11)

Least (T12)

Gonadal

**GENERAL VISCERAL AFFERENTS
RETURNING VIA SPLANCHNIC
NERVES TO SPINAL CORD**

**Coeliac trunk
to foregut**

**Superior mesenteric
artery to midgut**

**Inferior mesenteric
artery to hindgut**

Green arrows indicate the GVAs returning on the splanchnic nerves (yellow) via the
sympathetic chain to the spinal cord from foregut, midgut and hindgut

PATHWAY FOR RETURNING GENERAL VISCERAL AFFERENTS (GVA)

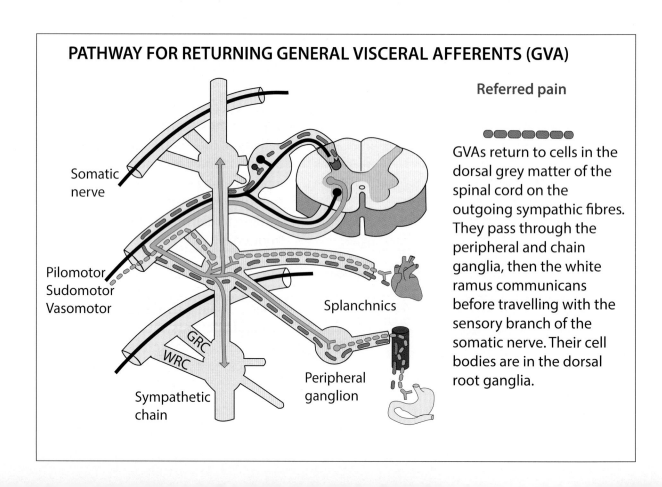

Somatic
nerve

Pilomotor
Sudomotor
Vasomotor

Splanchnics

GRC

WRC

Sympathetic
chain

Peripheral
ganglion

Referred pain

GVAs return to cells in the
dorsal grey matter of the
spinal cord on the
outgoing sympathic fibres.
They pass through the
peripheral and chain
ganglia, then the white
ramus communicans
before travelling with the
sensory branch of the
somatic nerve. Their cell
bodies are in the dorsal
root ganglia.

REFERRED ABDOMINAL AND LOWER CHEST PAIN

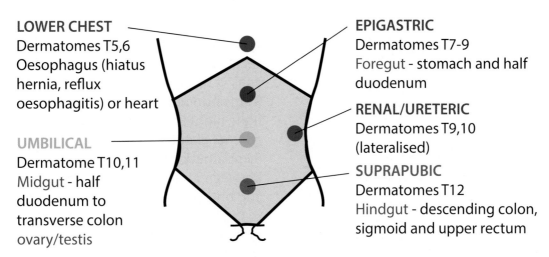

LOWER CHEST
Dermatomes T5,6
Oesophagus (hiatus hernia, reflux oesophagitis) or heart

UMBILICAL
Dermatome T10,11
Midgut - half duodenum to transverse colon ovary/testis

EPIGASTRIC
Dermatomes T7-9
Foregut - stomach and half duodenum

RENAL/URETERIC
Dermatomes T9,10
(lateralised)

SUPRAPUBIC
Dermatomes T12
Hindgut - descending colon, sigmoid and upper rectum

1. All pain is carried in **"general visceral afferents"** by the splanchnic sympathetics, via the sympathetic chain to the spinal cord.
2. It is then referred to the dermatome of that level.
3. All pain for the gastro-intestinal tract and related structures is felt in the midline because of its origin from the midline "gut tube".
4. Pain from the urinary tract can "lateralise" as it was formed bilaterally

REFERRED PAIN IN APPENDICITIS

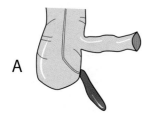

A

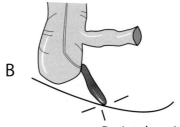

B

Parietal peritoneum

Sequence of events for pain of appendicitis
A. Inflammed appendix triggers general visceral afferents which return to the spinal cord in the lesser splanchnic nerves which supply the midgut. This pain is referred to dermatomes T10,11 - peri-umbilical. So the initial referred pain of appendicitis is felt around the umbilicus in the midline but is of a more generalised nature.
B. When the inflammed appendix touches and irritates the parietal peritoneum in the right iliac fossa, the pain is detected by local somatic nerves which supply this peritoneum. As it is now somatic pain it is more severe and localised. There will be acute tenderness and rebound tenderness to palpation

SYMPATHETIC THORACIC OUTFLOW

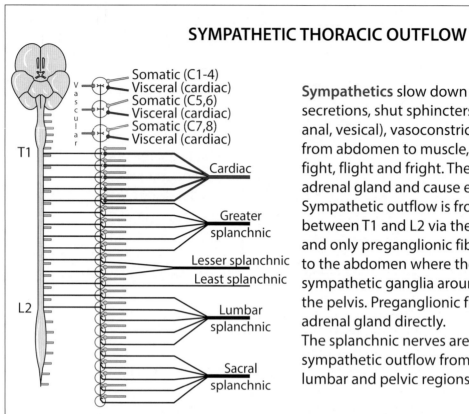

Sympathetics slow down gut activity, dry up secretions, shut sphincters (pylorus, internal anal, vesical), vasoconstrict to redirect blood from abdomen to muscle, heart and brain for fight, flight and fright. They also stimulate the adrenal gland and cause ejaculation. Sympathetic outflow is from the spinal cord between T1 and L2 via the sympathetic chain and only preganglionic fibres are distributed to the abdomen where they synapse in sympathetic ganglia around the aorta and in the pelvis. Preganglionic fibres reach the adrenal gland directly.

The splanchnic nerves are "reinforced" by sympathetic outflow from the chain in the lumbar and pelvic regions.

SUMMARY OF SYMPATHETIC DISTRIBUTION BEYOND CHAIN

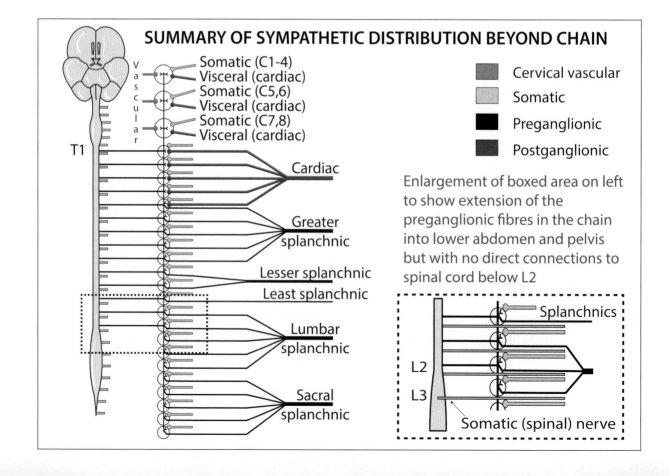

■ Cervical vascular
■ Somatic
■ Preganglionic
■ Postganglionic

Enlargement of boxed area on left to show extension of the preganglionic fibres in the chain into lower abdomen and pelvis but with no direct connections to spinal cord below L2

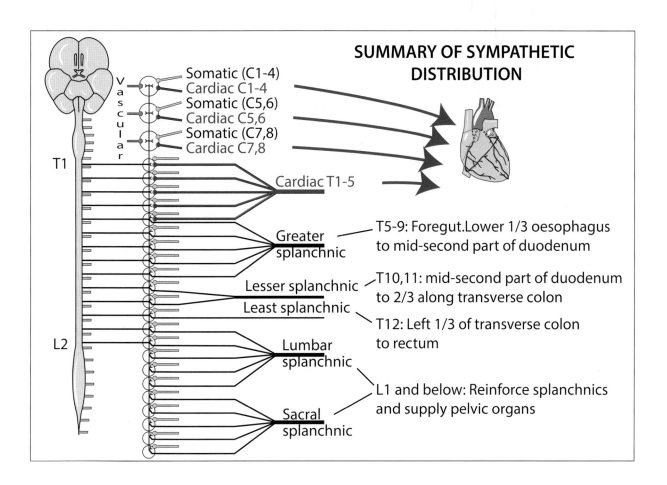

SUMMARY OF SYMPATHETIC DISTRIBUTION

Vascular

Somatic (C1-4)
Cardiac C1-4
Somatic (C5,6)
Cardiac C5,6
Somatic (C7,8)
Cardiac C7,8

T1

Cardiac T1-5

Greater splanchnic

T5-9: Foregut.Lower 1/3 oesophagus to mid-second part of duodenum

Lesser splanchnic

T10,11: mid-second part of duodenum to 2/3 along transverse colon

Least splanchnic

T12: Left 1/3 of transverse colon to rectum

L2

Lumbar splanchnic

L1 and below: Reinforce splanchnics and supply pelvic organs

Sacral splanchnic

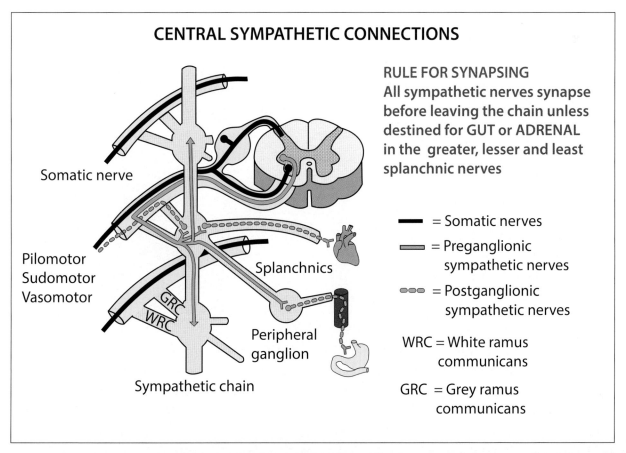

CENTRAL SYMPATHETIC CONNECTIONS

RULE FOR SYNAPSING
All sympathetic nerves synapse before leaving the chain unless destined for GUT or ADRENAL in the greater, lesser and least splanchnic nerves

Somatic nerve

Pilomotor
Sudomotor
Vasomotor

Splanchnics

GRC
WRC

Peripheral ganglion

Sympathetic chain

▬▬ = Somatic nerves

▬▬ = Preganglionic sympathetic nerves

●●● = Postganglionic sympathetic nerves

WRC = White ramus communicans

GRC = Grey ramus communicans

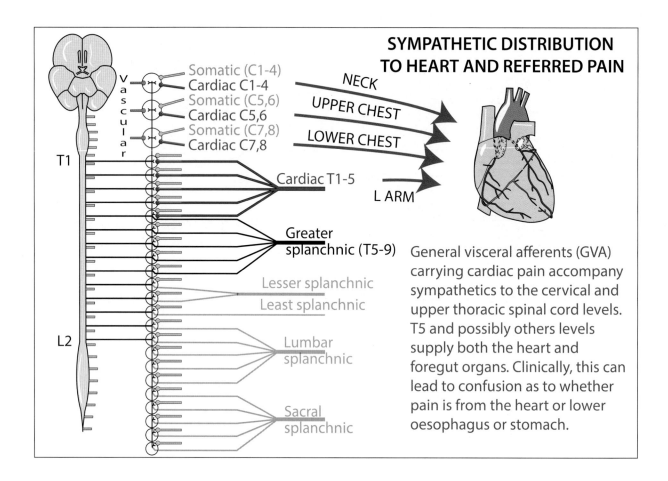

SYMPATHETIC DISTRIBUTION TO HEART AND REFERRED PAIN

Somatic (C1-4)
Cardiac C1-4
Somatic (C5,6)
Cardiac C5,6
Somatic (C7,8)
Cardiac C7,8

NECK
UPPER CHEST
LOWER CHEST

Cardiac T1-5

L ARM

Greater splanchnic (T5-9)

Lesser splanchnic
Least splanchnic

Lumbar splanchnic

Sacral splanchnic

T1
L2
Vascular

General visceral afferents (GVA) carrying cardiac pain accompany sympathetics to the cervical and upper thoracic spinal cord levels. T5 and possibly others levels supply both the heart and foregut organs. Clinically, this can lead to confusion as to whether pain is from the heart or lower oesophagus or stomach.

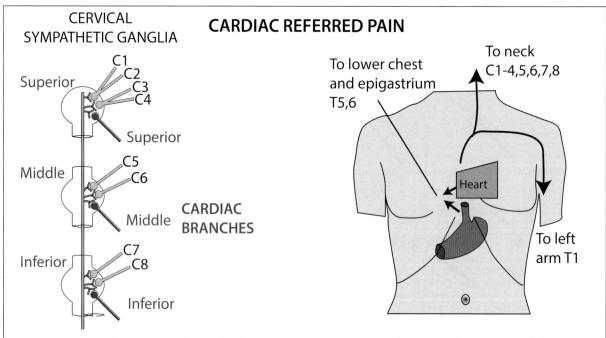

CERVICAL SYMPATHETIC GANGLIA

CARDIAC REFERRED PAIN

Superior
C1
C2
C3
C4
Superior

Middle
C5
C6
Middle

CARDIAC BRANCHES

Inferior
C7
C8
Inferior

To lower chest and epigastrium T5,6

To neck C1-4,5,6,7,8

Heart

To left arm T1

General visceral afferents from the heart return to the spinal cord on branches of the sympathetic chain. As there are cardiac branches from each of the cervical sympathetic ganglia and also from T1-5 in the upper thoracic chain, there can be referred pain to the dermatomes associated with these ganglia. C1-C8 dermatomes include the neck and upper limb

PARASYMPATHETIC CRANIOSACRAL OUTFLOW

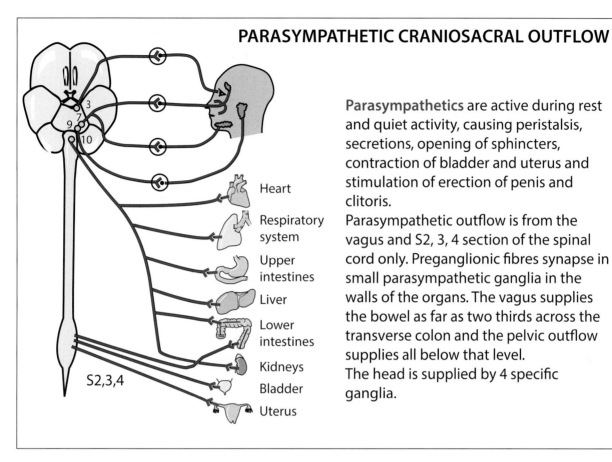

Heart

Respiratory system

Upper intestines

Liver

Lower intestines

Kidneys

Bladder

Uterus

S2,3,4

Parasympathetics are active during rest and quiet activity, causing peristalsis, secretions, opening of sphincters, contraction of bladder and uterus and stimulation of erection of penis and clitoris.

Parasympathetic outflow is from the vagus and S2, 3, 4 section of the spinal cord only. Preganglionic fibres synapse in small parasympathetic ganglia in the walls of the organs. The vagus supplies the bowel as far as two thirds across the transverse colon and the pelvic outflow supplies all below that level.

The head is supplied by 4 specific ganglia.

ABDOMINOPELVIC AUTONOMICS

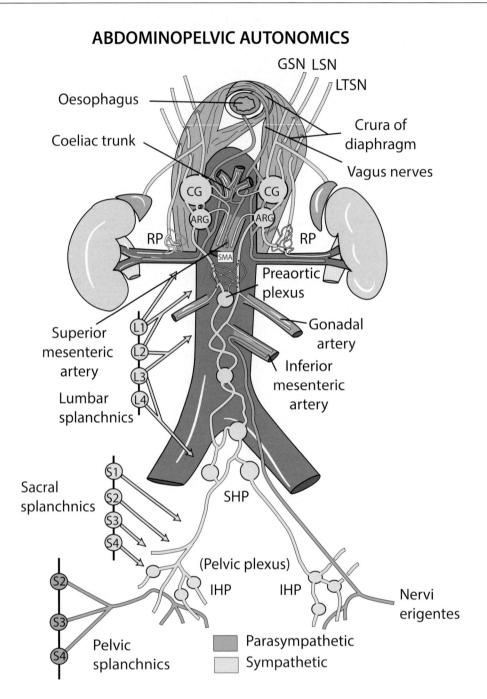

GSN LSN
LTSN

Oesophagus

Crura of diaphragm

Coeliac trunk

Vagus nerves

CG   CG

ARG   ARG

RP   RP

SMA

Preaortic plexus

Superior mesenteric artery

Gonadal artery

Inferior mesenteric artery

L1
L2
L3
L4

Lumbar splanchnics

S1

Sacral splanchnics

S2

S3

SHP

S4

(Pelvic plexus)

S2

IHP   IHP

Nervi erigentes

S3

S4

Pelvic splanchnics

Parasympathetic
Sympathetic

GSN: Greater splanchnic nerve   RP: Renal plexus
LRSN: Lesser splanchnic nerve   SHP: Superior hypogastric plexus
LTSN: Least splanchnic nerve   IHP: Inferior hypogastric plexus
CG: Coeliac ganglion   (The two IHPs together make
ARG: Aorticorenal ganglion   the pelvic plexus)

Other plexuses not shown: SRP: Suprarenal plexus. AAP:
Abdominal aortic plexus. IMP: Inferior mesenteric plexus

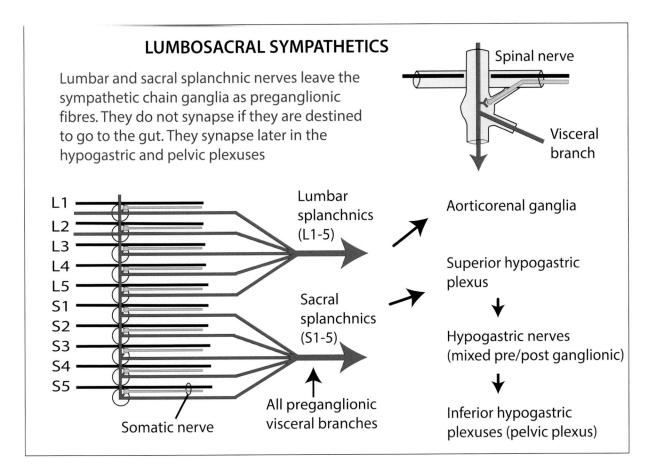

LUMBOSACRAL SYMPATHETICS

Lumbar and sacral splanchnic nerves leave the sympathetic chain ganglia as preganglionic fibres. They do not synapse if they are destined to go to the gut. They synapse later in the hypogastric and pelvic plexuses

Spinal nerve

Visceral branch

L1
L2
L3
L4
L5
S1
S2
S3
S4
S5

Somatic nerve

Lumbar splanchnics (L1-5)

Sacral splanchnics (S1-5)

All preganglionic visceral branches

Aorticorenal ganglia

Superior hypogastric plexus

Hypogastric nerves (mixed pre/post ganglionic)

Inferior hypogastric plexuses (pelvic plexus)

SECTION 5

Head and Neck

5.1 Skull Bones, Air Sinuses and Scalp

ANTERIOR VIEW OF SKULL BONES

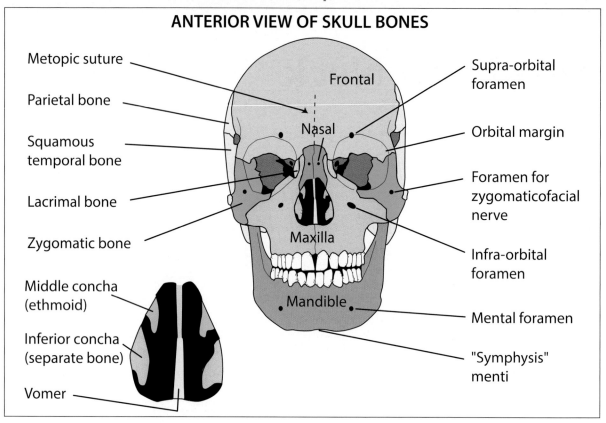

Metopic suture

Parietal bone

Squamous temporal bone

Lacrimal bone

Zygomatic bone

Middle concha (ethmoid)

Inferior concha (separate bone)

Vomer

Frontal

Nasal

Maxilla

Mandible

Supra-orbital foramen

Orbital margin

Foramen for zygomaticofacial nerve

Infra-orbital foramen

Mental foramen

"Symphysis" menti

LATERAL VIEW OF SKULL TO SHOW BONES AND OTHER FEATURES

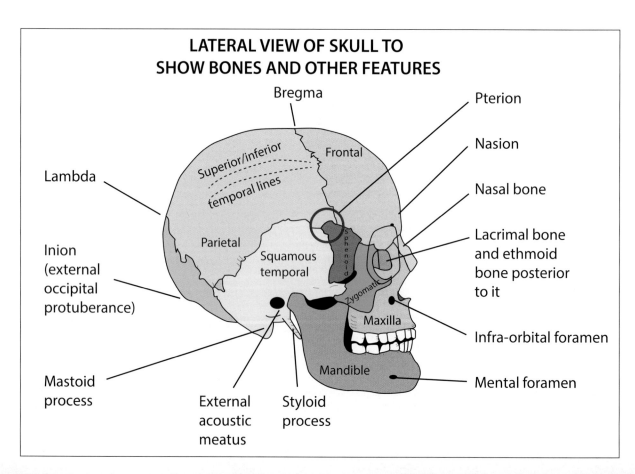

Bregma

Lambda

Inion (external occipital protuberance)

Mastoid process

Superior/inferior temporal lines

Frontal

Parietal

Squamous temporal

Sphenoid

Zygomatic

Maxilla

Mandible

External acoustic meatus

Styloid process

Pterion

Nasion

Nasal bone

Lacrimal bone and ethmoid bone posterior to it

Infra-orbital foramen

Mental foramen

INFERIOR VIEW OF SKULL TO SHOW BONES AND OTHER FEATURES

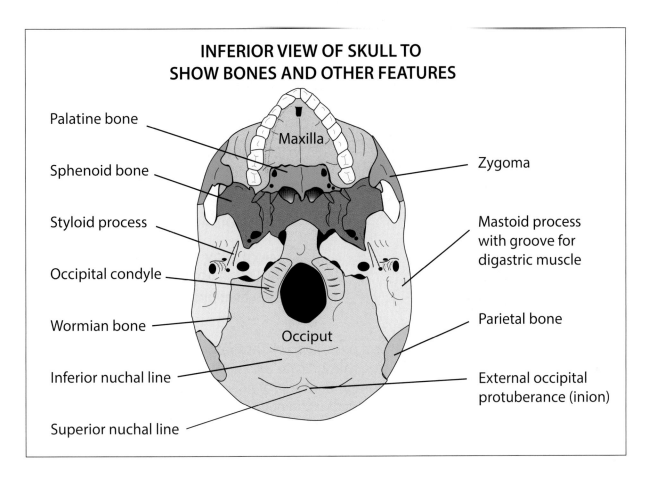

Palatine bone

Sphenoid bone

Styloid process

Occipital condyle

Wormian bone

Inferior nuchal line

Superior nuchal line

Maxilla

Zygoma

Mastoid process with groove for digastric muscle

Parietal bone

Occiput

External occipital protuberance (inion)

SKULL - LATERAL VIEW TO SHOW ZYGOMATIC BONE

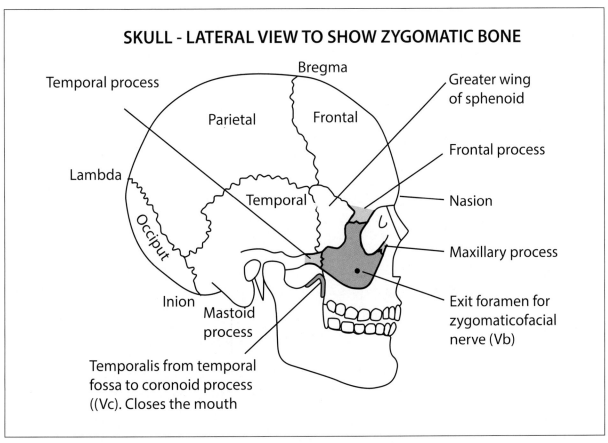

Temporal process

Bregma

Greater wing of sphenoid

Parietal

Frontal

Lambda

Frontal process

Temporal

Nasion

Occiput

Maxillary process

Inion

Mastoid process

Temporalis from temporal fossa to coronoid process ((Vc). Closes the mouth

Exit foramen for zygomaticofacial nerve (Vb)

PARANASAL SINUSES

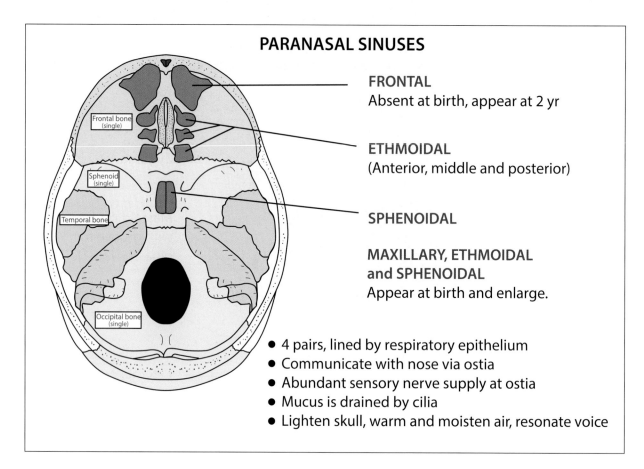

Frontal bone (single)

Sphenoid (single)

Temporal bone

Occipital bone (single)

FRONTAL
Absent at birth, appear at 2 yr

ETHMOIDAL
(Anterior, middle and posterior)

SPHENOIDAL

MAXILLARY, ETHMOIDAL and SPHENOIDAL
Appear at birth and enlarge.

- 4 pairs, lined by respiratory epithelium
- Communicate with nose via ostia
- Abundant sensory nerve supply at ostia
- Mucus is drained by cilia
- Lighten skull, warm and moisten air, resonate voice

ETHMOID BONE AND SINUSES
Schematic, likened to a catamaran

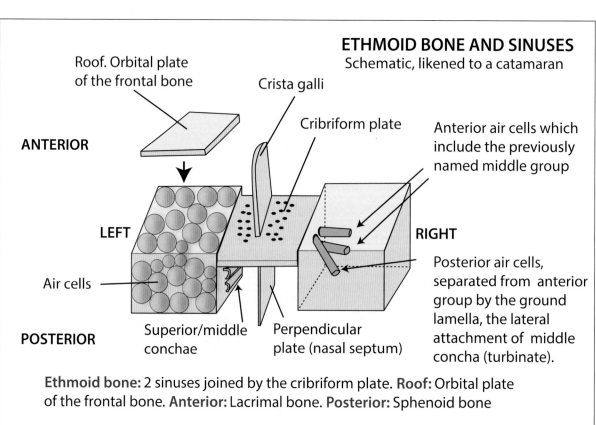

Roof. Orbital plate of the frontal bone

Crista galli

Cribriform plate

Anterior air cells which include the previously named middle group

ANTERIOR

LEFT

RIGHT

Air cells

Posterior air cells, separated from anterior group by the ground lamella, the lateral attachment of middle concha (turbinate).

POSTERIOR

Superior/middle conchae

Perpendicular plate (nasal septum)

Ethmoid bone: 2 sinuses joined by the cribriform plate. **Roof:** Orbital plate of the frontal bone. **Anterior:** Lacrimal bone. **Posterior:** Sphenoid bone

ETHMOIDAL SINUSES 2

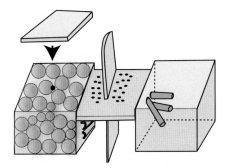

Ethmoidal sinuses: Lie between the orbit and nose in the lateral (labyrinthine) part of the bone. See image of lateral wall of nasal cavity for drainage sites.
Septa: Lie between 3-18 lots of air cells
Blood supply: Supra-orbital, anterior/posterior ethmoidal, sphenopalatine arteries
Lymph drainage: Submandibular and retropharyngeal nodes
Nerve: Supra-orbital (Va), Anterior ethmoidal (Va), lateral posterior superior nasal (Vb), posterior ethmoidal (Va) nerves

The ethmoid bone has many similarities to a catamaran:
2 bodies = hulls. Cribriform plate = deck. Crista galli = mast/sail.
Perpendicular plate = centreboard

FRONTAL SINUSES

Appear: 2 years; Unequal in size; Bony septum between them
Lie: Between orbit and anterior cranial fossa
Nerves: Supra-orbital and supratrochlear nerves
Blood supply: Supra-orbital and supratrochlear arteries
Lymph drainage: Submandibular nodes
Veins: Diploic and superior ophthalmic

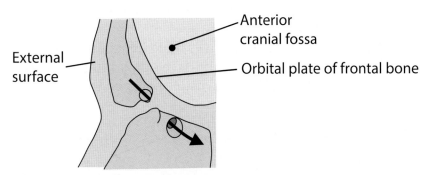

External surface

Anterior cranial fossa

Orbital plate of frontal bone

Drainage: To ostium (lower medial aspect), then to middle meatus via frontonasal canal (anterior end of hiatus semilunaris). May drain via infundibulum from anterior ethmoidal sinus

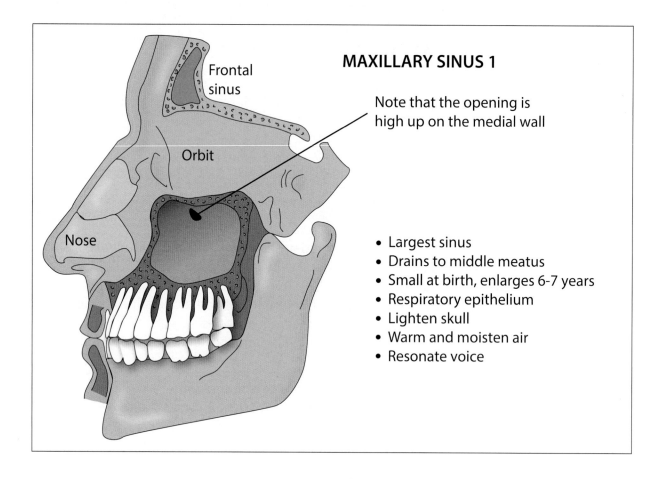

MAXILLARY SINUS 1

Frontal sinus

Orbit

Nose

Note that the opening is high up on the medial wall

- Largest sinus
- Drains to middle meatus
- Small at birth, enlarges 6-7 years
- Respiratory epithelium
- Lighten skull
- Warm and moisten air
- Resonate voice

MAXILLARY SINUS 2

Shape: Pyramidal

Walls: Anterior and posterior walls are maxilla

Drainage: Into posterior hiatus semilunaris of middle meatus. Ostium is 3-4mm, high on posterior end of nasal wall; may be a second ostium

Blood supply: Small arteries from facial, maxillary, infra-orbital and greater palatine

Lymph drainage: Submandibular glands

Nerve supply: Anterior/middle/posterior superior alveolar with secretomotor from pterygopalatine ganglion

Feature: The infra-orbital nerve lies in its ridge (junction of roof and anterior wall)

Note: The sinus is partially occupied by developing adult teeth in children. Removal of molar teeth in adults may lead to a fistula between the sinus and mouth

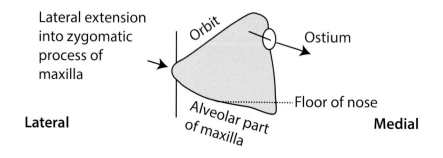

Lateral extension into zygomatic process of maxilla

Orbit

Ostium

Floor of nose

Alveolar part of maxilla

Lateral

Medial

SPHENOID BONE 1
POSTERIOR VIEW TO SHOW SINUSES

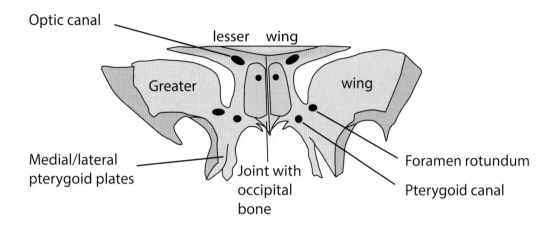

Optic canal

lesser   wing

Greater

wing

Medial/lateral
pterygoid plates

Joint with
occipital
bone

Foramen rotundum

Pterygoid canal

SPHENOIDAL SINUSES
Paired in body of sphenoid; **Septum:** Asymmetrical
If small: Then anterior to pituitary fossa; **If large:** Then beneath pituitary
fossa, extending posteriorly to basi-occiput and laterally into greater
wing; **Ostium:** In anterior wall, opening into spheno-ethmoidal recess

SPHENOID BONE 2
POSTERIOR VIEW TO SHOW SINUSES

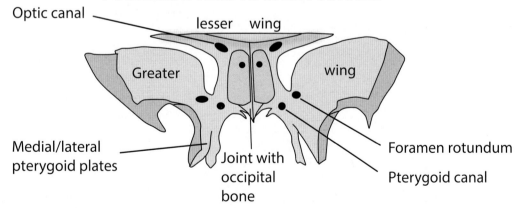

Optic canal

lesser   wing

Greater

wing

Medial/lateral
pterygoid plates

Joint with
occipital
bone

Foramen rotundum

Pterygoid canal

Lateral: Cavernous sinuses, internal carotid artery and maxillary nerve; **Posterior:**
Posterior cranial fossa and pons; **Inferior:** Roof of nasopharynx, nerve of pterygoid
canal and palatovaginal canal (containing pharyngeal branch of maxillary nerve);
Walls: Indented by pterygoid and palatovaginal canals, internal carotid artery and
maxillary nerve (Vb); **Nerve supply:** Posterior ethmoidal from maxillary and branches
of pterygopalatine ganglion; **Blood supply:** Posterior ethmoidal and sphenopalatine
branches of maxillary artery; **Lymph drainage:** Retropharyngeal

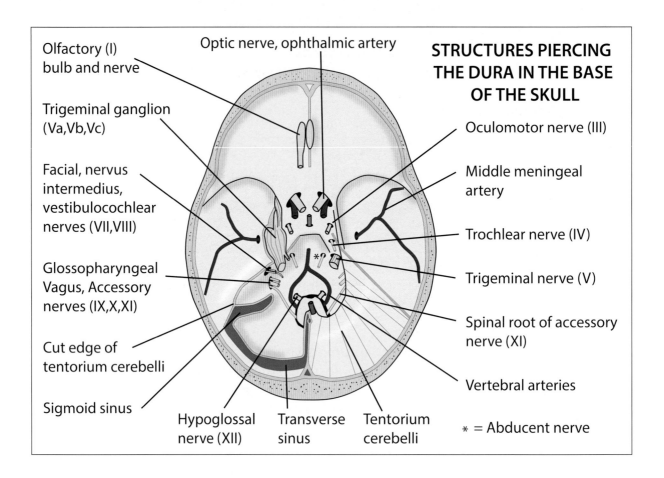

Olfactory (I) bulb and nerve

Optic nerve, ophthalmic artery

STRUCTURES PIERCING THE DURA IN THE BASE OF THE SKULL

Trigeminal ganglion (Va,Vb,Vc)

Facial, nervus intermedius, vestibulocochlear nerves (VII,VIII)

Glossopharyngeal Vagus, Accessory nerves (IX,X,XI)

Cut edge of tentorium cerebelli

Sigmoid sinus

Hypoglossal nerve (XII)

Transverse sinus

Tentorium cerebelli

Oculomotor nerve (III)

Middle meningeal artery

Trochlear nerve (IV)

Trigeminal nerve (V)

Spinal root of accessory nerve (XI)

Vertebral arteries

* = Abducent nerve

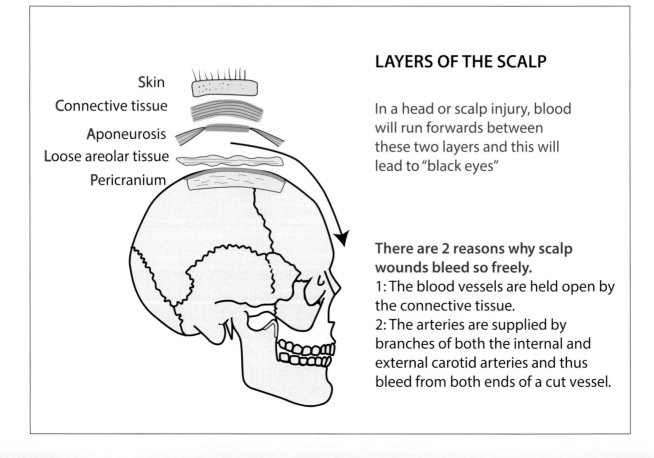

Skin
Connective tissue
Aponeurosis
Loose areolar tissue
Pericranium

LAYERS OF THE SCALP

In a head or scalp injury, blood will run forwards between these two layers and this will lead to "black eyes"

There are 2 reasons why scalp wounds bleed so freely.
1: The blood vessels are held open by the connective tissue.
2: The arteries are supplied by branches of both the internal and external carotid arteries and thus bleed from both ends of a cut vessel.

LAYERS OF SCALP

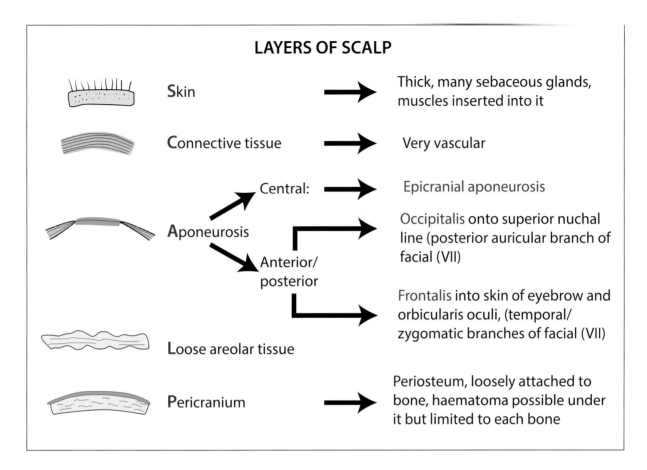

Skin ➡ Thick, many sebaceous glands, muscles inserted into it

Connective tissue ➡ Very vascular

Aponeurosis

Central: ➡ Epicranial aponeurosis

Anterior/posterior

➡ Occipitalis onto superior nuchal line (posterior auricular branch of facial (VII)

➡ Frontalis into skin of eyebrow and orbicularis oculi, (temporal/zygomatic branches of facial (VII)

Loose areolar tissue

Pericranium ➡ Periosteum, loosely attached to bone, haematoma possible under it but limited to each bone

SCALP - ARTERIES AND NERVES

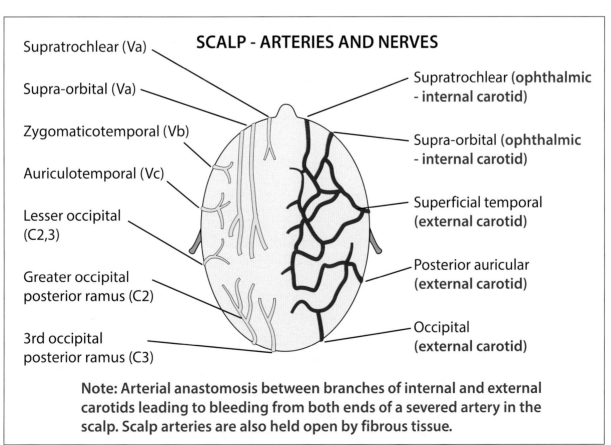

Supratrochlear (Va)

Supra-orbital (Va)

Zygomaticotemporal (Vb)

Auriculotemporal (Vc)

Lesser occipital (C2,3)

Greater occipital posterior ramus (C2)

3rd occipital posterior ramus (C3)

Supratrochlear (**ophthalmic - internal carotid**)

Supra-orbital (**ophthalmic - internal carotid**)

Superficial temporal (**external carotid**)

Posterior auricular (**external carotid**)

Occipital (**external carotid**)

Note: Arterial anastomosis between branches of internal and external carotids leading to bleeding from both ends of a severed artery in the scalp. Scalp arteries are also held open by fibrous tissue.

CORONAL SECTION OF SKULL, SCALP AND MENINGES IN MIDLINE

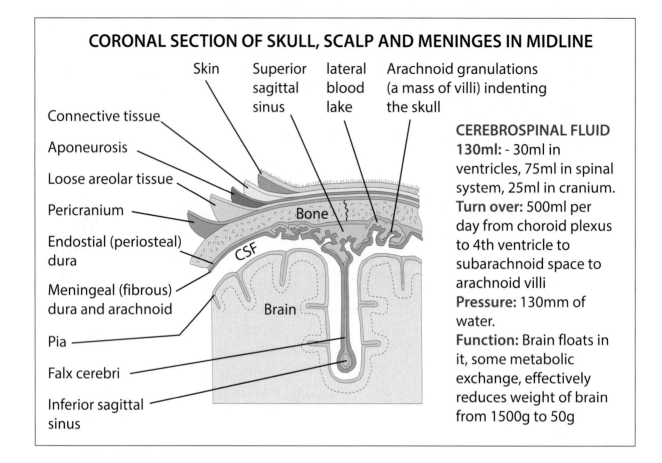

Skin Superior sagittal sinus lateral blood lake Arachnoid granulations (a mass of villi) indenting the skull

Connective tissue
Aponeurosis
Loose areolar tissue
Pericranium
Endostial (periosteal) dura
Meningeal (fibrous) dura and arachnoid
Pia
Falx cerebri
Inferior sagittal sinus

Bone

CSF

Brain

CEREBROSPINAL FLUID
130ml: - 30ml in ventricles, 75ml in spinal system, 25ml in cranium.
Turn over: 500ml per day from choroid plexus to 4th ventricle to subarachnoid space to arachnoid villi
Pressure: 130mm of water.
Function: Brain floats in it, some metabolic exchange, effectively reduces weight of brain from 1500g to 50g

5.2 Brain, Spine, Spinal Cord and Vessels

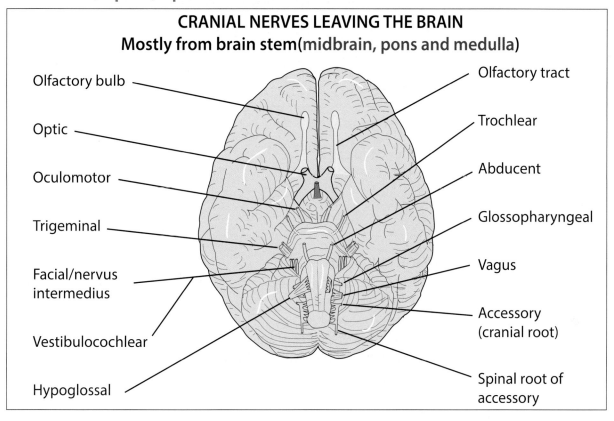

CRANIAL NERVES LEAVING THE BRAIN
Mostly from brain stem(midbrain, pons and medulla)

Olfactory bulb

Optic

Oculomotor

Trigeminal

Facial/nervus intermedius

Vestibulocochlear

Hypoglossal

Olfactory tract

Trochlear

Abducent

Glossopharyngeal

Vagus

Accessory (cranial root)

Spinal root of accessory

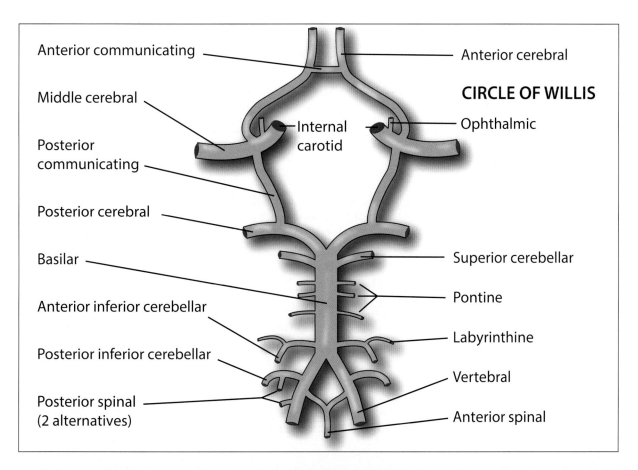

Anterior communicating

Middle cerebral

Posterior communicating

Posterior cerebral

Basilar

Anterior inferior cerebellar

Posterior inferior cerebellar

Posterior spinal (2 alternatives)

Internal carotid

Anterior cerebral

CIRCLE OF WILLIS

Ophthalmic

Superior cerebellar

Pontine

Labyrinthine

Vertebral

Anterior spinal

VERTEBRAL COLUMN - FEATURES AND CURVATURES

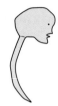

Primary curvature

Secondary curvatures (cervical and lumbar)

VERTEBRAE
- 7 cervical (atlas, axis and C7 are atypical)
- 12 thoracic
- 5 lumbar
- 5 sacral (fused)
- 4 coccygeal (3-5)

FUNCTIONS
- Weight bearing
- Movement of trunk
- Support for limbs
- Protection of spinal cord
- Production of blood
- Metabolic reserves (Calcium, etc)

WEIGHT BEARING
- Aided by: secondary lordosis
  40% bony wedge
  60% disc wedge
- Caused/held by: extensor spinal muscles
- Aided by: intervertebral discs (dampeners, resilience, compressible)

VERTEBRAL COLUMN - MOVEMENTS

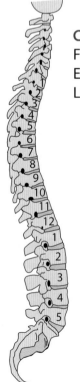
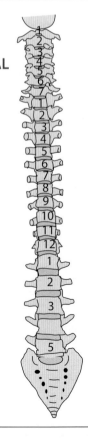

CERVICAL (7)
Flexion
Extension
Lateral flexion

ATLANTO-OCCIPITAL
Flexion/extension
ATLANTO-AXIAL
Rotation only

THORACIC (12)
Rotation only

LUMBAR (5)
Flexion/extension
Lateral flexion

SACRAL (5 FUSED)
No movement

Movements at facet and intervertebral joints are individually small but accumulatively considerable

RELATIONSHIP OF SPINAL CORD TO VERTEBRAL COLUMN

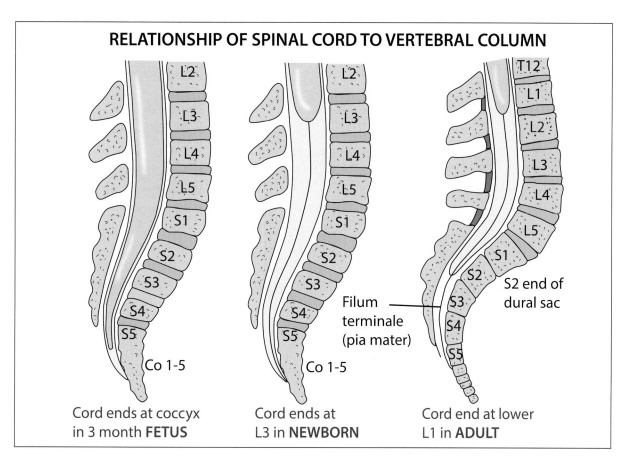

Cord ends at coccyx in 3 month **FETUS**

Cord ends at L3 in **NEWBORN**

Filum terminale (pia mater)

Cord end at lower L1 in **ADULT**

S2 end of dural sac

LUMBAR PUNCTURE AT L4/5 OR L3/4

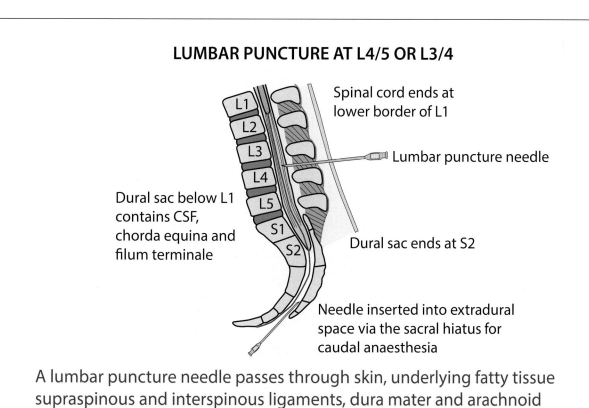

Spinal cord ends at lower border of L1

Lumbar puncture needle

Dural sac below L1 contains CSF, chorda equina and filum terminale

Dural sac ends at S2

Needle inserted into extradural space via the sacral hiatus for caudal anaesthesia

A lumbar puncture needle passes through skin, underlying fatty tissue supraspinous and interspinous ligaments, dura mater and arachnoid

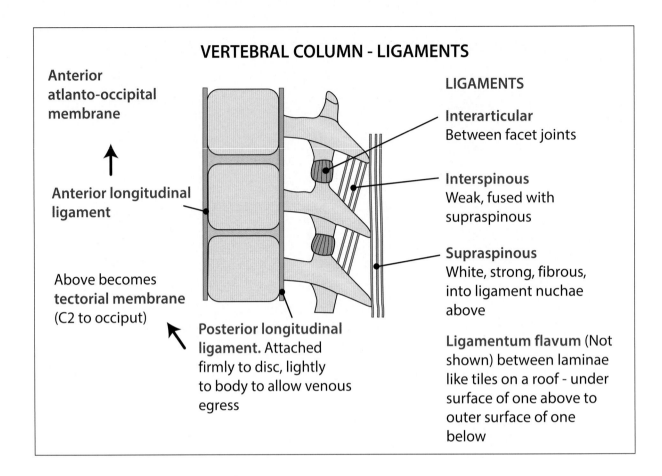

VERTEBRAL COLUMN - LIGAMENTS

Anterior atlanto-occipital membrane

Anterior longitudinal ligament

Above becomes tectorial membrane (C2 to occiput)

Posterior longitudinal ligament. Attached firmly to disc, lightly to body to allow venous egress

LIGAMENTS

Interarticular
Between facet joints

Interspinous
Weak, fused with supraspinous

Supraspinous
White, strong, fibrous, into ligament nuchae above

Ligamentum flavum (Not shown) between laminae like tiles on a roof - under surface of one above to outer surface of one below

ATLANTO-OCCIPITAL MEMBRANES

Posterior view

The posterior atlanto-occipital membrane is a separate membrane between the posterior arch of the atlas and the posterior rim of the foramen magnum. It could be regarded as an extension of the ligamentum flavum.

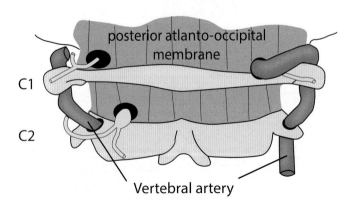

posterior atlanto-occipital membrane

C1

C2

Vertebral artery

The posterior longitudinal ligament , lying on the posterior aspects of all vertebrae, becomes the tectorial membrane between the atlas and the foramen magnum (not shown).

SPINAL COLUMN - VEINS AND SOME LIGAMENTS

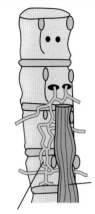

Basivertebral veins emerge from foramina (●) in posterior vertebral bodies and drain into **internal vertebral plexus** (anterior/posterior) which drains via **intervertebral segmental veins** (with nerve roots) into **external vertebral plexuses** which, in turn connect above and below diaphragm to inferior and superior vena cavae via vertebral, azygos, lumbar and lateral sacral veins. These veins are **VALVELESS,** thus cancer cells from thyroid, breast, kidney and prostate can easily enter the bones

The **posterior longitudinal ligament** attaches to discs only and not to the vertebral bodies so that there is free drainage of the basivertebral veins

Internal vertebral plexus

Posterior, external vertebral venous plexus

Internal vertebral venous plexus

Intervertebral veins: valveless and connect with portal and systemic systems. Allow retrograde spread of cancer cells

Lumbar vein and ascending lumbar vein

Basivertebral veins

Anterior, external vertebral venous plexus

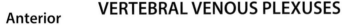

VERTEBRAL VENOUS PLEXUSES

Anterior

Posterior

External venous plexus. Anterior. Drain via vertebral bodies **VALVELESS**

 Drain to: cervical, azygos, ascending lumbar, lateral sacral veins

Drain to: intervertebral then to: vertebral, intercostal, lumbar, lateral sacral veins

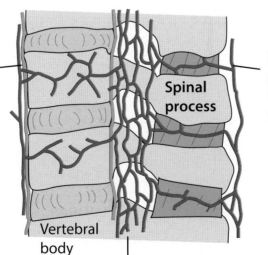

Spinal process

Vertebral body

External venous plexus. Posterior to ligamentum flavum. **VALVELESS**

Internal vertebral veins. One set of anterior and two sets of posterior. Around dura and posterior longitudinal ligament. **VALVELESS**. Communicate above with occipital and basilar sinuses, segmentally receive veins from spinal cord and basivertebral veins

A TYPICAL VERTEBRA

Each vertebra has:
A BODY: anteriorly
A VERTEBRAL ARCH: posteriorly
    Each arch has:
        2 pedicles, 2 laminae, a spinous process,
        a transverse process and a vertebral foramen

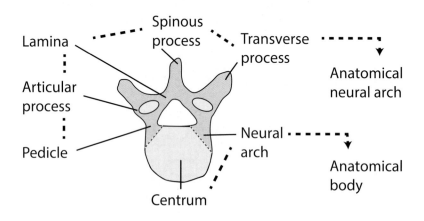

COSTAL ELEMENTS OF VERTEBRAE AT VARIOUS LEVELS

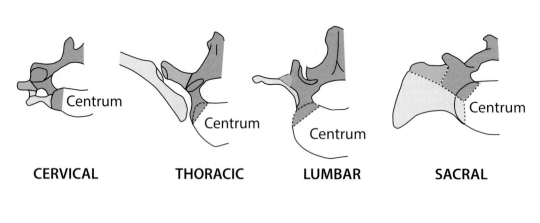

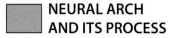 **CERVICAL**   **THORACIC**   **LUMBAR**   **SACRAL**

NEURAL ARCH AND ITS PROCESS   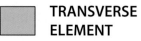 **TRANSVERSE ELEMENT**   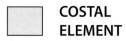 **COSTAL ELEMENT**

INTERVERTEBRAL DISCS
Secondary cartilaginous joint

BONE ⟷ HYALINE CARTILAGE ⟷ FIBRO-CARTILAGE ⟷ HYALINE CARTILAGE ⟷ BONE

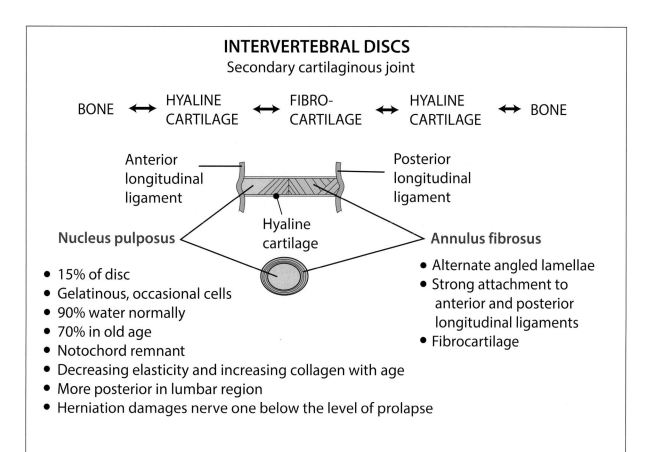

Anterior longitudinal ligament

Posterior longitudinal ligament

Hyaline cartilage

Nucleus pulposus

- 15% of disc
- Gelatinous, occasional cells
- 90% water normally
- 70% in old age
- Notochord remnant
- Decreasing elasticity and increasing collagen with age
- More posterior in lumbar region
- Herniation damages nerve one below the level of prolapse

Annulus fibrosus

- Alternate angled lamellae
- Strong attachment to anterior and posterior longitudinal ligaments
- Fibrocartilage

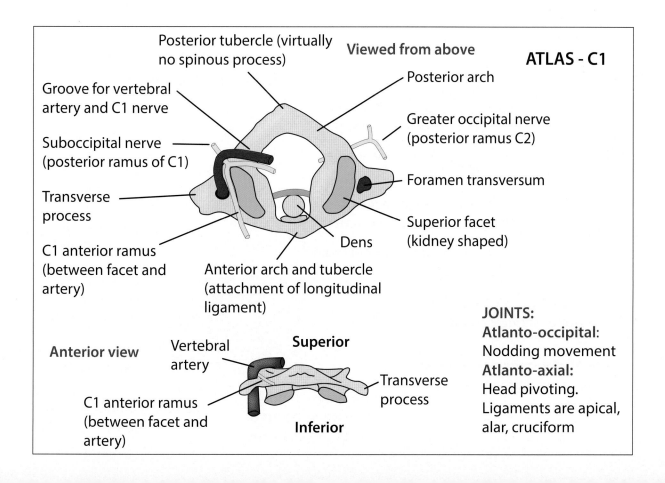

Posterior tubercle (virtually no spinous process)

Viewed from above

ATLAS - C1

Groove for vertebral artery and C1 nerve

Posterior arch

Suboccipital nerve (posterior ramus of C1)

Greater occipital nerve (posterior ramus C2)

Foramen transversum

Transverse process

Superior facet (kidney shaped)

C1 anterior ramus (between facet and artery)

Dens

Anterior arch and tubercle (attachment of longitudinal ligament)

Anterior view

Vertebral artery

Superior

Transverse process

C1 anterior ramus (between facet and artery)

Inferior

JOINTS:
Atlanto-occipital: Nodding movement
Atlanto-axial: Head pivoting. Ligaments are apical, alar, cruciform

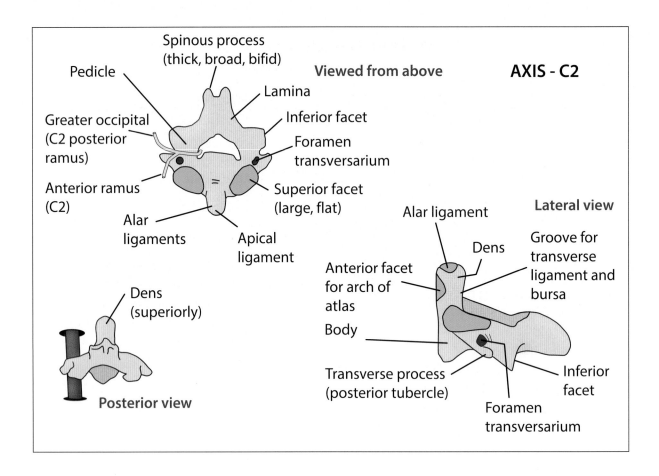

Viewed from above   **AXIS - C2**

Spinous process (thick, broad, bifid)

Pedicle

Lamina

Inferior facet

Greater occipital (C2 posterior ramus)

Foramen transversarium

Anterior ramus (C2)

Alar ligaments

Apical ligament

Superior facet (large, flat)

Lateral view

Alar ligament

Dens

Groove for transverse ligament and bursa

Anterior facet for arch of atlas

Body

Dens (superiorly)

Transverse process (posterior tubercle)

Foramen transversarium

Inferior facet

Posterior view

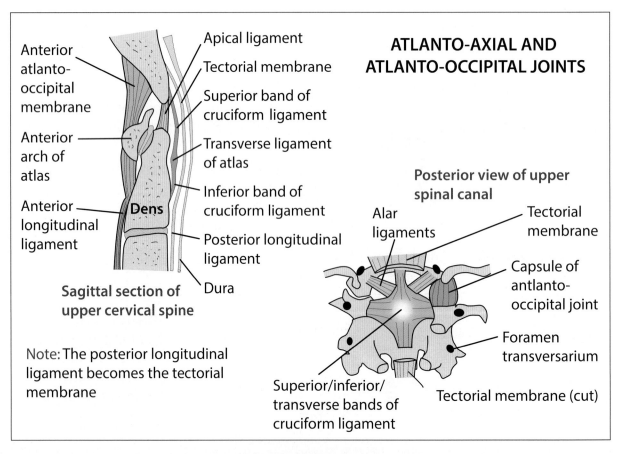

ATLANTO-AXIAL AND ATLANTO-OCCIPITAL JOINTS

Anterior atlanto-occipital membrane

Apical ligament

Tectorial membrane

Superior band of cruciform ligament

Anterior arch of atlas

Transverse ligament of atlas

Anterior longitudinal ligament

Dens

Inferior band of cruciform ligament

Posterior longitudinal ligament

Dura

Posterior view of upper spinal canal

Alar ligaments

Tectorial membrane

Capsule of antlanto-occipital joint

Foramen transversarium

Superior/inferior/transverse bands of cruciform ligament

Tectorial membrane (cut)

Sagittal section of upper cervical spine

Note: The posterior longitudinal ligament becomes the tectorial membrane

TYPICAL CERVICAL VERTEBRA

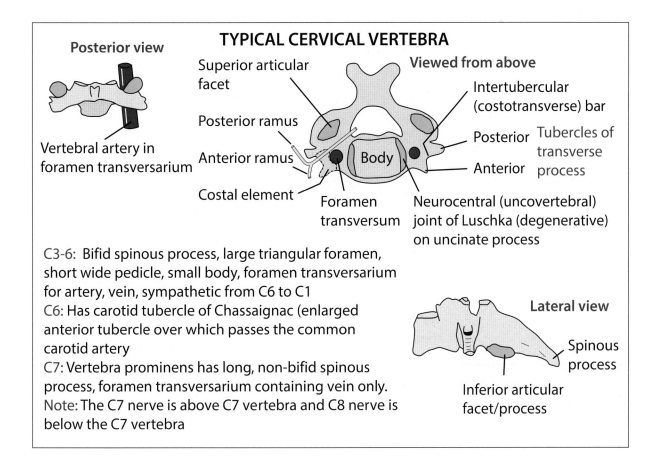

Posterior view

Vertebral artery in foramen transversarium

Viewed from above

Superior articular facet

Posterior ramus

Anterior ramus

Costal element

Foramen transversum

Body

Intertubercular (costotransverse) bar

Posterior — Tubercles of transverse process

Anterior

Neurocentral (uncovertebral) joint of Luschka (degenerative) on uncinate process

C3-6: Bifid spinous process, large triangular foramen, short wide pedicle, small body, foramen transversarium for artery, vein, sympathetic from C6 to C1

C6: Has carotid tubercle of Chassaignac (enlarged anterior tubercle over which passes the common carotid artery

C7: Vertebra prominens has long, non-bifid spinous process, foramen transversarium containing vein only.

Note: The C7 nerve is above C7 vertebra and C8 nerve is below the C7 vertebra

Lateral view

Spinous process

Inferior articular facet/process

THORACIC VERTEBRAE

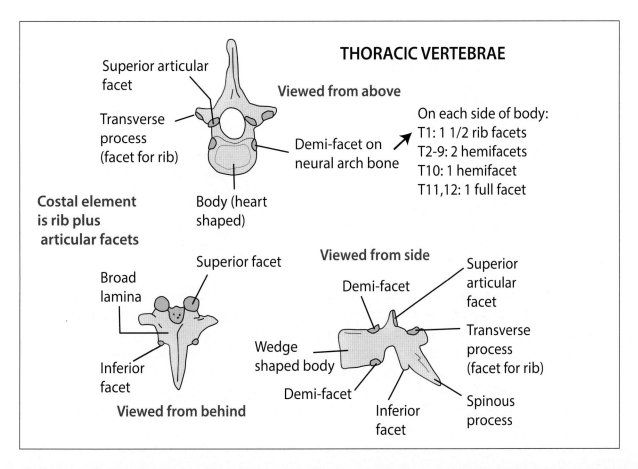

Superior articular facet

Transverse process (facet for rib)

Viewed from above

Demi-facet on neural arch bone

Body (heart shaped)

On each side of body:
T1: 1 1/2 rib facets
T2-9: 2 hemifacets
T10: 1 hemifacet
T11,12: 1 full facet

Costal element is rib plus articular facets

Broad lamina

Superior facet

Inferior facet

Viewed from behind

Viewed from side

Demi-facet

Wedge shaped body

Demi-facet

Inferior facet

Superior articular facet

Transverse process (facet for rib)

Spinous process

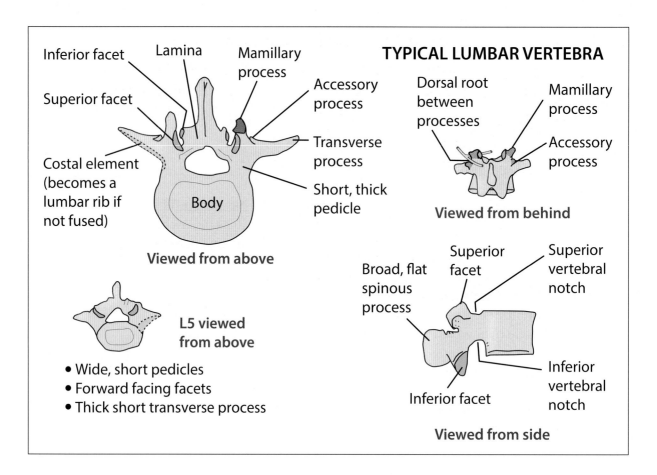

TYPICAL LUMBAR VERTEBRA

Inferior facet
Lamina
Mamillary process
Accessory process
Superior facet
Transverse process
Costal element (becomes a lumbar rib if not fused)
Body
Short, thick pedicle

Viewed from above

Dorsal root between processes
Mamillary process
Accessory process

Viewed from behind

L5 viewed from above
- Wide, short pedicles
- Forward facing facets
- Thick short transverse process

Broad, flat spinous process
Superior facet
Superior vertebral notch
Inferior facet
Inferior vertebral notch

Viewed from side

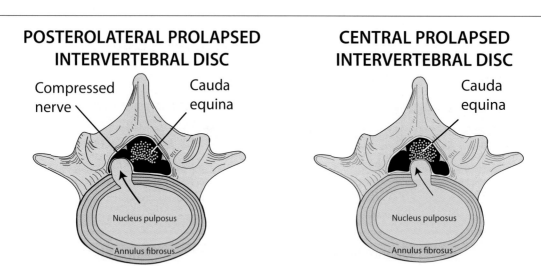

POSTEROLATERAL PROLAPSED INTERVERTEBRAL DISC

Compressed nerve
Cauda equina
Nucleus pulposus
Annulus fibrosus

CENTRAL PROLAPSED INTERVERTEBRAL DISC

Cauda equina
Nucleus pulposus
Annulus fibrosus

The softer **nucleus pulposus** is surrounded by a thick tough **annulus fibrosus.** The annulus weakens with age and causes it to rupture, usually posterolaterally, and the nucleus pulposus is squeezed out. Precipitating factors include bending and lifting which compress the anterior part of the disc and this pushes the nucleus pulposus posteriorly against the slightly thinner posterior wall of the annulus fibrosus.

In a **central prolapse** the cauda equina may be damaged and particularly vulnerable are the parasympathetic fibres (S2,3,4) which control bladder contraction leading to a presentation of retention of urine.

POSTEROLATERAL DISC PROLAPSE
(Direct pressure on a nerve)

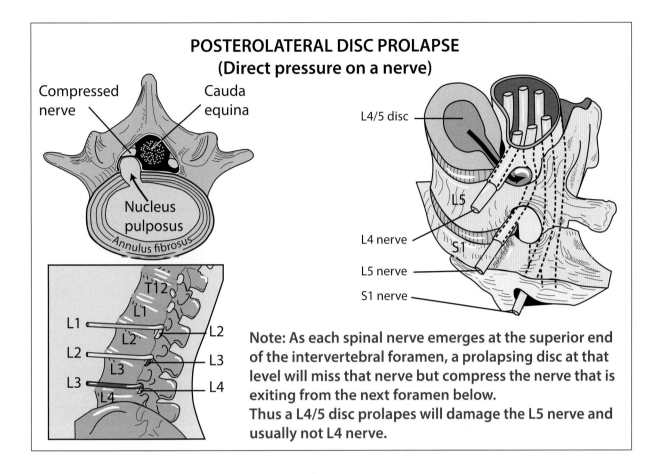

Compressed nerve

Cauda equina

Nucleus pulposus

Annulus fibrosus

T12
L1
L1
L2
L2
L2
L3
L3
L3
L4
L4

L4/5 disc

L5

L4 nerve

L5 nerve

S1 nerve

S1

Note: As each spinal nerve emerges at the superior end of the intervertebral foramen, a prolapsing disc at that level will miss that nerve but compress the nerve that is exiting from the next foramen below.

Thus a L4/5 disc prolapes will damage the L5 nerve and usually not L4 nerve.

SPINAL CORD - GENERAL

- Cord begins at lower medulla of brain stem
- Cord finishes at lower border of L1 vertebra
- 45cm long in an adult
- Covered by 3 layers of meninges and CSF

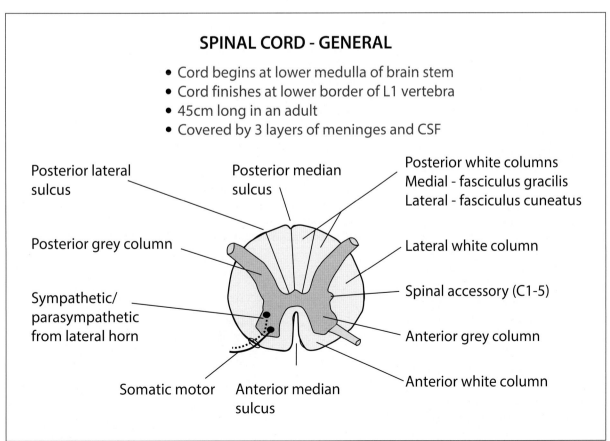

Posterior lateral sulcus

Posterior median sulcus

Posterior white columns
Medial - fasciculus gracilis
Lateral - fasciculus cuneatus

Posterior grey column

Lateral white column

Sympathetic/ parasympathetic from lateral horn

Spinal accessory (C1-5)

Anterior grey column

Somatic motor

Anterior median sulcus

Anterior white column

BLOOD SUPPLY OF SPINAL CORD

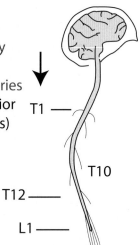

- One anterior spinal artery (from vertebral)
- Two posterior spinal arteries (from vertebral or posterior inferior cerebellar arteries)

T1

T10

T12

L1

- Ascending cervical arteries
- Deep cervical arteries

- Posterior intercostal arteries (at every level)

- Artery of Adamkiewicz
  A larger artery, usually from a left posterior intercostal artery between T9-12 (often T10)

- Lumbar arteries
- Lateral sacral arteries

All the above arteries enter via intervertebral foramina and anastomose with spinal arteries

BLOOD SUPPLY OF SPINAL CORD

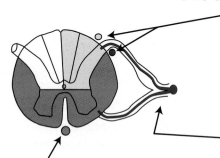

POSTERIOR SPINAL ARTERIES
- Arise at foramen magnum from posterior inferior cerebellar arteries (or vertebral)
- Lie anterior and posterior to posterior rootlets
- Run length of cord but poor anastomosis except at lower end of cord
- Supply own side of grey and white posterior columns

RADICULAR (FEEDER) ARTERIES
- Enter via intervertebral foramina and reinforce anterior and posterior spinal arteries and supply dorsal root ganglia
- Variable number at variable levels but largest is **Arteria Radicularis Magna**, usually at T10 or 11 (artery of Adamkiewicz)

ANTERIOR SPINAL ARTERY
- Single artery that arises from each vertebral artery at foramen magnum to run length of cord
- Usually larger than posterior spinal arteries but may be small.
- Supplies whole cord anterior to posterior grey columns, bilaterally

OTHER VESSELS
From vertebrals, deep and ascending cervicals, intercostals, lumbars and lateral sacrals. Note that all vessels anastomose under the pia mater in the periphery of the cord

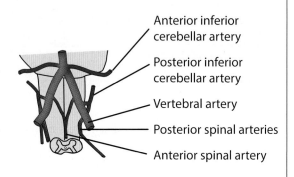

Anterior inferior cerebellar artery

Posterior inferior cerebellar artery

Vertebral artery

Posterior spinal arteries

Anterior spinal artery

SPINAL COLUMN - INTERNAL

The dural sac finishes at S2 but the **PIA MATER,** in the form of the filum terminale, continues below S2 and attaches to the back of the coccyx

The **DENTICULATE (dentate) ligament** is pia mater that connects the cord to the dura mater laterally between the exits sites for the nerves. It pierces the arachnoid mater. Note that the spinal roots of the accessory nerve (C1-5) emerge dorsal to the denticulate ligament, whereas the sensory roots emerge dorsal and the motor roots ventral to it.

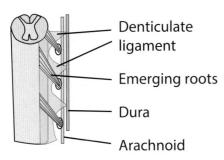

Denticulate ligament

Emerging roots

Dura

Arachnoid

SPINAL SUBARACHNOID SPACE
- Volume 75ml
- Tapped during spinal puncture or anaesthetic below L2

POSTERIOR ABDOMEN AND BACK

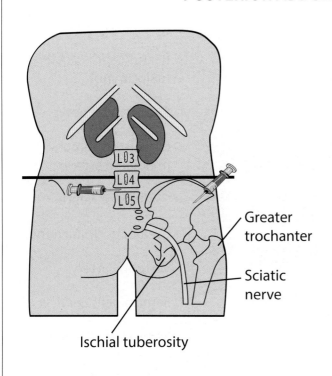

Greater trochanter

Sciatic nerve

Ischial tuberosity

Buttock injection
Intramuscular injections are given in the upper, outer (lateral) quadrant of the buttock to avoid the sciatic nerve which lies in the lower inner (medial) quadrant and passes inferiorly half way between the ischial tuberosity and the greater trochanter of the femur

Supracristal plane
A transverse line along the upper aspects of the iliac crests passing through the spinous process of the L4 vertebra. A useful aid in lumbar puncture for either the L3-4 or L4-5 spaces

PERIPHERAL NERVE INJURY

CAUSES: Direct trauma, ischaemia, traction, compression

CLASSIFICATION:

NEUROTMESIS: Complete or partial division of a nerve

AXONOTMESIS: Interuption of the axons without interuption of the sheath

NEUROPRAXIA: Bruising or concussion of a nerve without damage to the axon or sheath leading to temporary loss of function

CLASSIFICATION OF MUSCLE POWER

0. No contraction
1. Flicker or trace of contraction
2. Active movement, with gravity eliminated
3. Active movement against gravity
4. Active movement against gravity and resistance
5. Normal power

STRUCTURE OF A NERVE

Axon with myelin sheath and neurolemma which is composed of Schwann cells

Epineurium

Perineurium

SUBOCCIPITAL TRIANGLE 1

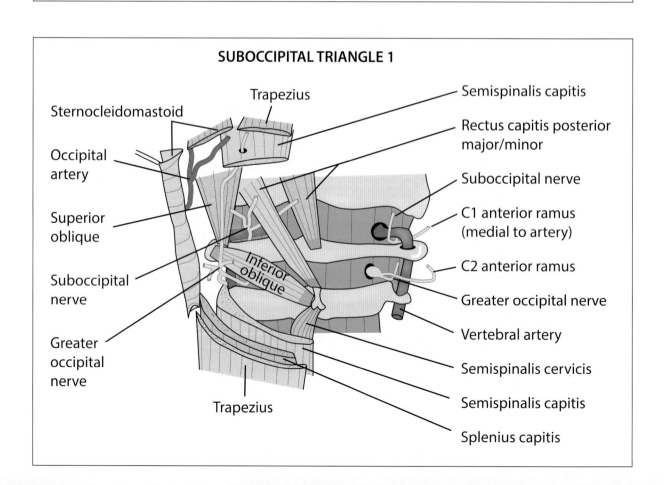

Sternocleidomastoid

Trapezius

Semispinalis capitis

Rectus capitis posterior major/minor

Suboccipital nerve

C1 anterior ramus (medial to artery)

C2 anterior ramus

Greater occipital nerve

Vertebral artery

Semispinalis cervicis

Semispinalis capitis

Splenius capitis

Occipital artery

Superior oblique

Suboccipital nerve

Greater occipital nerve

Inferior oblique

Trapezius

SUBOCCIPITAL TRIANGLE 2

SUBOCCIPITAL NERVE
- Posterior ramus of C1
- No skin distribution
- Rectus capitis posterior major/minor
- Superior/inferior obliques
- Semispinalis capitis

GREATER OCCIPITAL NERVE
- Posterior ramus of C2
- Semispinalis capitis
- Splenius capitis
- Inferior oblique via connection to C1
- Skin of posterior scalp

SUBOCCIPITAL TRIANGLE
Boundaries: Superior oblique, inferior oblique and rectus capitis posterior major
Floor: Posterior atlanto-occipital membrane, posterior arch of atlas
Contains: Vertebral artery and suboccipital nerve
In roof: Greater occipital nerve and occipital artery

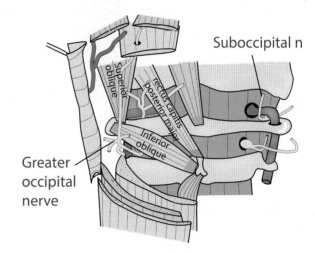

5.3   Intracranial Haemorrhages

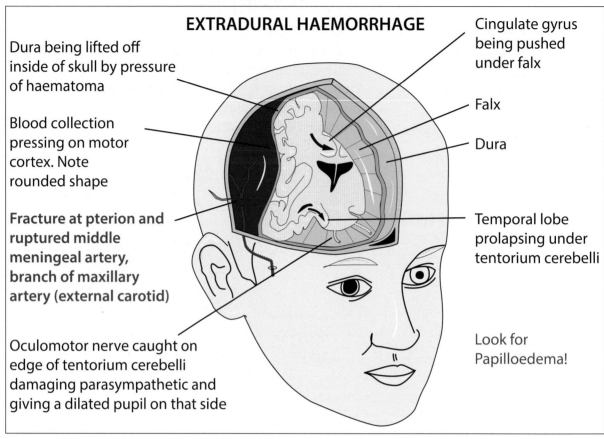

EXTRADURAL HAEMORRHAGE

Dura being lifted off inside of skull by pressure of haematoma

Blood collection pressing on motor cortex. Note rounded shape

Fracture at pterion and ruptured middle meningeal artery, branch of maxillary artery (external carotid)

Oculomotor nerve caught on edge of tentorium cerebelli damaging parasympathetic and giving a dilated pupil on that side

Cingulate gyrus being pushed under falx

Falx

Dura

Temporal lobe prolapsing under tentorium cerebelli

Look for Papilloedema!

EXTRADURAL HAEMORRHAGE

Haematoma is well rounded as it is arterial pressure lifting the endosteal dura from the inside of the skull. Note the position - deep to the pterion and the soft tissue swelling superficial to the fracture over it.
The midline structures have been shifted to the opposite side

As the endosteal dura is firmly attached to bone, the arterial bleed usually takes an hour or so to produce a haematoma of sufficient size to displace the brain and thus, clinically, there is typically a latent period before symptoms and signs appear

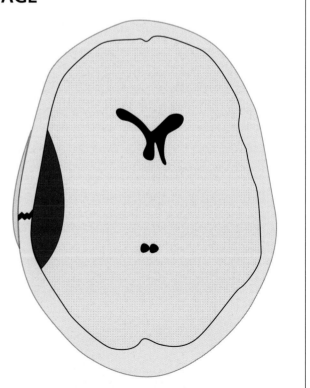

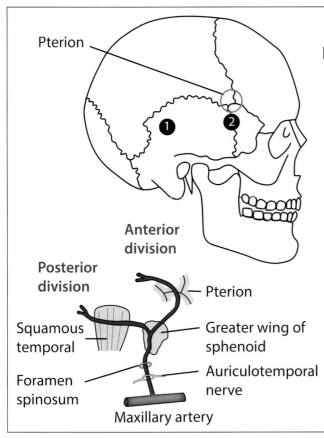

Pterion

Anterior
division

Posterior
division

Pterion

Squamous
temporal

Greater wing of
sphenoid

Foramen
spinosum

Auriculotemporal
nerve

Maxillary artery

BURR HOLES FOR EXTRADURAL HAEMORRHAGE

1. Surface marking for the posterior branch of the middle meningeal artery:
The crossing point of a line vertical from the mastoid process and a line horizontal from the outer canthus of the eye

2. Surface marking for the anterior branch of the middle meningeal artery:
3cm above the mid point of the zygomatic arch. (Just inferior to pterion)

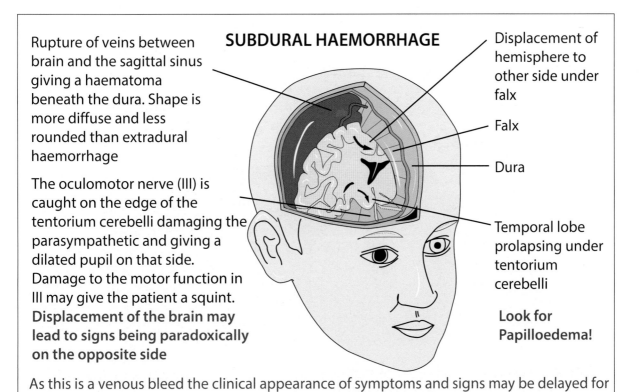

SUBDURAL HAEMORRHAGE

Rupture of veins between brain and the sagittal sinus giving a haematoma beneath the dura. Shape is more diffuse and less rounded than extradural haemorrhage

The oculomotor nerve (III) is caught on the edge of the tentorium cerebelli damaging the parasympathetic and giving a dilated pupil on that side. Damage to the motor function in III may give the patient a squint. **Displacement of the brain may lead to signs being paradoxically on the opposite side**

Displacement of hemisphere to other side under falx

Falx

Dura

Temporal lobe prolapsing under tentorium cerebelli

Look for Papilloedema!

As this is a venous bleed the clinical appearance of symptoms and signs may be delayed for days or even weeks. The veins are probably more likely to rupture in elderly people due to an element of brain shrinkage

SUBDURAL HAEMORRHAGE

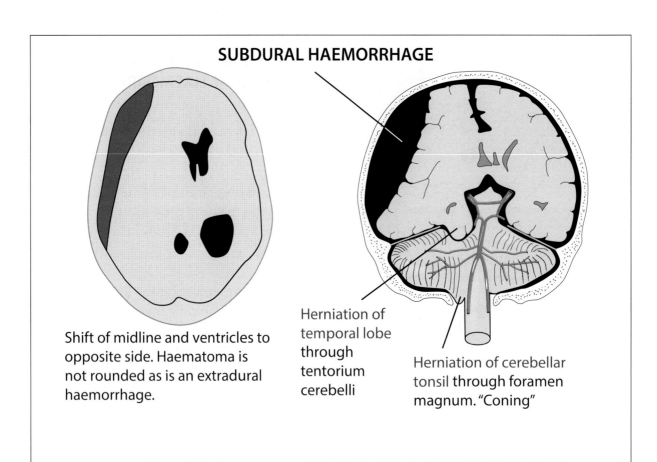

Shift of midline and ventricles to opposite side. Haematoma is not rounded as is an extradural haemorrhage.

Herniation of temporal lobe through tentorium cerebelli

Herniation of cerebellar tonsil through foramen magnum. "Coning"

SUBDURAL HAEMORRHAGE RUPTURE OF CEREBRAL VEINS

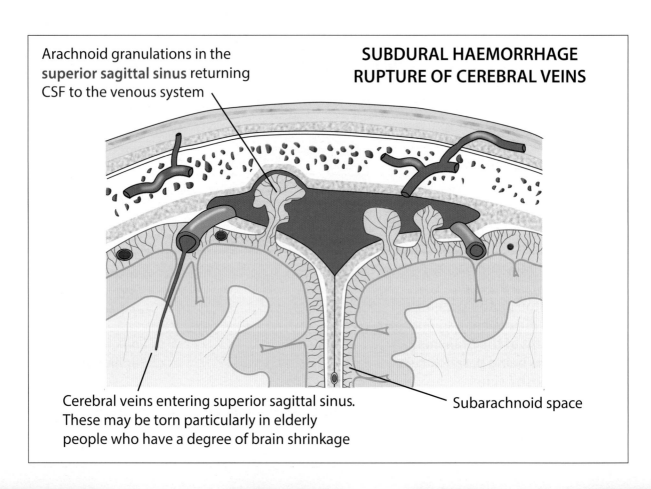

Arachnoid granulations in the **superior sagittal sinus** returning CSF to the venous system

Cerebral veins entering superior sagittal sinus. These may be torn particularly in elderly people who have a degree of brain shrinkage

Subarachnoid space

SUBARACHNOID HAEMORRHAGE
RUPTURE OF BERRY ANEURYSMS ON CIRCLE OF WILLIS

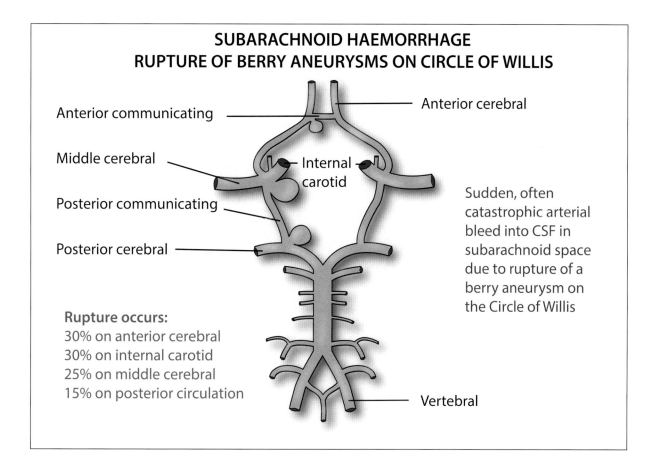

Anterior communicating

Anterior cerebral

Middle cerebral

Internal carotid

Posterior communicating

Posterior cerebral

Sudden, often catastrophic arterial bleed into CSF in subarachnoid space due to rupture of a berry aneurysm on the Circle of Willis

Rupture occurs:
30% on anterior cerebral
30% on internal carotid
25% on middle cerebral
15% on posterior circulation

Vertebral

5.4 Cranial Nerves in General and Skull Foramina

SIMPLE CLASSIFICATION OF CRANIAL NERVES

I	OLFACTORY	Special sense	Smell
II	OPTIC	Special sense	Sight
III	OCULOMOTOR	Somatic motor	Eye movements
IV	TROCHLEAR	Somatic motor	Eye movements
V	TRIGEMINAL	Somatic sensory	Sensory
		Branchiomotor	Muscles of mastication
VI	ABDUCENT	Somatic motor	Eye movements
VII	FACIAL	Branchiomotor	Muscles of facial expression
VIII	VESTIBULOCOCHLEAR	Special sense	Hearing/balance
IX	GLOSSOPHARYNGEAL	Somatic sensory	Oropharynx
		Branchiomotor	Stylopharyneus(single muscle)
X	VAGUS	Parasympathetic	Heart to colon
		Branchiomotor (from XI)	Palate, larynx
XI	ACCESSORY	Somatic motor	Sternomastoid, trapezius
		Branchiomotor (to vagus)	To vagus
XII	HYPOGLOSSAL	Somatic motor	Tongue

FUNCTIONS OF THE CRANIAL NERVES

I OLFACTORY

Special sense for smell

II OPTIC

Special sense for sight

III OCULOMOTOR

Somatic motor for muscles of eye

Carries parasympathetic to ciliary ganglion

IV TROCHLEAR

Somatic motor for muscles of eye

V TRIGEMINAL

Somatic sensory for face, sinuses, eye, nose

Branchiomotor for muscles of mastication

Carries all postganglionic parasympathetic to end organs

VI ABDUCENT

Somatic motor for muscles of eye

VII FACIAL

Branchiomotor for muscles of facial expression

Taste

Small sensation to external ear

Carries parasympathetic to submandibular and pterygopalatine ganglia

VIII VESTIBULOCOCHLEAR

Special sense for hearing and balance

IX GLOSSOPHARYNGEAL

Somatic sensory to oropharynx

Branchiomotor for stylopharyngeus

Taste in oropharynx

Baroreception

Carries parasympathetic to otic ganglion

X VAGUS

Parasympathetic down to left of transverse colon

Somatic sensation to ear, larynx and pharynx

Taste in vallecula

Baroreception

Branchiomotor (from XI) to muscles of palate, pharynx, larynx

XI ACCESSORY

Somatic motor to sternomastoid and trapezius

Branchiomotor transferred to vagus (see above)

XII HYPOGLOSSAL

Somatic motor for tongue muscles - (except palatoglossus - pharyngeal

plexus (IX, X sympathetic)

CRANIAL NERVES: NUCLEI AND FIBRES

	Somatic motor (Skeletal muscle)	Branchiomotor (Special visceral)	Parasympathetic (General visceral)	General visceral sensory	Special visceral sensory	Somatic sensory (Skin & membranes)	Special senses
I							Smell Limbic system
II							Sight: lateral geniculate body
III	Nu: Oculomotor recti (sup,med,inf) inf oblique, levator palpebrae superioris		Nu: Edinger-Westphal Ganglion: Ciliary; ciliary body and muscle, sphincter pupillae				
IV	Nu: Trochlear superior oblique						
V		Nu: Motor of trigeminal muscles of mastication, mylohyoid, anterior belly digastric, tensor palati and tensor tympani				Nu: Sensory of V Mesencephalic for proprioception: Main for touch: Spinal for pain/temp for face, orbit, tongue	
VI	Nu: Abducent lateral rectus						
VII		Nu: Facial muscles of facial expression, buccinator, post belly of digastric, stylohyoid, stapedius	Nu: Superior salivary Ganglion: Pterygopalatine; and submandibular lacrimal, submandibular, and palatine glands		Nu: Solitarius Chorda tympani for taste: anterior tongue	Nu: Sensory of V some skin of external auditory meatus and tympanic membrane	
VIII							2 nu: hearing 4 nu: equilibrium
IX		Nu: Ambiguus stylopharyngeus	Nu: Inferior salivary Ganglion: Otic; parotid, glands in post tongue and oropharynx		Nu: Solitarius taste: post tongue, vallate papillae, oropharynx, baro/chemoreceptors	Nu: Sensory of V post tongue, palate, pharynx, tonsil, middle ear	
X		Vagus carries and distributes fibres from cranial nucleus of XI	Nu: Dorsal motor of vagus cardiac and visceral muscles of thorax and abdomen	Nu: Solitarius from heart, lungs and abdo. viscera	Nu: Solitarius Taste: vallecula and epiglottis; baro/chemoreceptors	Nu: Sensory of V skin of post/inf auricle, ext auditory meatus: pharynx and larynx	
XI	Spinal Nu: Lat roots C1-5 Sternomastoid and trapezius	Cranial Nu: Ambiguus muscles of pharynx, larynx, palate, upper oesophagus via vagus					
XII	Nu: Hypoglossal muscles of tongue except palatoglossus						

PATHWAYS OF PARASYMPATHETIC NERVES ASSOCIATED WITH CRANIAL NERVES

Cranial nerve	Central nucleus	Nerve carrying preganglionic fibres	Pathway and foramen	Site of ganglion	Name of ganglion	Nerve (V) carrying postganglionic fibres	Organs supplied
III	Edinger- Westphal (mid brain)	III via n to inferior oblique	Cavernous sinus to SOF to orbit	Between optic nerve and lateral rectus in apex of orbit	Ciliary	Nasociliary and short ciliary (Va)	Ciliary m for accommodation. Circular m of pupil for constriction
VII	Superior salivary (pons)	NI to VII to greater petrosal n to n of pterygoid canal	IAM to middle ear to MCF to pterygoid canal	Ptergyopalatine fossa	Pterygopalatine	Maxillary n brs (Vb) and zygomatico-temporal to lacrimal n (Va)	Mucosal glands of nose, nasopharynx and soft palate. Lacrimal gland
VII	Superior salivary (pons)	NI to chorda tympani to lingual n	IAM to middle ear to petrotympanic fissure to ITF	Below lingual nerve on hyoglossus	Submandibular	Lingual (Vc)	Submandibular, sublingual and ant lingual salivary glands
IX	Inferior salivary (medulla)	IX to tympanic br to lesser petrosal n	Middle ear to MCF to foramen ovale	Below foramen ovale on n to tensor tympani/palati	Otic	Auriculotemporal (Vc)	Parotid salivary gland
IX	Inferior salivary (medulla)	Pharyngeal and laryngeal branches	Direct to oropharynx and posterior third of tongue	In relevant mucosa			Mucosal glands of oropharynx and post third of tongue
X	Dorsal motor (medulla)	X - Vagus	Cardiac brs in neck then thorax and abdomen	On target organs			Viscera of thorax and abdomen down to transverse colon

Ant = Anterior. Br(s) = Branch(es). IAM = Internal auditory meatus. ITF = Infratemporal fossa. M = Muscle:
MCF = Middle cranial fossa N = Nerve. NI = Nervus intermedius. Post = Posterior. SOF = Superior orbital fissure

CRANIAL NERVES LEAVING THE BRAIN
MOSTLY FROM BRAIN STEM
(Mid brain, pons and medulla)

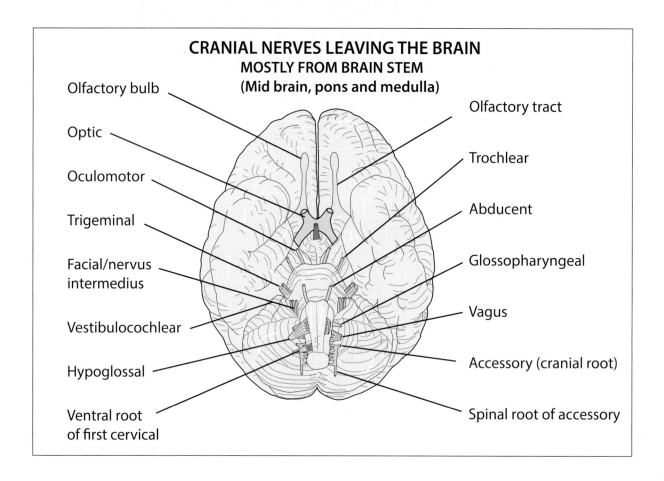

Olfactory bulb

Optic

Oculomotor

Trigeminal

Facial/nervus intermedius

Vestibulocochlear

Hypoglossal

Ventral root of first cervical

Olfactory tract

Trochlear

Abducent

Glossopharyngeal

Vagus

Accessory (cranial root)

Spinal root of accessory

CRANIAL NERVES LEAVING THE BRAIN - 1

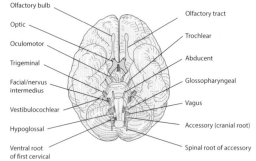

OLFACTORY: Enters brain just anterior to midbrain in region of anterior perforating substance and septal areas. To hypothalamic region via anterior perforating substance and septal areas.

OPTIC: Enters brain just anterior to midbrain to reach lateral geniculate body, pretectal nucleus and superior colliculus for eye reflexes. To occipital cortex.

OCULOMOTOR: Emerges from brain stem, medial to cerebral peduncle.

TROCHLEAR: Emeges dorsally from brain stem just below inferior colliculus and winds around cerebral peduncle just superior to pons. Pierces free edge of tentorium to enter cavernous sinus just posterior to oculomotor. (Nucleus in floor of cerebral aqueduct. Decussates just before emerging).

TRIGEMINAL: Emerges ventral surface of pons, near upper border between pons and pyramid of medulla oblongata.

CRANIAL NERVES LEAVING THE BRAIN - 2

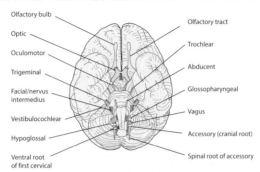

ABDUCENT: Emerges in sulcus between pons and pyramid of medulla oblongata.

FACIAL: Emerges lower border of pons, lateral to recess between inferior olive and inferior cerebral peduncle.

VESTIBULOCOCHLEAR: Emerges in a groove between pons and medulla, posterior to facial, anterior to inferior cerebral peduncle.

GLOSSOPHARYNGEAL: Emerges as 3 or 4 rootlets from upper medulla in groove between olive and inferior cerebral peduncle, superior to vagus.

VAGUS: Emerges as 8-10 rootlets from medulla in groove between olive and inferior cerebral peduncle, below glossopharyngeal.

ACCESSORY: Emerges 4-5 rootlets from side of medulla in groove between olive and inferior cerebral peduncle, below vagus.

HYPOGLOSSAL: Emerges by 10-15 rootlets in sulcus between pyramid and olive.

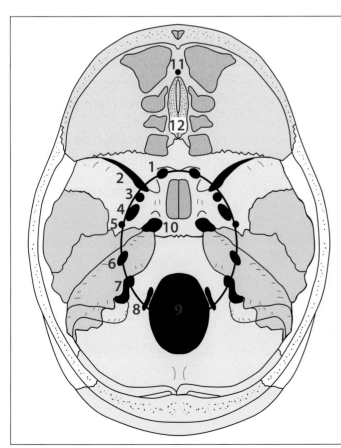

FORAMINA ON AN OVAL LINE

1   Optic canal
2   Superior orbital fissure
3   Foramen rotundum
4   Foramen ovale
5   Foramen spinosum
6   Internal acoustic (auditory) meatus
7   Jugular foramen
8   Hypoglossal canal
9   Foramen magnum

FORAMINA NOT ON OVAL LINE

10   Foramen lacerum
11   Foramen caecum (single midline)
12   Cribriform plate of ethmoid

EXIT FORAMINA BASE OF SKULL

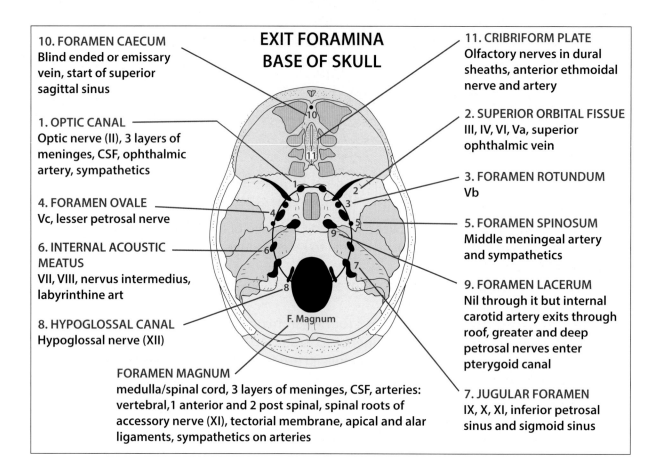

10. FORAMEN CAECUM
Blind ended or emissary vein, start of superior sagittal sinus

1. OPTIC CANAL
Optic nerve (II), 3 layers of meninges, CSF, ophthalmic artery, sympathetics

4. FORAMEN OVALE
Vc, lesser petrosal nerve

6. INTERNAL ACOUSTIC MEATUS
VII, VIII, nervus intermedius, labyrinthine art

8. HYPOGLOSSAL CANAL
Hypoglossal nerve (XII)

FORAMEN MAGNUM
medulla/spinal cord, 3 layers of meninges, CSF, arteries: vertebral,1 anterior and 2 post spinal, spinal roots of accessory nerve (XI), tectorial membrane, apical and alar ligaments, sympathetics on arteries

11. CRIBRIFORM PLATE
Olfactory nerves in dural sheaths, anterior ethmoidal nerve and artery

2. SUPERIOR ORBITAL FISSUE
III, IV, VI, Va, superior ophthalmic vein

3. FORAMEN ROTUNDUM
Vb

5. FORAMEN SPINOSUM
Middle meningeal artery and sympathetics

9. FORAMEN LACERUM
Nil through it but internal carotid artery exits through roof, greater and deep petrosal nerves enter pterygoid canal

7. JUGULAR FORAMEN
IX, X, XI, inferior petrosal sinus and sigmoid sinus

FORAMINA IN THE BASE OF THE SKULL

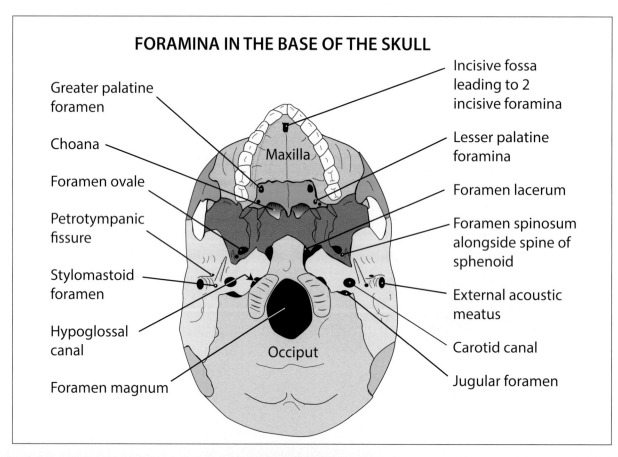

Greater palatine foramen

Choana

Foramen ovale

Petrotympanic fissure

Stylomastoid foramen

Hypoglossal canal

Foramen magnum

Incisive fossa leading to 2 incisive foramina

Lesser palatine foramina

Foramen lacerum

Foramen spinosum alongside spine of sphenoid

External acoustic meatus

Carotid canal

Jugular foramen

Maxilla

Occiput

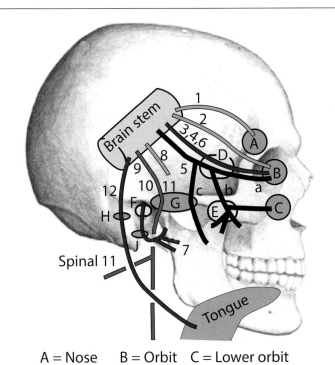

CRANIAL NERVES FROM BRAIN TO END ORGAN

The purpose of this figure is to show how some cranial nerves pass directly to their end organ (1,2,5c,8,9,10,11,12) whilst others pass through well defined cavities such as the cavernous sinus (3,4,5a,5b,6) or the pterygopalatine fossa (5b). For purposes of remembering the likely exit from the skull of cranial nerves, they can be grouped into those that pass to the nose (1), to the orbit (2,3,4,5a,6), to the front of the face (5b) and through the base of the skull (5c,7,9,10,11,12)

A = Nose   B = Orbit   C = Lower orbit
D = Cavernous sinus   E = Pterygopalatine fossa
F = Middle ear   G = Base of skull
H = Hypoglossal canal   J = Stylomastoid foramen

RULES FOR CORTICAL CONTROL OF CRANIAL NERVES

GENERAL RULE FOR CRANIAL NERVES

1st EXCEPTION - LOWER FACE
(spinal nerves also shown as this is the norm for them)

2nd EXCEPTION - SPINAL ROOT OF ACCESSORY NERVE
(to sternomastoid)

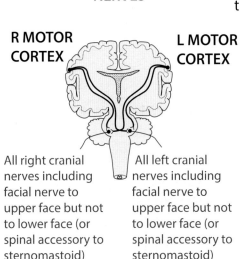

R MOTOR CORTEX   L MOTOR CORTEX

All right cranial nerves including facial nerve to upper face but not to lower face (or spinal accessory to sternomastoid)

All left cranial nerves including facial nerve to upper face but not to lower face (or spinal accessory to sternomastoid)

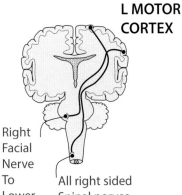

L MOTOR CORTEX

Right Facial Nerve To Lower Face

All right sided Spinal nerves

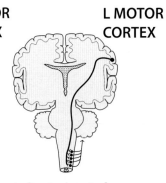

L MOTOR CORTEX

Left spinal root of Accessory nerve (C1-5) to left sternomastoid. Similarly on right

"BILATERAL" (CONTRALATERAL AND IPSILATERAL)

"UNILATERAL" (CONTRALATERAL)

"UNILATERAL" (IPSILATERAL)

PHARYNGEAL (BRANCHIAL) DERIVATIVES

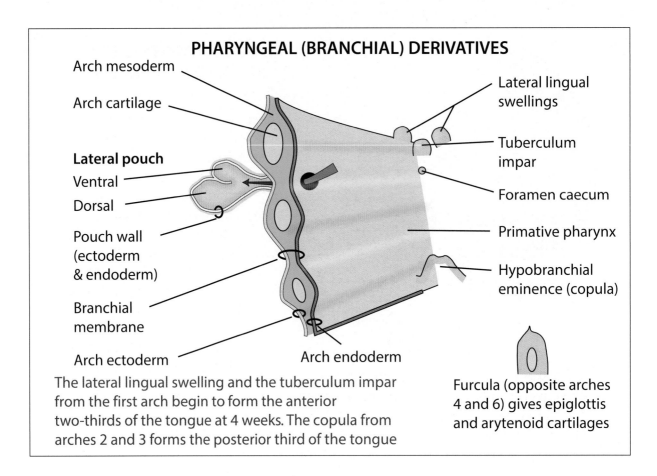

Arch mesoderm

Arch cartilage

Lateral pouch

Ventral

Dorsal

Pouch wall
(ectoderm
& endoderm)

Branchial
membrane

Arch ectoderm

Arch endoderm

Lateral lingual
swellings

Tuberculum
impar

Foramen caecum

Primative pharynx

Hypobranchial
eminence (copula)

The lateral lingual swelling and the tuberculum impar
from the first arch begin to form the anterior
two-thirds of the tongue at 4 weeks. The copula from
arches 2 and 3 forms the posterior third of the tongue

Furcula (opposite arches
4 and 6) gives epiglottis
and arytenoid cartilages

BRANCHIAL ARCH NERVES

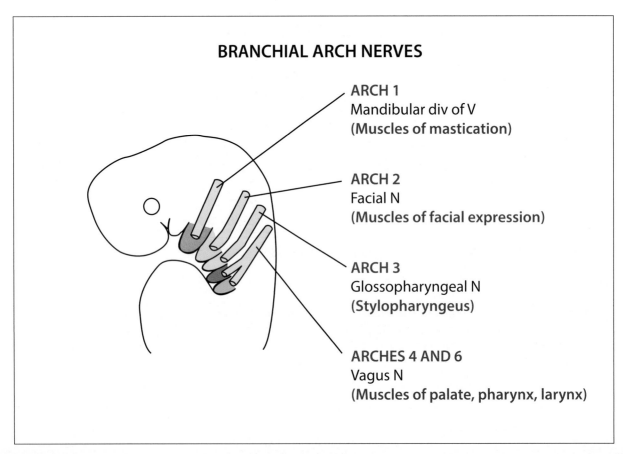

ARCH 1
Mandibular div of V
(Muscles of mastication)

ARCH 2
Facial N
(Muscles of facial expression)

ARCH 3
Glossopharyngeal N
(Stylopharyngeus)

ARCHES 4 AND 6
Vagus N
(Muscles of palate, pharynx, larynx)

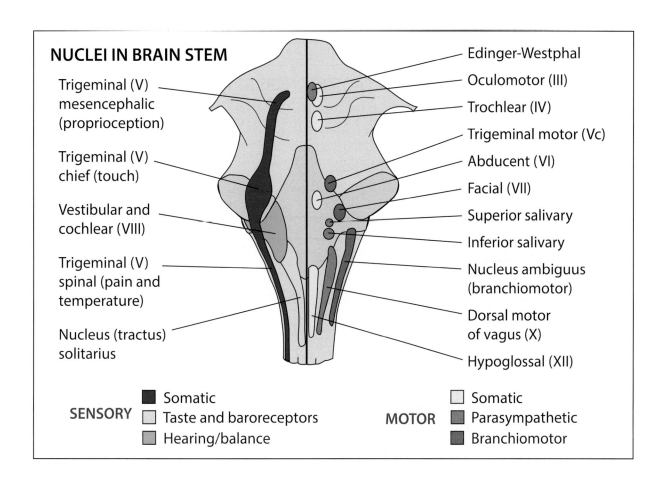

NUCLEI IN BRAIN STEM

Trigeminal (V)
mesencephalic
(proprioception)

Trigeminal (V)
chief (touch)

Vestibular and
cochlear (VIII)

Trigeminal (V)
spinal (pain and
temperature)

Nucleus (tractus)
solitarius

Edinger-Westphal

Oculomotor (III)

Trochlear (IV)

Trigeminal motor (Vc)

Abducent (VI)

Facial (VII)

Superior salivary

Inferior salivary

Nucleus ambiguus
(branchiomotor)

Dorsal motor
of vagus (X)

Hypoglossal (XII)

SENSORY
■ Somatic
☐ Taste and baroreceptors
▨ Hearing/balance

MOTOR
☐ Somatic
▨ Parasympathetic
■ Branchiomotor

5.5 Cranial Nerves I, V, VII

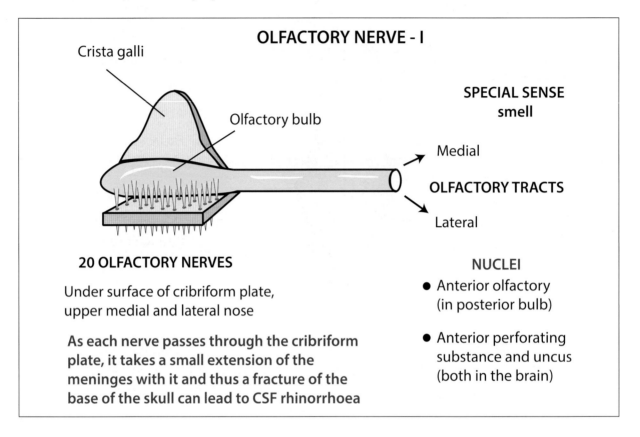

OLFACTORY NERVE - I

Crista galli

Olfactory bulb

SPECIAL SENSE
smell

Medial

OLFACTORY TRACTS

Lateral

20 OLFACTORY NERVES

Under surface of cribriform plate, upper medial and lateral nose

As each nerve passes through the cribriform plate, it takes a small extension of the meninges with it and thus a fracture of the base of the skull can lead to CSF rhinorrhoea

NUCLEI
- Anterior olfactory (in posterior bulb)

- Anterior perforating substance and uncus (both in the brain)

FIBRES IN, AND CARRIED BY, THE FACIAL NERVE - VII

Main Nerve
MOTOR: Muscles of facial expression plus 4 more muscles: stapedius, stylohyoid, posterior belly of digastric and occipitalis

In Nervus Intermedius
PARASYMPATHETIC: Secretomotor fibres from the superior salivary nucleus to be carried in the greater petrosal nerve for "hayfever glands" and in chorda tympani for the submandibular and sublingual glands.

TASTE: In greater petrosal nerve from the palate. In chorda tympani from the anterior 2/3 of tongue. Cell bodies in geniculate ganglion

SOMATIC SENSORY: Small area of skin in external auditory meatus and drum. (Ramsey Hunt Syndrome - recrudescence of varicella (chickenpox virus) giving herpes zoster/shingles). Cell bodies in geniculate ganglion

RIGHT FACIAL NERVE - VII
(in its simplest form to muscles of facial expression)

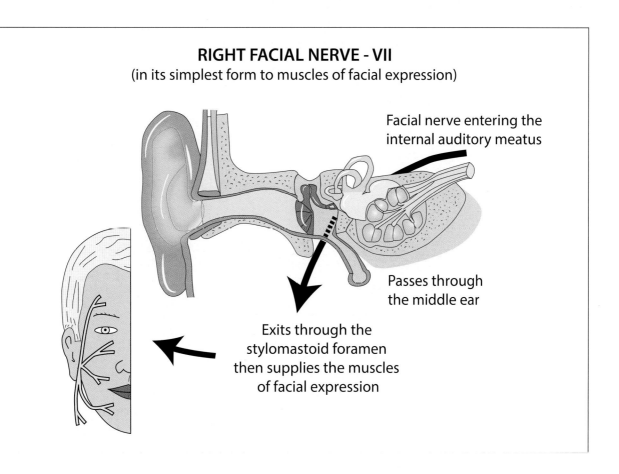

Facial nerve entering the internal auditory meatus

Passes through the middle ear

Exits through the stylomastoid foramen then supplies the muscles of facial expression

FACIAL NERVE - VII

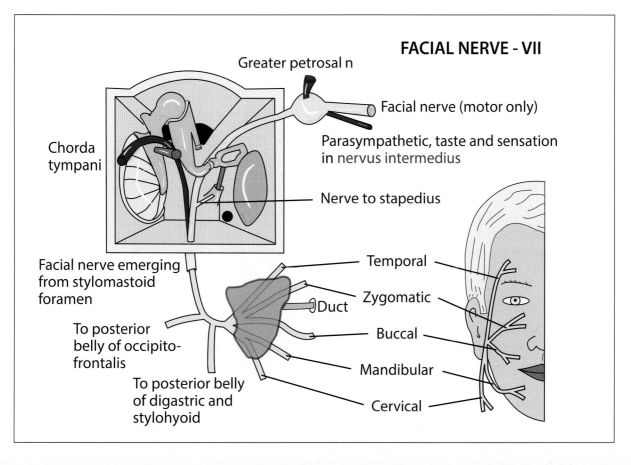

Greater petrosal n

Facial nerve (motor only)

Parasympathetic, taste and sensation in nervus intermedius

Nerve to stapedius

Chorda tympani

Facial nerve emerging from stylomastoid foramen

To posterior belly of occipito-frontalis

To posterior belly of digastric and stylohyoid

Duct

Temporal

Zygomatic

Buccal

Mandibular

Cervical

MUSCLES OF FACIAL EXPRESSION

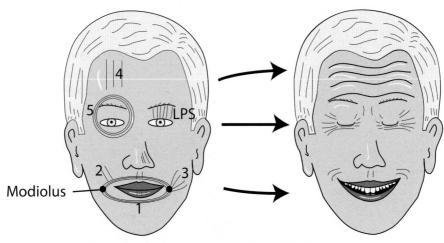

Modiolus

1. Close lips - obicularis oris. Facial (VII)
2. Smile - risorius, levator anguli oris Facial (VII)
3. Blow out cheeks - buccinator Facial (VII)
4. Wrinkle forehead - Frontalis Facial (VII)
5. Close eyes - obicularis oculi Facial (VII)
**Note: Eyes are opened by levator palpebrae superioris (LPS),
not a muscle of facial expresssion (Oculomotor and sympathetic)**

FACIAL NERVE: MOTOR SUPPLY TO MUSCLES OF FACIAL EXPRESSION

Facial nerve branches:
Temporal: Frontalis and procerus
Zygomatic 1: Eye and around orbit
Zygomatic 2: Mid face and smile
Buccal: Buccinator and upper lip
Mandibular: Lower lip and
    orbicularis oris
Cervical: Platysma
(Note: Proprioception is
supplied by trigeminal)

Temporal
Zygomatic
Buccal
Mandibular
Cervical

Mnemonic:
Two
Zebras
Befriended
My
Cat

Bell's Palsy
● Lower motor neurone
● All branches equally affected
● Variable recovery
● Unilateral

Stroke
● Upper motor neurone
● Lower face worse due to unilateral
  innervation

TESTING FOR FACIAL NERVE ACTION IN A NORMAL PATIENT - 1

3 functions are tested separately in turn:

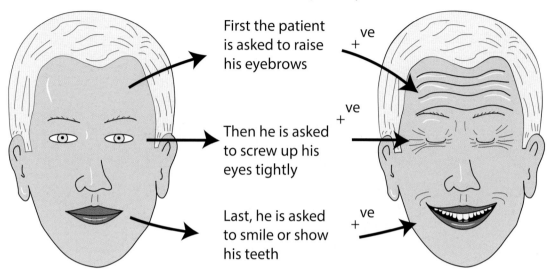

First the patient is asked to raise his eyebrows +ve

Then he is asked to screw up his eyes tightly +ve

Last, he is asked to smile or show his teeth +ve

ALL MOVEMENTS ARE NORMAL AND SYMMETRICAL

TESTING FOR FACIAL NERVE ACTION - 2

3 functions are tested separately in turn:

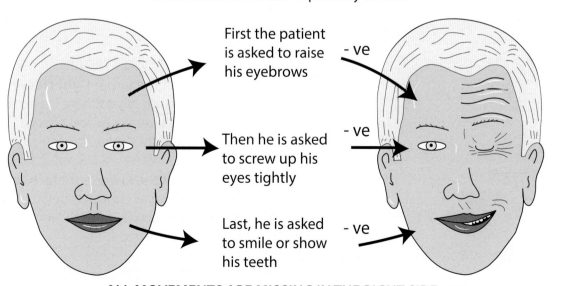

First the patient is asked to raise his eyebrows - ve

Then he is asked to screw up his eyes tightly - ve

Last, he is asked to smile or show his teeth - ve

**ALL MOVEMENTS ARE MISSING IN THE RIGHT SIDE
OF THE FACE INDICATING A "LOWER MOTOR LESION"
TYPICALLY A BELL'S PALSY**

TESTING FOR FACIAL NERVE ACTION - 3

3 functions are tested separately in turn:

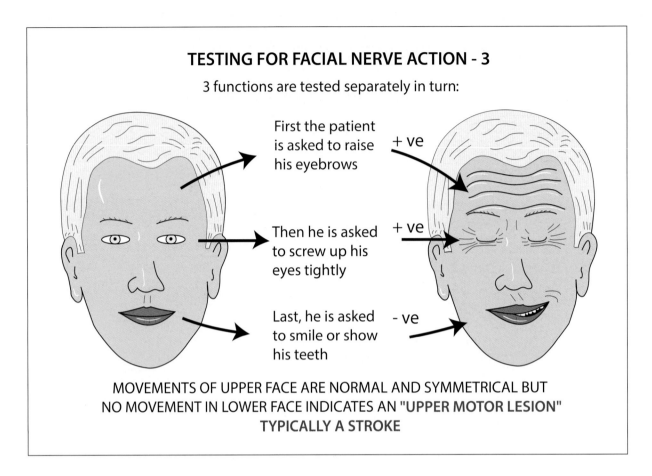

First the patient is asked to raise his eyebrows + ve

Then he is asked to screw up his eyes tightly + ve

Last, he is asked to smile or show his teeth - ve

MOVEMENTS OF UPPER FACE ARE NORMAL AND SYMMETRICAL BUT NO MOVEMENT IN LOWER FACE INDICATES AN "UPPER MOTOR LESION" TYPICALLY A STROKE

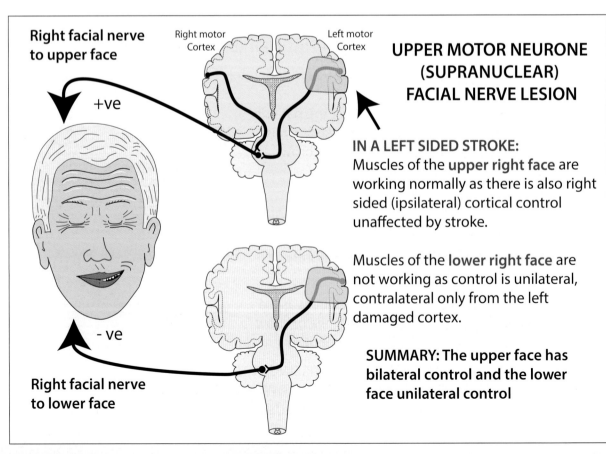

Right facial nerve to upper face

+ve

Right motor Cortex   Left motor Cortex

Right facial nerve to lower face

- ve

UPPER MOTOR NEURONE (SUPRANUCLEAR) FACIAL NERVE LESION

IN A LEFT SIDED STROKE:
Muscles of the **upper right face** are working normally as there is also right sided (ipsilateral) cortical control unaffected by stroke.

Muscles of the **lower right face** are not working as control is unilateral, contralateral only from the left damaged cortex.

SUMMARY: The upper face has bilateral control and the lower face unilateral control

SYMPTOMS AND SIGNS RELATED TO SITE OF LESION IN FACIAL NERVE - VII

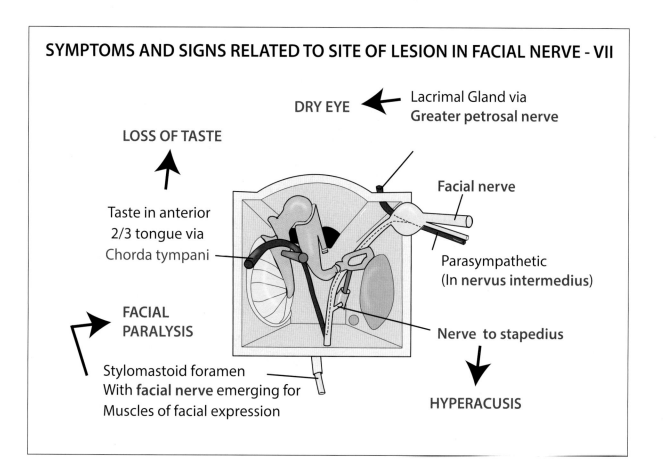

DRY EYE ← Lacrimal Gland via **Greater petrosal nerve**

LOSS OF TASTE

Taste in anterior 2/3 tongue via Chorda tympani

Facial nerve

Parasympathetic (In **nervus intermedius**)

FACIAL PARALYSIS

Nerve to stapedius

Stylomastoid foramen With **facial nerve** emerging for Muscles of facial expression

HYPERACUSIS

SENSORY DIVISIONS ON FACE OF TRIGEMINAL NERVE - V

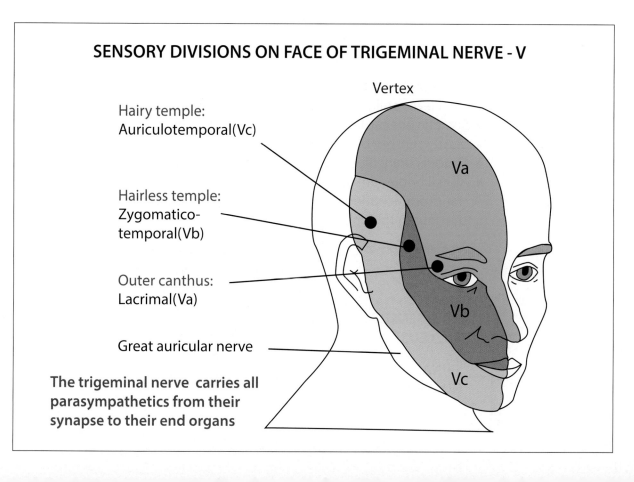

Vertex

Hairy temple: Auriculotemporal(Vc)

Hairless temple: Zygomatico-temporal(Vb)

Outer canthus: Lacrimal(Va)

Great auricular nerve

Va

Vb

Vc

The trigeminal nerve carries all parasympathetics from their synapse to their end organs

SENSORY DIVISIONS ON FACE OF TRIGEMINAL NERVE - V

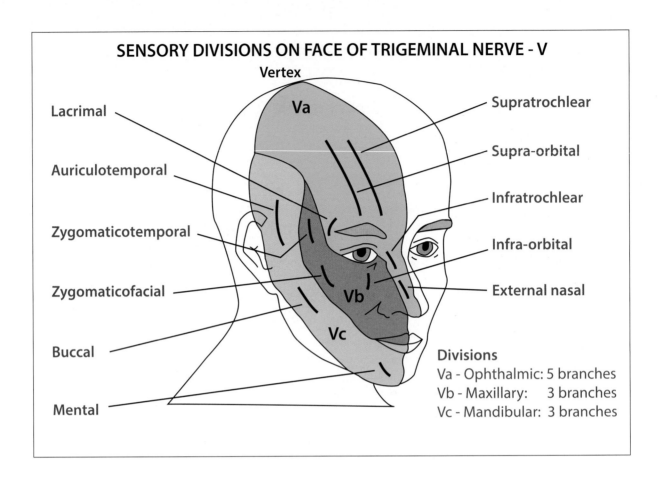

Vertex

Va

Lacrimal

Auriculotemporal

Zygomaticotemporal

Zygomaticofacial

Buccal

Mental

Supratrochlear

Supra-orbital

Infratrochlear

Infra-orbital

External nasal

Vb

Vc

Divisions
Va - Ophthalmic: 5 branches
Vb - Maxillary:　3 branches
Vc - Mandibular: 3 branches

TRIGEMINAL NERVE - V
(Extra notes)

- Nerve of the first pharyngeal arch
- 3 nuclei in brain stem (see below)
- Somatic but carries parasympathetic and sympathetic
- Mostly sensory but small motor branch in mandibular division
- Motor is branchiomotor (special visceral motor)
- All cell bodies are in the trigeminal ganglion EXCEPT
  for proprioception and these are in the mesencephalic
  nucleus in the brain stem

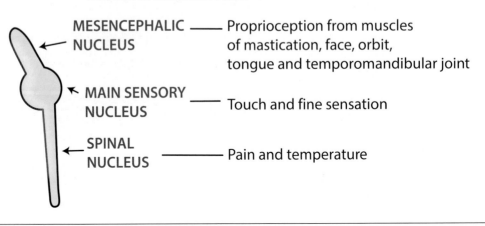

MESENCEPHALIC —— Proprioception from muscles
NUCLEUS　　　　　of mastication, face, orbit,
　　　　　　　　　tongue and temporomandibular joint

MAIN SENSORY
NUCLEUS　　　　　Touch and fine sensation

SPINAL
NUCLEUS　　　　　Pain and temperature

TRIGEMINAL GANGLION

- Posteriorly the ganglion is in Meckel's cave surrounded by CSF then anteriorly it is beneath the dura of the cavernous sinus
- The motor root runs beneath ganglion and exits foramen ovale with the lesser petrosal nerve and accessory meningeal artery, a branch of the maxillary, which supplies the ganglion as do branches of the internal carotid in the cavernous sinus
- The ganglion contains the sensory cell bodies

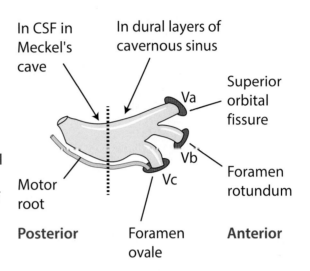

In CSF in Meckel's cave

In dural layers of cavernous sinus

Superior orbital fissure

Va

Vb

Foramen rotundum

Vc

Motor root

Posterior

Foramen ovale

Anterior

TRIGEMINAL NERVE - Vc - MOTOR FIBRES IN MANDIBULAR DIVISION

Muscles of mastication
Close the mouth
Temporalis
Masseter
Medial pterygoid
Opens the mouth
Lateral pterygoid

Four other Muscles
Tensor tympani
Tensor palati
Mylohyoid
Anterior belly of digastric

5.6 Cranial Nerves VIII, IX, X, XI, XII

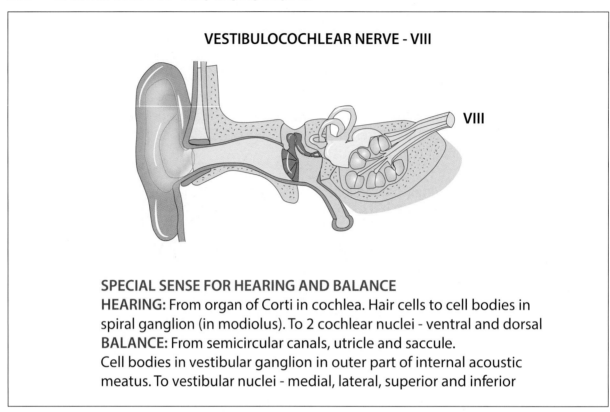

VESTIBULOCOCHLEAR NERVE - VIII

SPECIAL SENSE FOR HEARING AND BALANCE
HEARING: From organ of Corti in cochlea. Hair cells to cell bodies in spiral ganglion (in modiolus). To 2 cochlear nuclei - ventral and dorsal
BALANCE: From semicircular canals, utricle and saccule.
Cell bodies in vestibular ganglion in outer part of internal acoustic meatus. To vestibular nuclei - medial, lateral, superior and inferior

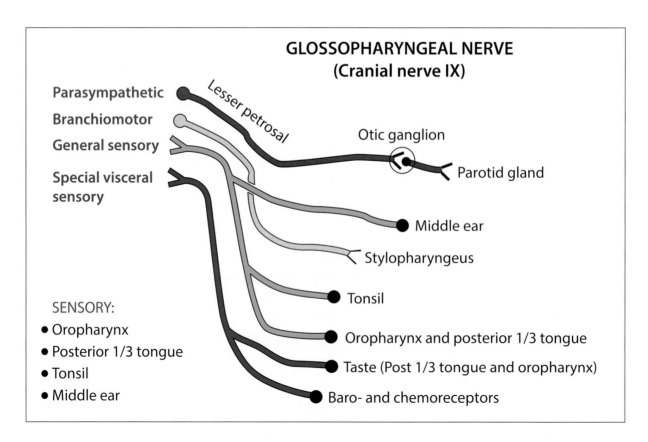

GLOSSOPHARYNGEAL NERVE
(Cranial nerve IX)

Parasympathetic
Branchiomotor
General sensory
Special visceral sensory

Lesser petrosal

Otic ganglion
Parotid gland
Middle ear
Stylopharyngeus
Tonsil
Oropharynx and posterior 1/3 tongue
Taste (Post 1/3 tongue and oropharynx)
Baro- and chemoreceptors

SENSORY:
- Oropharynx
- Posterior 1/3 tongue
- Tonsil
- Middle ear

ACCESSORY NERVE
(Cranial nerve XI - accessory to vagus)

BRANCHIOMOTOR

Cranial root
of accessory

Jugular
foramen

Vagus

Foramen
magnum

SOMATIC MOTOR

Spinal roots
of accessory
(C1-5)

Spinal roots to
sternomastoid and
trapezius

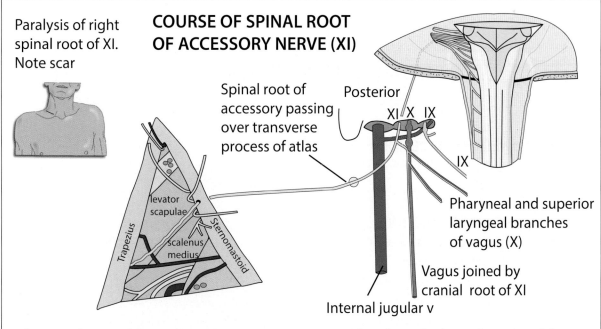

Paralysis of right
spinal root of XI.
Note scar

COURSE OF SPINAL ROOT
OF ACCESSORY NERVE (XI)

Spinal root of
accessory passing
over transverse
process of atlas

Posterior

XI X IX

IX

Trapezius

levator
scapulae

scalenus
medius

Sternomastoid

Pharyneal and superior
laryngeal branches
of vagus (X)

Vagus joined by
cranial root of XI

Internal jugular v

The spinal root of the accessory nerve arises as 5 rootlets from the lateral aspect of the ventral grey horn of C1-5 sections of the spinal cord. The rootlets combine to pass as a single nerve up through the foramen magnum. It then runs out through the jugular foramen with the cranial root. The cranial root joins the vagus and the spinal root passes through the posterior triangle supplying sternocleidomastoid and trapezius.

HYPOGLOSSAL NERVE
(Cranial nerve XII)
SOMATIC MOTOR

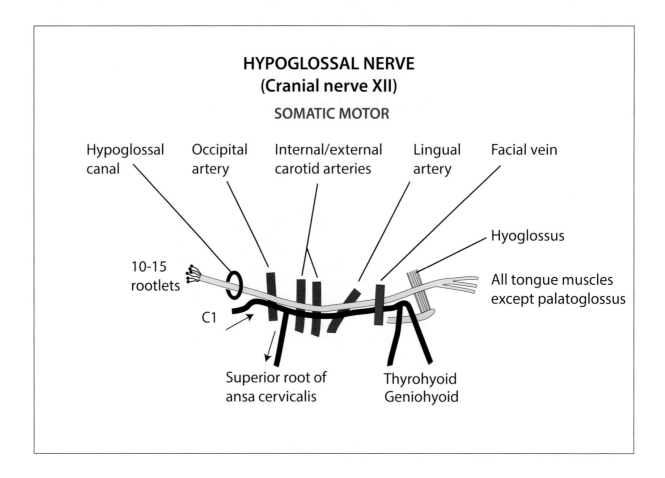

Hypoglossal canal

Occipital artery

Internal/external carotid arteries

Lingual artery

Facial vein

10-15 rootlets

C1

Hyoglossus

All tongue muscles except palatoglossus

Superior root of ansa cervicalis

Thyrohyoid Geniohyoid

HYPOGLOSSAL NERVE LESIONS

LOWER MOTOR LESION
Tongue protrudes towards side of the nerve lesion

UPPER MOTOR LESION
Tongue protrudes away from the side of the cerebral lesion

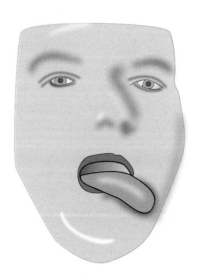

VAGUS EXITING RIGHT JUGULAR FORAMEN 1

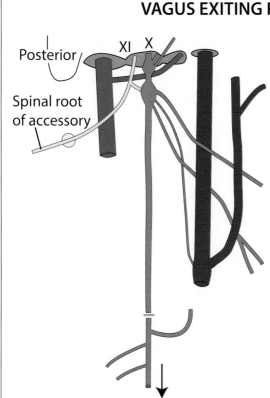

Vagus arises from 8-10 rootlets on medulla. Associated nuclei are:

1. Dorsal nucleus of vagus

General visceral efferent: parasympathetic to smooth muscle of bronchi, heart, oesophagus, intestine to transverse colon.

General visceral afferent (sensory) from above organs.

2. Nucleus ambiguus

Branchiomotor supply to striated muscle of palate, pharynx, larynx and upper oesophagus (these fibres originate from the cranial root of accessory).

3. Nucleus solitarius

Sensory for baroreceptors and taste.

4. Spinal nucleus of trigeminal nerve

All **somatic sensory** fibres in vagus end here.

VAGUS EXITING RIGHT JUGULAR FORAMEN 2

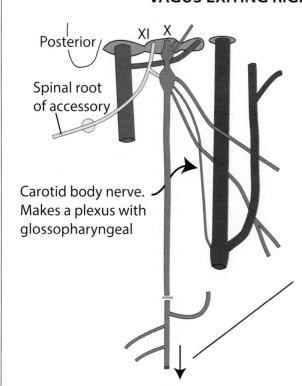

Superior vagal ganglion - cell bodies for:
1. **Meningeal branch.** Sensory to posterior cranial fossa
2. **Auricular branch.** Sensory to external auditory meatus and part of eardrum (communicates with VII)

Inferior vagal ganglion - cell bodies for:
1. **Special visceral afferent** (baroreceptors and taste)
2. **General visceral afferent** (detects stretch and inflammation in heart, lungs, abdominal contents , pharynx and larynx

Vagus continuing

Parasympathetic to pulmonary and oesophageal branches and to coeliac, hepatic and renal plexuses.

Carries **general visceral afferents** from all these organs

VAGUS EXITING RIGHT JUGULAR FORAMEN 3

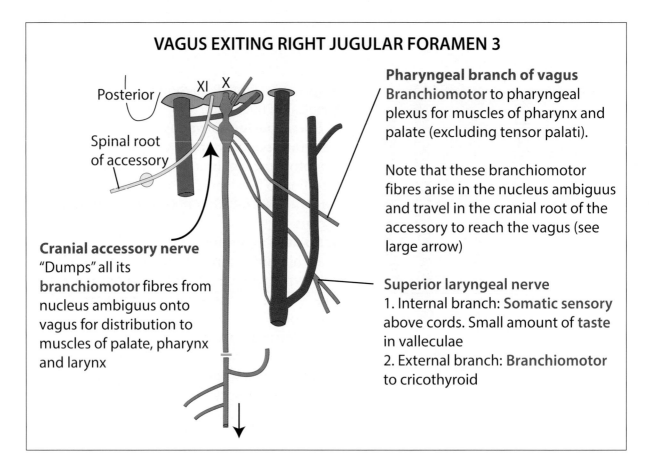

Posterior

XI X

Spinal root of accessory

Cranial accessory nerve
"Dumps" all its **branchiomotor** fibres from nucleus ambiguus onto vagus for distribution to muscles of palate, pharynx and larynx

Pharyngeal branch of vagus
Branchiomotor to pharyngeal plexus for muscles of pharynx and palate (excluding tensor palati).

Note that these branchiomotor fibres arise in the nucleus ambiguus and travel in the cranial root of the accessory to reach the vagus (see large arrow)

Superior laryngeal nerve
1. Internal branch: **Somatic sensory** above cords. Small amount of **taste** in valleculae
2. External branch: **Branchiomotor** to cricothyroid

VAGUS EXITING RIGHT JUGULAR FORAMEN 4

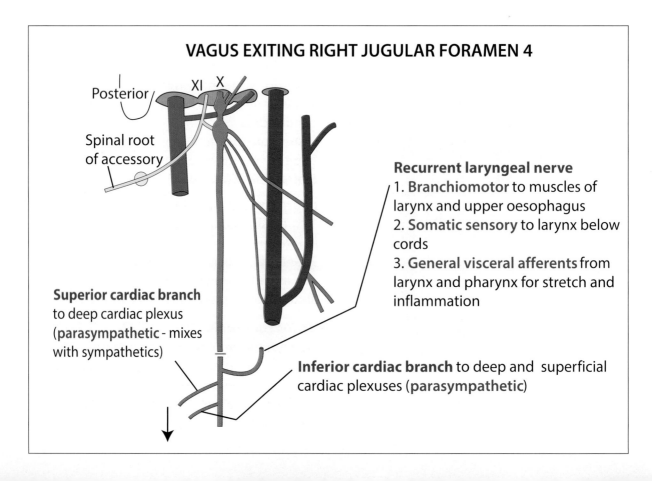

Posterior

XI X

Spinal root of accessory

Superior cardiac branch
to deep cardiac plexus (parasympathetic - mixes with sympathetics)

Recurrent laryngeal nerve
1. **Branchiomotor** to muscles of larynx and upper oesophagus
2. **Somatic sensory** to larynx below cords
3. **General visceral afferents** from larynx and pharynx for stretch and inflammation

Inferior cardiac branch to deep and superficial cardiac plexuses (**parasympathetic**)

SUMMARY OF RELATIONSHIPS AT RIGHT JUGULAR FORAMEN

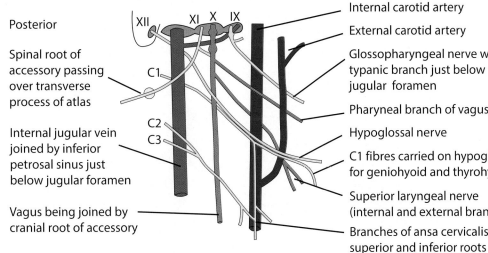

Posterior

Spinal root of accessory passing over transverse process of atlas

Internal jugular vein joined by inferior petrosal sinus just below jugular foramen

Vagus being joined by cranial root of accessory

Internal carotid artery

External carotid artery

Glossopharyngeal nerve with typanic branch just below the jugular foramen

Pharyneal branch of vagus

Hypoglossal nerve

C1 fibres carried on hypoglossal (XII) for geniohyoid and thyrohyoid

Superior laryngeal nerve (internal and external branches)

Branches of ansa cervicalis from its superior and inferior roots

Note:
1. Hyoglossal nerve passes lateral to internal and external carotid arteries
2. Superior laryngeal nerve passes medial to both arteries
3. Glossopharyngeal and pharyneal branch of vagus pass between them

RELATIONSHIPS OF VAGUS AND PHRENIC NERVES

IN NECK

Vagus nerve within carotid sheath

Right

Subclavian vessels

Phrenic nerve emerges from posterior to scalenus anterior to lie on its anterior surface, then off medial edge inferiorly

ENTERING THE THORAX

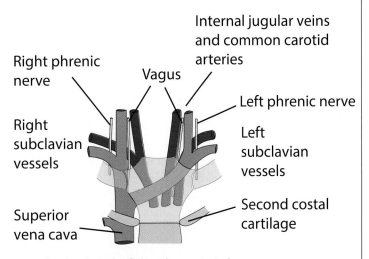

Right phrenic nerve

Vagus

Internal jugular veins and common carotid arteries

Left phrenic nerve

Right subclavian vessels

Left subclavian vessels

Superior vena cava

Second costal cartilage

At the level of the thoracic inlet, both vagus and phrenic nerves enter the thorax between the veins anteriorly and the arteries posteriorly

RELATIONSHIPS OF VAGUS AND PHRENIC NERVES

PASSING HILA OF LUNGS

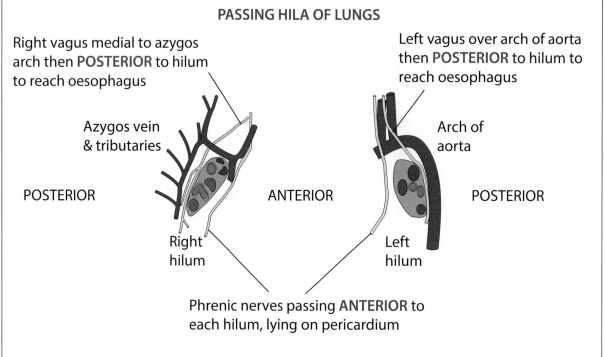

Right vagus medial to azygos arch then **POSTERIOR** to hilum to reach oesophagus

Left vagus over arch of aorta then **POSTERIOR** to hilum to reach oesophagus

Azygos vein & tributaries

Arch of aorta

POSTERIOR

ANTERIOR

POSTERIOR

Right hilum

Left hilum

Phrenic nerves passing **ANTERIOR** to each hilum, lying on pericardium

5.7   Rules and Nerve Supply of Muscles

All Muscles of:	Are supplied by:	Except:	Which is/are supplied instead by:
Pharynx	Pharyngeal plexus (IX, X, sympathetic)	Stylopharyngeus	Glossopharyngeal (IX)
		Cricopharyngeus	Recurrent laryngeal
Palate	Pharyngeal plexus (IX, X, sympathetic)	Tensor palati	Off nerve to medial pterygoid (Vc)
Tongue	Hypoglossal (XII)	Palatoglossus	Pharyngeal plexus
Mastication	Mandibular (Vc)	Buccinator	Facial (VII)
Larynx	Recurrent laryngeal (X)	Cricothyroid	External branch of superior laryngeal (X)
Facial expression and buccinator	Facial (VII)	Levator palpebrae superioris	Oculomotor (III) and sympathetic
Eye	Oculomotor (III)	Superior oblique	Trochlear (IV)
		Lateral rectus	Abducent (VI)
Strap group	Ansa cervicalis	Thyrohyoid	C1 fibres on hypoglossal

Muscles: all	Except
Strap muscles are supplied by ansa cervicalis	Thyrohyoid which is supplied by C_1 fibres carried on hypoglossal nerve
Muscles of mastication close jaw	Lateral pterygoid which opens it
Muscles of mastication are supplied by mandibular division of trigeminal nerve	Buccinator which is supplied by facial nerve
Muscles of facial expression (including buccinator) are supplied by facial nerve	Levator palpebrae superioris which is supplied by oculomotor (III) nerve and sympathetics
Veins: all	**Except**
Veins draining the thyroid gland enter internal jugular vein	Inferior thyroid veins enter left brachiocephalic vein
Palate: all	**Except**
Muscles of palate and pharynx originate outside pharynx	Levator palati which arises from petrous temporal bone within pharyngobasilar fascia
Muscles of palate are supplied by pharyngeal plexus (IX, X, sympathetic)	Tensor palati which is supplied by mandibular division of trigeminal nerve by a nerve branching off nerve to medial pterygoid (Vc)
Eye: all	**Except**
Nerves to muscles of eye pass through tendinous ring	Trochlear (IV) which passes above it
Extrinsic muscles of eye are supplied by oculomotor nerve (III)	Superior oblique which is supplied by trochlear nerve and lateral rectus which is supplied by abducent nerve (VI)
Extrinsic muscles of eye which are supplied by oculomotor nerve turn eye upwards or inwards	Inferior rectus which turns it downwards and inwards

Larynx: all	Except
Intrinsic muscles of larynx lie inside larynx	Cricothyroid which lies on outside of larynx
Intrinsic muscles of larynx close, shorten or tighten cords	Posterior crico-arytenoid which opens them
Intrinsic muscles of larynx open, close or loosen cords	Cricothyroid which tightens them
Muscles of larynx are supplied by recurrent laryngeal nerve	Cricothyroid which is supplied by external branch of superior laryngeal branch of vagus
Pharynx: all	Except
Muscles of pharynx are relaxed until a bolus arrives	Cricopharyngeus which is tonicallly closed but opens as a bolus approaches
Muscles of pharynx are supplied by pharyngeal plexus (IX, X, sympathetic)	Stylopharyngeus which is supplied by glossopharyngeal nerve and cricopharyngeus which is supplied by the recurrent laryngeal nerve
Sinuses: all	Except
Ethmoid sinuses open into middle meatus of nose	Posterior ethmoidal which opens into superior meatus
Paranasal air sinuses are present at birth	Frontal which appears at approximately age of 2 years
Skull foramina: all	Except
Important foramina leaving or entering base of skull from inside, lie on an oval which passes through foramen magnum and lesser wings of sphenoid	Cribriform plate of ethmoid, foramen lacerum and foramen caecum which do not lie on this oval
Pharyngeal arches: all	Except
Branchial arches give rise to several muscles	Third arch which has a single muscle - stylopharyngeus

Cranial nerves: all	Except
Cranial nerves have bilateral control from cortex	Facial nerve to lower face
Cranial nerves leave brain stem (midbrain, pons and medulla)	Olfactory (I) and Optic (II) which are extended brain tissue emerging further anteriorly
Branches of trigeminal nerve (V) enter cavernous sinus	Mandibular division
Cell bodies for taste lie in geniculate ganglion	Glossopharyngeal (IX) and vagus (X) which each have a sensory ganglion just below jugular foramen
Sensory fibres in trigeminal nerve (V) have their cell bodies (nuclei) in trigeminal ganglion	Proprioception which has its cell bodies in mesencephalic part of trigeminal nucleus in brain stem
Fibres in trigeminal nerve (V) pass through trigeminal ganglion	Motor fibres in its mandibular branch
Three main branches of trigeminal nerve (V) have three branches to skin	Ophthalmic branch which has five skin branches
Muscles of tongue are supplied by hypoglossal nerve (XII)	Palatoglossus which is supplied by pharyngeal plexus
Of the hypoglossal nerve (XII) passes lateral to all important structures in neck	Facial vein which passes lateral to the nerve

Autonomics: all	Except
Four parasympathetic ganglia in head supply salivary or mucous glands	Ciliary ganglion in the orbit which supplies eye with accommodation and pupillary constriction only
Postganglionic parasympathetic fibres are carried from their ganglion to their destination by branches of trigeminal nerve (V) which join at a parasympathetic ganglion	In the case of submandibular ganglion preganglionic parasympathetic fibres (in chorda tympani) are also carried TO ganglion by a branch of V (lingual nerve)
Sympathetic preganglionic fibres synapse before leaving sympathetic chain	Unless they are destined to supply abdominal contents or, specifically, the adrenal gland
Sympathetic fibres that pass through four parasympathetic ganglion in head are carried by internal carotid artery or its branches	Sympathetic fibres in submandibular and otic ganglia leave facial and middle meningeal arteries respectively
Other nerves: all	Except
Sensory cell bodies for sensory nerves lie outside the central nervous system	Proprioception for head which has its cell bodies in mesencephalic part of trigeminal nucleus in brain stem
Posterior rami of somatic nerves reach and supply skin	C1, L1, S1 do not reach skin
Nerves leave their intervertebral foramina below same named vertebral body	Upper 7 cervical nerves which exit above their same named bodies. C8 exits below C7 vertebra
Somatic cervical nerves emerge posterolateral to vertebral artery	Anterior ramus of C1 nerve which passes vertebral artery anteromedially

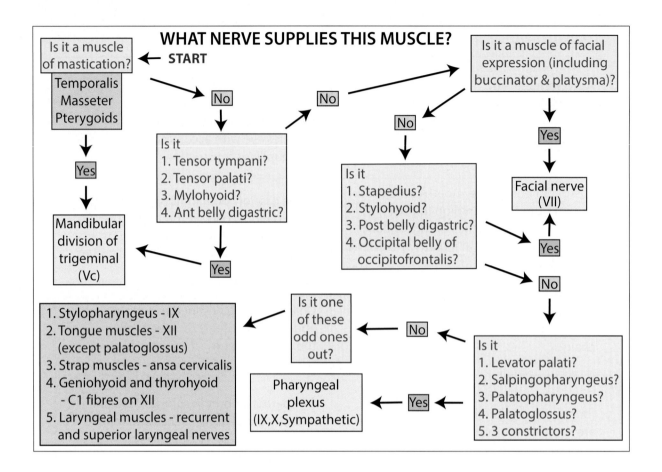

5.8 Eye Visual Pathways, CN III, IV, VI, Autonomics and Oculomotor Versus Horner's

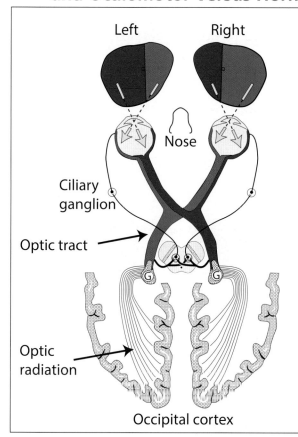

OPTIC NERVE - II

From the lateral geniculate bodies fibres pass in the optic radiations to the left and right occipital cortex where the images arrive inverted (upside down). To initiate rapid reflexes at brain stem level, the incoming fibres from the eye must connect to the mid brain which lies near the optic tracts. These fibres from each optic tracts synapse with both Edinger Westphal nuclei so that all reflexes are bilateral. Parasympathetics from the Edinger Westphal nuclei synapse in the ciliary ganglia and then supply the sphincter pupillae muscles for constricting the pupils in the light reflex.

G= Lateral geniculate body

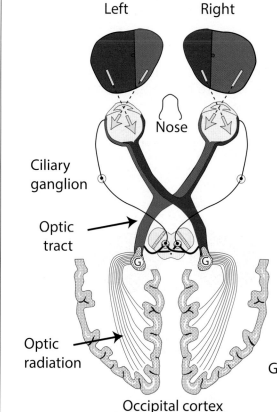

NORMAL VISUAL PATHWAYS

Light is detected on the retina and transmitted in the optic nerves to the chiasma where the fibres from the lateral field (medial retina) cross. The cell bodies are in the lateral geniculate body. Fibres continue to the occipital cortex via the optic radiations.

A small amount of the optic fibres enter the pretectal nuclei in the mid brain which are connected to the oculomotor and Edinger Westphal nuclei bilaterally to enable the consensual light reflex.

G= Lateral geniculate body

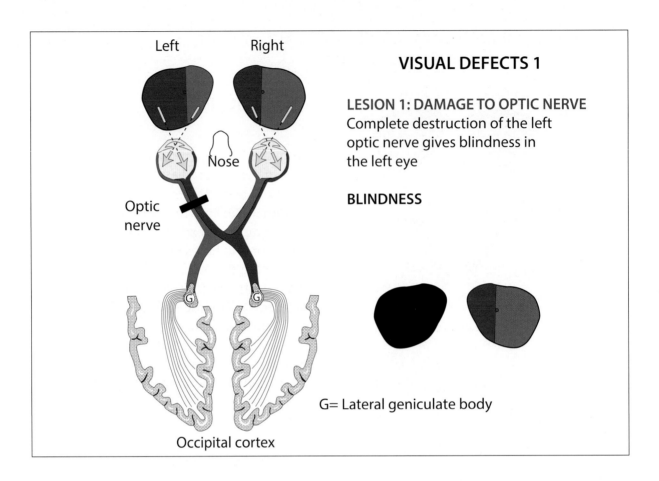

VISUAL DEFECTS 1

LESION 1: DAMAGE TO OPTIC NERVE
Complete destruction of the left optic nerve gives blindness in the left eye

BLINDNESS

G= Lateral geniculate body

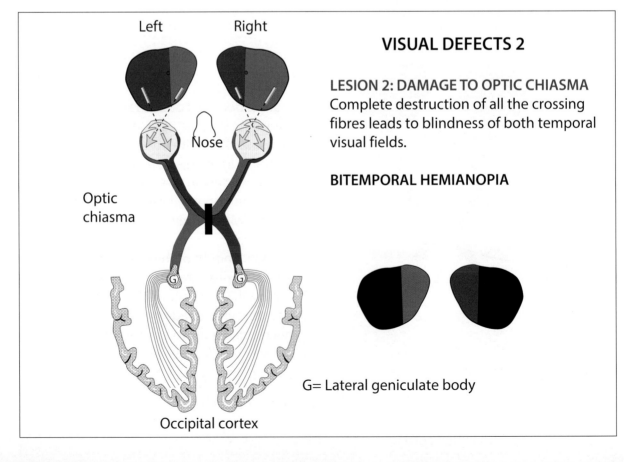

VISUAL DEFECTS 2

LESION 2: DAMAGE TO OPTIC CHIASMA
Complete destruction of all the crossing fibres leads to blindness of both temporal visual fields.

BITEMPORAL HEMIANOPIA

G= Lateral geniculate body

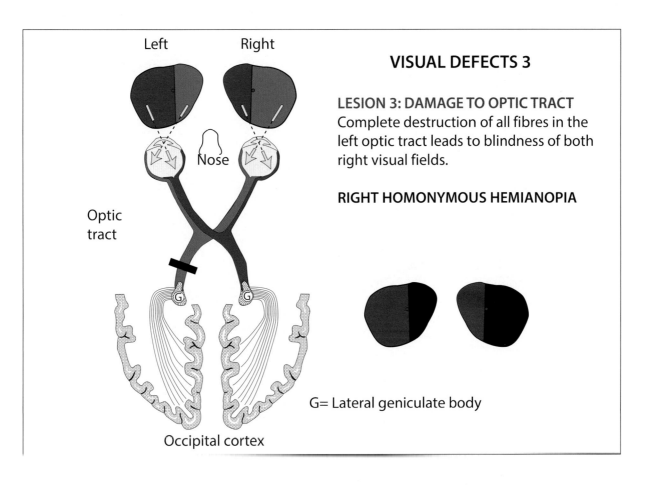

VISUAL DEFECTS 3

LESION 3: DAMAGE TO OPTIC TRACT
Complete destruction of all fibres in the left optic tract leads to blindness of both right visual fields.

RIGHT HOMONYMOUS HEMIANOPIA

G= Lateral geniculate body

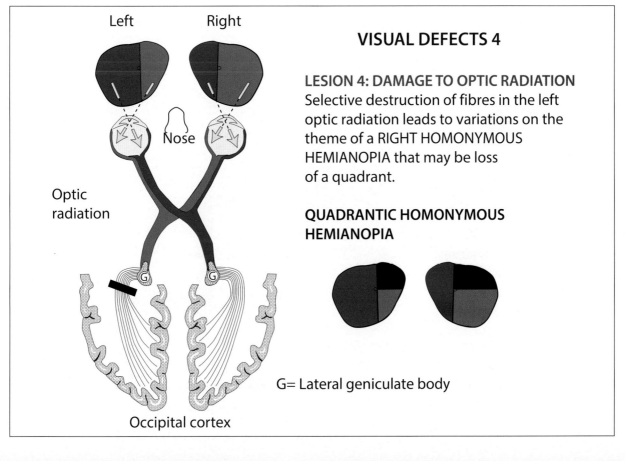

VISUAL DEFECTS 4

LESION 4: DAMAGE TO OPTIC RADIATION
Selective destruction of fibres in the left optic radiation leads to variations on the theme of a RIGHT HOMONYMOUS HEMIANOPIA that may be loss of a quadrant.

QUADRANTIC HOMONYMOUS HEMIANOPIA

G= Lateral geniculate body

NERVES: OCULOMOTOR - III, TROCHLEAR - IV, ABDUCENT - VI

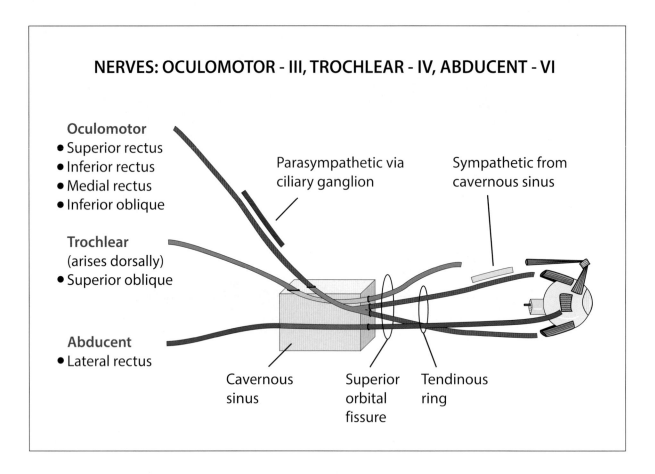

Oculomotor
- Superior rectus
- Inferior rectus
- Medial rectus
- Inferior oblique

Trochlear
(arises dorsally)
- Superior oblique

Abducent
- Lateral rectus

Parasympathetic via ciliary ganglion

Sympathetic from cavernous sinus

Cavernous sinus

Superior orbital fissure

Tendinous ring

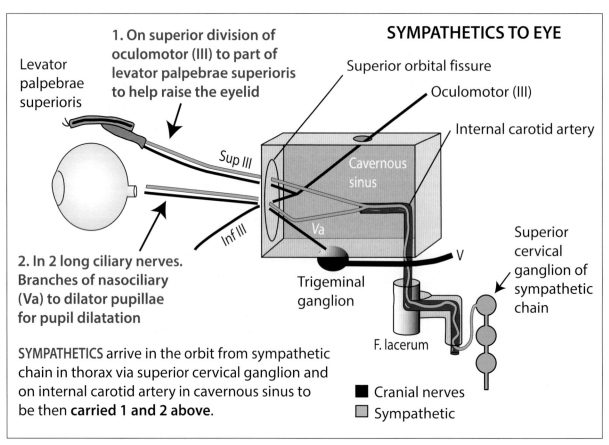

SYMPATHETICS TO EYE

Levator palpebrae superioris

1. On superior division of oculomotor (III) to part of levator palpebrae superioris to help raise the eyelid

Superior orbital fissure

Oculomotor (III)

Internal carotid artery

Sup III

Cavernous sinus

Inf III

Va

2. In 2 long ciliary nerves. Branches of nasociliary (Va) to dilator pupillae for pupil dilatation

Trigeminal ganglion

V

Superior cervical ganglion of sympathetic chain

F. lacerum

SYMPATHETICS arrive in the orbit from sympathetic chain in thorax via superior cervical ganglion and on internal carotid artery in cavernous sinus to be then **carried 1 and 2 above.**

■ Cranial nerves
■ Sympathetic

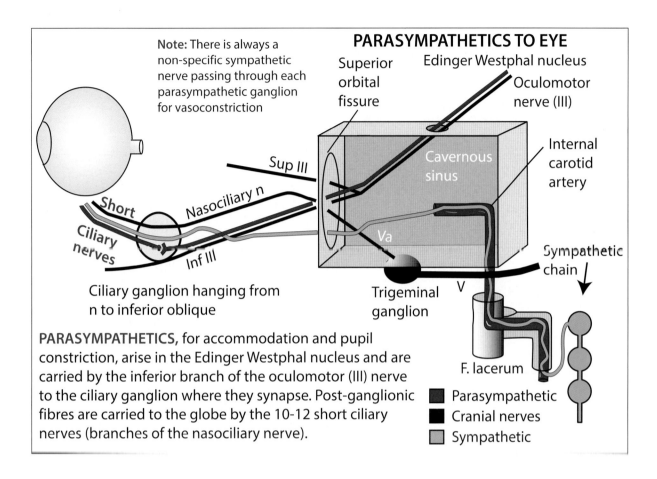

Note: There is always a non-specific sympathetic nerve passing through each parasympathetic ganglion for vasoconstriction

PARASYMPATHETICS TO EYE

Superior orbital fissure

Edinger Westphal nucleus

Oculomotor nerve (III)

Cavernous sinus

Internal carotid artery

Sup III

Short Ciliary nerves

Nasociliary n

Va

Inf III

V

Sympathetic chain

Trigeminal ganglion

Ciliary ganglion hanging from n to inferior oblique

F. lacerum

PARASYMPATHETICS, for accommodation and pupil constriction, arise in the Edinger Westphal nucleus and are carried by the inferior branch of the oculomotor (III) nerve to the ciliary ganglion where they synapse. Post-ganglionic fibres are carried to the globe by the 10-12 short ciliary nerves (branches of the nasociliary nerve).

■ Parasympathetic
■ Cranial nerves
■ Sympathetic

COMPARING HORNER'S SYNDROME WITH OCULOMOTOR LESION

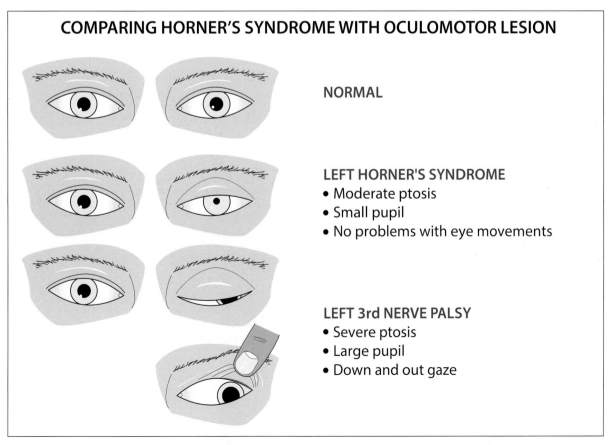

NORMAL

LEFT HORNER'S SYNDROME
• Moderate ptosis
• Small pupil
• No problems with eye movements

LEFT 3rd NERVE PALSY
• Severe ptosis
• Large pupil
• Down and out gaze

HORNER'S VERSUS OCULOMOTOR (III) NERVE LESION

LESION	PUPIL SIZE	PTOSIS	FACE	EYE MOVEMENTS
HORNER'S (loss of sympathetic)	SMALL	YES (mild)	DRY FLUSHED	NORMAL
Oculomotor (III)	LARGE (loss of parasympathetic)	YES (severe) (loss of somatic)	NORMAL	PATIENT LOOKS DOWNWARDS AND OUTWARDS (sole action of superior oblique and lateral rectus)

NOTE: Levator palpebrae superioris needs both sympathetic and somatic nerves to function correctly

5.9   Eye Lids, Orbit, Lacrimal Gland, Retina and Optic Nerve

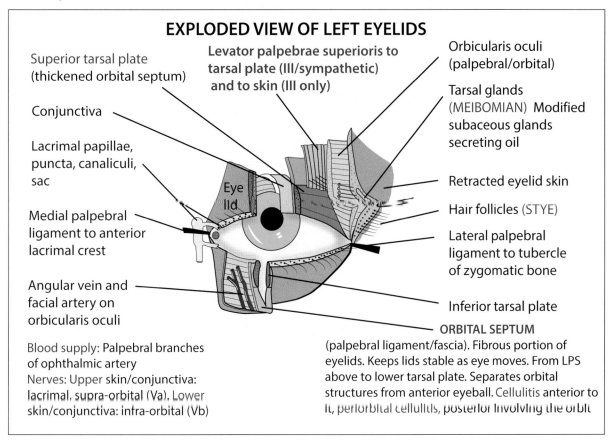

EXPLODED VIEW OF LEFT EYELIDS

Superior tarsal plate (thickened orbital septum)

Conjunctiva

Lacrimal papillae, puncta, canaliculi, sac

Medial palpebral ligament to anterior lacrimal crest

Angular vein and facial artery on orbicularis oculi

Levator palpebrae superioris to tarsal plate (III/sympathetic) and to skin (III only)

Eye lid

Orbicularis oculi (palpebral/orbital)

Tarsal glands (MEIBOMIAN) Modified subaceous glands secreting oil

Retracted eyelid skin

Hair follicles (STYE)

Lateral palpebral ligament to tubercle of zygomatic bone

Inferior tarsal plate

ORBITAL SEPTUM

Blood supply: Palpebral branches of ophthalmic artery
Nerves: Upper skin/conjunctiva: lacrimal, supra-orbital (Va), Lower skin/conjunctiva: infra-orbital (Vb)

(palpebral ligament/fascia). Fibrous portion of eyelids. Keeps lids stable as eye moves. From LPS above to lower tarsal plate. Separates orbital structures from anterior eyeball. Cellulitis anterior to it, periorbital cellulitis, posterior involving the orbit

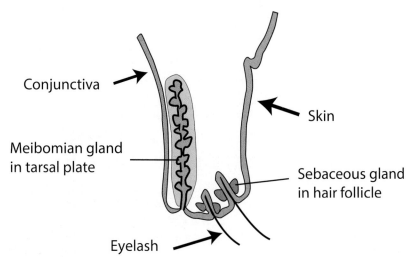

ANATOMY OF STYE AND MEIBOMIAN LESIONS

Conjunctiva

Meibomian gland in tarsal plate

Skin

Sebaceous gland in hair follicle

Eyelash

A **stye** is an infection of the sebaceous gland associated with a hair follicle.

If a **meibomian gland** become infected it becomes a **meibomian abscess**.
If the duct is simply blocked the gland becomes a **cyst (chalazion)**

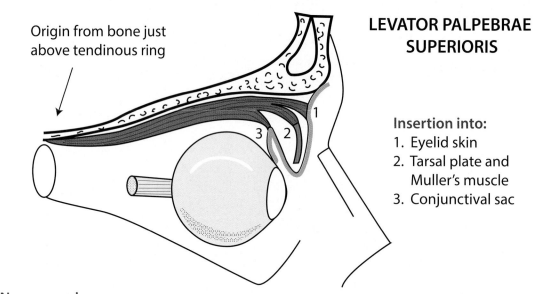

Origin from bone just above tendinous ring

LEVATOR PALPEBRAE SUPERIORIS

Insertion into:
1. Eyelid skin
2. Tarsal plate and Muller's muscle
3. Conjunctival sac

Nerve supply:
- Oculomotor (III) to all three insertions (somatic) so defect gives complete ptosis.
- Sympathetic to Muller's muscle to tarsal plate only (autonomic) so defect gives only partial ptosis.

Note: For levator palpebrae superioris to function correctly both somatic and sympathetic supply must be intact

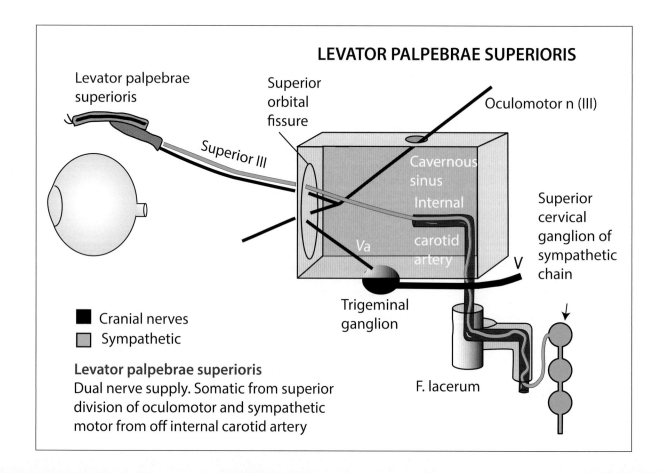

LEVATOR PALPEBRAE SUPERIORIS

Levator palpebrae superioris

Superior orbital fissure

Oculomotor n (III)

Superior III

Cavernous sinus

Internal

carotid artery

Va

Superior cervical ganglion of sympathetic chain

V

Trigeminal ganglion

F. lacerum

■ Cranial nerves
▨ Sympathetic

Levator palpebrae superioris
Dual nerve supply. Somatic from superior division of oculomotor and sympathetic motor from off internal carotid artery

BONES OF RIGHT ORBIT

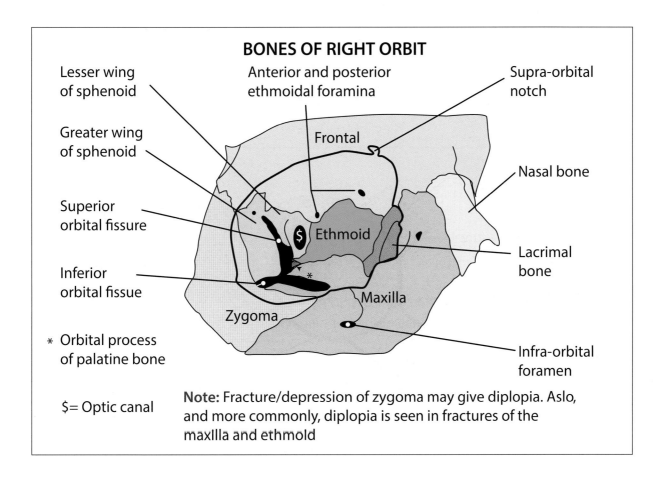

Lesser wing of sphenoid

Greater wing of sphenoid

Superior orbital fissure

Inferior orbital fissue

Anterior and posterior ethmoidal foramina

Frontal

Ethmoid

Zygoma

Maxilla

Supra-orbital notch

Nasal bone

Lacrimal bone

Infra-orbital foramen

* Orbital process of palatine bone

\$= Optic canal

Note: Fracture/depression of zygoma may give diplopia. Aslo, and more commonly, diplopia is seen in fractures of the maxilla and ethmoid

STRUCTURES PASSING THROUGH RIGHT SUPERIOR/INFERIOR ORBITAL FISSURES

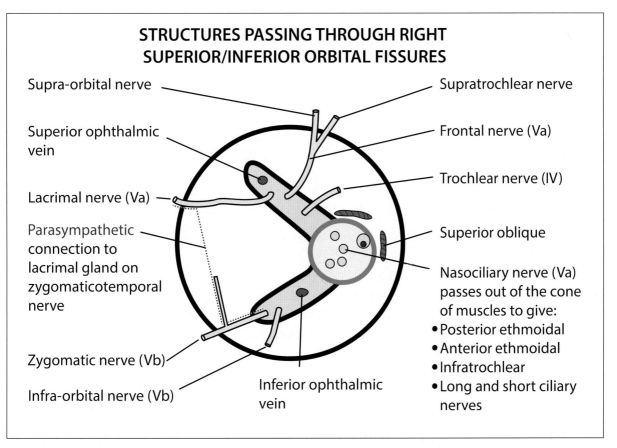

Supra-orbital nerve

Superior ophthalmic vein

Lacrimal nerve (Va)

Parasympathetic connection to lacrimal gland on zygomaticotemporal nerve

Zygomatic nerve (Vb)

Infra-orbital nerve (Vb)

Inferior ophthalmic vein

Supratrochlear nerve

Frontal nerve (Va)

Trochlear nerve (IV)

Superior oblique

Nasociliary nerve (Va) passes out of the cone of muscles to give:
- Posterior ethmoidal
- Anterior ethmoidal
- Infratrochlear
- Long and short ciliary nerves

STRUCTURES PASSING THROUGH RIGHT TENDINOUS RING

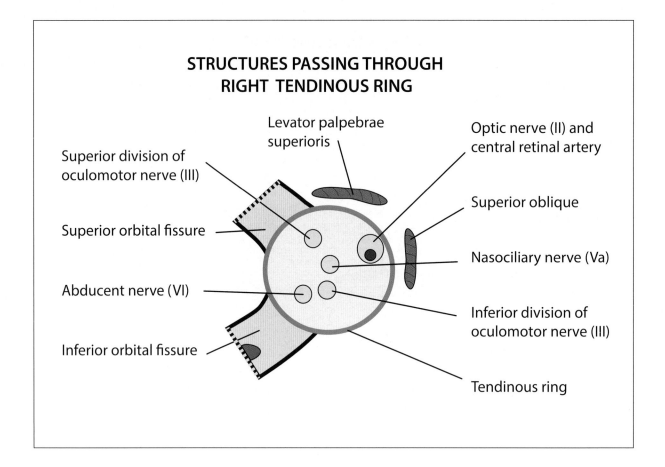

Levator palpebrae superioris

Superior division of oculomotor nerve (III)

Superior orbital fissure

Abducent nerve (VI)

Inferior orbital fissure

Optic nerve (II) and central retinal artery

Superior oblique

Nasociliary nerve (Va)

Inferior division of oculomotor nerve (III)

Tendinous ring

ORBITS FROM ABOVE

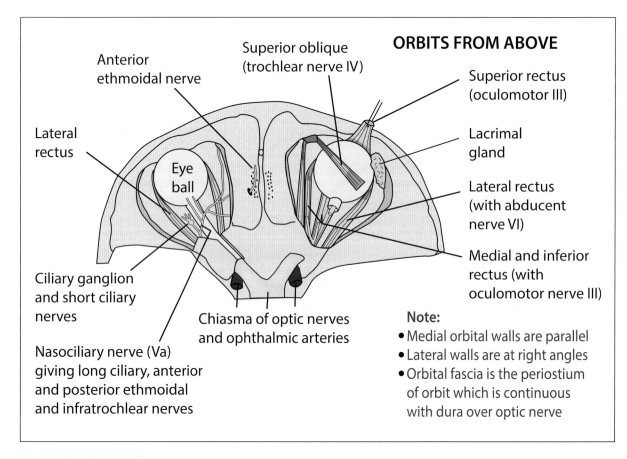

Anterior ethmoidal nerve

Superior oblique (trochlear nerve IV)

Lateral rectus

Eye ball

Superior rectus (oculomotor III)

Lacrimal gland

Lateral rectus (with abducent nerve VI)

Medial and inferior rectus (with oculomotor nerve III)

Ciliary ganglion and short ciliary nerves

Chiasma of optic nerves and ophthalmic arteries

Nasociliary nerve (Va) giving long ciliary, anterior and posterior ethmoidal and infratrochlear nerves

Note:
- Medial orbital walls are parallel
- Lateral walls are at right angles
- Orbital fascia is the periostium of orbit which is continuous with dura over optic nerve

LACRIMAL GLAND

Serous gland in lateral roof of orbit. 10-12 ducts draining into lateral/superior fornix of conjunctiva. Tears swept medially by progressive lid closure.
Blinking: By palpebral part of obicularis oculi (no tear spill)
Screwing up: By orbital part of obicularis oculi (tears spill and lacrimal sac is squeezed)
Lacrimal sac has palpebral fibres of orbicularis oculi inserting into it to open it and to suck in tears. Lacrimal lake lies above it. lacrimal duct is 2cm long, drains into inferior meatus of lateral wall of nose and its mucosal folds are valvular to stop air ascending
Nerve supply: Secretomotor. Superior salivary nucleus to facial nerve to greater petrosal nerve to pterygopalatine ganglion to zygomatic branch of maxillary division of trigeminal (Vb) to zygomaticotemporal nerve to connecting branch in orbit to lacrimal nerve (Va) to gland

Looking down into right orbit

RIGHT OPHTHALMIC ARTERY
(viewed from above)

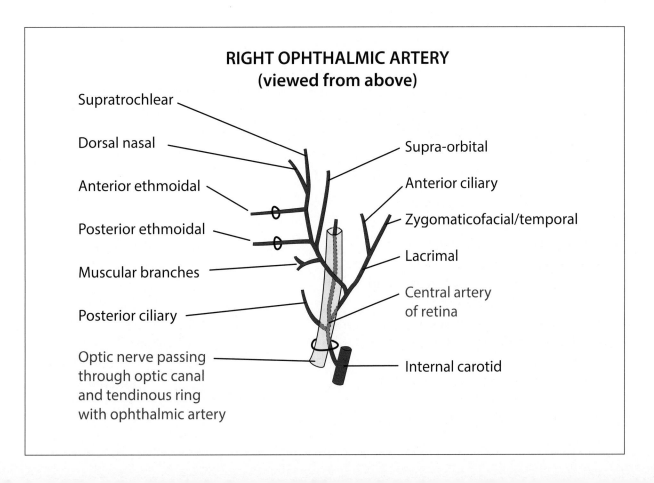

Supratrochlear

Dorsal nasal

Anterior ethmoidal

Posterior ethmoidal

Muscular branches

Posterior ciliary

Optic nerve passing through optic canal and tendinous ring with ophthalmic artery

Supra-orbital

Anterior ciliary

Zygomaticofacial/temporal

Lacrimal

Central artery of retina

Internal carotid

EYE - OPTIC NERVE AND ITS COVERINGS

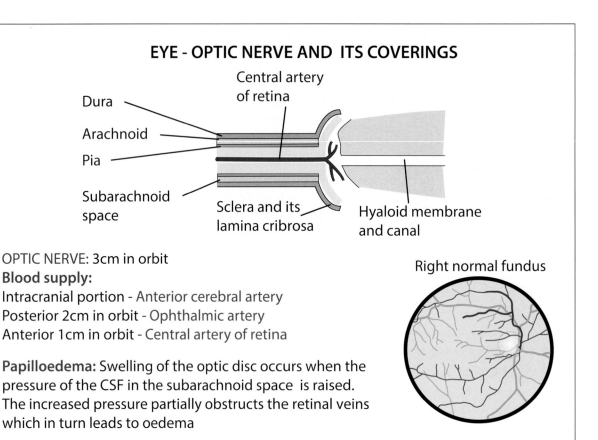

Right normal fundus

OPTIC NERVE: 3cm in orbit
Blood supply:
Intracranial portion - Anterior cerebral artery
Posterior 2cm in orbit - Ophthalmic artery
Anterior 1cm in orbit - Central artery of retina

Papilloedema: Swelling of the optic disc occurs when the pressure of the CSF in the subarachnoid space is raised. The increased pressure partially obstructs the retinal veins which in turn leads to oedema

FASCIAL COVERINGS OF EYE

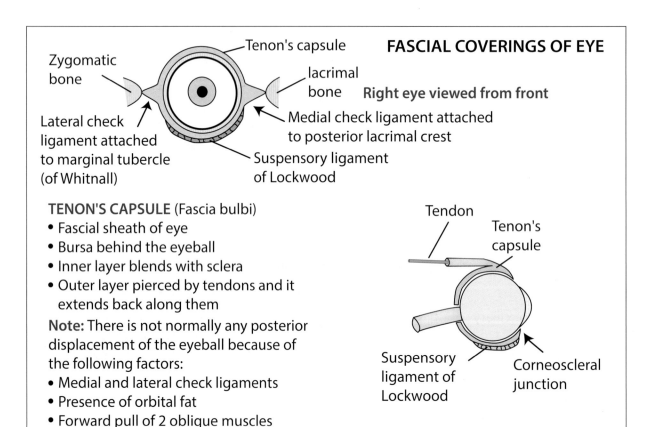

Right eye viewed from front

TENON'S CAPSULE (Fascia bulbi)
• Fascial sheath of eye
• Bursa behind the eyeball
• Inner layer blends with sclera
• Outer layer pierced by tendons and it extends back along them

Note: There is not normally any posterior displacement of the eyeball because of the following factors:
• Medial and lateral check ligaments
• Presence of orbital fat
• Forward pull of 2 oblique muscles

CILIARY BODY AND ANTERIOR EYEBALL

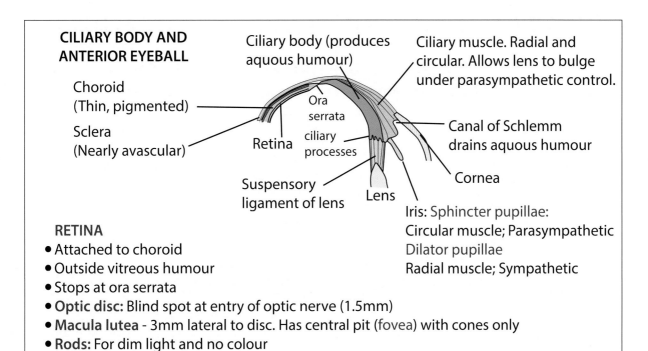

Choroid
(Thin, pigmented)

Sclera
(Nearly avascular)

Ciliary body (produces aquous humour)

Ora serrata

Retina

ciliary processes

Suspensory ligament of lens

Lens

Ciliary muscle. Radial and circular. Allows lens to bulge under parasympathetic control.

Canal of Schlemm drains aquous humour

Cornea

Iris: Sphincter pupillae:
Circular muscle; Parasympathetic
Dilator pupillae
Radial muscle; Sympathetic

RETINA

- Attached to choroid
- Outside vitreous humour
- Stops at ora serrata
- **Optic disc:** Blind spot at entry of optic nerve (1.5mm)
- **Macula lutea** - 3mm lateral to disc. Has central pit (fovea) with cones only
- **Rods:** For dim light and no colour
- **Cones:** For colour. Very sensitive
- **Fundus:** Entry of optic nerve and vessels. Seen with ophthalmoscope at back of eye
- **Blood supply:** Central artery of retina. Central veins to superior ophthalmic veins

5.10 Eye Light and Near Reactions, Eye Movements and Pupil Control

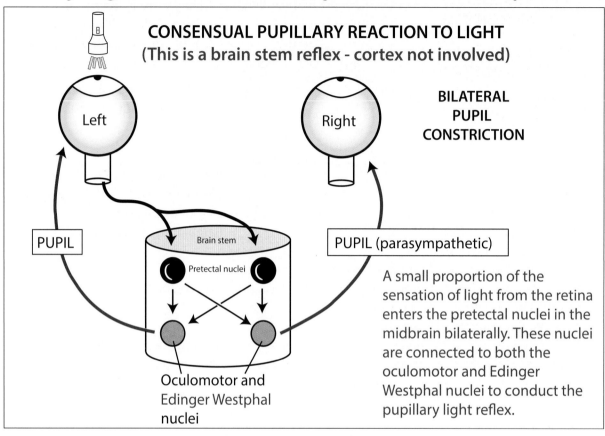

CONSENSUAL PUPILLARY REACTION TO LIGHT
(This is a brain stem reflex - cortex not involved)

Left

Right

BILATERAL PUPIL CONSTRICTION

PUPIL

Brain stem

Pretectal nuclei

PUPIL (parasympathetic)

Oculomotor and Edinger Westphal nuclei

A small proportion of the sensation of light from the retina enters the pretectal nuclei in the midbrain bilaterally. These nuclei are connected to both the oculomotor and Edinger Westphal nuclei to conduct the pupillary light reflex.

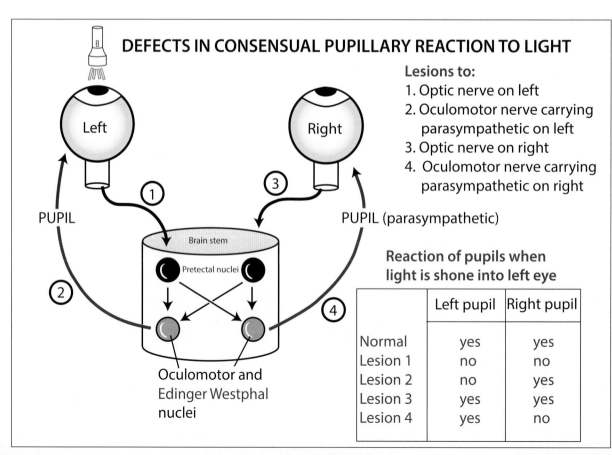

DEFECTS IN CONSENSUAL PUPILLARY REACTION TO LIGHT

Left

Right

Lesions to:
1. Optic nerve on left
2. Oculomotor nerve carrying parasympathetic on left
3. Optic nerve on right
4. Oculomotor nerve carrying parasympathetic on right

PUPIL

Brain stem

Pretectal nuclei

PUPIL (parasympathetic)

Oculomotor and Edinger Westphal nuclei

Reaction of pupils when light is shone into left eye

	Left pupil	Right pupil
Normal	yes	yes
Lesion 1	no	no
Lesion 2	no	yes
Lesion 3	yes	yes
Lesion 4	yes	no

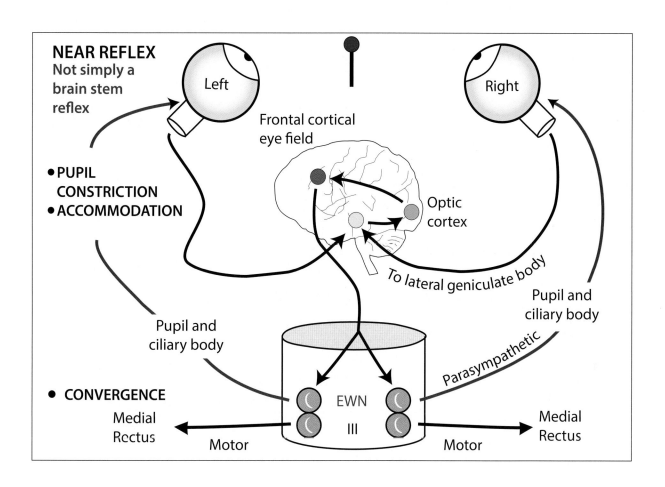

NEAR REFLEX
Not simply a brain stem reflex

- **PUPIL CONSTRICTION**
- **ACCOMMODATION**

Left

Right

Frontal cortical eye field

Optic cortex

To lateral geniculate body

Pupil and ciliary body

Pupil and ciliary body

Parasympathetic

- **CONVERGENCE**

Medial Rectus

Motor

EWN

III

Motor

Medial Rectus

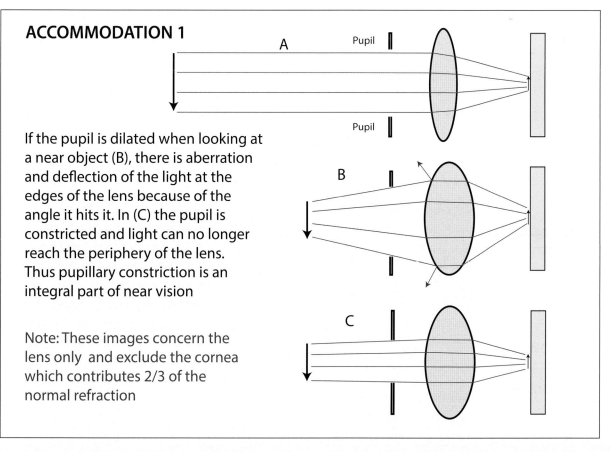

ACCOMMODATION 1

A

Pupil

Pupil

B

C

If the pupil is dilated when looking at a near object (B), there is aberration and deflection of the light at the edges of the lens because of the angle it hits it. In (C) the pupil is constricted and light can no longer reach the periphery of the lens. Thus pupillary constriction is an integral part of near vision

Note: These images concern the lens only and exclude the cornea which contributes 2/3 of the normal refraction

ACCOMMODATION 2

Ciliary muscle relaxed

Ciliary muscle contracting

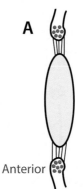

A

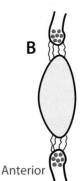

B

When the ciliary muscle is relaxed the suspensory ligaments holding the lens are tight (A) and they pull the lens into its elongated form.

When the ciliary muscle is contracting, as when looking at near objects, the suspensory ligaments are loose and the lens bulges to its natural shape (B). In this bulging state the increased refraction of the light allows focussing on the retina.

During accommodation there is a little diminution of the diameter of the lens and the bulging is predominantly anterior.

Anterior

Anterior

Suspensory ligaments tight

Suspensory ligaments loose

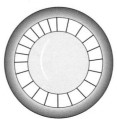

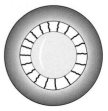

EYE MOVEMENTS PRODUCED BY INDIVIDUAL ISOLATED MUSCLES

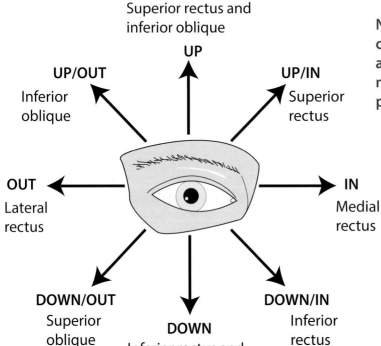

Superior rectus and inferior oblique

UP

UP/OUT
Inferior oblique

UP/IN
Superior rectus

OUT
Lateral rectus

IN
Medial rectus

DOWN/OUT
Superior oblique

DOWN
Inferior rectus and superior oblique

DOWN/IN
Inferior rectus

Note: This is not relevant to clinical testing but simply and indication of what movement each muscle can produce if acting alone

Note: Because of the obliquity of the orbit, the superior and inferior recti pull the eye medially as well as superiorly and inferiorly. Thus the inferior oblique and superior oblique are needed in combination with the recti to move the eye directly upwards and downwards.

CLINICAL TESTING OF EXTRA-OCULAR MUSCLES

Right eye

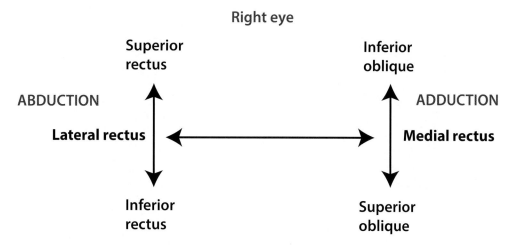

The patient is asked to look inwards (adduct the eye) and whilst adducted, asked to look upwards and downwards. Then these movements are repeated whilst looking outwards (abduction). The muscles that are tested are indicated above. In addition the superior oblique can be tested as indicated in a separate image

OBLIQUE PULL OF SUPERIOR AND INFERIOR RECTI

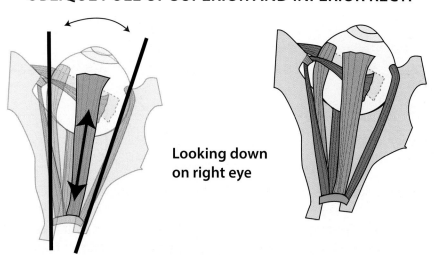

Looking down on right eye

The orbit does not face directly forward but obliquely outwards. This results in the pull of the superior and inferior recti muscles being upwards and downwards but also INWARDS

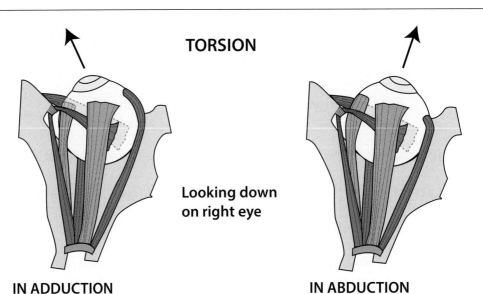

TORSION

Looking down on right eye

IN ADDUCTION

Superior rectus elevates and intorts
Inferior rectus depresses and extorts
Superior oblique turns eye down and out only
Inferior oblique turns eye up and out only

IN ABDUCTION

Superior rectus elevates only
Inferior rectus depresses only
Superior oblique turns eye down and out and intorts
Inferior oblique turns eye up and out and extorts

ACTION AND TESTING OF SUPERIOR OBLIQUE

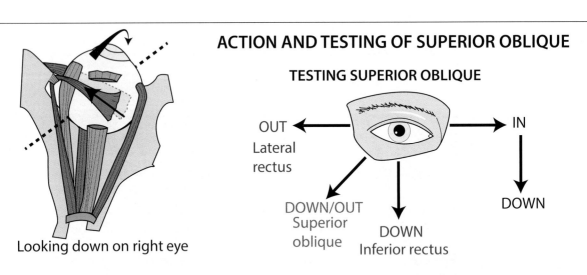

TESTING SUPERIOR OBLIQUE

OUT
Lateral rectus

IN

DOWN/OUT
Superior oblique

DOWN
Inferior rectus

DOWN

Looking down on right eye

Acting alone, superior oblique (S.O.) turns the eye down and out. But it cannot be tested by asking the patient to look down and out because a combination of lateral and inferior rectus could also achieve this. These muscle are negated by turning the eye inwards and downwards. When the eye is thus turned the only muscle that can turn the eye down is superior oblique.

Clinically S.O. is tested by tilting the head. If the right S.O. is not functioning, tilting to the right provokes vertical double vision. This diplopia should be counteracted by intorsion mediated by superior rectus and S.O. If S.O. is defective, superior rectus causes excessive elevation resulting in diplopia.

EXTRINSIC EYE MUSCLES OF THE
RIGHT EYE IN POSTERIOR ORBIT

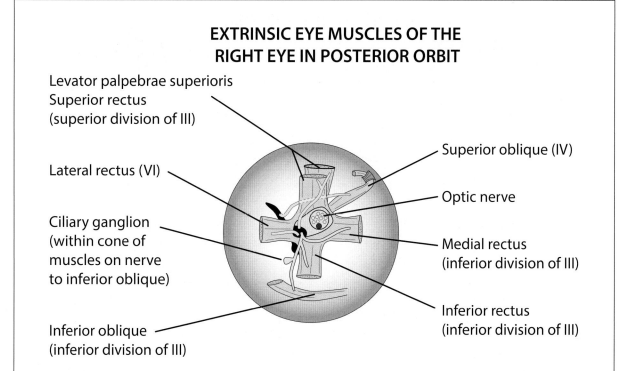

Levator palpebrae superioris
Superior rectus
(superior division of III)

Lateral rectus (VI)

Ciliary ganglion
(within cone of
muscles on nerve
to inferior oblique)

Inferior oblique
(inferior division of III)

Superior oblique (IV)

Optic nerve

Medial rectus
(inferior division of III)

Inferior rectus
(inferior division of III)

HORNER'S SYNDROME

Left Horner's Syndrome
• Ptosis
• Small pupil
• Dry flushed face
• Apparent enophthalmos

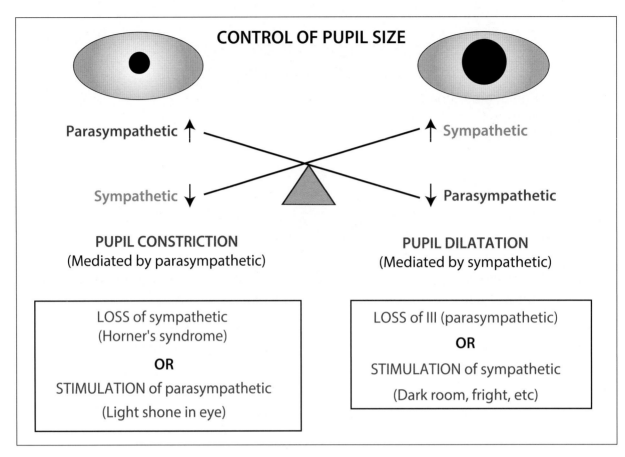

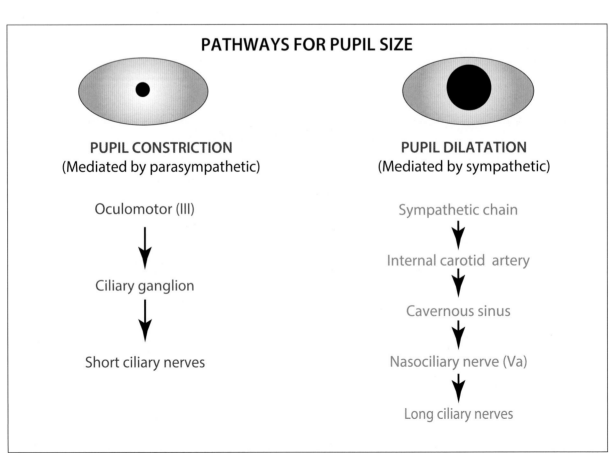

SIZE OF PUPIL AND REACTION TO LIGHT

CAUSES

SMALL PUPIL
normal reaction to light

Old age; Horner's syndrome; Pontine lesion

SMALL PUPIL
impaired reaction to light

Opiates; pilocarpine drops for glaucoma; diabetes; Argyll-Robertson pupil of neurosyphilis (accommodation but no reaction to light)

LARGE PUPIL
normal reaction to light

Normal finding in children

LARGE PUPIL
impaired reaction to light

Atropine drops; Optic and oculomotor nerve lesions; Holmes Adie pupil (myotonic pupil with slow contriction to light and slow dilatation in dark); post anoxia

5.11   Outer, Middle and Inner Ear

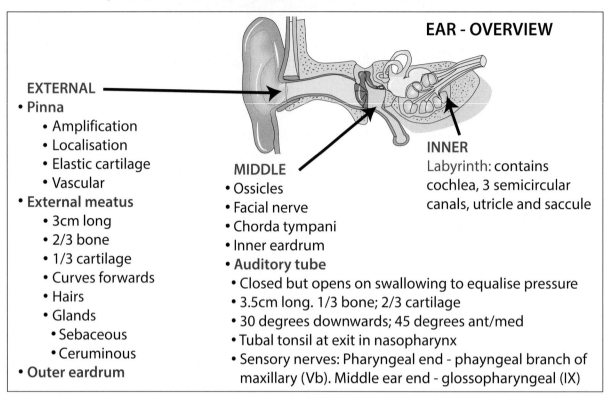

EAR - OVERVIEW

EXTERNAL
• Pinna
   • Amplification
   • Localisation
   • Elastic cartilage
   • Vascular
• External meatus
   • 3cm long
   • 2/3 bone
   • 1/3 cartilage
   • Curves forwards
   • Hairs
   • Glands
      • Sebaceous
      • Ceruminous
• Outer eardrum

MIDDLE
• Ossicles
• Facial nerve
• Chorda tympani
• Inner eardrum
• **Auditory tube**
 • Closed but opens on swallowing to equalise pressure
 • 3.5cm long. 1/3 bone; 2/3 cartilage
 • 30 degrees downwards; 45 degrees ant/med
 • Tubal tonsil at exit in nasopharynx
 • Sensory nerves: Pharyngeal end - phayngeal branch of maxillary (Vb). Middle ear end - glossopharyngeal (IX)

INNER
Labyrinth: contains cochlea, 3 semicircular canals, utricle and saccule

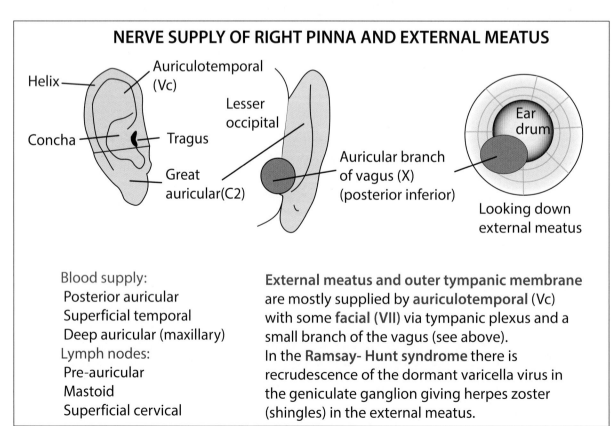

NERVE SUPPLY OF RIGHT PINNA AND EXTERNAL MEATUS

Helix

Auriculotemporal (Vc)

Concha

Tragus

Lesser occipital

Great auricular(C2)

Auricular branch of vagus (X) (posterior inferior)

Ear drum

Looking down external meatus

Blood supply:
   Posterior auricular
   Superficial temporal
   Deep auricular (maxillary)
Lymph nodes:
   Pre-auricular
   Mastoid
   Superficial cervical

External meatus and outer tympanic membrane are mostly supplied by **auriculotemporal** (Vc) with some **facial (VII)** via tympanic plexus and a small branch of the vagus (see above).
In the **Ramsay- Hunt syndrome** there is recrudescence of the dormant varicella virus in the geniculate ganglion giving herpes zoster (shingles) in the external meatus.

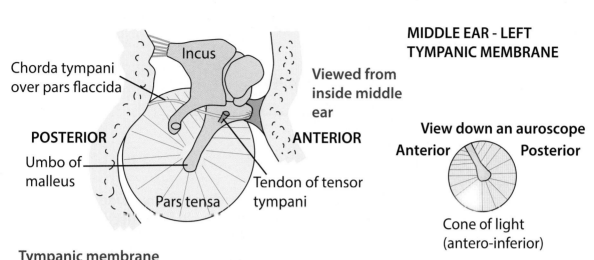

MIDDLE EAR - LEFT TYMPANIC MEMBRANE

Viewed from inside middle ear

View down an auroscope

Anterior   Posterior

Cone of light (antero-inferior)

Tympanic membrane
- 1cm diameter. Pearly grey and shiny
- **3 layers: Inner:** Mucosal surface of low columnar epithelium embryologically from first pouch. **Middle:** Fibrous. **Outer:** Squamous surface embryologically from first cleft.
- 55 degrees to horizontal. Concave outwards. Faces downwards, forwards and laterally
- Pulled inwards by tensor tympani
- **Sensory supply: Inner** - glossopharyngeal (IX). **Outer** - auriculotemporal (Vc)
- Vibrates with incoming sound. Needs equal air pressure on each side of it

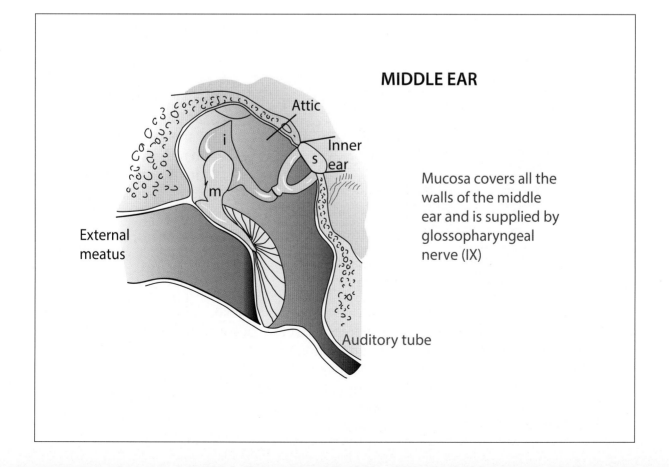

MIDDLE EAR

Mucosa covers all the walls of the middle ear and is supplied by glossopharyngeal nerve (IX)

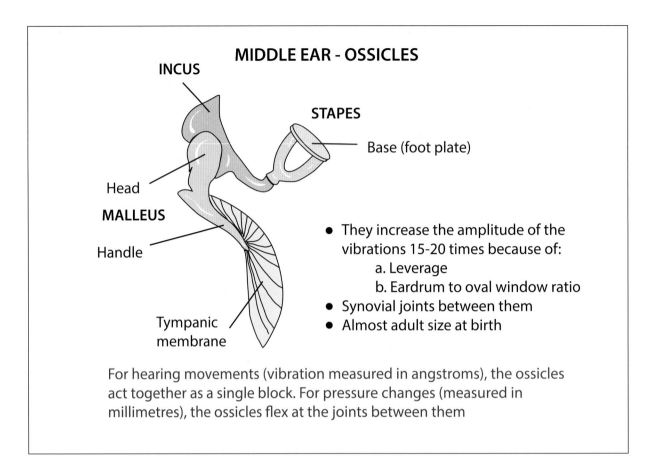

MIDDLE EAR - OSSICLES

INCUS

STAPES

Base (foot plate)

Head

MALLEUS

Handle

Tympanic
membrane

- They increase the amplitude of the
  vibrations 15-20 times because of:
    - a. Leverage
    - b. Eardrum to oval window ratio
- Synovial joints between them
- Almost adult size at birth

For hearing movements (vibration measured in angstroms), the ossicles
act together as a single block. For pressure changes (measured in
millimetres), the ossicles flex at the joints between them

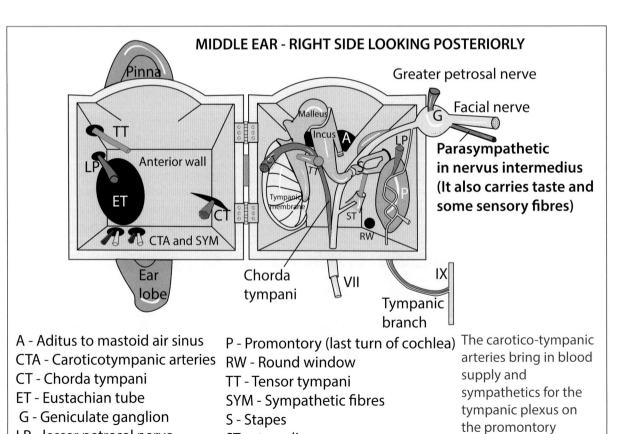

MIDDLE EAR - RIGHT SIDE LOOKING POSTERIORLY

Pinna

Greater petrosal nerve

Facial nerve

Malleus

Incus

A

LP

G

TT

LP

**Parasympathetic
in nervus intermedius
(It also carries taste and
some sensory fibres)**

Anterior wall

ET

TT

S

P

Tympanic
membrane

ST

RW

CT

CTA and SYM

Ear
lobe

Chorda
tympani

VII

IX

Tympanic
branch

A - Aditus to mastoid air sinus
CTA - Caroticotympanic arteries
CT - Chorda tympani
ET - Eustachian tube
 G - Geniculate ganglion
LP - lesser petrosal nerve

P - Promontory (last turn of cochlea)
RW - Round window
TT - Tensor tympani
SYM - Sympathetic fibres
S - Stapes
ST - stapedius

The carotico-tympanic
arteries bring in blood
supply and
sympathetics for the
tympanic plexus on
the promontory

MIDDLE EAR - AUDITORY (EUSTACHIAN) TUBE

NOTES
- 3-3.5cm long. Develops from 1st pharyngeal pouch
- **Arterial supply:** Ascending pharyngeal and middle meningeal
- **Angles:** 30 degrees downwards, 45 degrees anteromedially
- Tubal tonsil at exit in nasopharynx
- 1/3 bone: 2/3 cartilage
- **Opens:** On swallowing to equalise pressure
- **Mucosa:** Valve- like
- **Sensation: Lower part:** Pharyngeal branch of maxillary nerve (Vb). **Upper part:** Glossopharyngeal (IX) (hence referred pain to middle ear from tonsils and oropharynx)
- **Columnar epithelium:** Bony part in petrous temporal bone
- **Ciliated columnar epithelium:** Cartilaginous part in squamotympanic fissure
- **Muscles for opening:** Salpingopharyngeus, levator palati, tensor palati

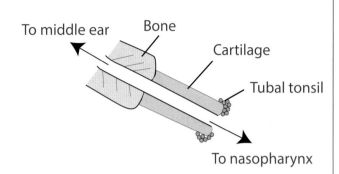

MIDDLE EAR - AUDITORY (EUSTACHIAN) TUBE - EFFECT OF BLOCKAGE

Eardrum Normal concavity

External meatus

Normal air absorption

P

P

Mastoid air cells

Middle ear

Normal air in and out on swallowing/ yawning

Eardrum about to burst

P

P

Bacteria in

Pus

Pus

Blocked tube (eg virus)

Effects of blocked auditory tube:
1. At first air is still absorbed - drum sucked in more. 2. Giving poor ossicle/drum movement - deafness. 3. Then viral/bacterial exudate becomes infected. 4. Middle ear +/- mastoid air cells fill with pus (otitis media). 5. Then pressure rises - drum bulges outwards, may burst. 6. Infection may spread to - inner ear, venous sinuses, extradural, subdural, meninges, brain abscess.
7. **THEN EITHER:**
a. Drains and heals or b. Becomes chronic, +/- glue ear or cholesteatoma or c. Persistent perforation of drum, +/- necrosis of ossicles

RINNE TEST FOR INDIVIDUAL EAR DEAFNESS

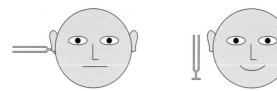

To compare AIR to BONE conduction in the RIGHT ear, the vibrating tuning fork is held first against the mastoid bone, then outside the external meatus. The patient is asked which position produces the louder sound. If it is louder at the meatus then AIR conduction (AC) is better than BONE conduction (BC). The RINNE test is positive. The Rinne test will be positive both in a patient with normal hearing and in a patient with sensori-neural loss

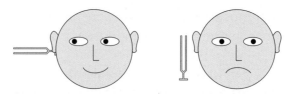

In **CONDUCTIVE LOSS** sound is heard louder via BONE than in AIR. Rinne negative

WEBER TEST FOR WHEN THERE IS DEAFNESS IN ONLY ONE EAR

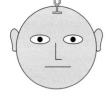

The vibrating tuning fork is placed on the patient's forehead in the midline and asked in which ear the sound is louder

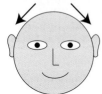

The normal response is to hear equally in the two ears

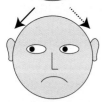

If there is a **CONDUCTIVE LOSS** in the RIGHT ear, the sound will be heard louder in the RIGHT (deaf) ear by passing through bone to the inner ear, free of any ambient (background) noise. The likely explanation is that an ear with a conductive deafness is protected from any ambient sounds whereas the other ear is not.

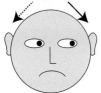

If the patient has a **SENSORI-NEURAL LOSS** in the RIGHT ear the sound will be heard louder in the normal ear

INNER EAR - BONY LABYRINTH

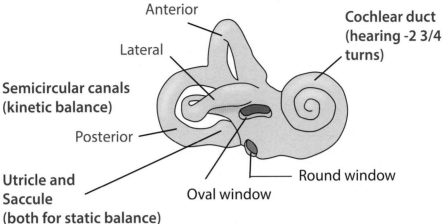

Anterior

Lateral

**Semicircular canals
(kinetic balance)**

Posterior

**Utricle and
Saccule
(both for static balance)**

Oval window

Round window

**Cochlear duct
(hearing -2 3/4
turns)**

Semicircular canals sense angular
acceleration such as fairground rides.
Utricle and saccule sense horizontal and
vertical acceleraton such as fast cars and
lifts (elevators).

- Full size at birth
- In petrous temporal bone
- One continuous cavity
- For hearing and balance
- Vestibulocochlear nerve
- **Blood:** Labyrinthine artery

INNER EAR - (Cochlea straightened out to aid understanding)

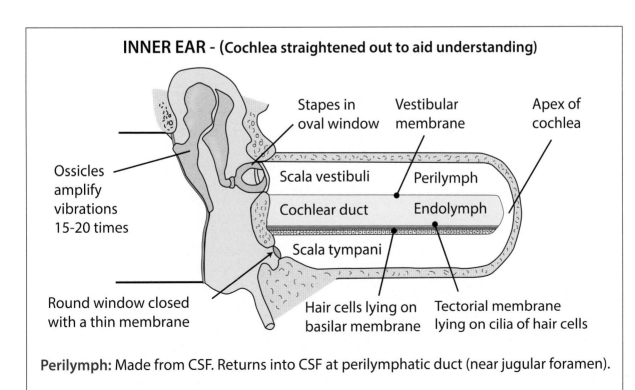

Ossicles
amplify
vibrations
15-20 times

Round window closed
with a thin membrane

Stapes in
oval window

Scala vestibuli

Cochlear duct

Scala tympani

Hair cells lying on
basilar membrane

Vestibular
membrane

Perilymph

Endolymph

Tectorial membrane
lying on cilia of hair cells

Apex of
cochlea

Perilymph: Made from CSF. Returns into CSF at perilymphatic duct (near jugular foramen).

Endolymph: Made in vascular part of membranous layer. Returns by being absorbed by
epithelium of endolympatic sac

INNER EAR - (Cochlea straightened out to aid understanding)

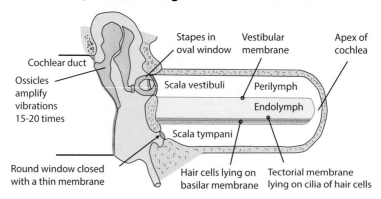

Cochlear duct

Ossicles amplify vibrations 15-20 times

Round window closed with a thin membrane

Stapes in oval window

Vestibular membrane

Apex of cochlea

Scala vestibuli

Perilymph

Endolymph

Scala tympani

Hair cells lying on basilar membrane

Tectorial membrane lying on cilia of hair cells

HEARING CONDUCTION

Sound waves → Pinna → External meatus → Tympanic membrane → Ossicles →

Round window → Vibrations in perilymph → Travelling wave in basilar membrane →

Outer hair cells - mechanically amplify the localised wave peak → Nearby inner hair cells

depolarise selected cochlear neurones → Auditory cortex via vestibulocochlear nerve (VIII)

Tonotopic organisation means that low pitches are perceived
at the apex of the cochlear spiral and high pitches at the base

5.12   Mouth and Mandible

ORAL CAVITY - MOUTH

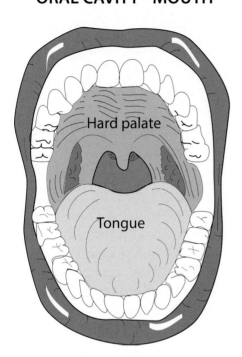

Hard palate

Tongue

Stratified squamous epithelium
Pierced by salivary gland ducts
Nerve: Buccal and mental
Vestibule: Between teeth and gums,
empted by buccinator

TEETH: 32. All but molars erupted by 13yrs.
Incisors 8
Canines 4
Premolars 8
Molars 8 (erupt approx 18yrs)
Deciduous: erupt 7-24 months
Teeth Ns: Superior alveolar (Vb)
                    Inferior alveolar (Vc)

**PALATINE TONSIL BETWEEN
PALATOGLOSSAL AND
PALATOPHARYNGEAL ARCHES**

RIGHT PALATINE TONSIL
(viewed from above)

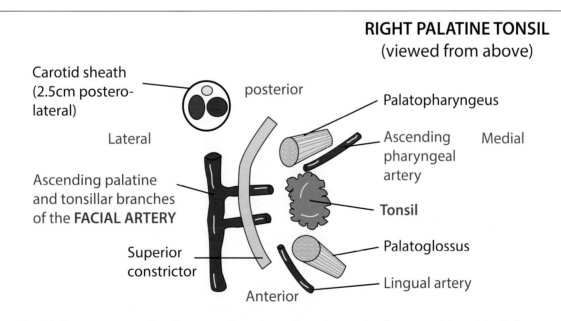

Carotid sheath
(2.5cm postero-
lateral)

posterior

Palatopharyngeus

Lateral

Ascending
pharyngeal
artery

Medial

Ascending palatine
and tonsillar branches
of the **FACIAL ARTERY**

Tonsil

Superior
constrictor

Palatoglossus

Lingual artery

Anterior

Lymphoid tissue: In tonsillar fossa with 20 tonsillar crypts. **Surface marking:** Medial to lower masseter. **Between:** Palatoglossal and palatopharyngeal arches.
Superior: Soft palate. **Inferior:** Tongue. **Lateral:** Capsule, superior constrictor, facial artery and branches. **Lymph:** Deep cervical and jugulodigastric. **Veins:** Pharyngeal plexus of veins. **Nerves:** Glossopharyngeal (referred pain to middle ear)

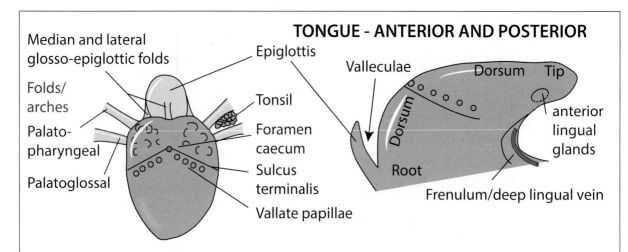

TONGUE - ANTERIOR AND POSTERIOR

Median and lateral glosso-epiglottic folds
Folds/arches
Palato-pharyngeal
Palatoglossal
Epiglottis
Tonsil
Foramen caecum
Sulcus terminalis
Vallate papillae

Valleculae
Dorsum
Tip
Dorsum
Root
anterior lingual glands
Frenulum/deep lingual vein

POSTERIOR 1/3
Oropharynx. smooth mucosa for swallowing. No papillae. Lingual tonsil. Serous/mucous glands
Taste/general sensation:
Glossopharyngeal nerve (IX)
Artery: Lingual
Lymph nodes: Jugulo-omohyoid and deep cervical

ANTERIOR 2/3
Oral cavity. Papillae (filiform, fungiform and vallate) for grip/taste. Stratified, keratinising squamous epithelium. Glands on tip and sides only
General sensation: Lingual (Vc)
Artery: Lingual
Lymph nodes: Tip - submental bilateral. Dorsum - unilateral to submandibular

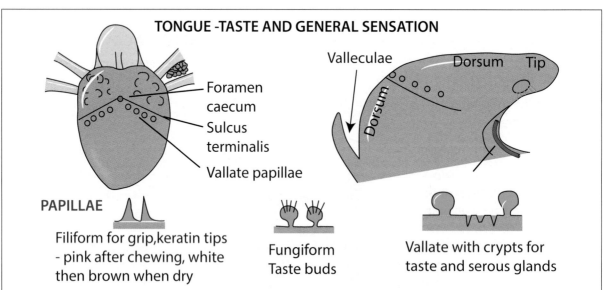

TONGUE -TASTE AND GENERAL SENSATION

Foramen caecum
Sulcus terminalis
Vallate papillae

Valleculae
Dorsum
Tip
Dorsum

PAPILLAE

Filiform for grip,keratin tips - pink after chewing, white then brown when dry

Fungiform
Taste buds

Vallate with crypts for taste and serous glands

TASTE: There are fungiform papillae throughout the anterior 2/3 of the tongue, supplied by the chorda tympani. The vallate papillae are aligned just anterior to the sulcus terminalis and, although they are in the anterior 2/3 of the tongue, they are supplied by the glossopharyngeal nerve (IX). There are also fungiform papillae in the arches lateral to the posterior third of the tongue (but not on its surface) which are also supplied by the glossopharyngeal nerve (IX). There are also a few taste buds in the vallecula supplied by the internal branch of the superior laryngeal nerve.

TONGUE - SENSATION AND TASTE (SUMMARY)

	SOMATIC SENSATION	TASTE	SECRETOMOTOR
ANTERIOR 2/3	Lingual (Vc)	Chorda tympani carried by VII	Chorda tympani carried by VII to anterior lingual glands
POSTERIOR 1/3 + VALLATE PAPILLAE	Glosso-pharyngeal (IX)	Glosso-pharyngeal (IX)	Glosso-pharyngeal (IX)
VALLECULAE	Glosso-pharyngeal (IX)	Internal branch of superior laryngeal nerve (X)	Glosso-pharyngeal (IX)

Note: Sympathetic supply to tongue is from superior cervical ganglion via lingual artery

TONGUE - MUSCLES

All tongue muscles are supplied by the hypoglossal nerve except palatoglossus which is supplied by the pharyngeal plexus (IX, X and sympathetic)

Hyoglossus: Hypoglossal nerve (XII)
Genioglossus: Hypoglossal nerve (XII)
Styloglossus: Hypoglossal nerve (XII)
Palatoglossus: Pharyngeal plexus (IX, X and sympathetic)
Intrinsic muscles: Hypoglossal nerve (XII)

Note: The intrinsic muscles of the tongue (Superior/inferior longitudinal, transverse and vertical) are not attached to bone)

TONGUE - BLOOD SUPPLY AND LYMPH DRAINAGE

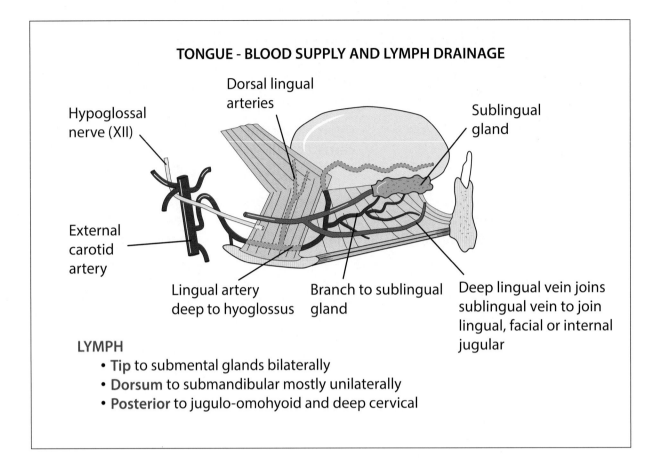

Dorsal lingual arteries

Hypoglossal nerve (XII)

Sublingual gland

External carotid artery

Lingual artery deep to hyoglossus

Branch to sublingual gland

Deep lingual vein joins sublingual vein to join lingual, facial or internal jugular

LYMPH
- **Tip** to submental glands bilaterally
- **Dorsum** to submandibular mostly unilaterally
- **Posterior** to jugulo-omohyoid and deep cervical

HARD PALATE

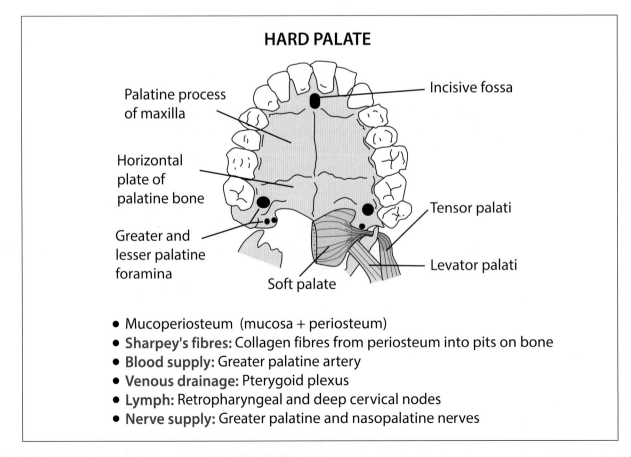

Palatine process of maxilla

Incisive fossa

Horizontal plate of palatine bone

Greater and lesser palatine foramina

Tensor palati

Levator palati

Soft palate

- Mucoperiosteum (mucosa + periosteum)
- **Sharpey's fibres:** Collagen fibres from periosteum into pits on bone
- **Blood supply:** Greater palatine artery
- **Venous drainage:** Pterygoid plexus
- **Lymph:** Retropharyngeal and deep cervical nodes
- **Nerve supply:** Greater palatine and nasopalatine nerves

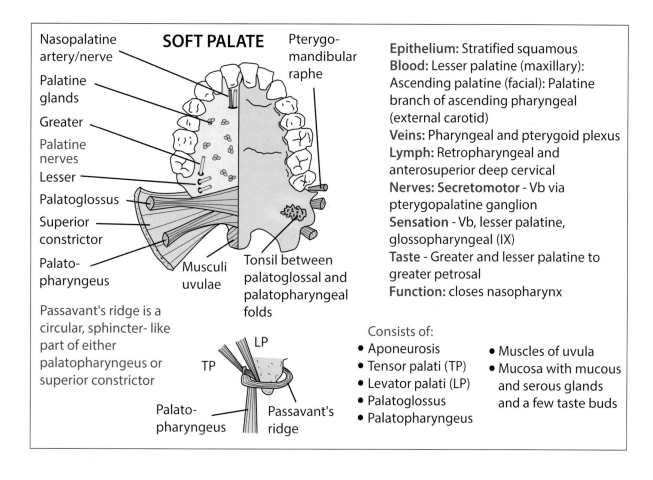

SOFT PALATE

Nasopalatine artery/nerve

Palatine glands

Greater

Palatine nerves

Lesser

Palatoglossus

Superior constrictor

Palato-pharyngeus

Musculi uvulae

Pterygo-mandibular raphe

Tonsil between palatoglossal and palatopharyngeal folds

Epithelium: Stratified squamous
Blood: Lesser palatine (maxillary): Ascending palatine (facial): Palatine branch of ascending pharyngeal (external carotid)
Veins: Pharyngeal and pterygoid plexus
Lymph: Retropharyngeal and anterosuperior deep cervical
Nerves: Secretomotor - Vb via pterygopalatine ganglion
Sensation - Vb, lesser palatine, glossopharyngeal (IX)
Taste - Greater and lesser palatine to greater petrosal
Function: closes nasopharynx

Passavant's ridge is a circular, sphincter- like part of either palatopharyngeus or superior constrictor

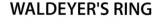

LP

TP

Palato-pharyngeus

Passavant's ridge

Consists of:
- Aponeurosis
- Tensor palati (TP)
- Levator palati (LP)
- Palatoglossus
- Palatopharyngeus

- Muscles of uvula
- Mucosa with mucous and serous glands and a few taste buds

WALDEYER'S RING

An interrupted circle of protective lymphoid tissue at the upper ends of the respiratory and alimentary tracts

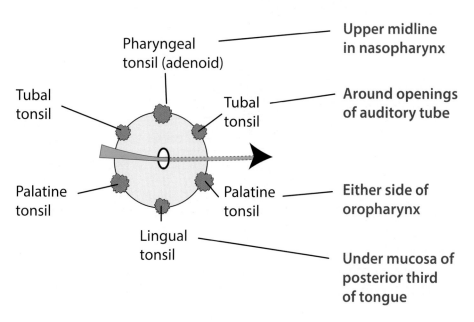

Pharyngeal tonsil (adenoid)

Tubal tonsil

Tubal tonsil

Palatine tonsil

Palatine tonsil

Lingual tonsil

Upper midline in nasopharynx

Around openings of auditory tube

Either side of oropharynx

Under mucosa of posterior third of tongue

PTERYGOMANDIBULAR RAPHÉ

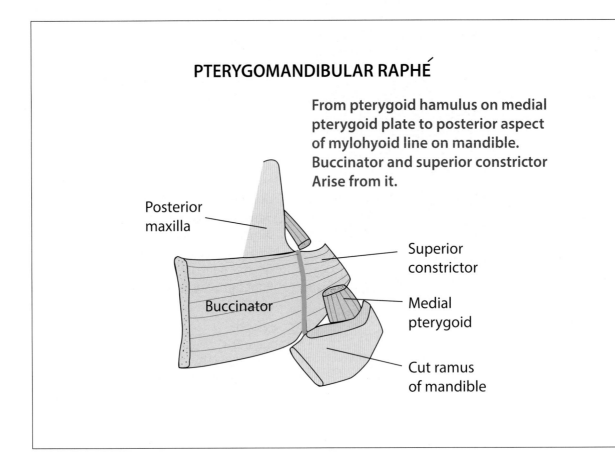

From pterygoid hamulus on medial pterygoid plate to posterior aspect of mylohyoid line on mandible. Buccinator and superior constrictor Arise from it.

Posterior maxilla

Buccinator

Superior constrictor

Medial pterygoid

Cut ramus of mandible

BUCCINATOR 1

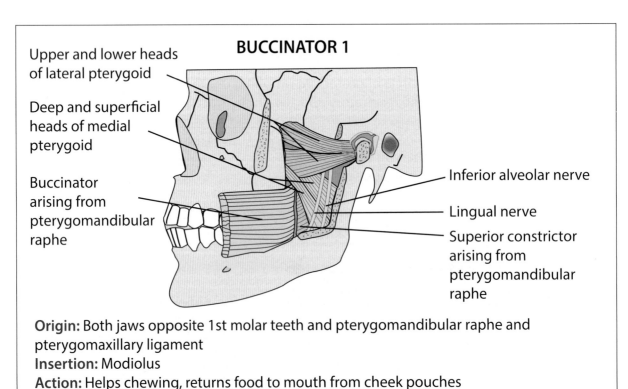

Upper and lower heads of lateral pterygoid

Deep and superficial heads of medial pterygoid

Buccinator arising from pterygomandibular raphe

Inferior alveolar nerve

Lingual nerve

Superior constrictor arising from pterygomandibular raphe

Origin: Both jaws opposite 1st molar teeth and pterygomandibular raphe and pterygomaxillary ligament
Insertion: Modiolus
Action: Helps chewing, returns food to mouth from cheek pouches
Nerve supply: Facial (VII) - buccal branches. Proprioceptive afferent fibres via buccal branch of Vc

BUCCINATOR 2
Viewed from medial aspect of mandible

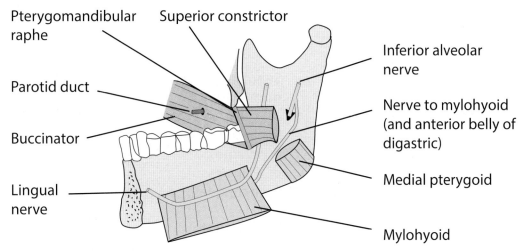

Pterygomandibular raphe

Superior constrictor

Parotid duct

Buccinator

Lingual nerve

Inferior alveolar nerve

Nerve to mylohyoid (and anterior belly of digastric)

Medial pterygoid

Mylohyoid

The pterygomandibular raphe is fibrous tissue extending from the pterygoid hamulus to the posterior end of the mylohyoid line. It is a landmark for dentists to anaesthetise the lingual nerve

MUSCLES OF TONGUE, MOUTH AND NECK

1. Tensor palati
2. Levator palati
3. Buccinator and superior contrictor from pterygo-mandibular raphe
4. Styloglossus
5. Stylopharyngeus
6. Rectus capitis lateralis
7. Stylohyoid
8. Inferior oblique
9. Middle constrictor
10. Thyropharyngeus
11. Transverse process of axis
12. Transverse process of atlas
13. Superior oblique
14. Hyoglossus
15. Genioglossus
16. Geniohyoid/mylohyoid
17. Cricothyroid
18. Thyrohyoid membrane

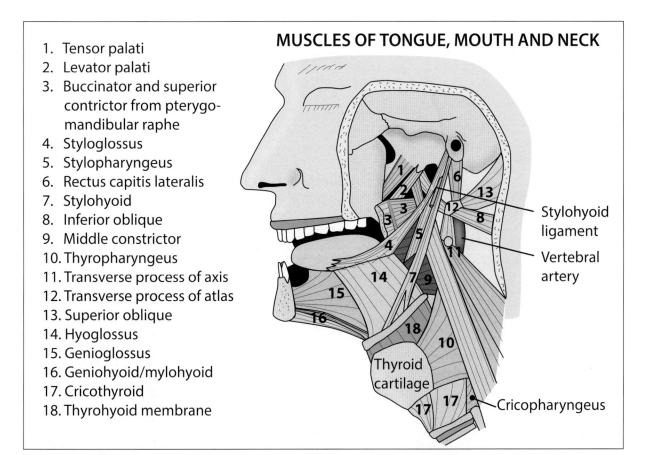

Stylohyoid ligament

Vertebral artery

Thyroid cartilage

Cricopharyngeus

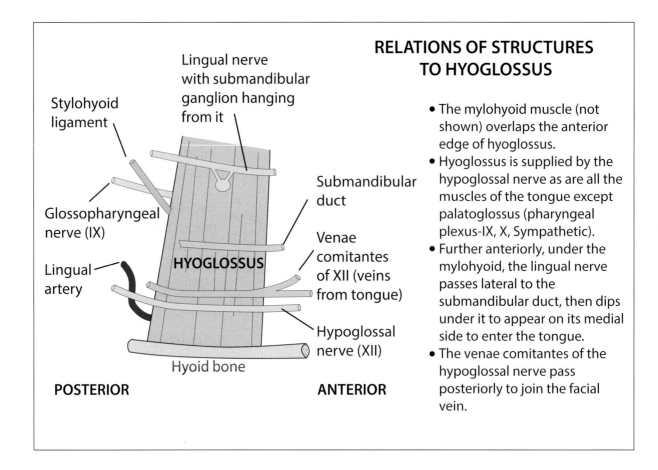

RELATIONS OF STRUCTURES TO HYOGLOSSUS

Stylohyoid ligament

Lingual nerve with submandibular ganglion hanging from it

Glossopharyngeal nerve (IX)

Lingual artery

HYOGLOSSUS

Submandibular duct

Venae comitantes of XII (veins from tongue)

Hypoglossal nerve (XII)

Hyoid bone

POSTERIOR

ANTERIOR

- The mylohyoid muscle (not shown) overlaps the anterior edge of hyoglossus.
- Hyoglossus is supplied by the hypoglossal nerve as are all the muscles of the tongue except palatoglossus (pharyngeal plexus-IX, X, Sympathetic).
- Further anteriorly, under the mylohyoid, the lingual nerve passes lateral to the submandibular duct, then dips under it to appear on its medial side to enter the tongue.
- The venae comitantes of the hypoglossal nerve pass posteriorly to join the facial vein.

INFERIOR ALVEOLAR NERVE: RELATIONS WITH MANDIBLE

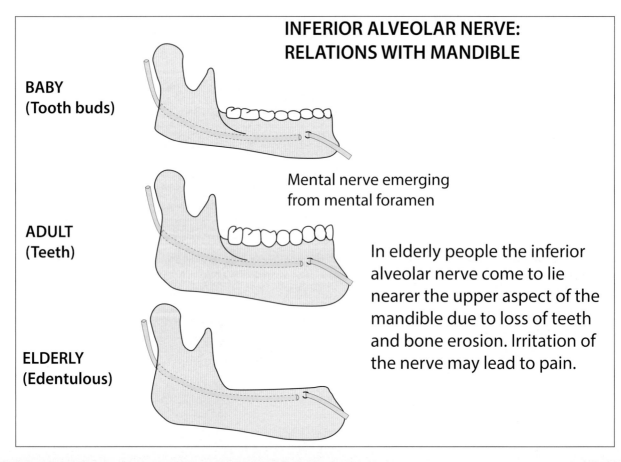

BABY (Tooth buds)

ADULT (Teeth)

ELDERLY (Edentulous)

Mental nerve emerging from mental foramen

In elderly people the inferior alveolar nerve come to lie nearer the upper aspect of the mandible due to loss of teeth and bone erosion. Irritation of the nerve may lead to pain.

TEMPOROMANDIBULAR JOINT

Articular tubercle

Lateral pterygoid

Disc

Lateral temporomandibular ligament

Capsule

Stylomandibular ligament. A thickening of the investing fascia of the neck

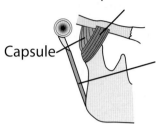

Synovial, condyloid, hemicylindrical, atypical (fibrocartilage on surfaces)
Fibrocartilaginous disc, synovial membrane lines capsule
Nerve: Auriculotemporal and nerve to masseter
Between: Mandible and mandibular fossa of squamous temporal bone
Disc: Moves forward with head of mandible
Capsule: Attached to neck of mandible and articular tubercle. Strong but lax at rest
Lateral temporomandibular ligament: Zygomatic arch to posterior neck and ramus of mandible. Fuses with capsule, lax at rest, tightens with any movement

MOVEMENTS OF TEMPOROMANDIBULAR JOINT

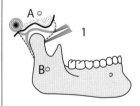

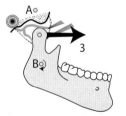

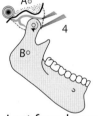

Points A and B are the 2 ends of the sphenomandibular ligament which is isometric at all joint positions. Axis for opening is through lingula (B)

First few degrees of opening are rotation only in lower cavity.

Majority of opening is rotation in lower joint cavity but with anterior displacement of head of mandible in upper joint cavity onto articular tubercle by action of lateral pterygoid

Last few degrees of opening are by further rotation in lower joint cavity only

Spine of sphenoid

Lingula of mandible

Sphenomandibular ligament

THE JOINT IS MOST STABLE WHEN CLOSED

PAROTID REGION AND MASSETER

Definition: Anterior and inferior to ear
Features: Masseter and parotid gland

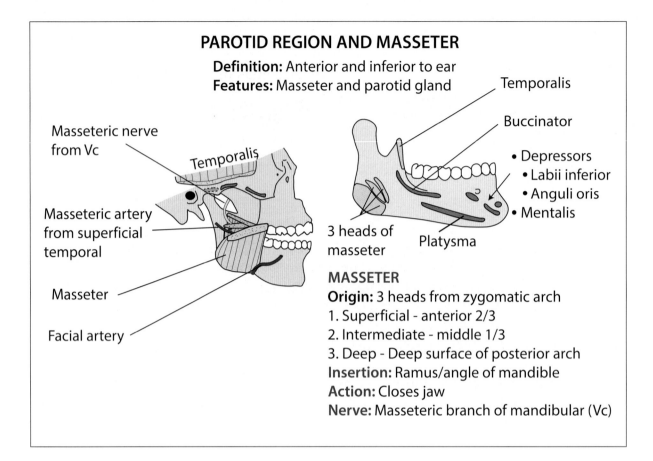

Masseteric nerve from Vc

Temporalis

Masseteric artery from superficial temporal

Masseter

Facial artery

Temporalis

Buccinator

• Depressors
  • Labii inferior
  • Anguli oris
• Mentalis

3 heads of masseter

Platysma

MASSETER
Origin: 3 heads from zygomatic arch
1. Superficial - anterior 2/3
2. Intermediate - middle 1/3
3. Deep - Deep surface of posterior arch
Insertion: Ramus/angle of mandible
Action: Closes jaw
Nerve: Masseteric branch of mandibular (Vc)

TEETH - 1

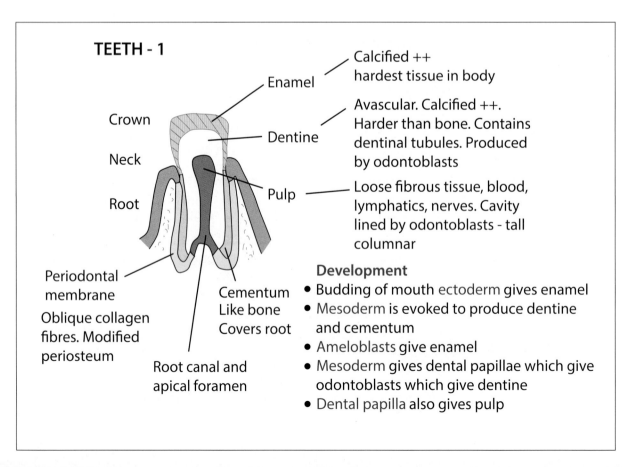

Crown

Neck

Root

Enamel — Calcified ++ hardest tissue in body

Dentine — Avascular. Calcified ++. Harder than bone. Contains dentinal tubules. Produced by odontoblasts

Pulp — Loose fibrous tissue, blood, lymphatics, nerves. Cavity lined by odontoblasts - tall columnar

Periodontal membrane

Oblique collagen fibres. Modified periosteum

Cementum Like bone Covers root

Root canal and apical foramen

Development
• Budding of mouth ectoderm gives enamel
• Mesoderm is evoked to produce dentine and cementum
• Ameloblasts give enamel
• Mesoderm gives dental papillae which give odontoblasts which give dentine
• Dental papilla also gives pulp

TEETH - 3

NERVE AND BLOOD SUPPLY

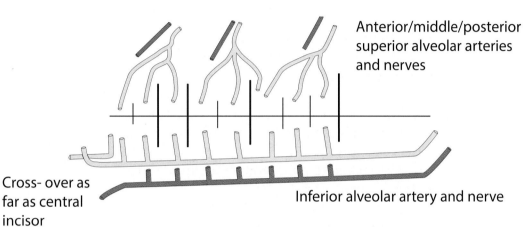

Anterior/middle/posterior superior alveolar arteries and nerves

Cross-over as far as central incisor

Inferior alveolar artery and nerve

Note: The further posterior that anaesthesia is needed the more a nerve block is required and the less efficient is local infiltration because of bone porosity

TEETH - 2

	INCISOR	CANINE	PREMOLAR		MOLAR	
ADULT NUMBER	2	1	2		3	
			lower	upper	lower	upper
ROOTS	1	1	1st and 2nd:1	1st:2 2nd: 1	2	3
CUSPS	1	1	2		5	4

TOTAL IN ADULTS 8 X 2 =16 X 2 = 32

ERUPTIONS	Incisors	Canines	Premolars	Molars	
Deciduous (5x2=10x2=20)	7 8	18		12 24	months
	6 9	18		12 24	
Permanent	7 8	11	9 10	6 12 18+	years
	7 8	11	9 10	6 12 18+	

5.13 Nose and Face

EXTERNAL NOSE AND NASAL CAVITY

EXTERNAL NOSE is fibrofatty tissue supported by 5 cartilages and two small bones

NASAL CAVITY   **For:**
- Breathing (stops during swallowing)
- Warming, moistening and filtering the air
- Sense of smell
  Structure:
- Conchae and sinuses increase the surface area, the epithelium is vascular, there are cilia and mucus is secreted
  Nerve supply:
- External nasal (terminal anterior ethmoidal) Va
- Supratrochlear (frontal) Va
- Infratrochlear (nasociliary) Va
- Infra-orbital (maxillary) Vb
  Blood supply:
- Dorsal nasal (ophthalmic)
- External nasal (anterior ethmoidal)
- Facial (lateral nasal and septal branches)

NASAL CAVITY - coronal view

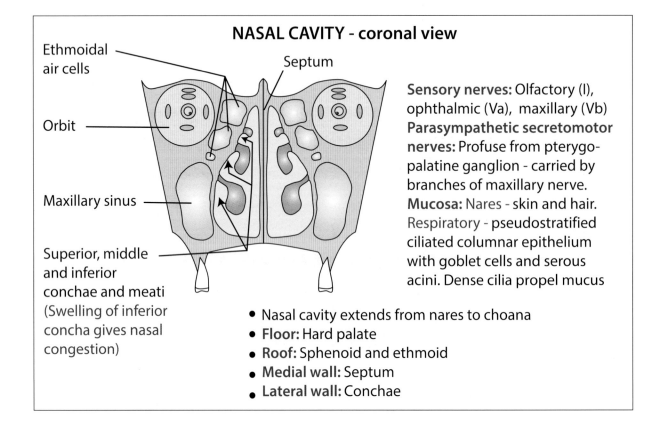

Ethmoidal air cells

Septum

Orbit

Maxillary sinus

Superior, middle and inferior conchae and meati
(Swelling of inferior concha gives nasal congestion)

Sensory nerves: Olfactory (I), ophthalmic (Va), maxillary (Vb)
Parasympathetic secretomotor nerves: Profuse from pterygo-palatine ganglion - carried by branches of maxillary nerve.
Mucosa: Nares - skin and hair. Respiratory - pseudostratified ciliated columnar epithelium with goblet cells and serous acini. Dense cilia propel mucus

- Nasal cavity extends from nares to choana
- **Floor:** Hard palate
- **Roof:** Sphenoid and ethmoid
- **Medial wall:** Septum
- **Lateral wall:** Conchae

NASAL CAVITY

Venous drainage

Anterior - to face

Posterior - to pterygoid plexus. Also via ethmoidal veins to ophthalmic and inferior cerebral veins. 1% via foramen caecum to superior sagittal sinus

Lymphatic drainage of lateral wall and septum

Posterior: To retropharyngeal and to anterior/ superior deep cervical nodes. **Anterior:** To submandibular nodes

Lining

Respiratory epithelium - pseudostratified ciliated columnar with mucous cells and very vascular

Olfactory epithelium - ciliated nerve cells, yellowish, on roof and septum, under superior concha and in spheno-ethmoidal recess

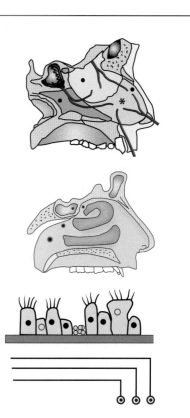

BLOOD SUPPLY OF LATERAL WALL OF NOSE

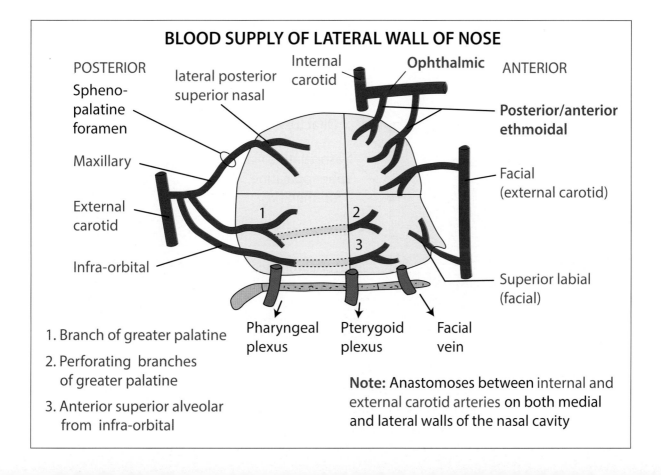

POSTERIOR

Spheno-palatine foramen

lateral posterior superior nasal

Internal carotid

Ophthalmic

ANTERIOR

Maxillary

External carotid

Infra-orbital

Posterior/anterior ethmoidal

Facial (external carotid)

Superior labial (facial)

Pharyngeal plexus

Pterygoid plexus

Facial vein

1. Branch of greater palatine

2. Perforating branches of greater palatine

3. Anterior superior alveolar from infra-orbital

Note: Anastomoses between internal and external carotid arteries on both medial and lateral walls of the nasal cavity

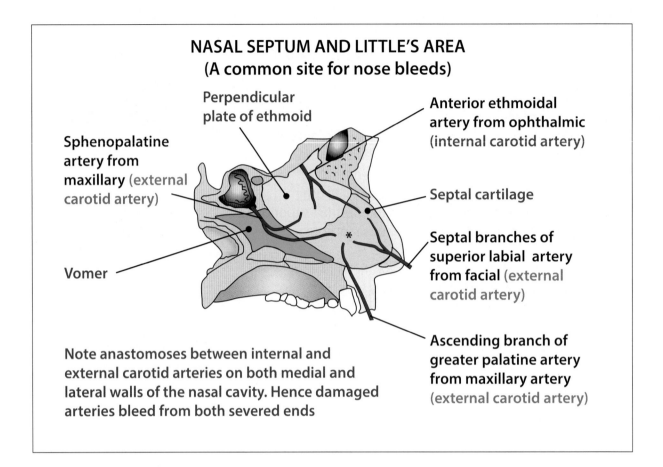

NASAL SEPTUM AND LITTLE'S AREA
(A common site for nose bleeds)

Perpendicular plate of ethmoid

Anterior ethmoidal artery from ophthalmic (internal carotid artery)

Sphenopalatine artery from maxillary (external carotid artery)

Septal cartilage

Vomer

Septal branches of superior labial artery from facial (external carotid artery)

Ascending branch of greater palatine artery from maxillary artery (external carotid artery)

Note anastomoses between internal and external carotid arteries on both medial and lateral walls of the nasal cavity. Hence damaged arteries bleed from both severed ends

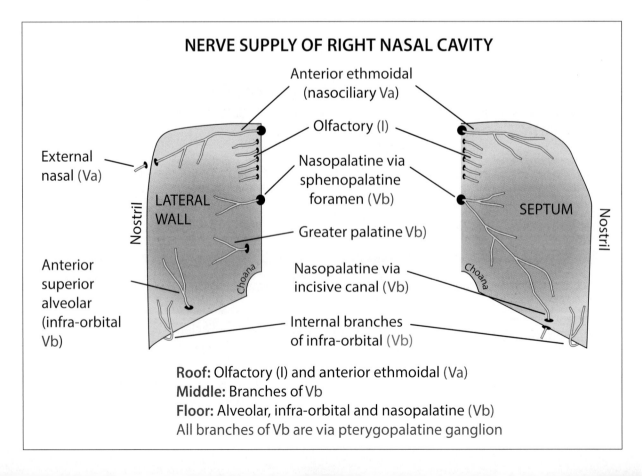

NERVE SUPPLY OF RIGHT NASAL CAVITY

Anterior ethmoidal (nasociliary Va)

Olfactory (I)

External nasal (Va)

Nasopalatine via sphenopalatine foramen (Vb)

LATERAL WALL

SEPTUM

Nostril

Nostril

Greater palatine Vb)

Anterior superior alveolar (infra-orbital Vb)

Choana

Choana

Nasopalatine via incisive canal (Vb)

Internal branches of infra-orbital (Vb)

Roof: Olfactory (I) and anterior ethmoidal (Va)
Middle: Branches of Vb
Floor: Alveolar, infra-orbital and nasopalatine (Vb)
All branches of Vb are via pterygopalatine ganglion

LATERAL WALL OF LEFT NASAL CAVITY

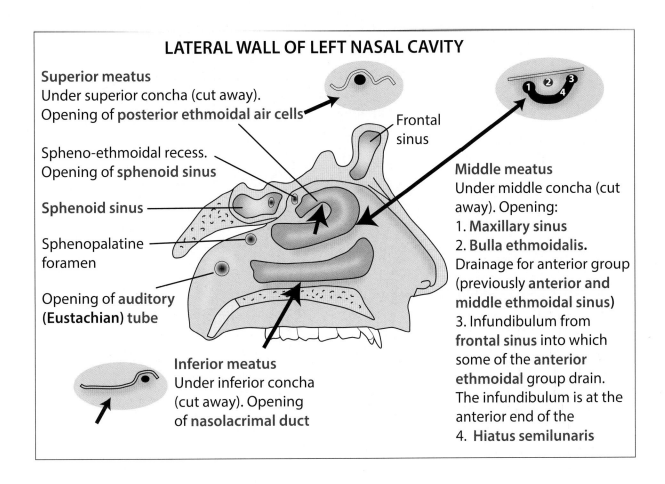

Superior meatus
Under superior concha (cut away).
Opening of **posterior ethmoidal air cells**

Spheno-ethmoidal recess.
Opening of **sphenoid sinus**

Sphenoid sinus

Sphenopalatine foramen

Opening of auditory (Eustachian) tube

Frontal sinus

Inferior meatus
Under inferior concha (cut away). Opening of **nasolacrimal duct**

Middle meatus
Under middle concha (cut away). Opening:
1. **Maxillary sinus**
2. **Bulla ethmoidalis.**
Drainage for anterior group (previously **anterior and middle ethmoidal sinus**)
3. Infundibulum from **frontal sinus** into which some of the **anterior ethmoidal** group drain. The infundibulum is at the anterior end of the
4. **Hiatus semilunaris**

MUSCLES OF FACIAL EXPRESSION

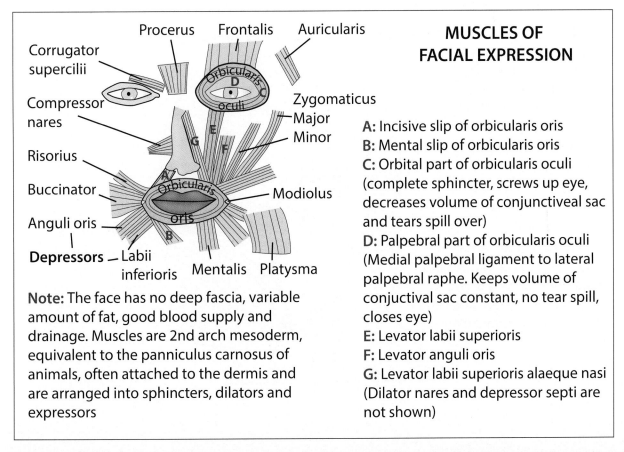

Corrugator supercilii
Procerus
Frontalis
Auricularis
Compressor nares
Zygomaticus
— Major
— Minor
Risorius
Buccinator
Modiolus
Anguli oris
Depressors — Labii inferioris
Mentalis
Platysma

A: Incisive slip of orbicularis oris
B: Mental slip of orbicularis oris
C: Orbital part of orbicularis oculi (complete sphincter, screws up eye, decreases volume of conjunctiveal sac and tears spill over)
D: Palpebral part of orbicularis oculi (Medial palpebral ligament to lateral palpebral raphe. Keeps volume of conjuctival sac constant, no tear spill, closes eye)
E: Levator labii superioris
F: Levator anguli oris
G: Levator labii superioris alaeque nasi (Dilator nares and depressor septi are not shown)

Note: The face has no deep fascia, variable amount of fat, good blood supply and drainage. Muscles are 2nd arch mesoderm, equivalent to the panniculus carnosus of animals, often attached to the dermis and are arranged into sphincters, dilators and expressors

FACE: ARTERIAL SUPPLY AND VENOUS DRAINAGE

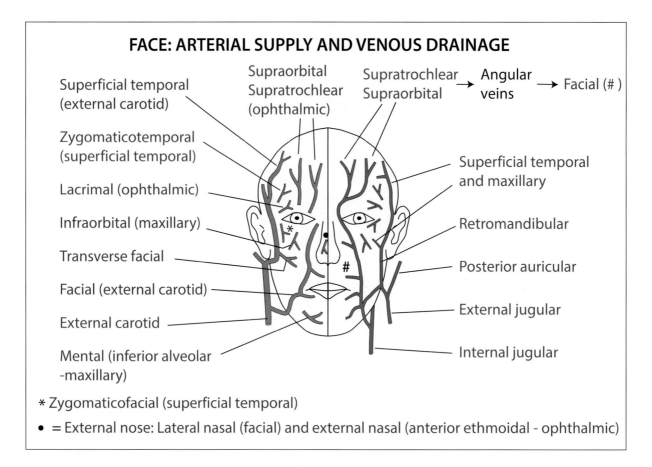

Superficial temporal (external carotid)

Zygomaticotemporal (superficial temporal)

Lacrimal (ophthalmic)

Infraorbital (maxillary)

Transverse facial

Facial (external carotid)

External carotid

Mental (inferior alveolar -maxillary)

Supraorbital Supratrochlear (ophthalmic)

Supratrochlear Supraorbital → Angular veins → Facial (#)

Superficial temporal and maxillary

Retromandibular

Posterior auricular

External jugular

Internal jugular

* Zygomaticofacial (superficial temporal)

• = External nose: Lateral nasal (facial) and external nasal (anterior ethmoidal - ophthalmic)

VESSELS ON FACE - VENOUS ANASTOMOSES

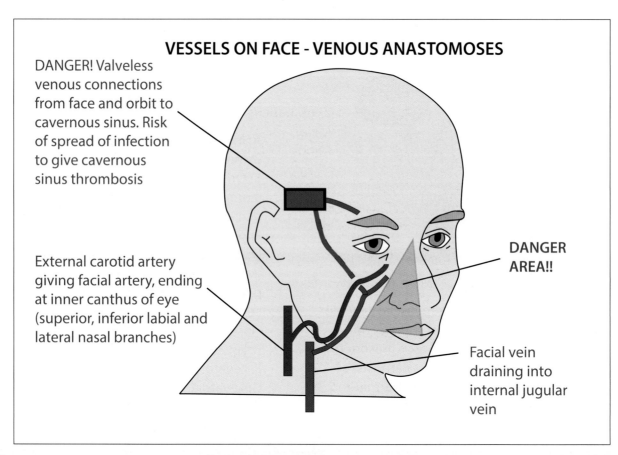

DANGER! Valveless venous connections from face and orbit to cavernous sinus. Risk of spread of infection to give cavernous sinus thrombosis

External carotid artery giving facial artery, ending at inner canthus of eye (superior, inferior labial and lateral nasal branches)

DANGER AREA!!

Facial vein draining into internal jugular vein

PTERYGOID PLEXUS CONNECTIONS - DIAGRAMMATIC ONLY

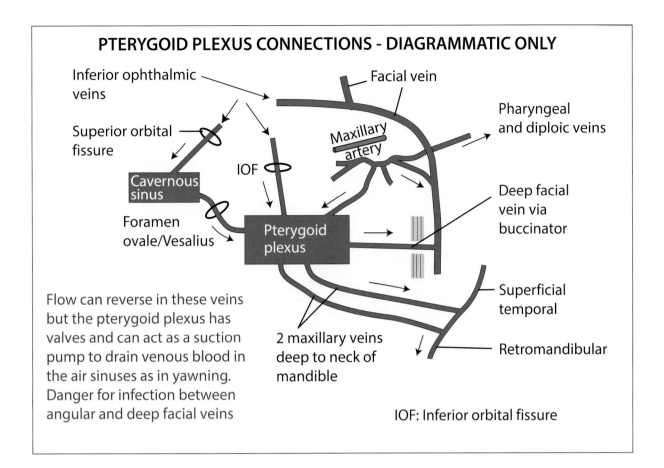

Inferior ophthalmic veins

Superior orbital fissure

Cavernous sinus

Foramen ovale/Vesalius

IOF

Facial vein

Maxillary artery

Pharyngeal and diploic veins

Deep facial vein via buccinator

Pterygoid plexus

Superficial temporal

Retromandibular

2 maxillary veins deep to neck of mandible

Flow can reverse in these veins but the pterygoid plexus has valves and can act as a suction pump to drain venous blood in the air sinuses as in yawning. Danger for infection between angular and deep facial veins

IOF: Inferior orbital fissure

5.14 Neck Fascia, Vessels and General Anatomy

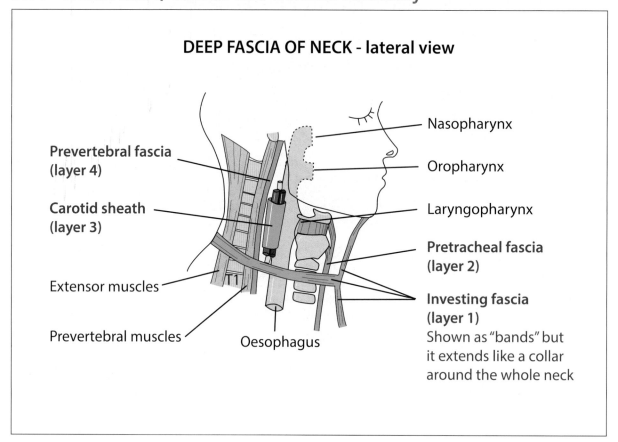

DEEP FASCIA OF NECK - lateral view

Prevertebral fascia
(layer 4)

Carotid sheath
(layer 3)

Extensor muscles

Prevertebral muscles

Oesophagus

Nasopharynx

Oropharynx

Laryngopharynx

**Pretracheal fascia
(layer 2)**

**Investing fascia
(layer 1)**
Shown as "bands" but
it extends like a collar
around the whole neck

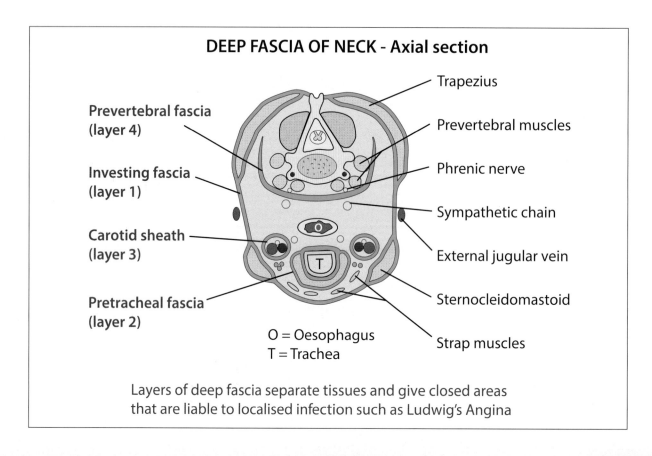

DEEP FASCIA OF NECK - Axial section

Prevertebral fascia
(layer 4)

Investing fascia
(layer 1)

Carotid sheath
(layer 3)

Pretracheal fascia
(layer 2)

Trapezius

Prevertebral muscles

Phrenic nerve

Sympathetic chain

External jugular vein

Sternocleidomastoid

Strap muscles

O = Oesophagus
T = Trachea

Layers of deep fascia separate tissues and give closed areas
that are liable to localised infection such as Ludwig's Angina

INVESTING LAYER OF DEEP FASCIA OF NECK

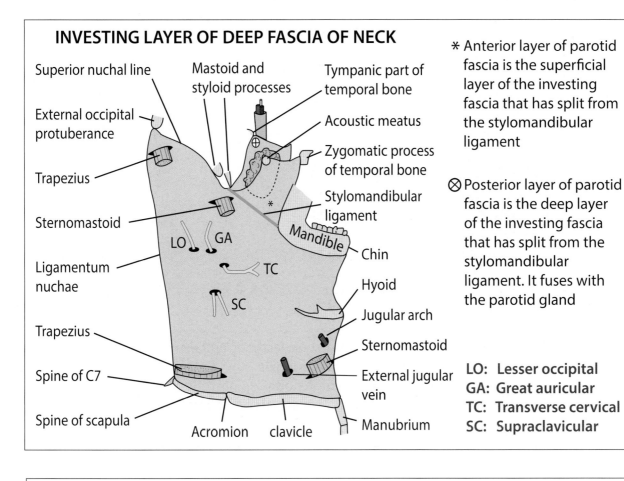

Superior nuchal line

External occipital protuberance

Trapezius

Sternomastoid

Ligamentum nuchae

Trapezius

Spine of C7

Spine of scapula

Mastoid and styloid processes

Tympanic part of temporal bone

Acoustic meatus

Zygomatic process of temporal bone

Stylomandibular ligament

Mandible

Chin

Hyoid

Jugular arch

Sternomastoid

External jugular vein

Acromion   clavicle

Manubrium

LO   GA

TC

SC

* Anterior layer of parotid fascia is the superficial layer of the investing fascia that has split from the stylomandibular ligament

⊗ Posterior layer of parotid fascia is the deep layer of the investing fascia that has split from the stylomandibular ligament. It fuses with the parotid gland

LO: Lesser occipital
GA: Great auricular
TC: Transverse cervical
SC: Supraclavicular

PRETRACHEAL PART OF DEEP FASCIA OF NECK

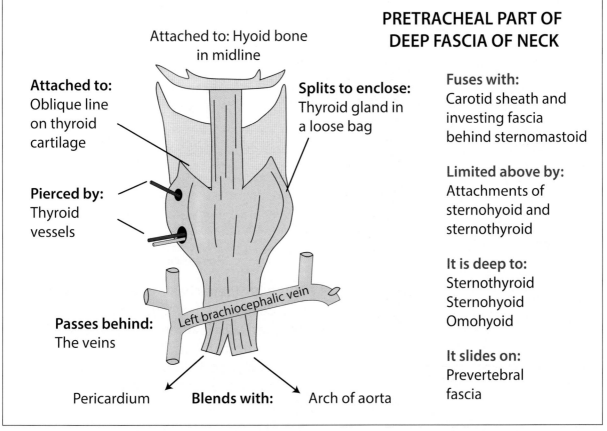

Attached to: Hyoid bone in midline

Attached to: Oblique line on thyroid cartilage

Pierced by: Thyroid vessels

Passes behind: The veins

Splits to enclose: Thyroid gland in a loose bag

Left brachiocephalic vein

Pericardium   **Blends with:**   Arch of aorta

Fuses with: Carotid sheath and investing fascia behind sternomastoid

Limited above by: Attachments of sternohyoid and sternothyroid

It is deep to: Sternothyroid Sternohyoid Omohyoid

It slides on: Prevertebral fascia

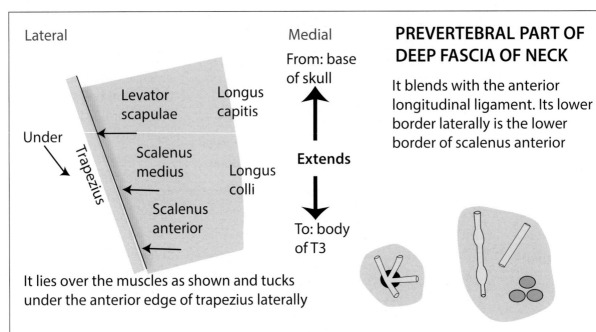

Lateral

Levator scapulae

Longus capitis

Under

Trapezius

Scalenus medius

Longus colli

Scalenus anterior

Medial

From: base of skull

Extends

To: body of T3

PREVERTEBRAL PART OF DEEP FASCIA OF NECK

It blends with the anterior longitudinal ligament. Its lower border laterally is the lower border of scalenus anterior

It lies over the muscles as shown and tucks under the anterior edge of trapezius laterally

Pierced by these nerves: Great auricular, lesser occipital, transverse cervical, supraclavicular, inferior root of ansa cervicalis
Lying on it: Sympathetic chain, lymph nodes, spinal root of accessory nerve
Deep to it: Cervical plexus, trunks of brachial plexus, 3rd part of subclavian artery, phrenic nerve

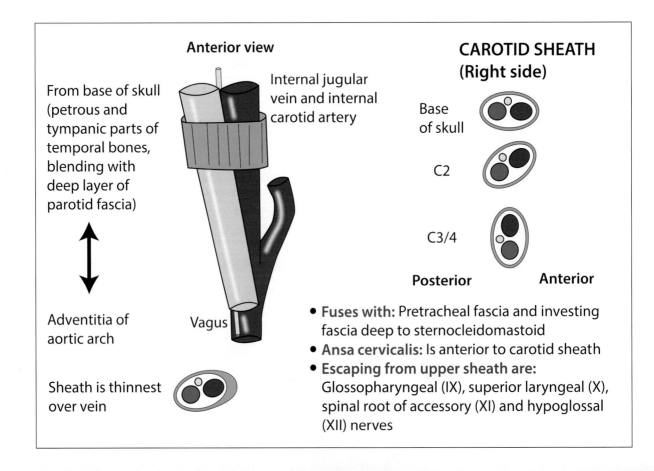

Anterior view

From base of skull (petrous and tympanic parts of temporal bones, blending with deep layer of parotid fascia)

Internal jugular vein and internal carotid artery

Vagus

Adventitia of aortic arch

Sheath is thinnest over vein

CAROTID SHEATH (Right side)

Base of skull

C2

C3/4

Posterior   Anterior

- **Fuses with:** Pretracheal fascia and investing fascia deep to sternocleidomastoid
- **Ansa cervicalis:** Is anterior to carotid sheath
- **Escaping from upper sheath are:** Glossopharyngeal (IX), superior laryngeal (X), spinal root of accessory (XI) and hypoglossal (XII) nerves

TISSUE SPACES IN THE NECK

PREVERTEBRAL SPACE
Closed space behind prevertebral fascia which allows infection to track down into axilla via the axillary sheath which is, itself, part of the prevertebral fascia which has been dragged off by the subclavian artery as it emerges from behind scalenus anterior

RETROPHARYNGEAL SPACE
Immediately anterior to prevertebral fascia. Below, it extends behind oesophagus to diaphragm via superior and then posterior mediastinum. Infection may spread from here, laterally, behind the carotid sheath into the posterior triangle

PARAPHARYNGEAL SPACE
Lateral continuation of retropharyngeal space

SUBMANDIBULAR SPACE
Extends superiorly to the investing layer of deep cervical fascia, between hyoid and mandible to mucous membrane of floor of mouth. Contains mylohyoid muscle, sublingual gland superior to this muscle and submandibular gland hooking around its posterior border. Infection here gives cellulitis known as **LUDWIG'S ANGINA**

INTERNAL AND EXTERNAL CAROTID ARTERIES AND BIFURCATION

External carotid branches:
1. Ascending pharyneal
2. Superior thyroid
3. Lingual
4. Facial
5. Occipital
6. Posterior auricular
7. Superficial temporal
8. Maxillary

The bifurcation is at the level of C4 - upper thyroid cartilage

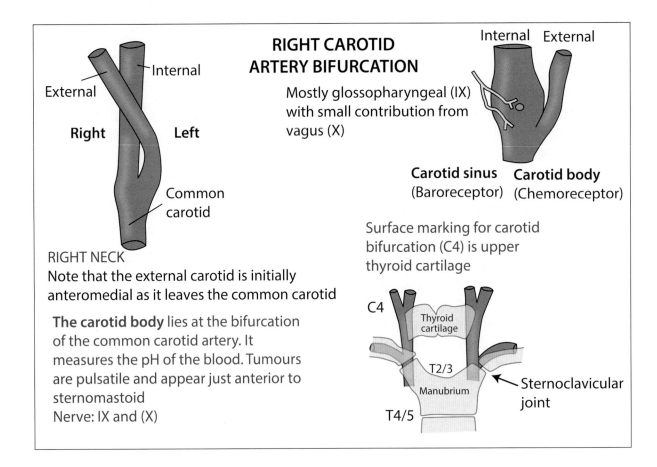

RIGHT CAROTID ARTERY BIFURCATION

External

Internal

Right

Left

Common carotid

Internal   External

Mostly glossopharyngeal (IX) with small contribution from vagus (X)

Carotid sinus (Baroreceptor)   **Carotid body** (Chemoreceptor)

RIGHT NECK
Note that the external carotid is initially anteromedial as it leaves the common carotid

The carotid body lies at the bifurcation of the common carotid artery. It measures the pH of the blood. Tumours are pulsatile and appear just anterior to sternomastoid
Nerve: IX and (X)

Surface marking for carotid bifurcation (C4) is upper thyroid cartilage

C4

Thyroid cartilage

T2/3

Manubrium

Sternoclavicular joint

T4/5

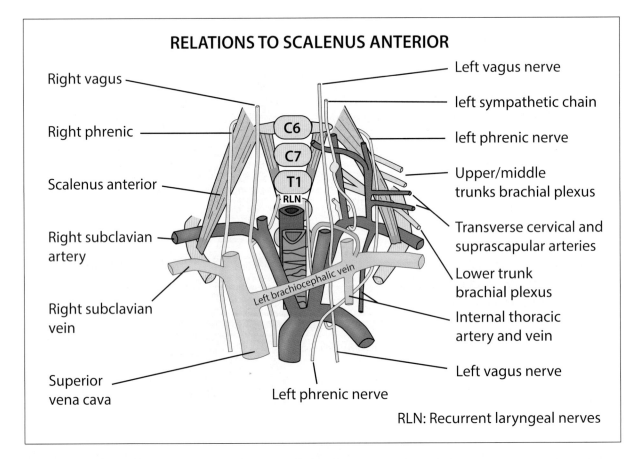

RELATIONS TO SCALENUS ANTERIOR

Right vagus

Right phrenic

Scalenus anterior

Right subclavian artery

Right subclavian vein

Superior vena cava

C6

C7

T1

RLN

Left brachiocephalic vein

Left phrenic nerve

Left vagus nerve

left sympathetic chain

left phrenic nerve

Upper/middle trunks brachial plexus

Transverse cervical and suprascapular arteries

Lower trunk brachial plexus

Internal thoracic artery and vein

Left vagus nerve

RLN: Recurrent laryngeal nerves

RELATIONS OF THE BIFURCATION OF THE CAROTID ARTERIES 1

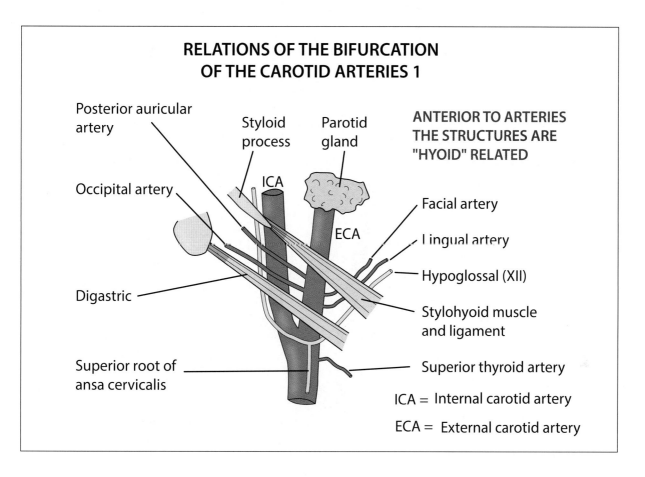

Posterior auricular artery

Styloid process

Parotid gland

ICA

ECA

Occipital artery

Digastric

Superior root of ansa cervicalis

ANTERIOR TO ARTERIES THE STRUCTURES ARE "HYOID" RELATED

Facial artery

Lingual artery

Hypoglossal (XII)

Stylohyoid muscle and ligament

Superior thyroid artery

ICA = Internal carotid artery

ECA = External carotid artery

RELATIONS OF THE BIFURCATION OF THE CAROTID ARTERIES 2

POSTERIOR TO ARTERIES THE STRUCTURES ARE "LARYNX" RELATED

BETWEEN ARTERIES THE STRUCTURES ARE TONGUE/PHARYNX" RELATED

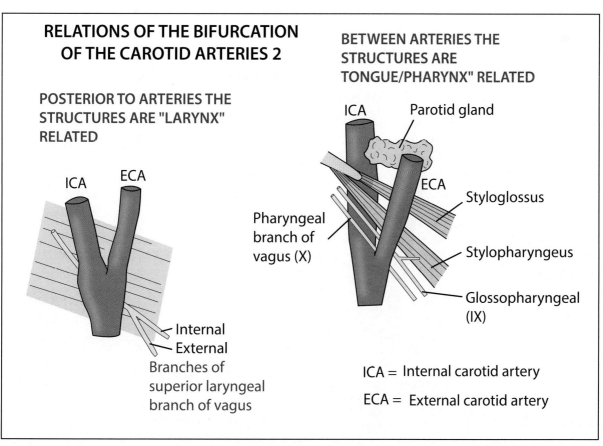

ICA

ECA

ICA

Parotid gland

ECA

Styloglossus

Stylopharyngeus

Glossopharyngeal (IX)

Pharyngeal branch of vagus (X)

Internal

External

Branches of superior laryngeal branch of vagus

ICA = Internal carotid artery

ECA = External carotid artery

SURFACE ANATOMY OF JUGULAR VEINS

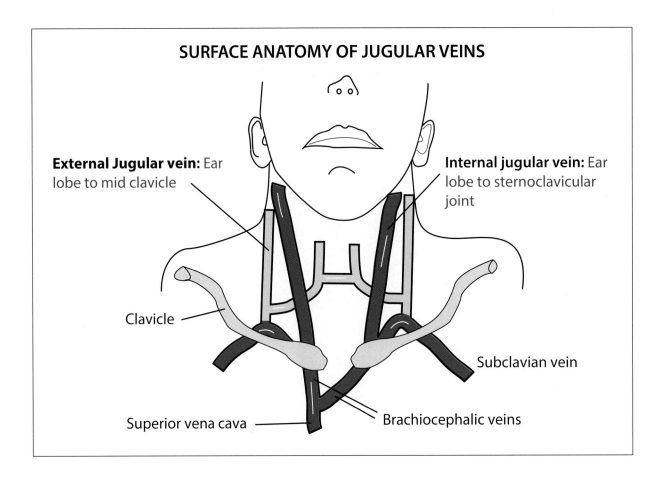

External Jugular vein: Ear lobe to mid clavicle

Internal jugular vein: Ear lobe to sternoclavicular joint

Clavicle

Subclavian vein

Superior vena cava

Brachiocephalic veins

RIGHT INTERNAL AND EXTERNAL JUGULAR VEINS

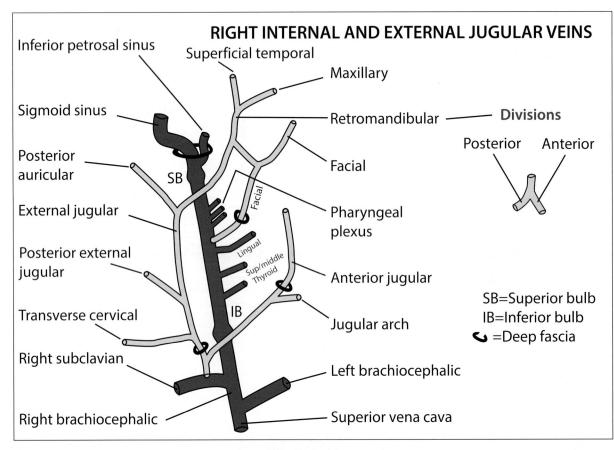

Inferior petrosal sinus

Superficial temporal

Maxillary

Sigmoid sinus

Retromandibular — **Divisions**

Posterior   Anterior

Posterior auricular

SB

Facial

External jugular

Facial

Pharyngeal plexus

Posterior external jugular

Lingual

Sup/middle Thyroid

Anterior jugular

Transverse cervical

IB

Jugular arch

SB=Superior bulb
IB=Inferior bulb
↰ =Deep fascia

Right subclavian

Left brachiocephalic

Right brachiocephalic

Superior vena cava

CERVICAL PLEXUS

Great auricular nerve should not be confused with:
Posterior auricular branch of facial (VII)-(motor to occipitalis)
OR
Auriculotemporal branch of mandibular (Vc) (sensory to hairy temple)

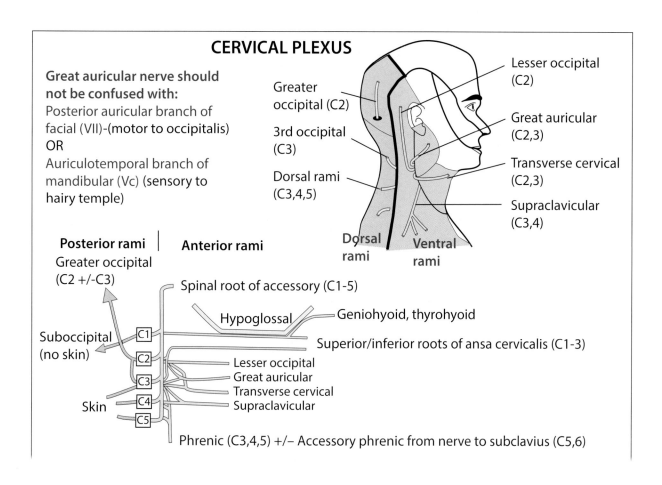

Greater occipital (C2)

3rd occipital (C3)

Dorsal rami (C3,4,5)

Lesser occipital (C2)

Great auricular (C2,3)

Transverse cervical (C2,3)

Supraclavicular (C3,4)

Dorsal rami

Ventral rami

Posterior rami	Anterior rami

Greater occipital (C2 +/-C3)

Spinal root of accessory (C1-5)

Hypoglossal

Geniohyoid, thyrohyoid

Suboccipital (no skin)

Superior/inferior roots of ansa cervicalis (C1-3)

Lesser occipital
Great auricular
Transverse cervical
Supraclavicular

Skin

C1
C2
C3
C4
C5

Phrenic (C3,4,5) +/– Accessory phrenic from nerve to subclavius (C5,6)

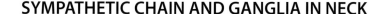

SYMPATHETIC CHAIN AND GANGLIA IN NECK

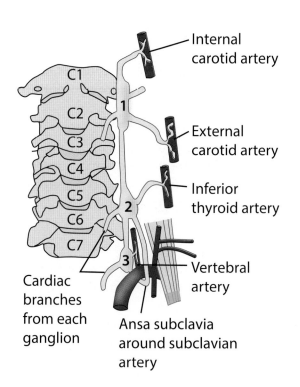

Internal carotid artery

External carotid artery

Inferior thyroid artery

Vertebral artery

Cardiac branches from each ganglion

Ansa subclavia around subclavian artery

1. SUPERIOR CERVICAL GANGLION
Anterior to lateral mass C1 and C2. 3cm long. 4 somatic branches. (C1-4). Branches to internal and external carotid arts

2. MIDDLE CERVICAL GANGLION
At C6, medial to carotid tubercle. Anterior to vertebral artery. 2 somatic branches. (C5,6). Branches to inferior thyroid and subclavian arteries

3. INFERIOR CERVICAL GANGLION
At C7, behind vertebral artery. 1cm x 0.5cm on neck of 1st rib. 2 somatic branches. (C7,8). Branches to vertebral artery

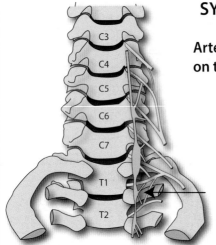

SYMPATHETIC CHAIN IN LOWER NECK

Arterial spasm may result from irritation of sympathetics on the subclavian artery from a cervical rib

SYMPATHECTOMY

Treatment of Raynaud's phenomenon by cutting the preganglionic sympathetic fibres at T2 and T3 to increase the blood flow to the fingers by preventing vasoconstriction

Small pupil
Mild ptosis
Flushed face
Dry face
Apparent enophthalmos

LEFT HORNER'S SYNDROME

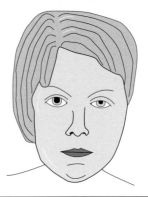

LYMPH NODES IN THE HEAD AND NECK

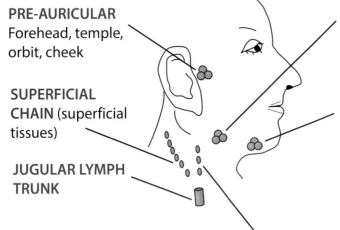

PRE-AURICULAR
Forehead, temple, orbit, cheek

SUPERFICIAL CHAIN (superficial tissues)

JUGULAR LYMPH TRUNK

SUBMANDIBULAR
Forehead, frontal and maxillary sinuses, anterior nose, upper lip, lower face, tongue and floor of mouth

SUBMENTAL
Chin, tip of tongue. Tip of tongue and posterior 1/3 drain bilaterally. There is also overlap across the midline in the anterior 2/3

DEEP CERVICAL CHAIN (Deeper tissues -thyroid, larynx, tonsil, etc)
Jugulodigastric (upper group): Between sternomastoid, angle of jaw and posterior digastric)
Jugulo-omohyoid (lower group): Above inferior belly of omohyoid, behind jugular vein, under posterior border of sternomastoid

VERTEBRAL LEVELS OF STRUCTURES

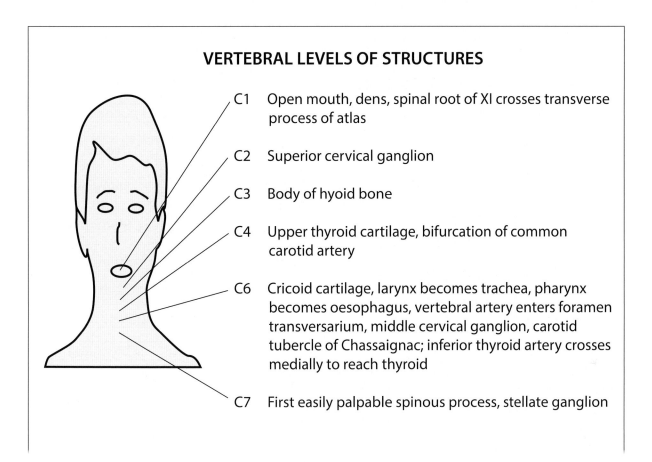

C1   Open mouth, dens, spinal root of XI crosses transverse process of atlas

C2   Superior cervical ganglion

C3   Body of hyoid bone

C4   Upper thyroid cartilage, bifurcation of common carotid artery

C6   Cricoid cartilage, larynx becomes trachea, pharynx becomes oesophagus, vertebral artery enters foramen transversarium, middle cervical ganglion, carotid tubercle of Chassaignac; inferior thyroid artery crosses medially to reach thyroid

C7   First easily palpable spinous process, stellate ganglion

PREVERTEBRAL MUSCLES

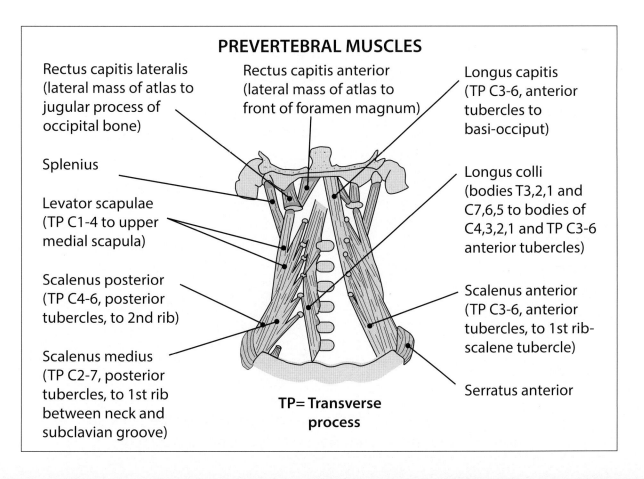

Rectus capitis lateralis (lateral mass of atlas to jugular process of occipital bone)

Splenius

Levator scapulae (TP C1-4 to upper medial scapula)

Scalenus posterior (TP C4-6, posterior tubercles, to 2nd rib)

Scalenus medius (TP C2-7, posterior tubercles, to 1st rib between neck and subclavian groove)

Rectus capitis anterior (lateral mass of atlas to front of foramen magnum)

Longus capitis (TP C3-6, anterior tubercles to basi-occiput)

Longus colli (bodies T3,2,1 and C7,6,5 to bodies of C4,3,2,1 and TP C3-6 anterior tubercles)

Scalenus anterior (TP C3-6, anterior tubercles, to 1st rib-scalene tubercle)

Serratus anterior

TP= Transverse process

5.15 Neck Triangles, Muscles, Thyroid and Parathyroid Glands

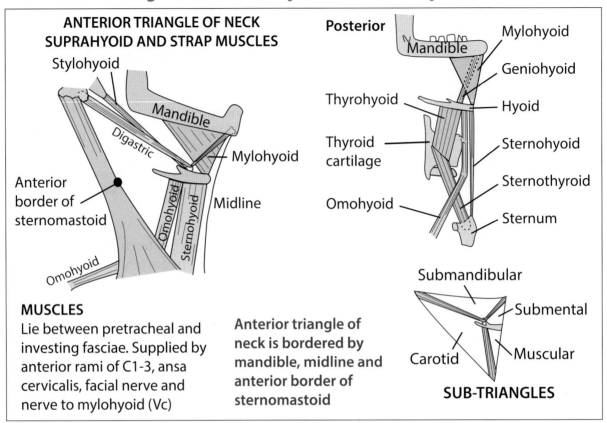

ANTERIOR TRIANGLE OF NECK SUPRAHYOID AND STRAP MUSCLES

Stylohyoid
Mandible
Digastric
Mylohyoid
Anterior border of sternomastoid
Omohyoid
Sternohyoid
Midline
Omohyoid

Posterior
Mandible
Mylohyoid
Geniohyoid
Thyrohyoid
Hyoid
Thyroid cartilage
Sternohyoid
Sternothyroid
Omohyoid
Sternum

MUSCLES
Lie between pretracheal and investing fasciae. Supplied by anterior rami of C1-3, ansa cervicalis, facial nerve and nerve to mylohyoid (Vc)

Anterior triangle of neck is bordered by mandible, midline and anterior border of sternomastoid

Submandibular
Submental
Carotid
Muscular
SUB-TRIANGLES

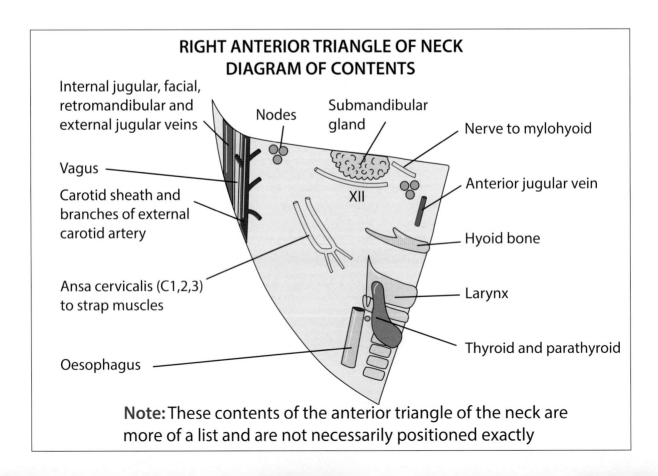

RIGHT ANTERIOR TRIANGLE OF NECK DIAGRAM OF CONTENTS

Internal jugular, facial, retromandibular and external jugular veins
Nodes
Submandibular gland
Nerve to mylohyoid

Vagus
XII
Anterior jugular vein

Carotid sheath and branches of external carotid artery
Hyoid bone

Ansa cervicalis (C1,2,3) to strap muscles
Larynx

Oesophagus
Thyroid and parathyroid

Note: These contents of the anterior triangle of the neck are more of a list and are not necessarily positioned exactly

POSTERIOR TRIANGLE OF NECK

Boundaries: Posterior border of sternocleidomastoid, anterior border of trapezius, middle 1/3 clavicle.
Shape: Spiral.
Roof: Investing fascia, platysma, external jugular vein.
Floor: Prevertebral fascia covering muscles, subclavian artery, trunks of brachial plexus and cervical plexus.
Contents:
Arteries: Occipital, superficial cervical, suprascpular.
Veins: Transverse cervical, suprascapular, external jugular.
Nerves: Branches of cervical plexus, spinal root of accessory.
Muscles: Omohyoid with its sling.
Lymph nodes: Occipital (rubella/scalp infections), supraclavicular (part of the deep chain)

Note: Each sternomastoid acting alone gives flexion and lateral rotation but acting together they give protrusion of head
Nerve: Spinal root of accessory (C1-5)

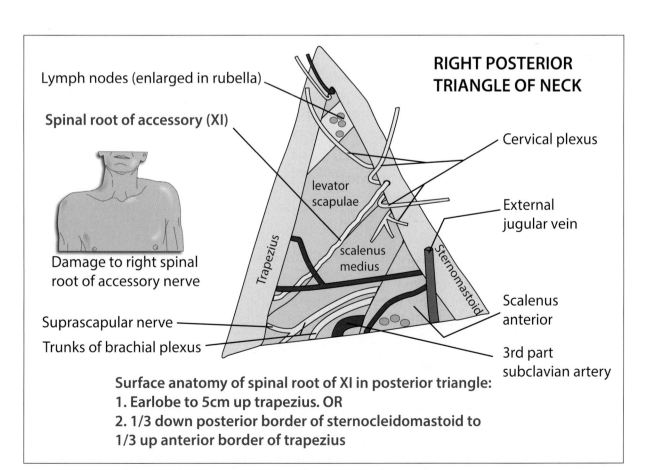

RIGHT POSTERIOR TRIANGLE OF NECK

Lymph nodes (enlarged in rubella)

Spinal root of accessory (XI)

Cervical plexus

levator scapulae

External jugular vein

Trapezius

scalenus medius

Sternomastoid

Damage to right spinal root of accessory nerve

Scalenus anterior

Suprascapular nerve

Trunks of brachial plexus

3rd part subclavian artery

Surface anatomy of spinal root of XI in posterior triangle:
1. Earlobe to 5cm up trapezius. OR
2. 1/3 down posterior border of sternocleidomastoid to 1/3 up anterior border of trapezius

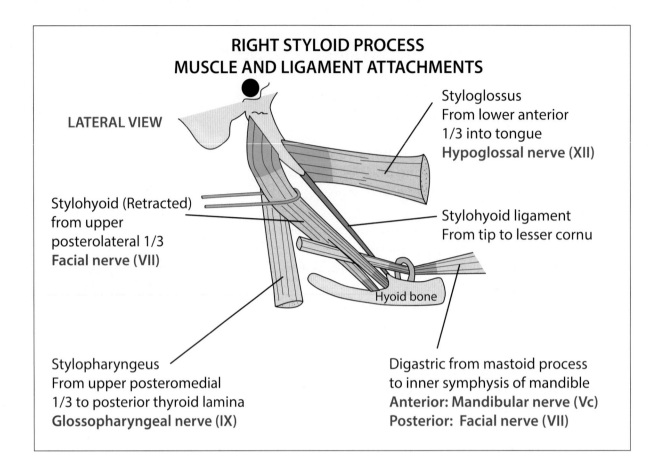

RIGHT STYLOID PROCESS
MUSCLE AND LIGAMENT ATTACHMENTS

LATERAL VIEW

Styloglossus
From lower anterior
1/3 into tongue
Hypoglossal nerve (XII)

Stylohyoid (Retracted)
from upper
posterolateral 1/3
Facial nerve (VII)

Stylohyoid ligament
From tip to lesser cornu

Hyoid bone

Stylopharyngeus
From upper posteromedial
1/3 to posterior thyroid lamina
Glossopharyngeal nerve (IX)

Digastric from mastoid process
to inner symphysis of mandible
Anterior: Mandibular nerve (Vc)
Posterior: Facial nerve (VII)

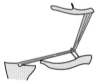

OMOHYOID
Transverse suprascapular ligament
via clavicle to hyoid
Nerve: 2 branches from ansa cervicalis (C1-3)

NECK MUSCLES 1

STYLOHYOID
Posterior base of styloid
process to hyoid
Nerve: Facial nerve (VII)

GENIOHYOID
Inferior mental (genial) spine
on mandible to hyoid
Nerve: C1 fibres on hypoglossal

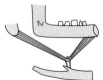

DIGASTRIC
Digastric notch on mastoid process, via sling on hyoid
to digastric fossa on posterior of anterior mandible
Nerve: Anterior belly - nerve to mylohyoid (Vc)
            Posterior belly - facial nerve (VII)

NECK MUSCLES 2

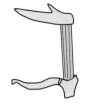

STERNOHYOID
Superior/lateral/posterior manubrium to hyoid
Nerve: Ansa cervicalis (C1-3)

THYROHYOID
Oblique line on thyroid cartilage to hyoid
Nerve: C1 fibres on hypoglossal

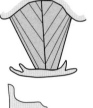

MYLOHYOID
Mylohyoid line on inner mandible. 3/4 into midline raphé, rest into hyoid
Nerve: Nerve to mylohyoid (Vc)

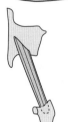

STERNOTHYROID
Posterior manubrium to oblique line on thyroid cartilage
Nerve: Ansa cervicalis (C1-3)

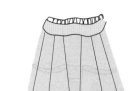

PLATYSMA
(Panniculus carnosus)
Deep fascia posterior to breasts to inferior border of mandible
Nerve: Cervical branch of facial (VII)

HYOID BONE AND ATTACHMENTS

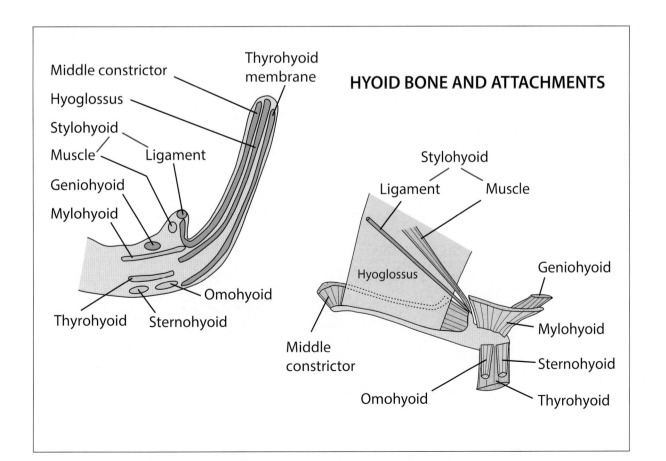

Middle constrictor
Hyoglossus
Stylohyoid
Muscle
Geniohyoid
Mylohyoid
Thyrohyoid membrane
Ligament
Thyrohyoid
Sternohyoid
Omohyoid

Stylohyoid
Ligament
Muscle
Hyoglossus
Middle constrictor
Omohyoid
Geniohyoid
Mylohyoid
Sternohyoid
Thyrohyoid

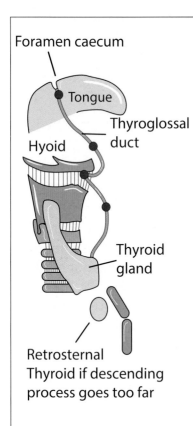

Foramen caecum
Tongue
Hyoid
Thyroglossal duct
Thyroid gland
Retrosternal Thyroid if descending process goes too far

THRYOID DEVELOPMENT
THYROGLOSSAL CYST AND FISTULA

The thyroid grows down from the tongue as a bilobed diverticulum connected back to the tongue by the thyroglossal duct. This duct solidifies and then usually disappears but can leave **thyroglossal cysts, fistulae or "rests"** (ectopic bits of thyroid) on the way in the **midline**. They move on swallowing or protruding the tongue. Radioactive scans show thyroid tissue even if it is ectopically placed.

LINGUAL THYROID

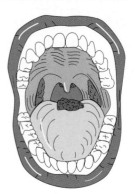

● Sites of thyroglossal cysts, remnant thyroid tissue (lingual thyroid), fistulae, sinuses and pyramidal lobe.

THYROID GLAND - AXIAL SECTION AT C7

Relations of thyroid gland
Posterior: Prevertebral fascia, carotid sheath, parathyroids, trachea
Medial: Recurrent laryngeal nerve, trachea, larynx, oesophagus
Anterior: Pretracheal fascia, sternohyoid, sternothyroid, venous arch

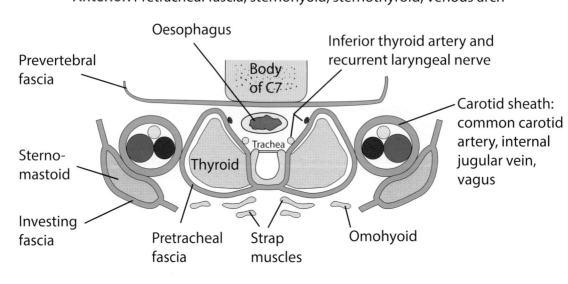

Prevertebral fascia
Oesophagus
Body of C7
Inferior thyroid artery and recurrent laryngeal nerve
Carotid sheath: common carotid artery, internal jugular vein, vagus
Sterno-mastoid
Trachea
Thyroid
Investing fascia
Pretracheal fascia
Strap muscles
Omohyoid

THYROID GLAND - GENERAL AND BLOOD SUPPPLY

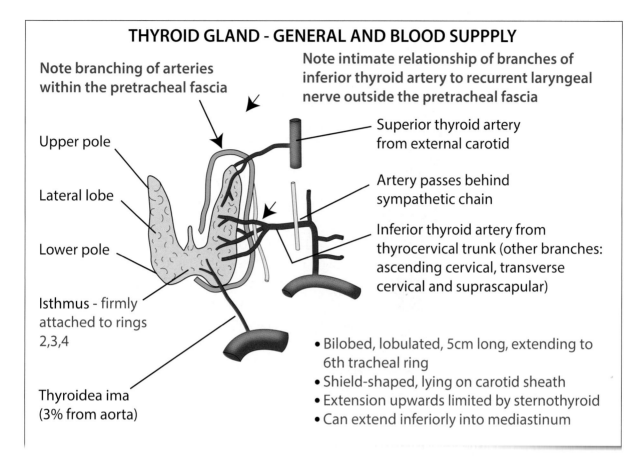

Note branching of arteries within the pretracheal fascia

Note intimate relationship of branches of inferior thyroid artery to recurrent laryngeal nerve outside the pretracheal fascia

Upper pole

Lateral lobe

Lower pole

Isthmus - firmly attached to rings 2,3,4

Thyroidea ima (3% from aorta)

Superior thyroid artery from external carotid

Artery passes behind sympathetic chain

Inferior thyroid artery from thyrocervical trunk (other branches: ascending cervical, transverse cervical and suprascapular)

- Bilobed, lobulated, 5cm long, extending to 6th tracheal ring
- Shield-shaped, lying on carotid sheath
- Extension upwards limited by sternothyroid
- Can extend inferiorly into mediastinum

VARIATIONS IN RELATIONSHIPS OF RECURRENT LARYNGEAL NERVE TO INFERIOR THYROID ARTERY

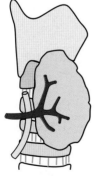

Deep to artery

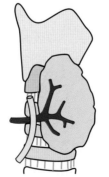

Superficial to artery

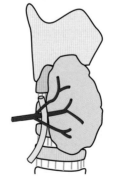

In amongst artery

Risks of surgery
- To parathyroid glands
- To recurrent laryngeal nerve when ligating inferior thyroid artery and to external branch of superior laryngeal nerve (cricothyroid muscle) when ligating superior thyroid artery

Note: The right recurrent laryngeal nerve can enter larynx directly from the vagus and not pass around subclavian artery

THYROID GLAND AND STRAP MUSCLES

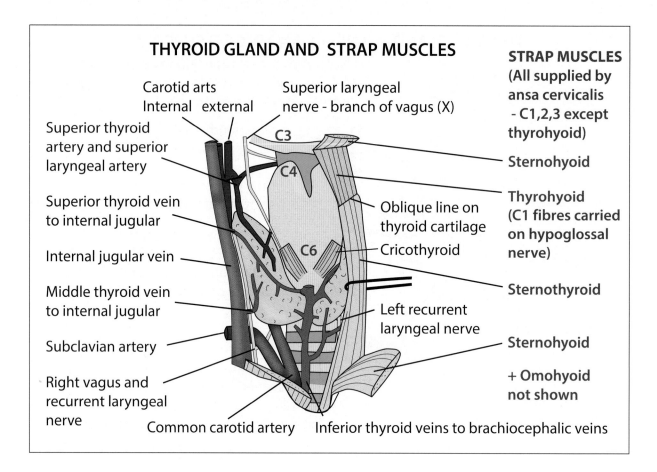

Carotid arts
Internal external

Superior laryngeal
nerve - branch of vagus (X)

Superior thyroid
artery and superior
laryngeal artery

Superior thyroid vein
to internal jugular

Internal jugular vein

Middle thyroid vein
to internal jugular

Subclavian artery

Right vagus and
recurrent laryngeal
nerve

C3

C4

C6

Oblique line on
thyroid cartilage

Cricothyroid

Left recurrent
laryngeal nerve

Common carotid artery

Inferior thyroid veins to brachiocephalic veins

STRAP MUSCLES
(All supplied by
ansa cervicalis
- C1,2,3 except
thyrohyoid)

Sternohyoid

Thyrohyoid
(C1 fibres carried
on hypoglossal
nerve)

Sternothyroid

Sternohyoid

+ Omohyoid
not shown

ANSA CERVICALIS

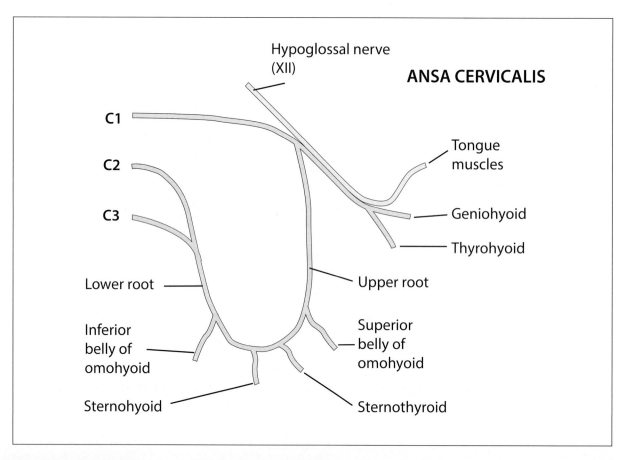

Hypoglossal nerve
(XII)

C1

C2

C3

Lower root

Inferior
belly of
omohyoid

Sternohyoid

Tongue
muscles

Geniohyoid

Thyrohyoid

Upper root

Superior
belly of
omohyoid

Sternothyroid

PARATHYROID GLANDS

Posterior view of thyroid gland

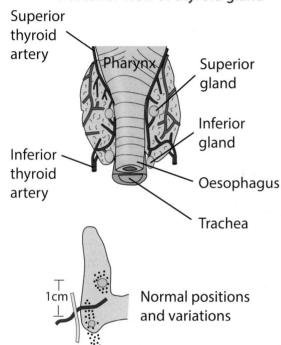

Superior thyroid artery

Pharynx

Superior gland

Inferior gland

Inferior thyroid artery

Oesophagus

Trachea

1cm

Normal positions and variations

- 4 (3-6) pinkish/brown 50mg glands.
- 6x3x2mm
- **Usually lie:** Within pretracheal fascia
  Superior: Less variation in position
  Inferior: More variation, even into upper mediastinum
- **Blood supply:** Inferior thyroid arteries
- **Nerves:** Sympathetics on arteries for vasoconstriction
- **Function:** Produce parathormone (PTH), increases tubular reabsorption of calcium, decrease tubular reabsorption of phosphate/bicarbonate, mobilise calcium from bones to give hypercalcaemia and hypercalciuria

5.16   Parotid and Submandibular Glands

PAROTID GLAND

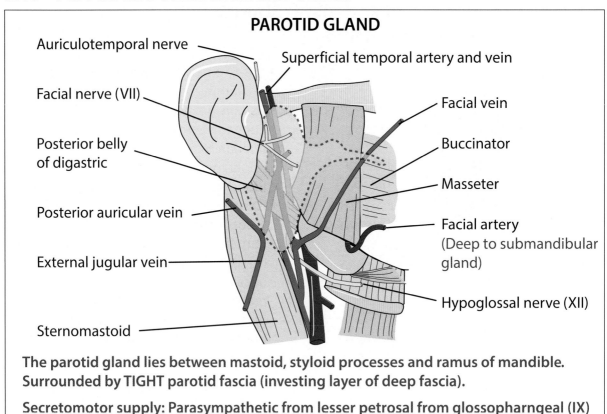

Auriculotemporal nerve

Superficial temporal artery and vein

Facial nerve (VII)

Facial vein

Posterior belly of digastric

Buccinator

Masseter

Posterior auricular vein

Facial artery (Deep to submandibular gland)

External jugular vein

Hypoglossal nerve (XII)

Sternomastoid

The parotid gland lies between mastoid, styloid processes and ramus of mandible. Surrounded by TIGHT parotid fascia (investing layer of deep fascia).

Secretomotor supply: Parasympathetic from lesser petrosal from glossopharngeal (IX)

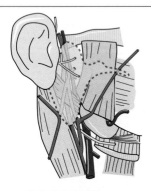

RELATIONS:
Posterior
Sternocleidomastoid
Mastoid process
Superior
External acoustic meatus
Temporomandibular joint
Anterior
Angle of mandible
Medial pterygoid plate
Masseter
Stylomandibular ligament

PAROTID GLAND

Serous secretions: Produces amylase, water, Ig factors (lubricates and aids oral hygiene). **Parts:** Has an upper and lower pole, lateral, anterior and deep surfaces
In gland: Facial nerve, retromandibular vein, external carotid artery, lymph nodes and fibres of auriculotemporal nerve
Deep to gland: Mastoid process, sternomastoid, posterior belly of digastric, styloid process, stylohyoid ligament, styloglossus, stylopharyngeus and tempormandibular joint

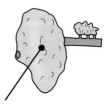

Lateral subcutaneous surface

MEDIAL SURFACE OF RIGHT PAROTID GLAND

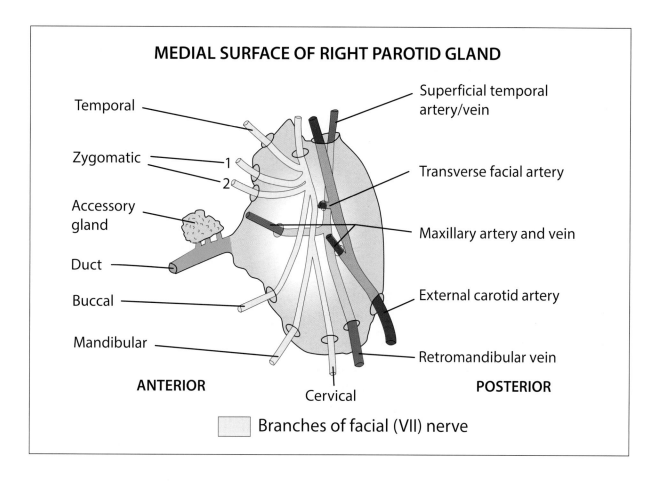

Temporal

Zygomatic
1
2

Accessory gland

Duct

Buccal

Mandibular

Superficial temporal artery/vein

Transverse facial artery

Maxillary artery and vein

External carotid artery

Retromandibular vein

ANTERIOR

Cervical

POSTERIOR

Branches of facial (VII) nerve

AXIAL SECTION OF RIGHT PAROTID GLAND

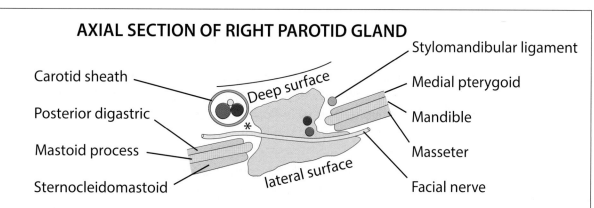

Carotid sheath

Posterior digastric

Mastoid process

Sternocleidomastoid

Deep surface

*

lateral surface

Stylomandibular ligament

Medial pterygoid

Mandible

Masseter

Facial nerve

- **Artery:** Branches of external carotid. **Vein:** Retromandibular
- **Lymph:** Pre-auricular to deep cervical
- **Nerves:** Secretomotor - via inferior salivary nucleus to glossopharyngeal nerve to its tympanic branch to lesser petrosal nerve to otic ganglion to auriculotemporal nerve. Sympathetics - via superior cervical ganglion and external carotid artery. Sensory - Auriculotemporal (Vc) and great auricular (C2)
- **Duct:** 5cm long, crosses masseter, pierces buccinator at 3rd molar and mucosa at 2nd molar

* Styloid process, stylohyoid, styloglossus, stylopharyngeus, stylohyoid and stylomandibular ligaments

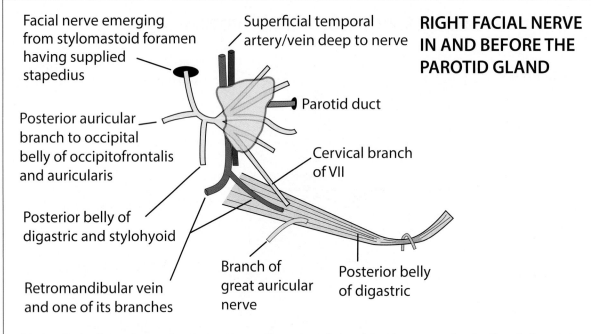

Facial nerve emerging from stylomastoid foramen having supplied stapedius

Superficial temporal artery/vein deep to nerve

RIGHT FACIAL NERVE IN AND BEFORE THE PAROTID GLAND

Parotid duct

Posterior auricular branch to occipital belly of occipitofrontalis and auricularis

Cervical branch of VII

Posterior belly of digastric and stylohyoid

Retromandibular vein and one of its branches

Branch of great auricular nerve

Posterior belly of digastric

Note: Only three important structures lie anterolateral to the posterior belly of digastric:-
- Cervical branch of facial nerve (VII)
- Branch of the retromandibular vein
- Branch of great auricular nerve (cervical plexus)

SUBMANDIBULAR GLAND

Secretions: Mixed - Mucous and serous
2 parts: Superficial - larger. Deep - smaller. Join behind posterior edge of mylohyoid
Duct: (Wharton's) 5cm long. First between mylohyoid and hyoglossus, then between sulingual gland and geniohyoid. **Opens:** In floor of mouth beside frenulum.
Develops: In ectoderm from a groove in the floor of mouth.
Produces: 70% of the saliva
Lymph nodes: In it and on it. Drain to submandibular glands.
Secretomotor supply: Chorda tympani from superior salivary nucleus carried on VII

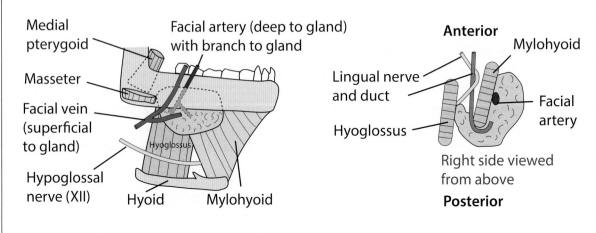

Medial pterygoid

Facial artery (deep to gland) with branch to gland

Anterior

Mylohyoid

Masseter

Lingual nerve and duct

Facial vein (superficial to gland)

Hyoglossus

Facial artery

Hyoglossus

Hypoglossal nerve (XII)

Hyoid

Mylohyoid

Right side viewed from above

Posterior

SUBMANDIBULAR AND SUBLINGUAL GLANDS
Coronal section

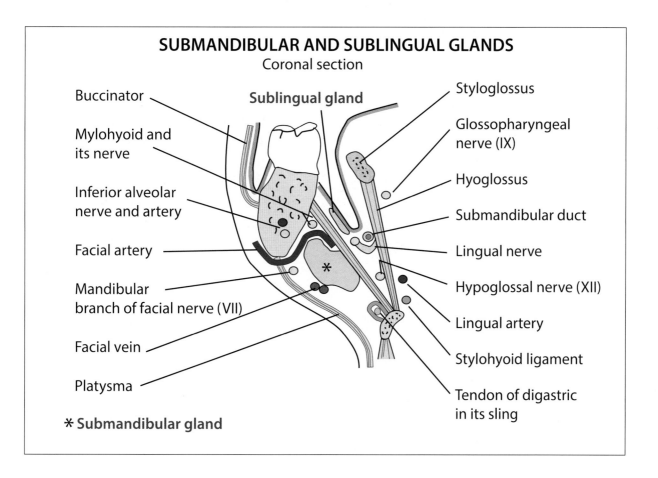

Buccinator

Mylohyoid and its nerve

Inferior alveolar nerve and artery

Facial artery

Mandibular branch of facial nerve (VII)

Facial vein

Platysma

Sublingual gland

Styloglossus

Glossopharyngeal nerve (IX)

Hyoglossus

Submandibular duct

Lingual nerve

Hypoglossal nerve (XII)

Lingual artery

Stylohyoid ligament

Tendon of digastric in its sling

* Submandibular gland

SUBLINGUAL GLAND

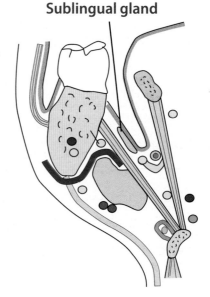

Sublingual gland

- Mucous gland
- Between mylohyoid and genioglossus
- 15 ducts - Half into submandibular duct; half into sublingual fold
- **Nerve supply:** Secretomotor via submandibular ganglion from chorda tympani; general sensation via lingual nerve (Vc)
- **Blood supply:** Lingual artery and branches of submental artery
- **Develops:** from a groove in floor of mouth that becomes a tunnel. Blind end proliferates (ectodermal) to give secreting acini
- **(Note: all salivary glands develop from epithelial lining of mouth)**

5.17   Larynx and Pharynx

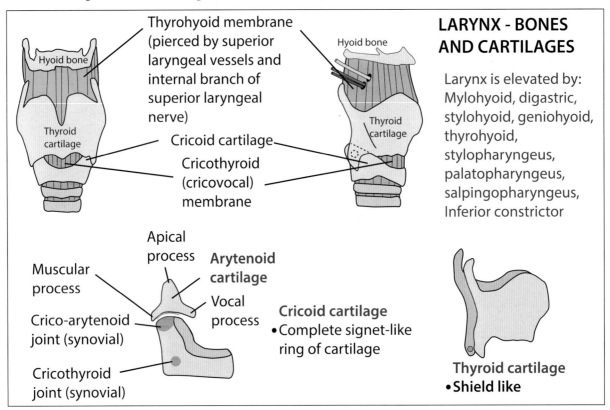

LARYNX - BONES AND CARTILAGES

Thyrohyoid membrane (pierced by superior laryngeal vessels and internal branch of superior laryngeal nerve)

Hyoid bone

Thyroid cartilage

Cricoid cartilage

Cricothyroid (cricovocal) membrane

Apical process

Arytenoid cartilage

Muscular process

Vocal process

Crico-arytenoid joint (synovial)

Cricothyroid joint (synovial)

Cricoid cartilage
• Complete signet-like ring of cartilage

Larynx is elevated by: Mylohyoid, digastric, stylohyoid, geniohyoid, thyrohyoid, stylopharyngeus, palatopharyngeus, salpingopharyngeus, Inferior constrictor

Thyroid cartilage
• **Shield like**

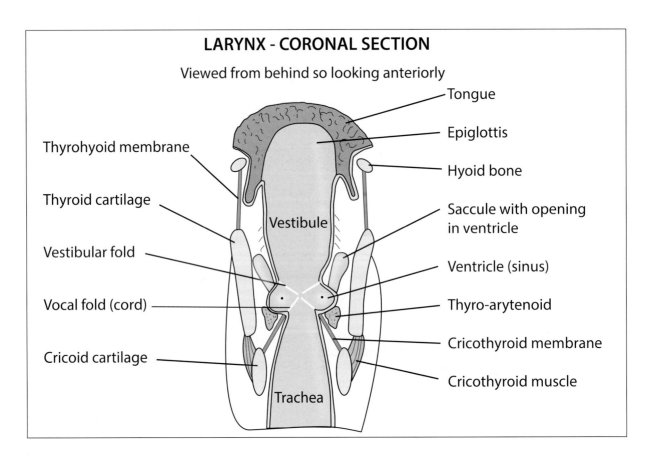

LARYNX - CORONAL SECTION

Viewed from behind so looking anteriorly

Thyrohyoid membrane

Thyroid cartilage

Vestibular fold

Vocal fold (cord)

Cricoid cartilage

Vestibule

Trachea

Tongue

Epiglottis

Hyoid bone

Saccule with opening in ventricle

Ventricle (sinus)

Thyro-arytenoid

Cricothyroid membrane

Cricothyroid muscle

LARYNX

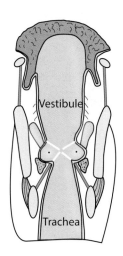

Mucosa: Pseudostratified ciliated columnar. Mucous glands in sinus. (Cords and upper epiglottis - stratified squamous)
Blood supply: Superior and inferior laryngeal arteries
Nerve supply:
Sensory above cords - Internal branch of superior laryngeal nerve from vagus (arch 4 nerves)
Sensory below cords - Recurrent laryngeal nerve branch of vagus (arch 6 nerves)
Motor to muscles: Nucleus ambiguus via cranial accessory nerve to vagus
Cricothyroid: External branch of superior laryngeal nerve.
All other laryngeal muscles (including upper oesophagus and cricopharyngeus): Recurrent laryngeal nerve
Lymphatic drainage:
Above cords: Upper deep cervical nodes
Below cords: Lower deep cervical nodes

LARYNX - INLET AND EPIGLOTTIS

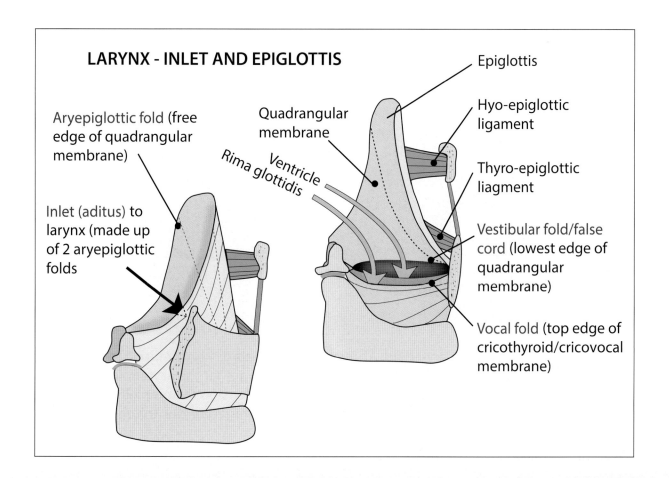

VOCAL CORDS AND CRICOTHYROID MEMBRANE

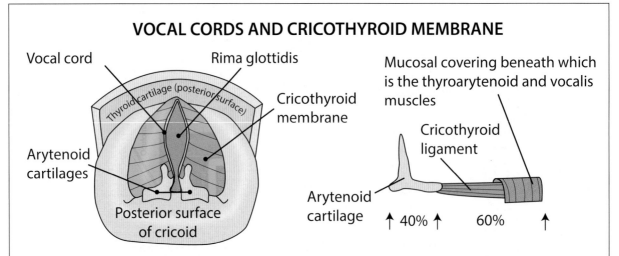

TRUE VOCAL CORDS are the free upper edges of the cricothyroid membrane (conus elasticus) where it is thickened to become the cricovocal liagment and covered with mucosa. The mucosa is pearly white and has no submucosa and thus in theory should not become oedematous, but in practice they do as in anaphylaxis and infection. 40% of the vocal cord is arytenoid cartilage: 60% is membrane. The cricothyroid membrane is attached around the inside of the ring of cricoid cartilage and has a free upper margin that is attached to the arytenoid cartilages posteriorly and to the posterior of the thyroid cartilage anteriorly

INTRINSIC MUSCLES OF THE LARYNX 1

Posterior view

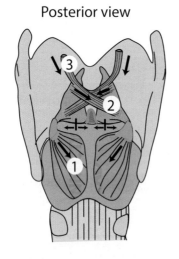

Posterior View

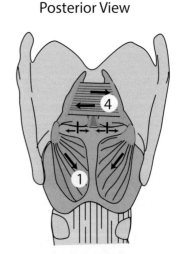

1. Posterior crico-arytenoid: **Abducts and open cords - only muscle to do so**
2. Oblique arytenoid: **Close cords by drawing together the arytenoids**
3. Aryepiglotticus: **Close aditus. They are the extension of aryepiglotticus**
4. Transverse arytenoid: **Close cords by drawing together the arytenoids**

INTRINSIC MUSCLES OF THE LARYNX 2

Looking down at cords

Lateral view

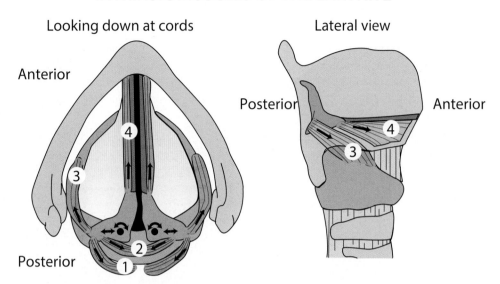

1. Posterior crico-arytenoid: **Open cords - only muscle to do so**
2. Transverse arytenoid: **Close cords**
3. Lateral crico-arytenoid: **Adduct and close cords by rotating arytenoids medially**
4. Thyro-arytenoid: **Loosen cords by pulling the thyroid cartilage towards the arytenoids**
4. Vocalis (part of thyro-arytenoid): **Alter shape and thickness of cords**

CRICOTHYROID MUSCLE

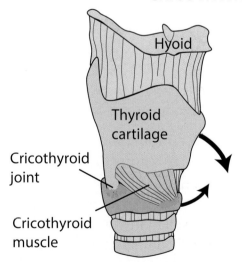

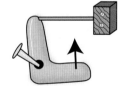 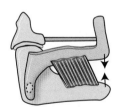

The action of cricothyroid can be likened to nailing an angle iron to the wall, as above, and levering it upwards. The attached cord will tighten

Only muscle of larynx that:
- Is outside the larynx
- Is supplied by external branch of superior laryngeal nerve
- Tightens(lengthens) the cords

Mucosa of larynx: Pseudostratified ciliated columnar BUT squamous over cords and top of epiglottis.
Lymphatic drainage:
Above cords - upper deep cervical nodes
Below cords - lower deep cervical nodes

VOCAL CORDS

CLOSED   OPEN

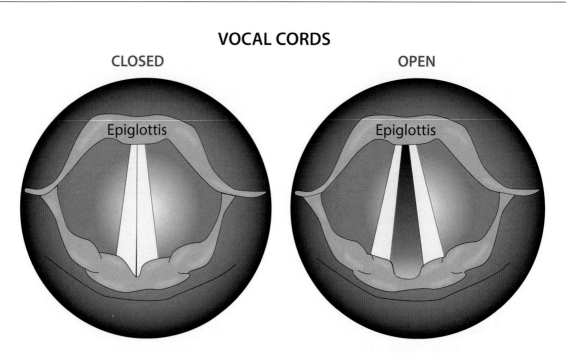

The vocal cords open by the arytenoid cartilages sliding down the slope of the cricoid cartilage and thus open as a "triangle" shape and not as a "diamond" shape

SEMON'S LAW: DAMAGE TO THE RECURRENT LARYNGEAL NERVE

RLN   CORDS   RLN   CORDS

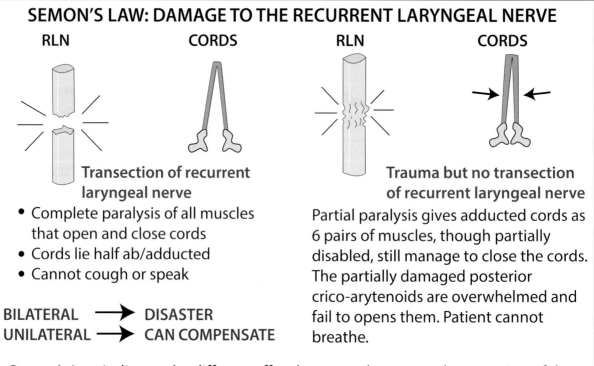

Transection of recurrent laryngeal nerve

- Complete paralysis of all muscles that open and close cords
- Cords lie half ab/adducted
- Cannot cough or speak

BILATERAL   ⟶   DISASTER

UNILATERAL ⟶   CAN COMPENSATE

Trauma but no transection of recurrent laryngeal nerve

Partial paralysis gives adducted cords as 6 pairs of muscles, though partially disabled, still manage to close the cords. The partially damaged posterior crico-arytenoids are overwhelmed and fail to opens them. Patient cannot breathe.

Semon's Law indicates the different effect between damage and transection of the recurrent laryngeal nerve as applicable to surgery in the region of this nerve (eg thyroidectomy or parathyroidectomy). It is probably more of a guide than a rule

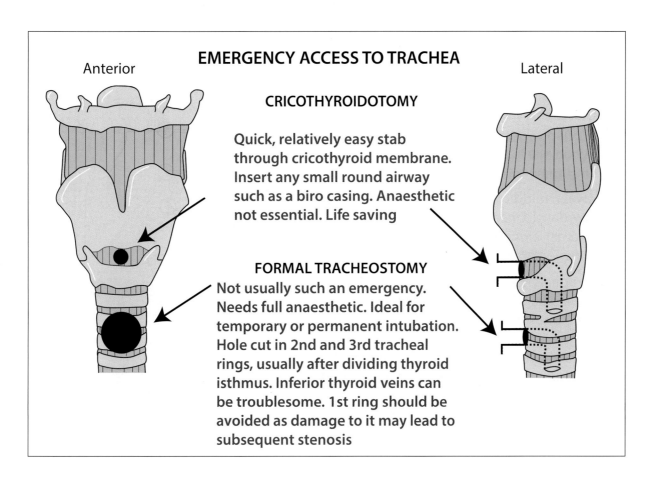

EMERGENCY ACCESS TO TRACHEA

Anterior

Lateral

CRICOTHYROIDOTOMY

Quick, relatively easy stab through cricothyroid membrane. Insert any small round airway such as a biro casing. Anaesthetic not essential. Life saving

FORMAL TRACHEOSTOMY

Not usually such an emergency. Needs full anaesthetic. Ideal for temporary or permanent intubation. Hole cut in 2nd and 3rd tracheal rings, usually after dividing thyroid isthmus. Inferior thyroid veins can be troublesome. 1st ring should be avoided as damage to it may lead to subsequent stenosis

PHARYNX - CARTOON OF MUSCLES AND PHARYNGOBASILAR FASCIA

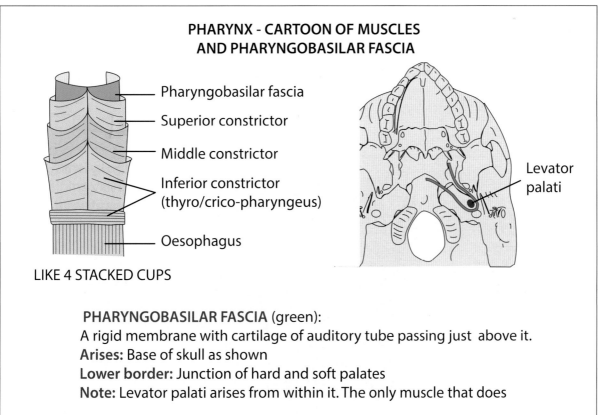

- Pharyngobasilar fascia
- Superior constrictor
- Middle constrictor
- Inferior constrictor (thyro/crico-pharyngeus)
- Oesophagus

Levator palati

LIKE 4 STACKED CUPS

PHARYNGOBASILAR FASCIA (green):
A rigid membrane with cartilage of auditory tube passing just above it.
Arises: Base of skull as shown
Lower border: Junction of hard and soft palates
Note: Levator palati arises from within it. The only muscle that does

PHARYNX - MUSCLES AND STRUCTURES ENTERING IT

Between superior and middle constrictors:
1. Glossopharyngeal nerve (IX)
2. Stylopharyngeus (IX)
3. Stylohyoid ligament
4. Lingual nerve (Vc)

Between middle and inferior constrictors:
5. Thyrohyoid membrane pierced by -
6. Internal laryngeal nerve
7. Superior laryngeal vessels

(Thyropharyngeus (8) is upper part that behaves like the other constrictors, closing on swallowing. Cricopharyngeus (9) is lower part - a sphincter that opens on swallowing. Between 2 parts is potential pharyngeal pouch (Dehiscence of Killian) (10)

Below inferior constrictor and passing upwards:
11. Recurrent laryngeal nerve
12. Inferior laryngeal vessels

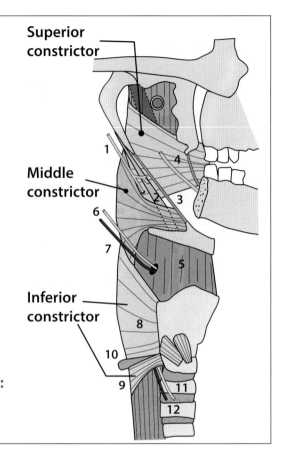

Superior constrictor

Middle constrictor

Inferior constrictor

STYLOID PROCESS MUSCLE AND LIGAMENT ATTACHMENTS POSTERIOR VIEW

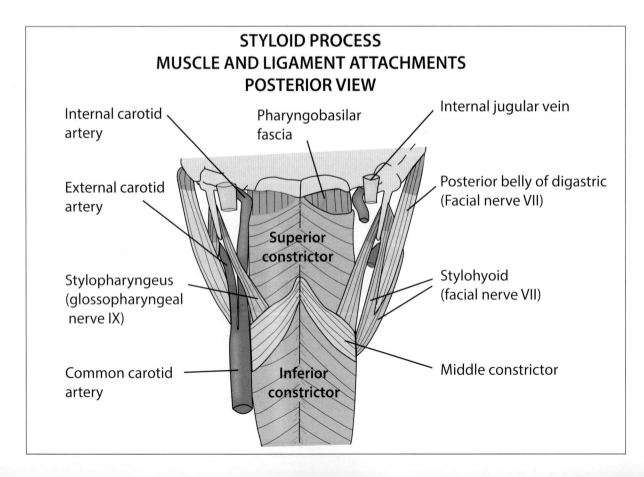

Internal carotid artery

External carotid artery

Stylopharyngeus (glossopharyngeal nerve IX)

Common carotid artery

Pharyngobasilar fascia

Superior constrictor

Inferior constrictor

Internal jugular vein

Posterior belly of digastric (Facial nerve VII)

Stylohyoid (facial nerve VII)

Middle constrictor

NASAL, ORAL AND LARYGOPHARYNX OPENED POSTERIORLY

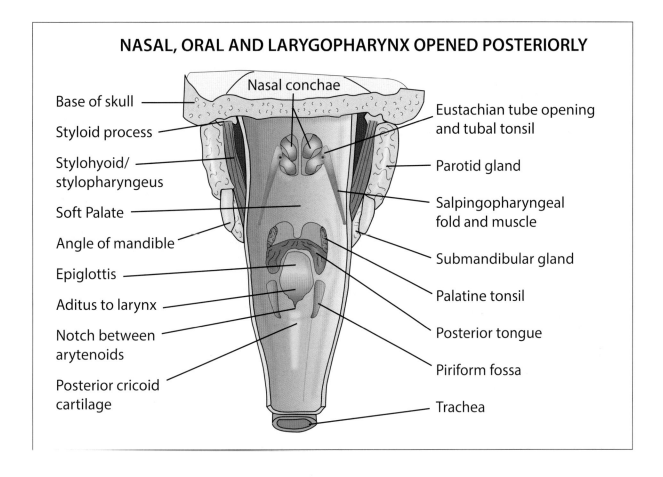

Base of skull

Styloid process

Stylohyoid/
stylopharyngeus

Soft Palate

Angle of mandible

Epiglottis

Aditus to larynx

Notch between
arytenoids

Posterior cricoid
cartilage

Nasal conchae

Eustachian tube opening
and tubal tonsil

Parotid gland

Salpingopharyngeal
fold and muscle

Submandibular gland

Palatine tonsil

Posterior tongue

Piriform fossa

Trachea

3 PARTS OF THE PHARYNX

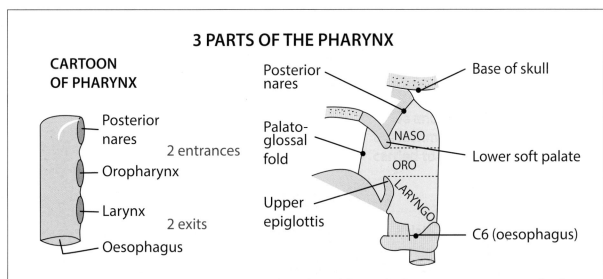

**CARTOON
OF PHARYNX**

Posterior
nares

2 entrances

Oropharynx

Larynx

2 exits

Oesophagus

Posterior
nares

Palato-
glossal
fold

Upper
epiglottis

Base of skull

NASO

Lower soft palate

ORO

LARYNGO

C6 (oesophagus)

- 5" (13cm) long fibromuscular tube suspended from skull. Anterior to prevertebral fascia like a mask applied to back of face
- **Extends:** From nose to C6 (oesophagus)
- **Walls:** Mucous membrane, fibrous submucosa, muscle and buccopharyngeal fascia
- **Muscles:** 3 constrictors + stylopharyngeus, palatopharyngeus, salpingopharyngeus
- **Note:** Levator palati is wholly intra-pharyngeal

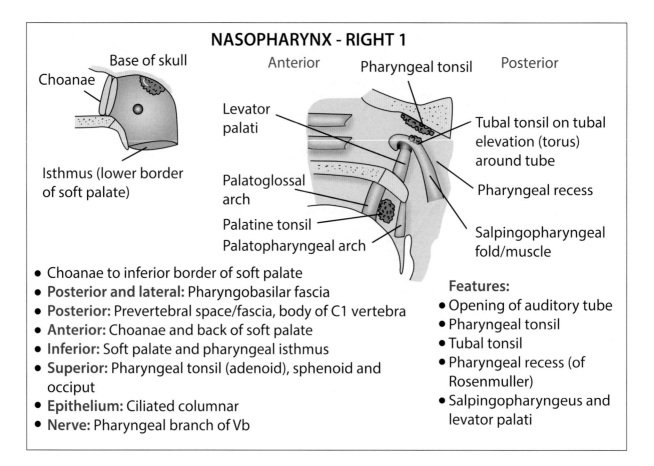

NASOPHARYNX - RIGHT 1

Base of skull

Choanae

Isthmus (lower border of soft palate)

Anterior — Pharyngeal tonsil — Posterior

Levator palati

Palatoglossal arch

Palatine tonsil

Palatopharyngeal arch

Tubal tonsil on tubal elevation (torus) around tube

Pharyngeal recess

Salpingopharyngeal fold/muscle

- Choanae to inferior border of soft palate
- **Posterior and lateral:** Pharyngobasilar fascia
- **Posterior:** Prevertebral space/fascia, body of C1 vertebra
- **Anterior:** Choanae and back of soft palate
- **Inferior:** Soft palate and pharyngeal isthmus
- **Superior:** Pharyngeal tonsil (adenoid), sphenoid and occiput
- **Epithelium:** Ciliated columnar
- **Nerve:** Pharyngeal branch of Vb

Features:
- Opening of auditory tube
- Pharyngeal tonsil
- Tubal tonsil
- Pharyngeal recess (of Rosenmuller)
- Salpingopharyngeus and levator palati

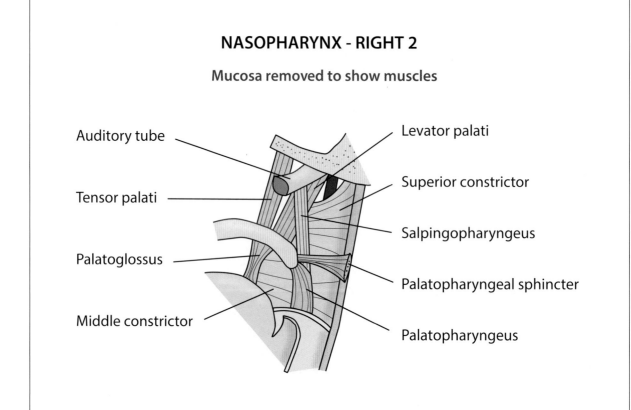

NASOPHARYNX - RIGHT 2

Mucosa removed to show muscles

Auditory tube

Tensor palati

Palatoglossus

Middle constrictor

Levator palati

Superior constrictor

Salpingopharyngeus

Palatopharyngeal sphincter

Palatopharyngeus

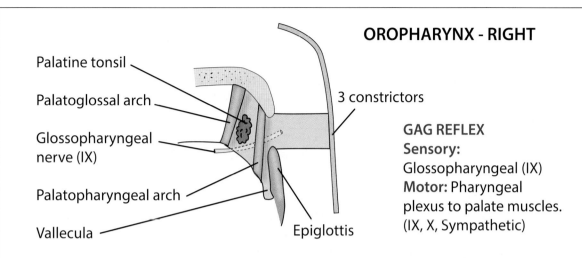

OROPHARYNX - RIGHT

Palatine tonsil

Palatoglossal arch

Glossopharyngeal nerve (IX)

Palatopharyngeal arch

Vallecula

3 constrictors

Epiglottis

GAG REFLEX
Sensory:
Glossopharyngeal (IX)
Motor: Pharyngeal
plexus to palate muscles.
(IX, X, Sympathetic)

- Lower border of soft palate to upper border of epiglottis
- **Anterior:** Posterior aspect of tongue and palatoglossal arch
- **Posterior:** 3 constrictors and C2/C3 vertebrae
- **Inferior:** Back of tongue, lingual tonsil and valleculae
- **Lateral:** Palatoglossal/palatopharyngeal arches, constrictors and palatine tonsil
- **Lining:** Squamous epithelium
- **Nerves:** Glossopharyngeal (IX) and internal laryngeal (X) in valleculae
- **Features:** Palatine tonsils, lingual tonsils, valleculae

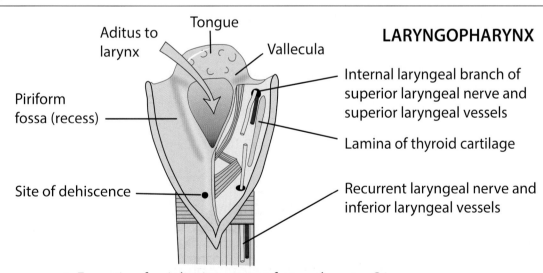

LARYNGOPHARYNX

Aditus to larynx

Tongue

Vallecula

Piriform fossa (recess)

Site of dehiscence

Internal laryngeal branch of superior laryngeal nerve and superior laryngeal vessels

Lamina of thyroid cartilage

Recurrent laryngeal nerve and inferior laryngeal vessels

- From tip of epiglottis to start of oesophagus - C6
- **Anterior:** Larynx, aditus, epiglottis
- **Posterior:** 3 constrictors, cricopharyngeus, vertebrae C4,5,6
- **Nerves:** Internal laryngeal branch of superior laryngeal nerve (X) and recurrent laryngeal nerve (X). (Some overlapping of supply in the laryngopharynx unlike in the larynx)
- **Lining:** Squamous non-keratinising epithelium
- **Features:** Aditus to larynx and piriform fossa

SWALLOWING

1. FOOD BOLUS MOVED BY TONGUE TO OROPHARYNX
Mylohyoid (Vc) lifts tongue - Tongue (XII) - Styloglossus - Muscles of mastication (Vc) - Buccinator (VII)
2. NASOPHARYNX CLOSES
Superior constrictor (PP- pharyngeal plexus) - Passavant's ridge (PP) - Tensor palati (Vc) - Levator palati (PP)
3. AUDITORY TUBE OPENS
Levator palati (PP) - Tensor palati (Vc) - Salpingopharyngeus (PP)
4. PHARYNX AND LARYNX MOVE UP TO HYOID
Happens before bolus arrives - Stylopharyngeus (IX) - Salpingopharyngeus (PP) - Palatopharyngeus (PP) - Inferior constrictor (PP)
5. OROPHARYNX KEPT CLOSED
Palatoglossus (PP) - Intrinsic muscles of tongue (XII) - Styloglossus (XII)
6. LARYNX CLOSES
Aryepiglotticus (X-RLN) - Cords close (X-RLN) - Epiglottis flaps
7. HYOID ELEVATES BRINGING PHARYNX/LARYNX UP MORE
Stylohyoid (VII)
8. HYPOPHARYNX OPENS
Cricopharyngeus/upper oesophagus relax (X-RLN)
9. HYOID, LARYNX AND PHARYNX MOVE DOWN TOGETHER
Elastic recoil
10. LARYNX AND PHARYNX MOVE DOWN FROM HYOID
Elastic recoil
11. PERISTALSIS
Striated muscle then smooth muscle of oesophagus (3-5cm/sec) (X-RLN)

ORDER OF EVENTS IN SUMMARY

LARYNX AND PHARYNX MOVE UP TO HYOID

LARYNX, PHARYNX AND HYOID MOVE UP

LARYNX, PHARYNX AND HYOID MOVE DOWN

LARYNX AND PHARYNX MOVE DOWN FROM HYOID

VASCULAR SUPPLY TO PHARYNX

ARTERIAL SUPPLY FROM EXTERNAL CAROTID

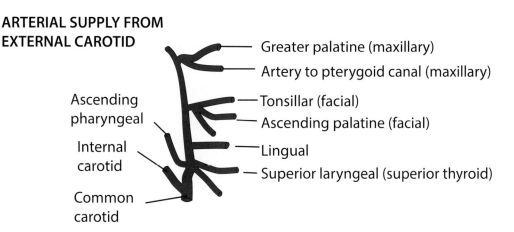

Greater palatine (maxillary)
Artery to pterygoid canal (maxillary)
Ascending pharyngeal
Tonsillar (facial)
Ascending palatine (facial)
Internal carotid
Lingual
Superior laryngeal (superior thyroid)
Common carotid

VENOUS DRAINAGE
Plexus on middle constrictor draining to:
Pterygoid plexus
Internal jugular vein
Lower pharynx to inferior thyroid veins

NERVES OF THE PHARYNX

PHARYNGEAL PLEXUS
On posterior wall of pharynx.
IX (glossopharyngeal) sensory only.
X (pharyngeal branch of vagus).
Branchiomotor fibres from nucleus ambiguus via cranial accessory (XI)
Sympathetic - vasocontrictor only

Supplies →

Levator palati
Salpingopharyngeus
Palatopharyngeus
Palatoglossus
3 constrictors
Striated oesophagus

GLOSSOPHARYNGEAL (IX) → Stylopharyngeus (motor)
Oropharynx/valleculae (sensation)

RECURRENT LARYNGEAL (X) → Cricopharyngeus
Upper oesophagus

PHARYNGEAL BRANCH OF MAXILLARY (VB)
via pterygopalatine ganglion and palatovaginal canal

Nasopharynx (sensation)

INTERNAL BRANCH OF SUPERIOR LARYNGEAL (X)

Sensation/taste vallecula and upper pharynx

RECURRENT LARYNGEAL (X)

Laryngopharynx

5.18 Autonomic Nervous System, in General, Sympathetic and Parasympathetic

NEURONS

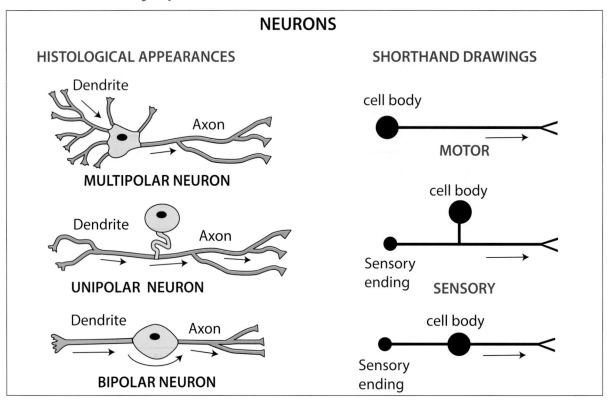

HISTOLOGICAL APPEARANCES

Dendrite

Axon

MULTIPOLAR NEURON

Dendrite

Axon

UNIPOLAR NEURON

Dendrite

Axon

BIPOLAR NEURON

SHORTHAND DRAWINGS

cell body

MOTOR

cell body

Sensory ending

SENSORY

cell body

Sensory ending

PERIPHERAL NERVOUS SYSTEM

SOMATIC
(Voluntary control)
Motor: Voluntary muscles
Sensory: Localisable

AUTONOMIC
(Involuntary, largely unconscious control)
Motor: Smooth muscle, secretions (glandular, sweat, digestive). Sensory: General visceral afferent and special visceral afferent (taste and baroreception). General, vague, usually midline, poorly-localisable sensation

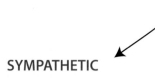

SYMPATHETIC

Urgent activities: "Flight, Fight, Fright"
• Increases heart rate, raises blood pressure
• Dilates bronchi
• Dilated pupil
• Raises eyelids
• Vasoconstricts (vasomotor) diverting blood to muscles
• Sweat (sudomotor)
• Erect hairs on skin (pilomotor)
• Stimulates adrenalin from adrenal gland
• Stimulates ejaculation
• Closes sphincters, inhibits peristalsis

PARASYMPATHETIC

Quiet activities: "Rest and Digest"
• Stimulates secretions (salivary, mucous)
• Slows heart, minimises blood pressure
• Constricts bronchi
• Constricts pupil
• Stimulates gut peristalsis
• Opens sphincters
• Contracts bladder
• Contracts uterus
• Accommodates the eye
• Erects the penis and clitoris

EMERGENCE OF NERVES FROM CENTRAL NERVOUS SYSTEM

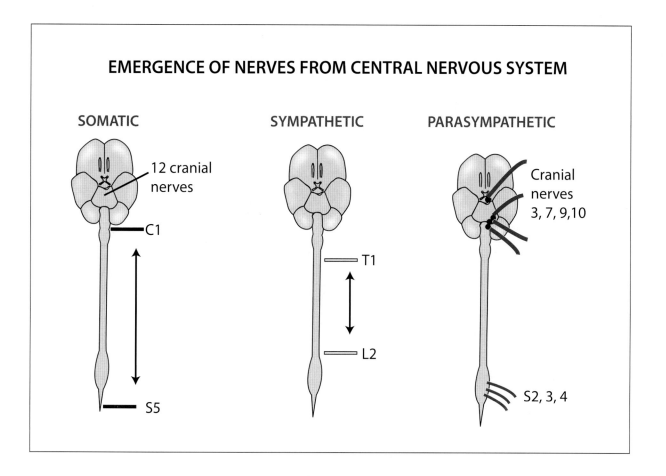

SOMATIC

12 cranial nerves

C1

S5

SYMPATHETIC

T1

L2

PARASYMPATHETIC

Cranial nerves 3, 7, 9,10

S2, 3, 4

AUTONOMIC NERVOUS SYSTEM

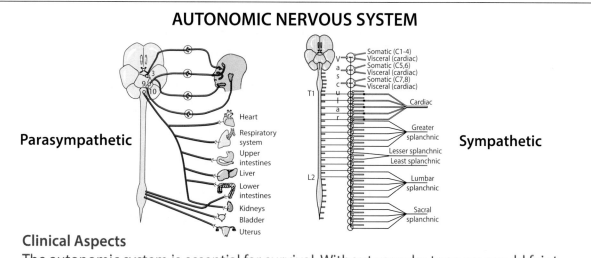

Parasympathetic

Heart
Respiratory system
Upper intestines
Liver
Lower intestines
Kidneys
Bladder
Uterus

Somatic (C1-4)
Visceral (cardiac)
Somatic (C5,6)
Visceral (cardiac)
Somatic (C7,8)
Visceral (cardiac)

Cardiac

Greater splanchnic
Lesser splanchnic
Least splanchnic

Lumbar splanchnic

Sacral splanchnic

Sympathetic

Clinical Aspects

The autonomic system is essential for survival. Without vascular tone we would faint every time we stood up. There would be no intestinal activity to digest and absorb food and no increase in heart rate with exercise. Without sexual activity there would be no continuation of the species!

Deliberate destruction of the nerves is sometimes necessary. For instance in excessive sweating, sympathetic nerves can be cut selectively or the parasympathetics (vagus nerves) can be cut to decrease acid production in the stomach. Referred pain, for example from the appendix or gonads, is explicable in terms of general visceral sensory fibres carried in the autonomic system.

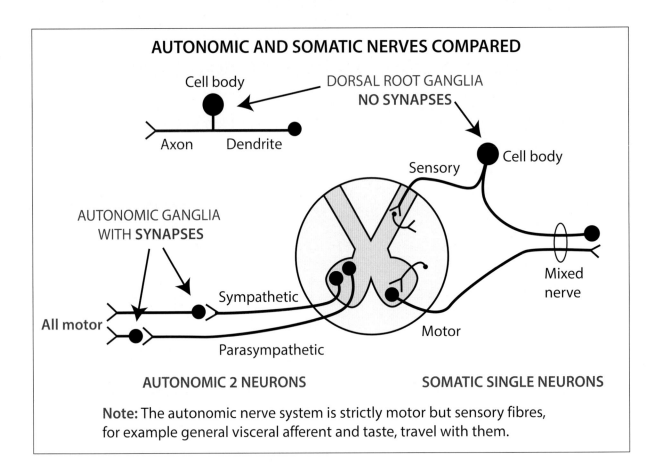

AUTONOMIC AND SOMATIC NERVES COMPARED

Cell body

DORSAL ROOT GANGLIA
NO SYNAPSES

Axon   Dendrite

Sensory   Cell body

AUTONOMIC GANGLIA
WITH **SYNAPSES**

Mixed nerve

Sympathetic

All motor

Parasympathetic

Motor

AUTONOMIC 2 NEURONS   **SOMATIC SINGLE NEURONS**

Note: The autonomic nerve system is strictly motor but sensory fibres,
for example general visceral afferent and taste, travel with them.

AUTONOMIC NERVOUS ACTIONS
ANTAGONISTIC VERSUS INDEPENDENT ACTIONS

SYMPATHETIC	ANTAGONISTIC	PARASYMPATHETIC
Speeds heart		Slows heart
Dilates bronchi		Constricts bronchi
Dilates pupil		Constricts pupil

SYMPATHETIC	INDEPENDENT	PARASYMPATHETIC
Raises eyelids		Eye accommodation
Stimulates ejaculation		Erection of penis/clitoris

HITCHHIKING PRINCIPLE 1

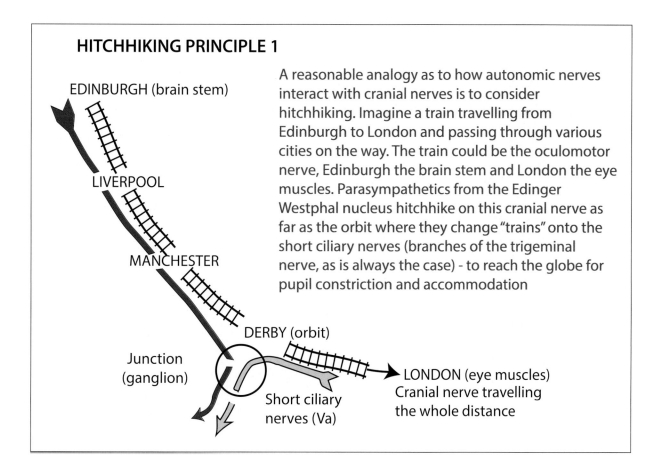

EDINBURGH (brain stem)

LIVERPOOL

MANCHESTER

DERBY (orbit)

Junction (ganglion)

Short ciliary nerves (Va)

LONDON (eye muscles)
Cranial nerve travelling the whole distance

A reasonable analogy as to how autonomic nerves interact with cranial nerves is to consider hitchhiking. Imagine a train travelling from Edinburgh to London and passing through various cities on the way. The train could be the oculomotor nerve, Edinburgh the brain stem and London the eye muscles. Parasympathetics from the Edinger Westphal nucleus hitchhike on this cranial nerve as far as the orbit where they change "trains" onto the short ciliary nerves (branches of the trigeminal nerve, as is always the case) - to reach the globe for pupil constriction and accommodation

HITCHHIKING PRINCIPLE 2

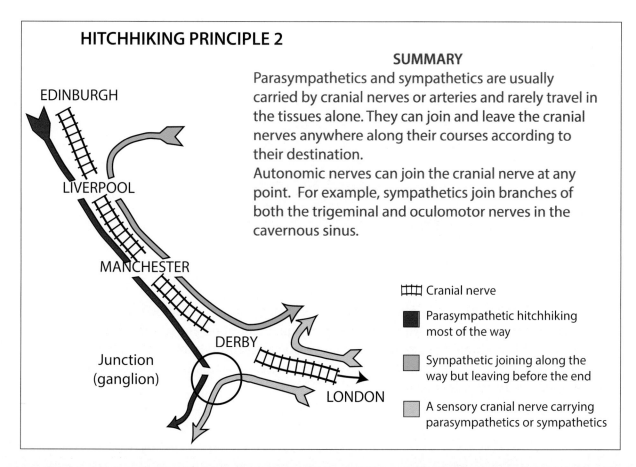

EDINBURGH

LIVERPOOL

MANCHESTER

DERBY

Junction (ganglion)

LONDON

SUMMARY

Parasympathetics and sympathetics are usually carried by cranial nerves or arteries and rarely travel in the tissues alone. They can join and leave the cranial nerves anywhere along their courses according to their destination.

Autonomic nerves can join the cranial nerve at any point. For example, sympathetics join branches of both the trigeminal and oculomotor nerves in the cavernous sinus.

Cranial nerve

Parasympathetic hitchhiking most of the way

Sympathetic joining along the way but leaving before the end

A sensory cranial nerve carrying parasympathetics or sympathetics

3 TYPES OF GANGLIA

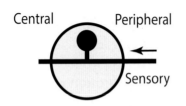

Central | Peripheral

Sensory

A SENSORY GANGLION has cell bodies only and NO synapses.

Examples:
- Posterior (dorsal) root
- Trigeminal
- Glossopharyngeal
- Geniculate
- Vagal

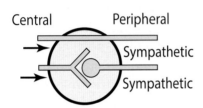

Central | Peripheral

Sympathetic

Sympathetic

A SYMPATHETIC GANGLION has either a synapse or a fibre passing through it which will synapse later.

Examples:
- Sympathetic chain
- Sympathetic peripheral ganglia (coeliac, renal, superior mesenteric)

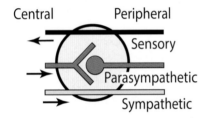

Central | Peripheral

Sensory

Parasympathetic

Sympathetic

A PARASYMPATHETIC GANGLION has parasympathetic nerves synapsing and both a somatic sensory and a sympathetic nerve passing through it. Examples:
- Ciliary
- Pterygopalatine
- Submandibular
- Otic

PARASYMPATHETIC GANGLIA

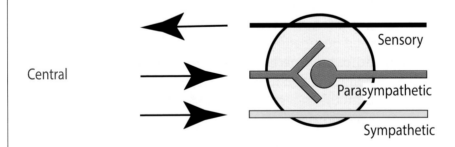

Central

Sensory

Parasympathetic

Sympathetic

Peripheral

All the PARASYMPATHETIC GANGLIA (ciliary, pterygopalatine, submandibular and otic) have the same pattern of a synapse of the parasympathetic fibres and passing through the ganglion is a branch of the trigeminal nerve (somatic sensory) which carries the parasympathetics to their destination. In addition there is a sympathetic fibre passing through for vasoconstriction only.

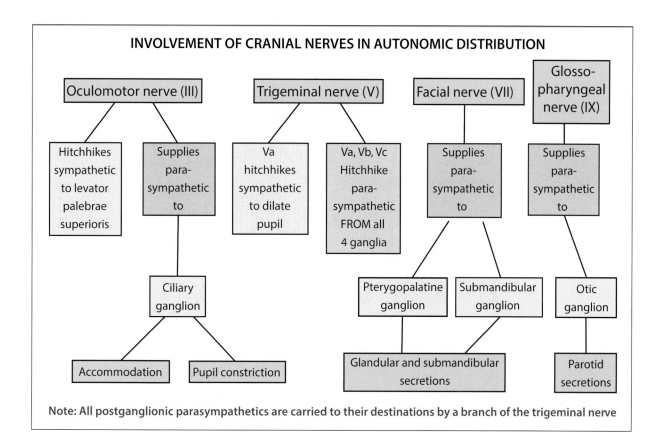

INVOLVEMENT OF CRANIAL NERVES IN AUTONOMIC DISTRIBUTION

Oculomotor nerve (III)
- Hitchhikes sympathetic to levator palebrae superioris
- Supplies para-sympathetic to
  - Ciliary ganglion
    - Accommodation
    - Pupil constriction

Trigeminal nerve (V)
- Va hitchhikes sympathetic to dilate pupil
- Va, Vb, Vc Hitchhike para-sympathetic FROM all 4 ganglia

Facial nerve (VII)
- Supplies para-sympathetic to
  - Pterygopalatine ganglion
  - Submandibular ganglion
    - Glandular and submandibular secretions

Glosso-pharyngeal nerve (IX)
- Supplies para-sympathetic to
  - Otic ganglion
    - Parotid secretions

Note: All postganglionic parasympathetics are carried to their destinations by a branch of the trigeminal nerve

AUTONOMIC CONNECTIONS IN THE HEAD

n/ns: Nerve/nerves
TP: Tensor palati
TT: Tensor tympani
V: Divisions of trigeminal nerve
Va - Ophthalmic
Vb - Maxillary
Vc - Mandibular
F - Foramen
br: Branch

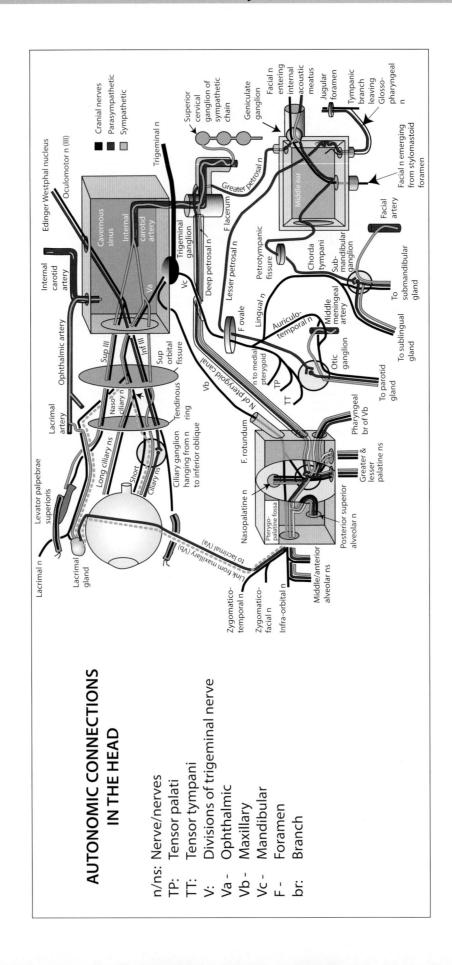

Cranial nerves
Parasympathetic
Sympathetic

SUMMARY OF SYMPATHETIC DISTRIBUTION BEYOND CHAIN

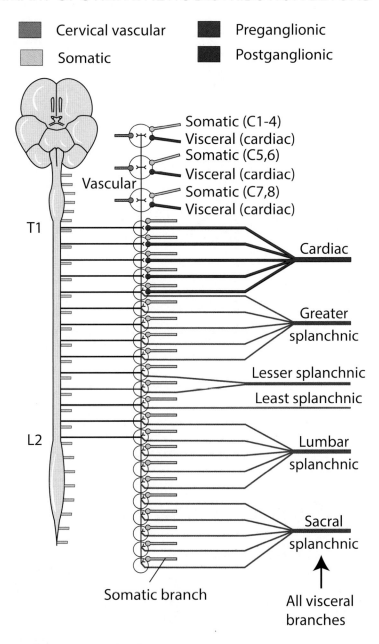

Cervical vascular

Somatic

Preganglionic

Postganglionic

Somatic (C1-4)
Visceral (cardiac)
Somatic (C5,6)
Visceral (cardiac)
Somatic (C7,8)
Visceral (cardiac)

Vascular

T1

Cardiac

Greater
splanchnic

Lesser splanchnic

Least splanchnic

L2

Lumbar
splanchnic

Sacral
splanchnic

Somatic branch

All visceral
branches

Functions of the sympathetic nerves
Homeostasis (skin): Sudomotor, pilomotor, vasomotor carried on spinal and cranial nerves.
Homeostasis (other): Vasomotor only, on any convenient nerve or vessel
Specific (to organs): Heart and bronchi. Via splanchnics to all abdominal organs including adrenals, sphincters and pelvic organs. Via superior cervical ganglion to head for pupil dilatation and raising the eyelids.

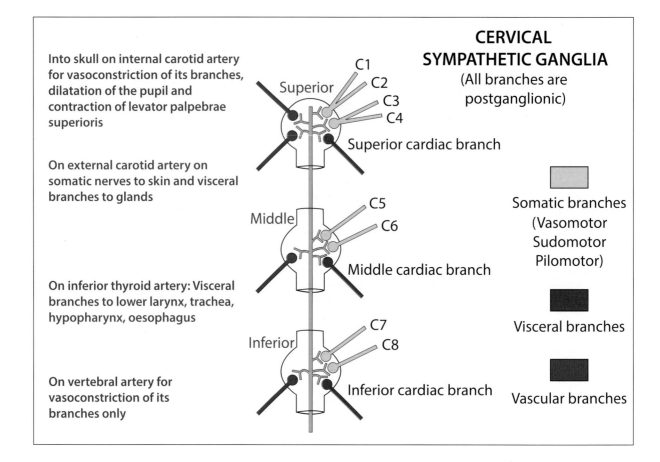

CERVICAL SYMPATHETIC GANGLIA
(All branches are postganglionic)

Into skull on internal carotid artery for vasoconstriction of its branches, dilatation of the pupil and contraction of levator palpebrae superioris

On external carotid artery on somatic nerves to skin and visceral branches to glands

On inferior thyroid artery: Visceral branches to lower larynx, trachea, hypopharynx, oesophagus

On vertebral artery for vasoconstriction of its branches only

Superior

Middle

Inferior

C1
C2
C3
C4

Superior cardiac branch

C5
C6

Middle cardiac branch

C7
C8

Inferior cardiac branch

Somatic branches (Vasomotor Sudomotor Pilomotor)

Visceral branches

Vascular branches

SYMPATHETICS IN PARASYMPATHETIC GANGLIA

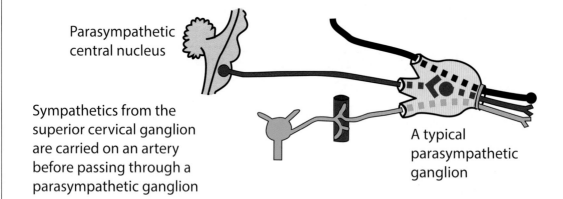

Parasympathetic central nucleus

Sympathetics from the superior cervical ganglion are carried on an artery before passing through a parasympathetic ganglion

A typical parasympathetic ganglion

There are always sympathetic fibres passing through each of the parasympathetic ganglia. They arise from the internal carotid for the ciliary and pterygopalatine ganglia and branches of the external carotid for the submandibular and otic ganglia. They do not synapse in these parasympathetic ganglia as they have already synapsed in the superior cervical ganglion. They supply vasoconstriction to the end organs and NEVER have special functions such as pupillary dilatation

AUTONOMIC OUTFLOW

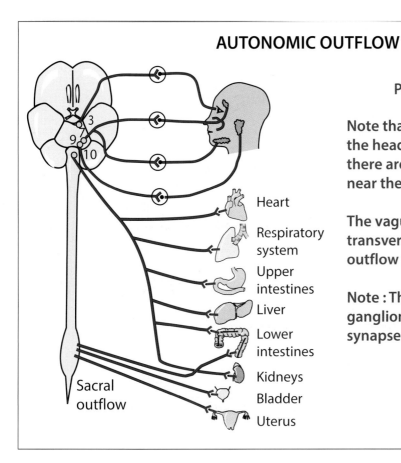

Heart

Respiratory system

Upper intestines

Liver

Lower intestines

Kidneys

Bladder

Uterus

Sacral outflow

PARASYMPATHETIC

Note that there are 4 specific ganglia in the head but in the rest of the body there are small peripheral ganglia on or near the end-organs.

The vagus reaches to the left side of the transverse colon and then the sacral outflow (S2, 3, 4) takes over.

Note : The ratio of pre- to post-ganglionic fibres in a parasympathetic synapse is 1:1

PATTERN OF PARASYMPATHETICS IN HEAD

Va To ciliary ganglion then on via nasociliary

Vb To pterygopalatine ganglion then on via maxillary or lacrimal

Vc To submandibular ganglion then on via lingual. Or to otic ganglion then on via auriculotemporal

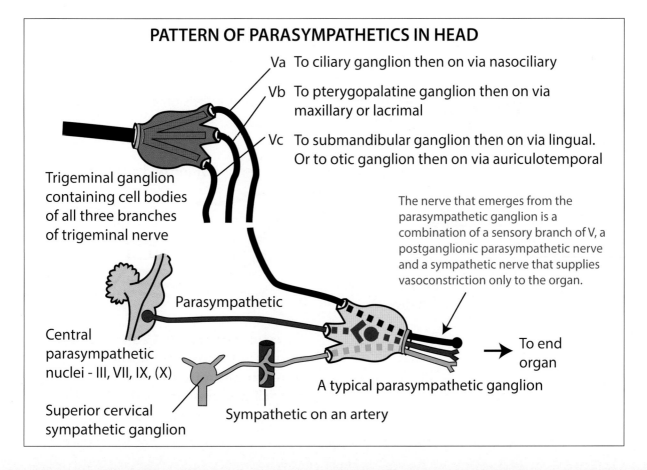

Trigeminal ganglion containing cell bodies of all three branches of trigeminal nerve

The nerve that emerges from the parasympathetic ganglion is a combination of a sensory branch of V, a postganglionic parasympathetic nerve and a sympathetic nerve that supplies vasoconstriction only to the organ.

Parasympathetic

Central parasympathetic nuclei - III, VII, IX, (X)

To end organ

A typical parasympathetic ganglion

Superior cervical sympathetic ganglion

Sympathetic on an artery

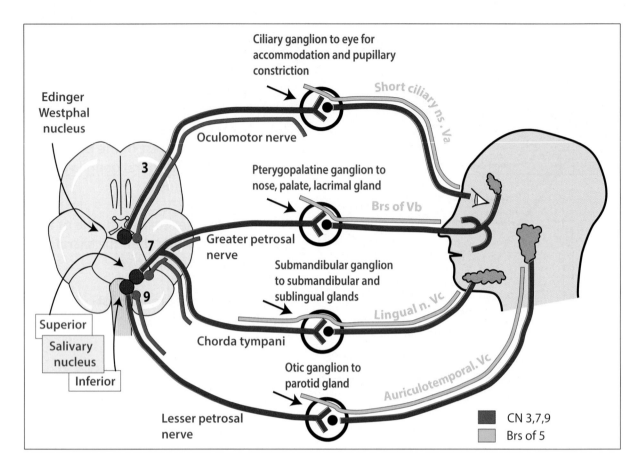

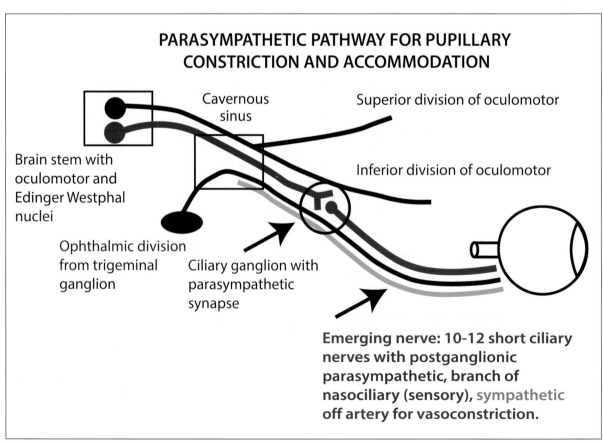

PARASYMPATHETIC PATHWAY FOR PUPILLARY CONSTRICTION AND ACCOMMODATION

PARASYMPATHETIC PATHWAY TO SUBMANDIBULAR AND SUBLINGUAL GLANDS

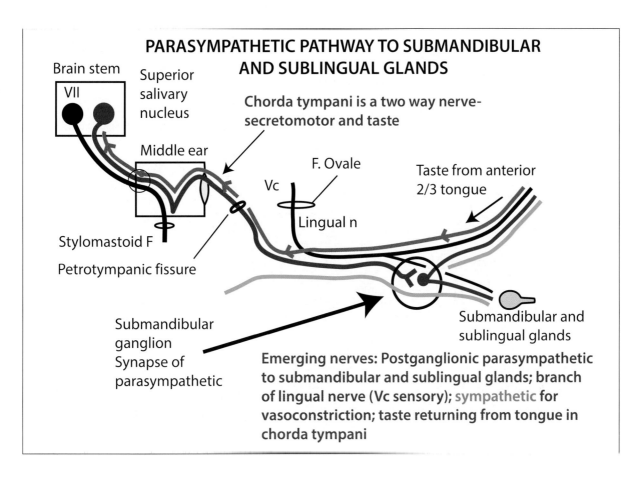

Brain stem

VII

Superior salivary nucleus

Chorda tympani is a two way nerve- secretomotor and taste

Middle ear

F. Ovale

Vc

Taste from anterior 2/3 tongue

Lingual n

Stylomastoid F

Petrotympanic fissure

Submandibular ganglion
Synapse of parasympathetic

Submandibular and sublingual glands

Emerging nerves: Postganglionic parasympathetic to submandibular and sublingual glands; branch of lingual nerve (Vc sensory); sympathetic for vasoconstriction; taste returning from tongue in chorda tympani

PARASYMPATHETIC PATHWAY TO NOSE, SINUSES, AND LACRIMAL GLAND

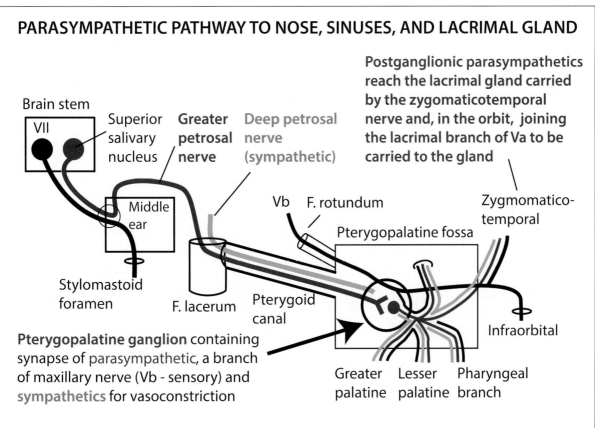

Postganglionic parasympathetics reach the lacrimal gland carried by the zygomaticotemporal nerve and, in the orbit, joining the lacrimal branch of Va to be carried to the gland

Brain stem

VII

Superior salivary nucleus

Greater petrosal nerve

Deep petrosal nerve (sympathetic)

Vb   F. rotundum

Pterygopalatine fossa

Zygmomatico- temporal

Middle ear

Stylomastoid foramen

F. lacerum

Pterygoid canal

Infraorbital

Pterygopalatine ganglion containing synapse of parasympathetic, a branch of maxillary nerve (Vb - sensory) and sympathetics for vasoconstriction

Greater palatine

Lesser palatine

Pharyngeal branch

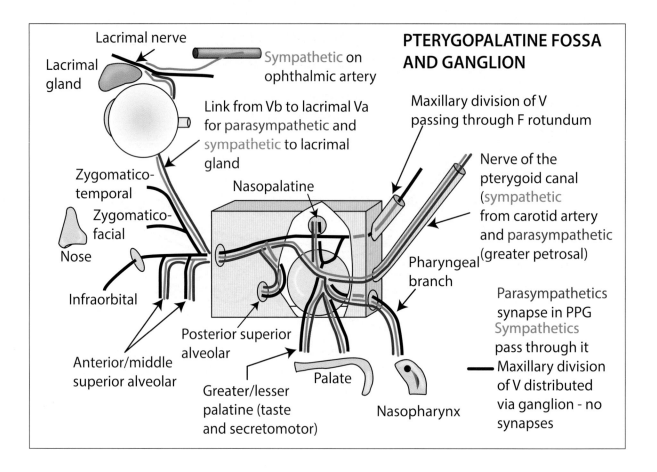

PTERYGOPALATINE FOSSA AND GANGLION

Lacrimal nerve

Lacrimal gland

Sympathetic on ophthalmic artery

Link from Vb to lacrimal Va for parasympathetic and sympathetic to lacrimal gland

Zygomatico-temporal

Zygomatico-facial

Nose

Nasopalatine

Infraorbital

Anterior/middle superior alveolar

Posterior superior alveolar

Greater/lesser palatine (taste and secretomotor)

Palate

Maxillary division of V passing through F rotundum

Nerve of the pterygoid canal (sympathetic from carotid artery and parasympathetic (greater petrosal)

Pharyngeal branch

Nasopharynx

Parasympathetics synapse in PPG
Sympathetics pass through it
— Maxillary division of V distributed via ganglion - no synapses

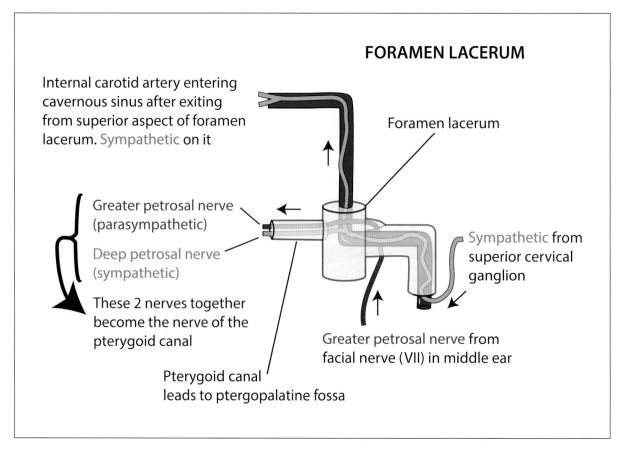

FORAMEN LACERUM

Internal carotid artery entering cavernous sinus after exiting from superior aspect of foramen lacerum. Sympathetic on it

Greater petrosal nerve (parasympathetic)

Deep petrosal nerve (sympathetic)

These 2 nerves together become the nerve of the pterygoid canal

Foramen lacerum

Sympathetic from superior cervical ganglion

Greater petrosal nerve from facial nerve (VII) in middle ear

Pterygoid canal leads to ptergopalatine fossa

TASTE FROM THE PALATE

Taste returns from the palate in the greater and lesser palatine nerves via the pterygopalatine ganglion (not synapsing) and then to the greater petrosal nerve to reach its cell bodies in the **geniculate ganglion** in the middle ear. Passes centrally to the tractus solitarius

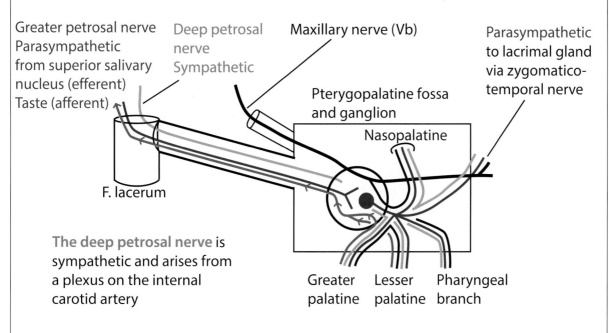

Greater petrosal nerve
Parasympathetic from superior salivary nucleus (efferent)
Taste (afferent)

Deep petrosal nerve
Sympathetic

Maxillary nerve (Vb)

Parasympathetic to lacrimal gland via zygomatico-temporal nerve

Pterygopalatine fossa and ganglion

Nasopalatine

F. lacerum

The deep petrosal nerve is sympathetic and arises from a plexus on the internal carotid artery

Greater palatine   Lesser palatine   Pharyngeal branch

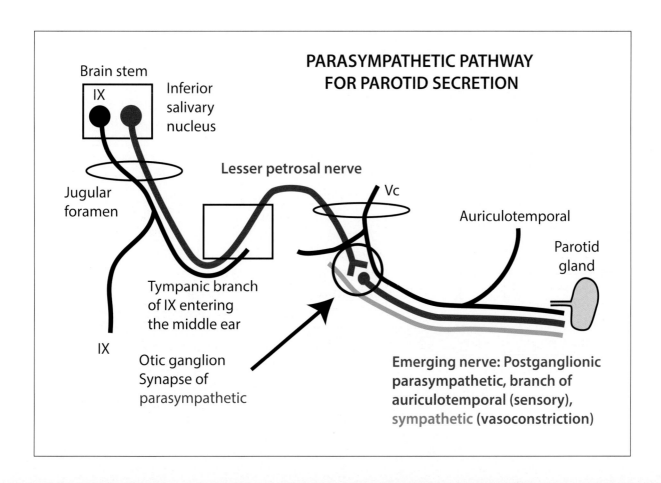

PARASYMPATHETIC PATHWAY FOR PAROTID SECRETION

Brain stem
IX
Inferior salivary nucleus

Lesser petrosal nerve

Vc

Auriculotemporal

Parotid gland

Jugular foramen

Tympanic branch of IX entering the middle ear

IX

Otic ganglion
Synapse of parasympathetic

Emerging nerve: Postganglionic parasympathetic, branch of auriculotemporal (sensory), sympathetic (vasoconstriction)

SUMMARY AND KEY POINTS OF PARASYMPATHETICS

- Parasympathetic output in the body is only carried by cranial nerves oculomotor (III), facial (VII), glossopharyngeal (IX) and vagus (X) and sacral segments S2,3,4.
- In the head it constricts the pupil, accommodates the eye and stimulates the salivary and lacrimal glands secrete. The vagus supplies the viscera as far as the left side of the transverse colon. Below that the supply is from S2,3,4 output.
- Each vagus nerve has two branches in the neck to the heart. There are further vagal branches to the heart and respiratory system in the chest and branches in the abdomen as far as the left transverse colon.
- The parasympathetics from S2,3,4 arise from cell bodies in the lateral horn of the spinal cord but emerge with the somatic motor nerves via the ventral horn. They join the pelvic plexus as the pelvic splanchnic nerves.
- True parasympathetic nerves are all motor. Sensory nerves within the parasympathetic system are general visceral afferent nerves that run with the parasympathetics but are not strictly part of the system.
- The vagus nerves and the output from S2,3,4 are all preganglionic fibres which all synapse in small peripheral ganglia on or near the organs of distribution.
- In the head there are four special parasympathetic ganglia (ciliary, pterygopalatine, submandibular and otic) for synapsing.
- There is no parasympathetic supply to limbs or gonads (ovaries and testes).

CHORDA TYMPANI

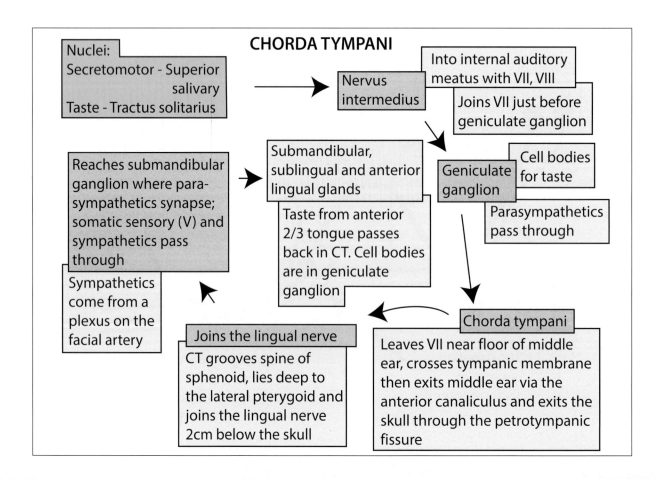

Nuclei:
Secretomotor - Superior salivary
Taste - Tractus solitarius

Nervus intermedius

Into internal auditory meatus with VII, VIII

Joins VII just before geniculate ganglion

Reaches submandibular ganglion where parasympathetics synapse; somatic sensory (V) and sympathetics pass through

Submandibular, sublingual and anterior lingual glands

Taste from anterior 2/3 tongue passes back in CT. Cell bodies are in geniculate ganglion

Geniculate ganglion

Cell bodies for taste

Parasympathetics pass through

Sympathetics come from a plexus on the facial artery

Joins the lingual nerve
CT grooves spine of sphenoid, lies deep to the lateral pterygoid and joins the lingual nerve 2cm below the skull

Chorda tympani
Leaves VII near floor of middle ear, crosses tympanic membrane then exits middle ear via the anterior canaliculus and exits the skull through the petrotympanic fissure

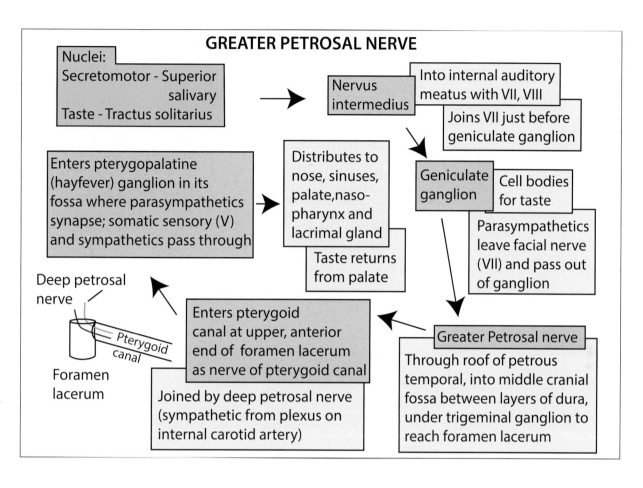

GREATER PETROSAL NERVE

Nuclei:
Secretomotor - Superior salivary
Taste - Tractus solitarius

Nervus intermedius

Into internal auditory meatus with VII, VIII

Joins VII just before geniculate ganglion

Enters pterygopalatine (hayfever) ganglion in its fossa where parasympathetics synapse; somatic sensory (V) and sympathetics pass through

Distributes to nose, sinuses, palate, nasopharynx and lacrimal gland

Taste returns from palate

Geniculate ganglion

Cell bodies for taste

Parasympathetics leave facial nerve (VII) and pass out of ganglion

Deep petrosal nerve

Pterygoid canal

Foramen lacerum

Enters pterygoid canal at upper, anterior end of foramen lacerum as nerve of pterygoid canal

Joined by deep petrosal nerve (sympathetic from plexus on internal carotid artery)

Greater Petrosal nerve

Through roof of petrous temporal, into middle cranial fossa between layers of dura, under trigeminal ganglion to reach foramen lacerum

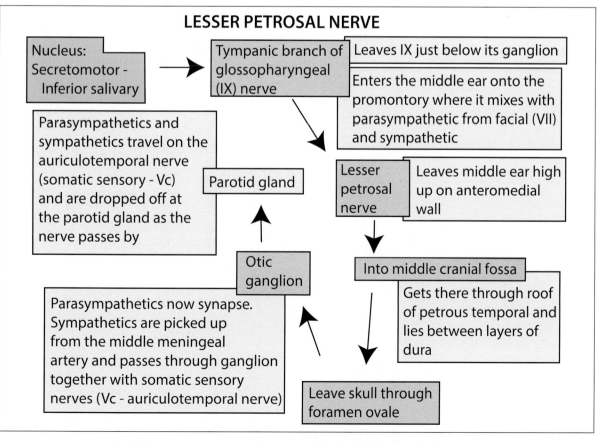

LESSER PETROSAL NERVE

Nucleus:
Secretomotor - Inferior salivary

Tympanic branch of glossopharyngeal (IX) nerve

Leaves IX just below its ganglion

Enters the middle ear onto the promontory where it mixes with parasympathetic from facial (VII) and sympathetic

Parasympathetics and sympathetics travel on the auriculotemporal nerve (somatic sensory - Vc) and are dropped off at the parotid gland as the nerve passes by

Parotid gland

Lesser petrosal nerve

Leaves middle ear high up on anteromedial wall

Otic ganglion

Into middle cranial fossa

Gets there through roof of petrous temporal and lies between layers of dura

Parasympathetics now synapse. Sympathetics are picked up from the middle meningeal artery and passes through ganglion together with somatic sensory nerves (Vc - auriculotemporal nerve)

Leave skull through foramen ovale

PARASYMPATHETIC PATHWAYS

Cranial nerve	Central nucleus	Nerve carrying preganglionic fibres	Pathway and foramen	Site of ganglion	Name of ganglion	Nerve carrying postganglionic fibres	Organ supplied
3	Edinger-Westphal (mid brain)	III via nerve to inferior oblique	Cavernous sinus to SOF to orbit	Between optic n and lateral rectus in apex of orbit	Ciliary	Nasociliary and short ciliary (Va)	Ciliary muscle for accommodation. Circular muscle for pupil constriction
7	Superior salivary (pons)	VII (NI) then greater petrosal	IAM to middle ear to MCF to pterygoid canal	Pterygopalatine fossa	Pterygo-palatine	Maxillary brs (Vb) Zygomatico-temporal to lacrimal (Va)	Mucous glands in nose, naso-pharynx soft palate Lacrimal gland
7	Superior salivary (pons)	VII (NI) then CT to lingual nerve	IAM to middle ear to petrotypanic fissure to ITF	Below lingual nerve on hyoglossus	Sub-mandibular	Lingual (Vc)	Sublingual and Submandibular salivary glands
9	Inferior salivary (medulla)	IX to tympanic branches to lesser petrosal	Middle ear to MCF to f ovale	Below formen ovale on nerve to tensor tympani/palati	Otic	Auriculo-temporal (Vc)	Parotid salivary gland
9		Pharyngeal and laryngeal branches	Direct to oropharynx and post 1/3 tongue	In relevant mucosa			Mucous glands oropharynx and post 1/3 tongue
10	Dorsal motor (medulla)	X (vagus)	Cardiac branches in neck. Thorax and abdomen	On target organs			Viscera of thorax and abdomen down to transverse colon

SOF = Superior orbital fissure   IAM = Internal auditory meatus   CT = Chorda tympani
NI = Nervus intermedius   IF = Infratemporal fossa   MCF = Middle cranial fossa

5.19 Temporal, Infratemporal and Pterygopalatine Fossae

RIGHT TEMPORAL FOSSA

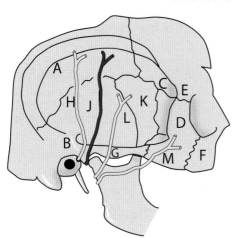

Medial to temporalis which is attached to, and below inferior temporal line (A)
Roof: Temporalis fascia
Posterior: Supramastoid crest (B)
Floor: Skull - pterion (C)
Anterior: Zygoma (D), zygomatic process of frontal bone (E) and zygomatic process of maxilla (F)
Inferior: Zygomatic arch and zygomatic process of temporal bone (G)

Contains: Temporalis, deep temporal arteries (maxillary), deep temporal nerves (Vc), Superficial temporal artery (external carotid). Auriculotemporal nerve (H) from mandibular nerve (Vc)
Other structures shown: Temporal bone (J), greater wing of sphenoid (K), Temporal branch of facial (VII) (L), zygomatic branch of facial (VII) (M)

INFRATEMPORAL FOSSA - BOUNDARIES

ROOF
- Infratemporal crest (greater wing of sphenoid)
- Squamous temporal

MEDIAL WALL
- Tensor palati
- Levator palati
- Superior constrictor
- Lateral pterygoid plate
- Pterygomaxillary fissure
- Maxilla

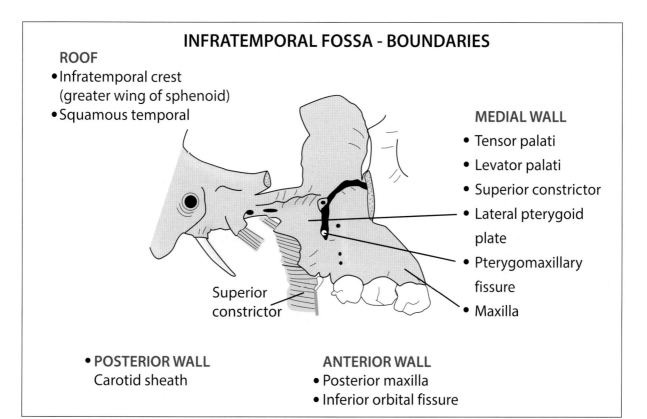

Superior constrictor

POSTERIOR WALL
Carotid sheath

ANTERIOR WALL
- Posterior maxilla
- Inferior orbital fissure

INFRATEMPORAL FOSSA - BOUNDARIES

- Base of skull
- Between pharynx and ramus of mandible

LATERAL WALL
Ramus of mandible
Coronoid process

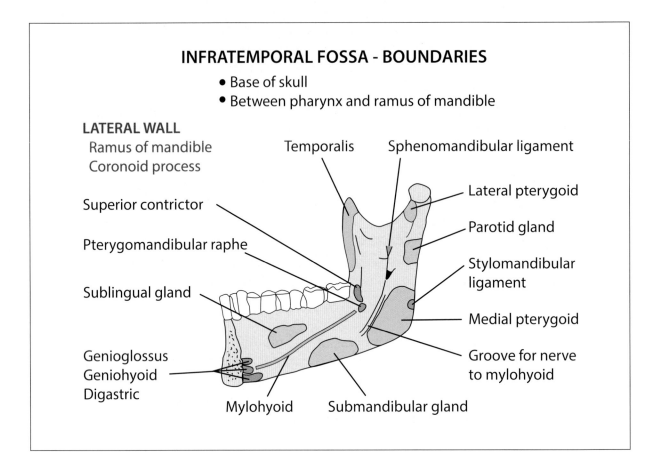

Temporalis

Sphenomandibular ligament

Superior contrictor

Pterygomandibular raphe

Sublingual gland

Genioglossus
Geniohyoid
Digastric

Lateral pterygoid

Parotid gland

Stylomandibular
ligament

Medial pterygoid

Groove for nerve
to mylohyoid

Mylohyoid

Submandibular gland

INFRATEMPORAL FOSSA

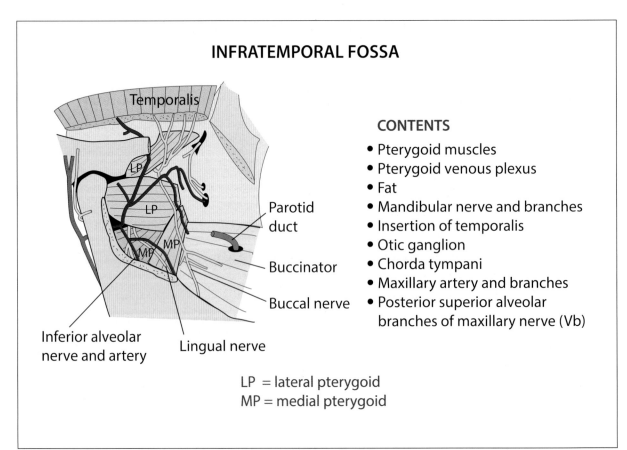

Temporalis

LP

LP

MP

MP

Parotid
duct

Buccinator

Buccal nerve

Inferior alveolar
nerve and artery

Lingual nerve

CONTENTS
- Pterygoid muscles
- Pterygoid venous plexus
- Fat
- Mandibular nerve and branches
- Insertion of temporalis
- Otic ganglion
- Chorda tympani
- Maxillary artery and branches
- Posterior superior alveolar
  branches of maxillary nerve (Vb)

LP = lateral pterygoid
MP = medial pterygoid

INFRATEMPORAL FOSSA - DEEP DISSECTION

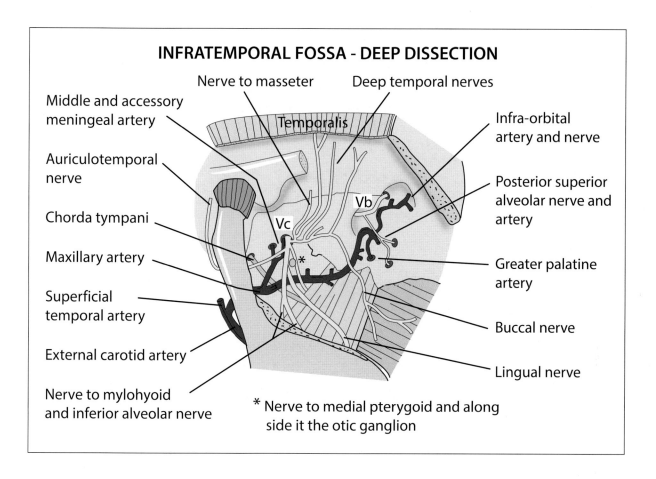

Nerve to masseter

Deep temporal nerves

Middle and accessory meningeal artery

Temporalis

Infra-orbital artery and nerve

Auriculotemporal nerve

Vb

Posterior superior alveolar nerve and artery

Chorda tympani

Vc

Maxillary artery

*

Greater palatine artery

Superficial temporal artery

Buccal nerve

External carotid artery

Lingual nerve

Nerve to mylohyoid and inferior alveolar nerve

* Nerve to medial pterygoid and along side it the otic ganglion

MAXILLARY DIVISION OF TRIGEMINAL NERVE IN PTERYGOPALATINE FOSSA

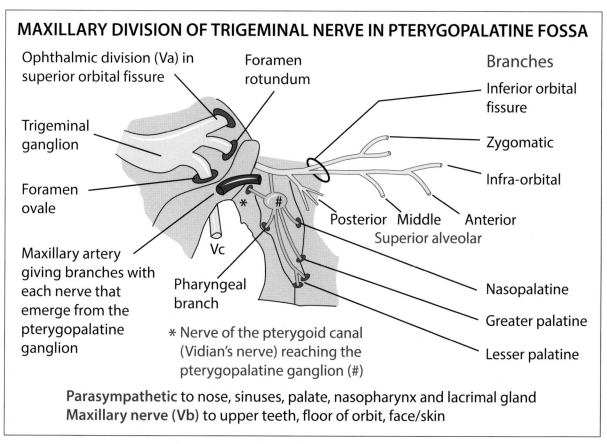

Ophthalmic division (Va) in superior orbital fissure

Foramen rotundum

Branches

Inferior orbital fissure

Trigeminal ganglion

Zygomatic

Infra-orbital

Foramen ovale

*

#

Maxillary artery giving branches with each nerve that emerge from the pterygopalatine ganglion

Vc

Posterior   Middle   Anterior
Superior alveolar

Pharyngeal branch

Nasopalatine

Greater palatine

* Nerve of the pterygoid canal (Vidian's nerve) reaching the pterygopalatine ganglion (#)

Lesser palatine

Parasympathetic to nose, sinuses, palate, nasopharynx and lacrimal gland
Maxillary nerve (Vb) to upper teeth, floor of orbit, face/skin

MANDIBULAR DIVISION OF TRIGEMINAL NERVE (Vc)
Foramen ovale to infratemporal fossa

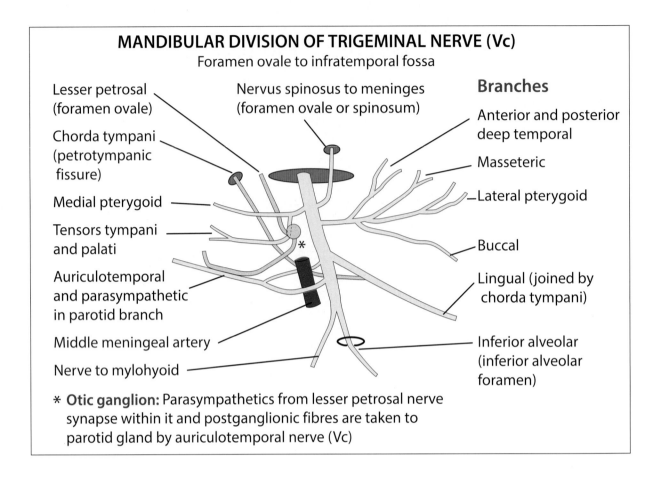

Lesser petrosal (foramen ovale)

Chorda tympani (petrotympanic fissure)

Medial pterygoid

Tensors tympani and palati

Auriculotemporal and parasympathetic in parotid branch

Middle meningeal artery

Nerve to mylohyoid

Nervus spinosus to meninges (foramen ovale or spinosum)

Branches

Anterior and posterior deep temporal

Masseteric

Lateral pterygoid

Buccal

Lingual (joined by chorda tympani)

Inferior alveolar (inferior alveolar foramen)

* **Otic ganglion:** Parasympathetics from lesser petrosal nerve synapse within it and postganglionic fibres are taken to parotid gland by auriculotemporal nerve (Vc)

MUSCLES OF MASTICATION

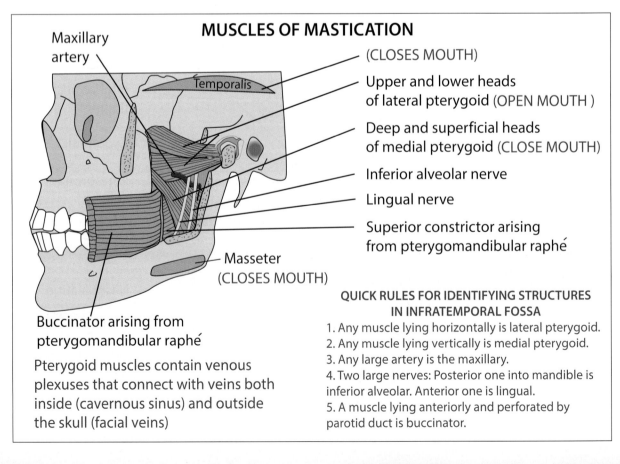

Maxillary artery

Temporalis

(CLOSES MOUTH)

Upper and lower heads of lateral pterygoid (OPEN MOUTH)

Deep and superficial heads of medial pterygoid (CLOSE MOUTH)

Inferior alveolar nerve

Lingual nerve

Superior constrictor arising from pterygomandibular raphé

Masseter (CLOSES MOUTH)

Buccinator arising from pterygomandibular raphé

Pterygoid muscles contain venous plexuses that connect with veins both inside (cavernous sinus) and outside the skull (facial veins)

QUICK RULES FOR IDENTIFYING STRUCTURES IN INFRATEMPORAL FOSSA
1. Any muscle lying horizontally is lateral pterygoid.
2. Any muscle lying vertically is medial pterygoid.
3. Any large artery is the maxillary.
4. Two large nerves: Posterior one into mandible is inferior alveolar. Anterior one is lingual.
5. A muscle lying anteriorly and perforated by parotid duct is buccinator.

MUSCLES OF MASTICATION

- Temporalis
- Masseter
- Medial pterygoid
- Lateral pterygoid

All supplied by:
- Mandibular division of Trigeminal (Vc)
- All derived from 1st pharyngeal arch

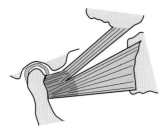

LATERAL PTERYGOID
Arises: 2 heads:
Upper - infratemporal surface sphenoid
Lower - lateral surface of lateral pterygoid plate
Inserts: pterygoid fossa below head of mandible, disc and capsule of temporomandibular joint
Action: protrudes jaw and opens mouth

MEDIAL PTERYGOID
Arises: 2 heads:
Deep - medial side of lateral pterygoid plate and fossa between plates
Superficial - smaller. Tuberosity of maxilla and pyramidal process of palatine bone
Inserts: Medial ramus of mandible
Action: pulls mandible upwards, forwards and medially (closes mouth and chews)

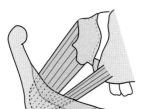

MAXILLARY ARTERY

In infratemporal fossa, within or lateral to superficial head of lateral pterygoid muscle (shown below)

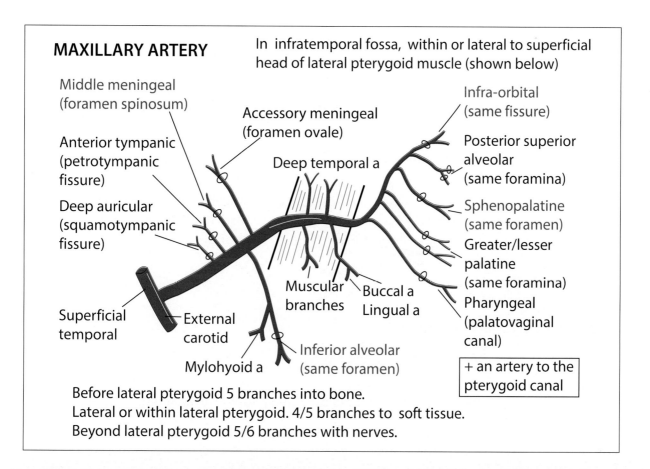

Middle meningeal (foramen spinosum)
Anterior tympanic (petrotympanic fissure)
Deep auricular (squamotympanic fissure)
Superficial temporal
External carotid
Mylohyoid a
Accessory meningeal (foramen ovale)
Deep temporal a
Muscular branches
Buccal a
Lingual a
Inferior alveolar (same foramen)
Infra-orbital (same fissure)
Posterior superior alveolar (same foramina)
Sphenopalatine (same foramen)
Greater/lesser palatine (same foramina)
Pharyngeal (palatovaginal canal)

+ an artery to the pterygoid canal

Before lateral pterygoid 5 branches into bone.
Lateral or within lateral pterygoid. 4/5 branches to soft tissue.
Beyond lateral pterygoid 5/6 branches with nerves.

LINGUAL NERVE: RELATION TO MUSCLES

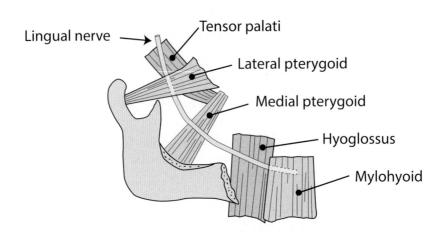

Lingual nerve — Tensor palati — Lateral pterygoid — Medial pterygoid — Hyoglossus — Mylohyoid

The lingual nerve can be considered as a "2-way nerve":
SENSORY: General sensory: Anterior 2/3 tongue
Taste (via chorda tympani): Anterior 2/3 tongue
MOTOR: Secretomotor (via chorda tympani): Submandibular and sublingual glands

SPHENOMANDIBULAR LIGAMENT RELATIONS

Structures that pass between sphenomandiblular ligament and mandible

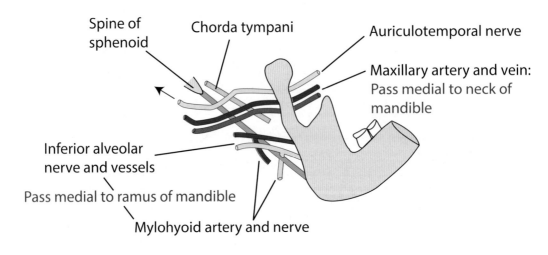

Spine of sphenoid — Chorda tympani — Auriculotemporal nerve — Maxillary artery and vein: Pass medial to neck of mandible

Inferior alveolar nerve and vessels
Pass medial to ramus of mandible

Mylohyoid artery and nerve

Note that nerve to mylohyoid often pierces the ligament

LIGAMENTS ASSOCIATED WITH MANDIBLE AND HYOID

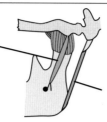

SPHENOMANDIBULAR LIGAMENT
Spine of sphenoid to lingula of mandible (1st arch remnant). Is the axis of rotation for opening of mouth

STYLOMANDIBULAR LIGAMENT
Specialised band of deep cervical fascia. Styloid process to angle of mandible. Is the postero-inferior aspect of the parotid fascia

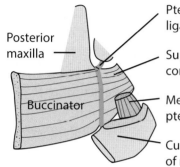

Posterior maxilla

Pterygomaxillary ligament

Superior constrictor

Buccinator

Medial pterygoid

Cut ramus of mandible

Styloglossus from lower anterior 1/3 of ligament

Middle constrictor

Hyoid bone

STYLOHYOID LIGAMENT
Tip of styloid process to lesser cornu of hyoid. 2nd arch remnant. Styloglossus from its upper end and middle constrictor from its lower end

PTERYGOMANDIBULAR RAPHÉ
Tendinous muscle fibres from pterygoid hamulus to posterior end of mylohyoid line. Medially: Buccal mucosa. From it: Superior constrictor posteriorly and buccinator anteriorly. Buccinator also extends onto pterygo-maxillary ligament to reach maxilla

RIGHT PTERYGOPALATINE FOSSA
Looking in from the lateral side

POSTERIOR

ANTERIOR

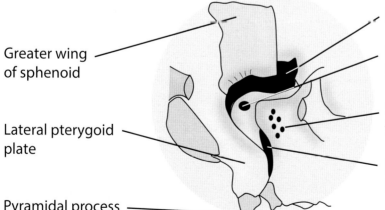

Greater wing of sphenoid

Lateral pterygoid plate

Pyramidal process of palatine bone

Inferior orbital fissure

Sphenopalatine foramen into lateral nose

Posterior superior alveolar foramina in posterior maxilla

Pterygomaxillary fissure

Lateral access into the fossa is via the pterygomaxillary fissure. Other entry and exit sites are shown on a separate illustration

PTERYGOPALATINE FOSSA - VIEWED FROM ABOVE

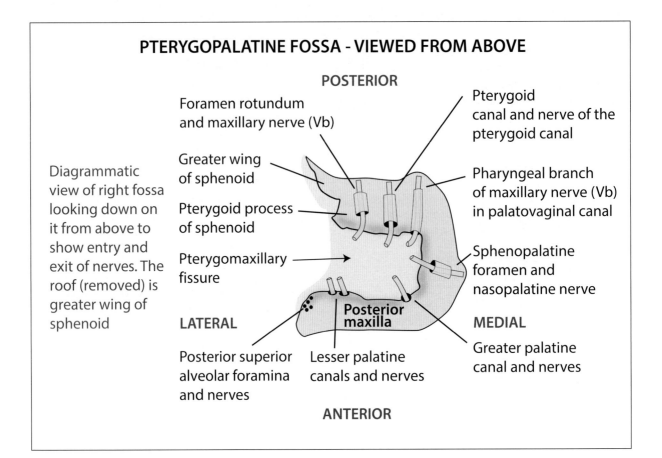

POSTERIOR

Foramen rotundum
and maxillary nerve (Vb)

Pterygoid
canal and nerve of the
pterygoid canal

Greater wing
of sphenoid

Diagrammatic
view of right fossa
looking down on
it from above to
show entry and
exit of nerves. The
roof (removed) is
greater wing of
sphenoid

Pterygoid process
of sphenoid

Pharyngeal branch
of maxillary nerve (Vb)
in palatovaginal canal

Pterygomaxillary
fissure

Sphenopalatine
foramen and
nasopalatine nerve

LATERAL

Posterior
maxilla

MEDIAL

Greater palatine
canal and nerves

Posterior superior
alveolar foramina
and nerves

Lesser palatine
canals and nerves

ANTERIOR

5.20   Cavernous Sinus and other Venous Sinuses

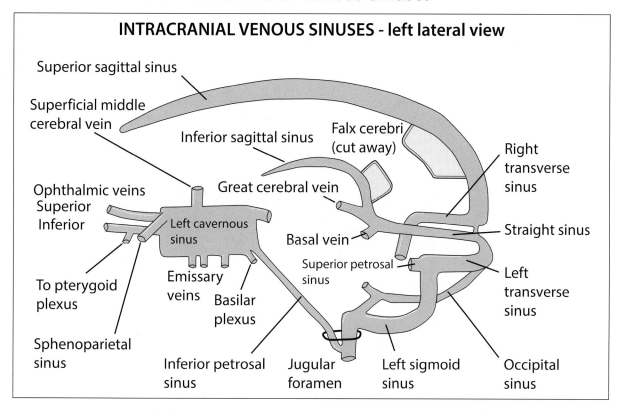

INTRACRANIAL VENOUS SINUSES - left lateral view

Superior sagittal sinus

Superficial middle cerebral vein

Inferior sagittal sinus

Falx cerebri (cut away)

Right transverse sinus

Ophthalmic veins
Superior
Inferior

Great cerebral vein

Left cavernous sinus

Basal vein

Straight sinus

Superior petrosal sinus

To pterygoid plexus

Emissary veins

Basilar plexus

Left transverse sinus

Sphenoparietal sinus

Inferior petrosal sinus

Jugular foramen

Left sigmoid sinus

Occipital sinus

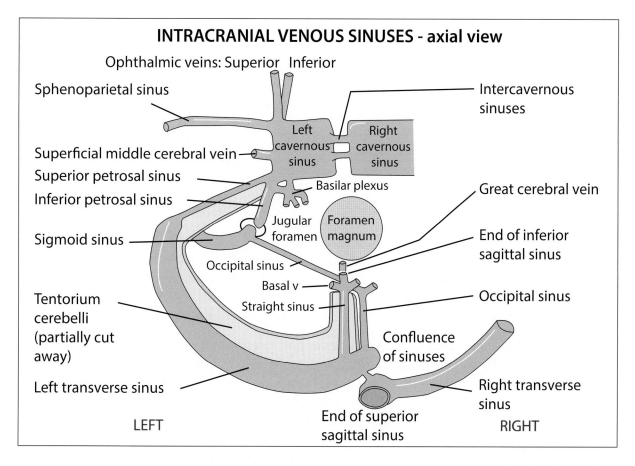

INTRACRANIAL VENOUS SINUSES - axial view

Ophthalmic veins: Superior   Inferior

Sphenoparietal sinus

Intercavernous sinuses

Left cavernous sinus

Right cavernous sinus

Superficial middle cerebral vein

Superior petrosal sinus

Inferior petrosal sinus

Basilar plexus

Great cerebral vein

Sigmoid sinus

Jugular foramen

Foramen magnum

End of inferior sagittal sinus

Occipital sinus

Tentorium cerebelli (partially cut away)

Basal v

Straight sinus

Occipital sinus

Confluence of sinuses

Left transverse sinus

Right transverse sinus

LEFT

End of superior sagittal sinus

RIGHT

LEFT CAVERNOUS SINUS

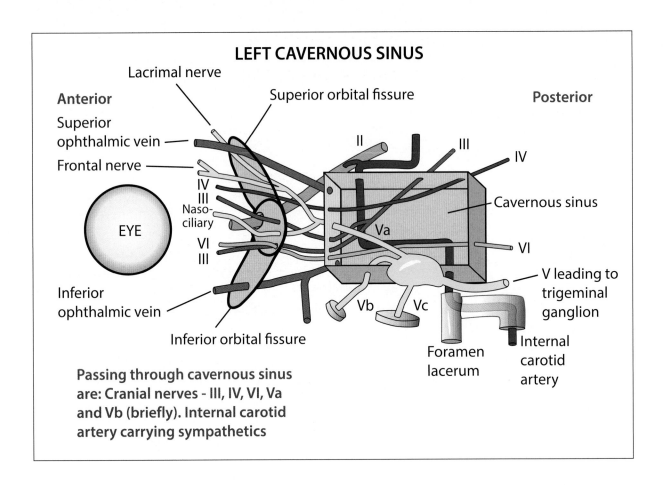

Lacrimal nerve

Superior orbital fissure

Anterior

Posterior

Superior ophthalmic vein

Frontal nerve

EYE

IV
III
Naso-ciliary

VI
III

Inferior ophthalmic vein

II

III

IV

Cavernous sinus

Va

VI

V leading to trigeminal ganglion

Vb   Vc

Internal carotid artery

Foramen lacerum

Inferior orbital fissure

Passing through cavernous sinus are: Cranial nerves - III, IV, VI, Va and Vb (briefly). Internal carotid artery carrying sympathetics

CAVERNOUS SINUS - CORONAL (TRANSVERSE) VIEW RIGHT SIDE LOOKING ANTERIORLY

In: Middle cranial fossa. **Alongside:** Body of the sphenoid. **Between:** Endosteal and meningeal dura. **Roof:** Anterior and posterior clinoid processes with uncus of temporal lobe and internal carotid artery on it, III and IV into it. **Lateral wall:** Dura, temporal lobe, III, IV, Va, Vb in wall. **Floor:** Greater wing of sphenoid. **Medial wall:** Dura over sphenoid, sella turcica, pituitary, sphenoid sinus.

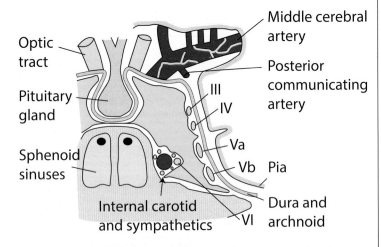

Optic tract

Pituitary gland

Sphenoid sinuses

V

Middle cerebral artery

Posterior communicating artery

III
IV

Va

Vb Pia

Internal carotid and sympathetics

VI

Dura and archnoid

Posterior wall: Dura of posterior fossa, superior and inferior petrosal sinuses, peduncle of brain. **Anterior wall:** Medial end of superior orbital fissure, ophthalmic veins, orbit. **Contains:** Internal carotid artery, VI and blood. **Draining into it:** Superior and inferior ophthalmic veins, intercavernous sinuses, sphenoparietal sinuses, superficial middle cerebral vein. **Draining out of it:** Superior and inferior petrosal sinuses, emissary veins to pterygoid plexus

6 RIGHT ANGLE BENDS OF THE INTERNAL CAROTID ARTERY

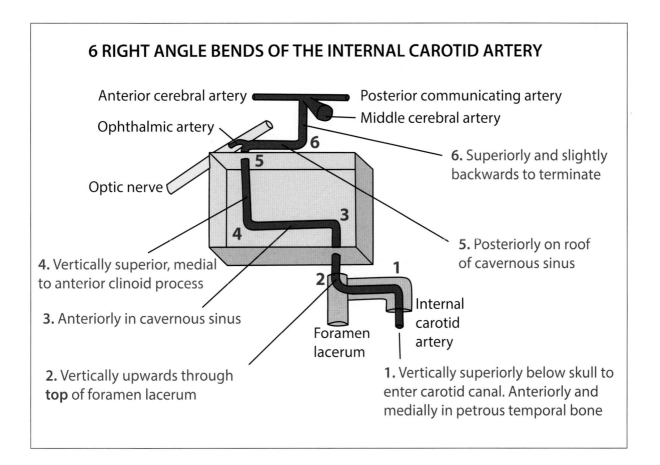

Anterior cerebral artery

Posterior communicating artery

Middle cerebral artery

Ophthalmic artery

Optic nerve

6. Superiorly and slightly backwards to terminate

5. Posteriorly on roof of cavernous sinus

4. Vertically superior, medial to anterior clinoid process

3. Anteriorly in cavernous sinus

2. Vertically upwards through **top** of foramen lacerum

Foramen lacerum

Internal carotid artery

1. Vertically superiorly below skull to enter carotid canal. Anteriorly and medially in petrous temporal bone